Ligaments of the Vertebral Column

Mehmet Turgut • R. Shane Tubbs
Ahmet T. Turgut • Joe Iwanaga
Fuyou Guo
Editors

Ligaments of the Vertebral Column

Embryology, Neuroanatomy, Function, Imaging, and Management

Springer

Editors
Mehmet Turgut
Department of Neurosurgery
Aydın Adnan Menderes University
Faculty of Medicine
Aydın, Aydın, Türkiye

Ahmet T. Turgut
Ankara, Türkiye

Fuyou Guo
Department of Neurosurgery
The First Affiliated Hospital of
Zhengzhou University
Zhengzhou, Henan, China

R. Shane Tubbs
Department of Neurosurgery
Tulane University
New Orleans, LA, USA

Joe Iwanaga
Department of Neurosurgery
Tulane University School of Medicine
New Orleans, LA, USA

ISBN 978-3-032-09069-0 ISBN 978-3-032-09070-6 (eBook)
https://doi.org/10.1007/978-3-032-09070-6

This Springer imprint is published by the registered company Springer Nature Switzerland AG
The registered company address is: Gewerbestrasse 11, 6330 Cham, Switzerland

Contents

Part I

History, Embryology, Histology, Neuroanatomy and Imaging of the Spinal Ligaments

History of the Spinal Ligaments

1

Nikolaos Syrmos and Mehmet Turgut

1.1 Introduction

Since early human records, knowledge of neuroanatomy and spinal anatomy has developed in concert with medicine as an autonomous science, along with the related terminology [1–6]. The evolution of neurosurgery as a medical discipline through the ages has been closely related to that of spine surgery [3–8]. More recent neurological and radiological studies of humans have provided a particularly well-understood and documented understanding of the spinal ligaments through both anatomical-morphological and physiological-functional investigations [4–9]. The spinal ligaments remain a crucial and challenging subject of study in anatomy, physiology, neuroanatomy, neurophysiology, neurosurgery, and spine surgery [6–12]. Their normal function is affected in many morbidities, diseases, degeneration, and traumas worldwide [5–10].

1.2 Ancient Period

In the papyrus of Edwin Smith, a medical treatise written in Egypt around 1700 BCE, we find accurate descriptions of spinal pathologies (sprains, fractures, dislocations, and other traumatic conditions). This demonstrates knowledge of the spine among ancient civilizations around the Mediterranean Sea (Egyptians, Greeks, Romans, etc.) [1–8]. The first edition of this important historical document was probably written by Imhotep, the chief physician to the ruler of Egypt, Zoser, during the Third Pharaonic Dynasty of the Old Kingdom Era, when the Great Pyramid was built (2600 to 2200 BCE). Subsequent copies of the document were made and studied by various authors until the American scientist Edwin Smith acquired it in 1862. The papyrus was donated to the Historical Scientific Society of New York City in 1906 [3–10].

Srimad Bhagwat Mahapuranam is an Indian text written between 1800 BCE and 3500 BCE. This document provides accurate descriptions of spinal deformations, offering evidence of the evolution of medicine in this region [1–8].

The first documented physician and the first pioneer of neurological and spinal surgery in

N. Syrmos (✉)
Aristotle University of Thessaloniki, Thessaloniki, Macedonia, Greece

Human Performance and Health, Master Science Program, Aristotle University of Thessaloniki, Thessaloniki, Macedonia, Greece

European Association of Neurosurgical Societies (EANS), Brussels, Belgium
e-mail: milanako76@yahoo.gr

M. Turgut
Department of Neurosurgery, Aydın Adnan Menderes University Faculty of Medicine, Aydın, Aydın, Türkiye

Department of Histology and Embryology, Aydın Adnan Menderes University Health Sciences Institute, Efeler, Aydın, Türkiye

M. Turgut et al. (eds.), *Ligaments of the Vertebral Column*,
https://doi.org/10.1007/978-3-032-09070-6_1

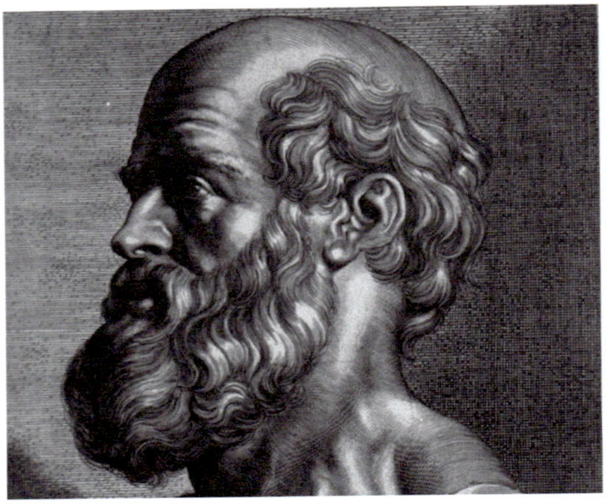

Fig. 1.1 Hippocrates of Kos (460–370 BC)

medical history was the Hellenic Hippocrates of Kos (460–370 BCE), who conducted anatomical and morphological studies and undertook surgical, neurosurgical, and spinal operations. His books describe numerous structures within the spinal segments, including the spinal ligaments [3–11]. He used a kind of local pressure-traction to treat spinal deformities in his patients (ΙΠΠΟΚΡΑΤΙΟ ΒΟΘΡΙΟ), with documented success. He helped many people with spinal problems improve their quality of life. He had many students (ΜΑΘΗΤΕΣ), and through them he transmitted the spirit of scientific study of the human spine, and of the human body [2–9] (Fig. 1.1).

1.3 Hellenic-Roman-Byzantine-Islamic Era

Alcmaeon of Croton (sixth century BCE) provided one of the first documented attempts to describe spinal structures and the spinal ligaments, utilizing the knowledge available during that period. Galen of Pergamon (131–201 BCE) was a skilled surgeon and anatomist of the Roman Empire [2–7] (Fig. 1.2). He and his pupils used neuro-anatomical and spinal terminology in the colloquial Hellenic language of his era. He provided detailed descriptions of the anatomical and physiological protective segments of the spinal cord, including the bones, ligaments (such as the posterior longitudinal ligament, PLL), and the meninges (dura and pia mater) [2–10]. Aurelius Cornelius Celsus of Rome (25 BCE- 50 CE) presented very accurate studies of spinal and spinal cord lesions. He became a well-known physician and scientific polymath after publishing his book "De Medicina." This work is believed to be the surviving section of a much larger series of scientific documents. We can find in it primitive and primary sources of various disciplines (medicine, dietetics, pharmacy, surgery, anatomy, physiology, and related fields). It is considered one of the most accurate sources of medical knowledge in the Roman Empire (IMPERO ROMANO) [3–10].

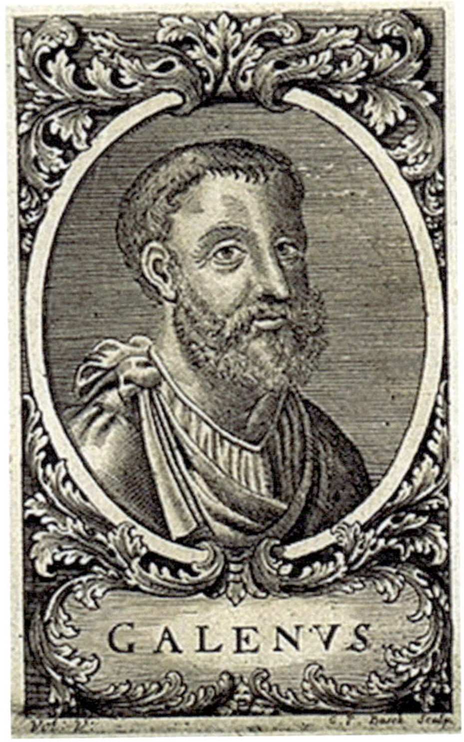

Fig. 1.2 Galen of Pergamon (131–201 BC)

The Arab physicians Avicenna (980–1037 CE) and Albucasis (936–1013 CE) codified the medical, neuro-anatomical, and spinal terminology of their period [5–11]. Paul of Aegina (625–690 CE) studied the works and scientific insights of Hippocrates, Galen, Celsus, Avicenna, and Albucasis to obtain accurate descriptions of the morphology and function of the human spine and its ligaments. He was the first to perform a laminectomy. Throughout his medical career, he endeavored to refine his understanding of spinal anatomy and the spinal segments [3–9].

1.3.1 Renaissance Period

Leonardo da Vinci (1452–1519) produced accurate documentation, descriptions, and drawings. In his studies (Tavole Anstomiche of Da Vinci, Codici di Leonardo) we have an accurate description of the spinal ligaments and a comprehensive effort to investigate spinal stability to manage spine instability better [2–10]. Leonardo da Vinci (15 April 1452 to 2 May 1519), born in Florence, Italy, was a brilliant polymath of the High Renaissance. He was simultaneously a renowned designer, painter, mechanic, inventor, engineer, scientist, theorist, sculptor, architect, anatomist, physiologist, and physician [4–11]. His fame rested initially on his various achievements in the arts. Later, he became well-known for his notebooks, which contain drawings and notes on various subjects, including the human body, medicine, spine anatomy, physiology, human motion, astronomy, painting, botanical designs, paleontology, and history [1–7]. Leonardo is recognized as a multi-science genius, the ideal representative of the Renaissance humanist spirit. Initially, he was educated in his hometown (Florence) by Andrea del Verrocchio, a famous sculptor and painter [2–8]. He began his scientific career in Florence; then he spent a long time in Milan under the protection of Ludovico Sforza, ruler of the Lombardia region in northern Italy. He worked in various Italian cities (Florence, Milan, Rome), all the while surrounded by a large following of students (STUDENTI) [3–10]. He accepted an invitation from Francis I and spent his final three years in France until he died in 1519. His many disciplines, and also other aspects of his life (interests, personal facts, scientific achievements, and empirical thinking) are still studied worldwide with great interest and admiration, making him one of the most frequently heard names and subjects in the entire scientific panorama [4–11] (Fig. 1.3).

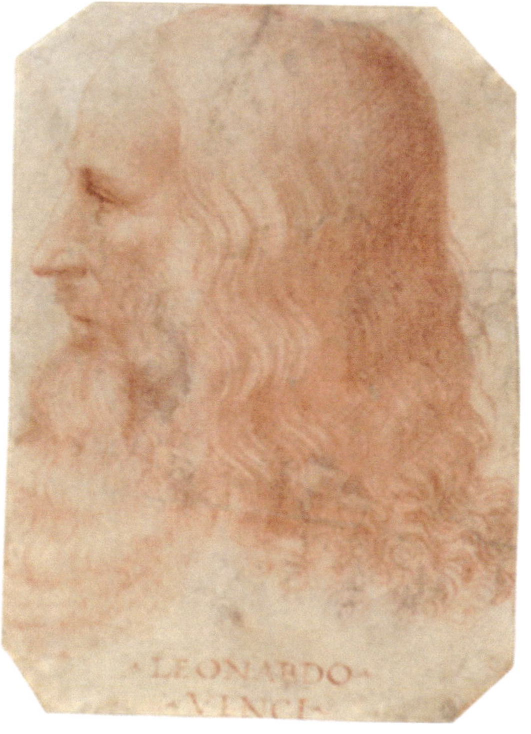

Fig. 1.3 Leonardo da Vinci (1452–1519)

Arantio (1530–1589) was an Italian physician, polymath, anatomist, and pioneer surgeon (Fig. 1.4). He studied human anatomy and spine morphology with his teacher, Andreas Vesalius (Andries van Wezel) (31 December 1514 to 15 October 1564), the so-called founder of modern human anatomy [3–10] (Figs. 1.5 and 1.6). Vesalius's home city was Brussels, which was then part of the Habsburg Netherlands [1–9]; he became a professor of Medicine at the University of Padua (Padova) in northern Italy (1537–1542). Later, he was appointed physician to the court of Emperor Charles the Fifth. Vesalius, through Andreas Vesalius and his other students, made significant contributions to the scientific knowledge of human anatomy and physiology (including the body, brain, spine, etc.) [2–8].

In 1675, René Descartes published a philosophical scientific work, "Tractus de Homine et de Formatione Foetus," providing a philosophical and mechanistic approach to the human body, a

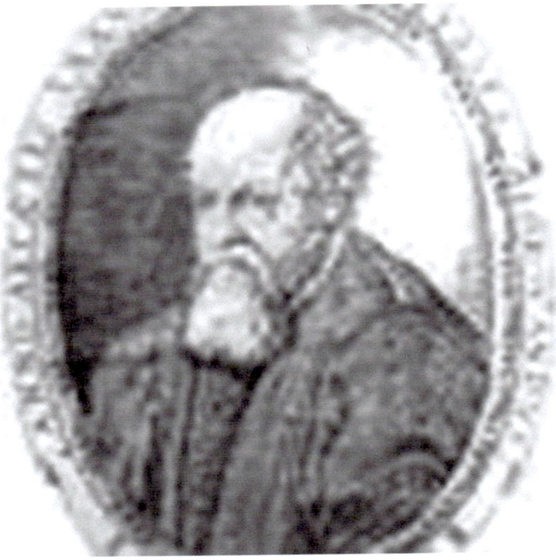

Fig. 1.4 Gulio Cesare Arantio (1530–1589)

kind of experimental physiological and anthropological study [4–11].

1.4 Contribution of Giovanni Borelli

Giovanni Borreli (1608–1679) is considered one of the fathers of scientific spine motion studies. He was a polymath from Naples (Napoli), Southern Italy, a mathematician, astronomist, physiologist, and anthropologist. He studied human anatomy, including spine function and motion through the spinal ligaments. In 1653, he became a professor in Naples, and then he moved to the University of Pisa in central Italy, where he developed a highly productive collaboration with

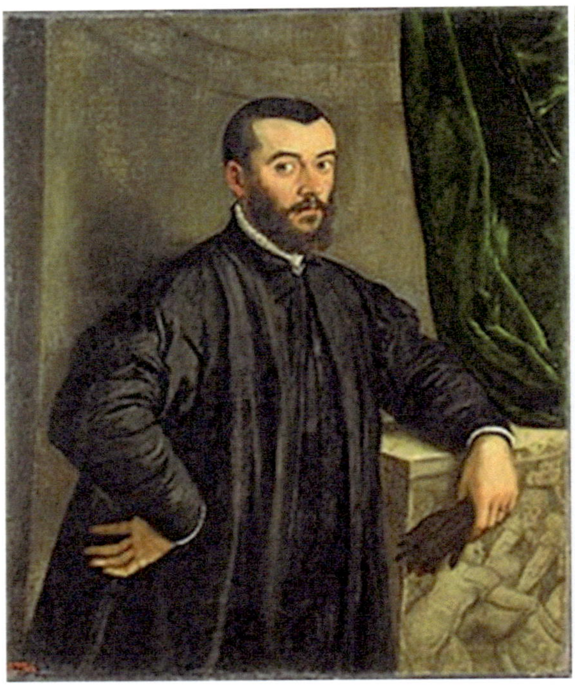

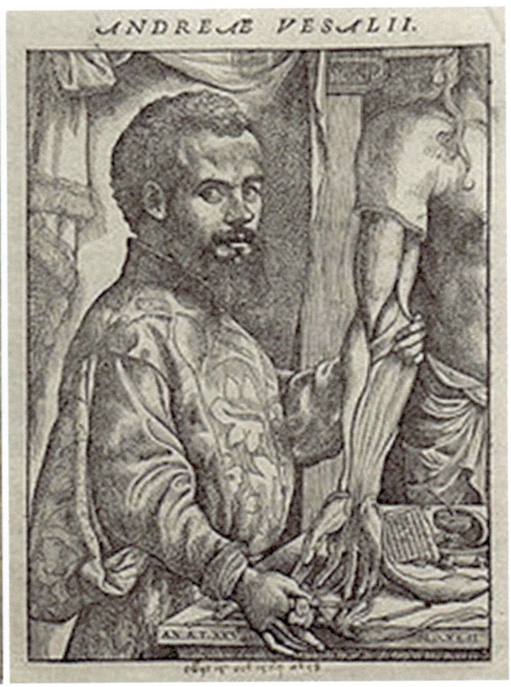

Figs. 1.5 and 1.6 Vesalius (1514–1564)

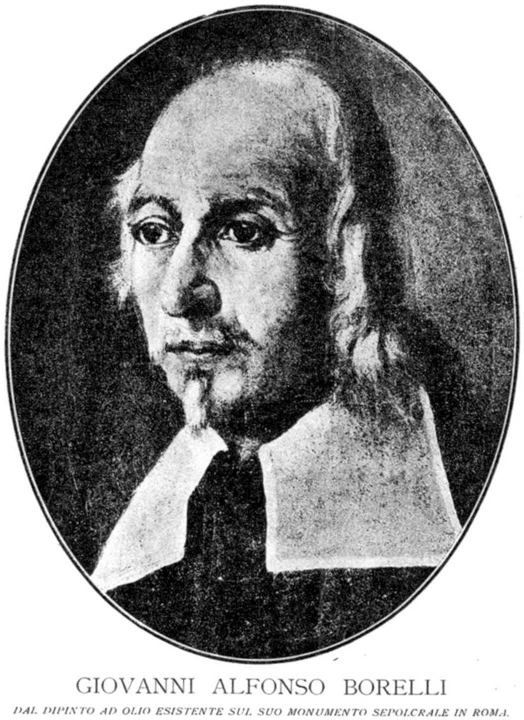
GIOVANNI ALFONSO BORELLI
DAL DIPINTO AD OLIO ESISTENTE SUL SUO MONUMENTO SEPOLCRALE IN ROMA.

Fig. 1.7 Giovanni Borelli (1608–1679)

another important scientist, Marcello Malpighi [7–15]. He published a major scientific work, "De Motu Animalium," concerning the internal and external movements of the human body (musculoskeletal, ligament and joint functions, motility, muscle actions, circulatory supply, etc.). His designs continue to provide valuable insights into spine motion and human biomechanics. His studies were only rediscovered and used in 1935 by the English historian, scientist, and scholar Friedrich Powels (4 January 1850 to 8 May 1904) [8–14] (Fig. 1.7).

1.5 Further Studies Regarding Spinal Ligaments

In 1646, Fabrizius Hildanus of Germany employed cervical traction to treat cervical dislocations, highlighting the crucial role of the spinal ligaments in his studies [8–14]. Leonhard Euler (1707–1783) developed a model of spine motion analysis, and Julius Wolff, a German orthopedic surgeon, performed bone studies to establish better explanations of the kinematic function of the human spine and the support provided by the spinal ligaments [9–13]. Hermet Burrel in Boston City Hospital made seminal observations about spine motility, spine performance, and spinal cord functions through the anatomical segments, including the spinal ligaments [8–14]. Samuel Haughton developed new methods for "drop" hanging at Newgate Gaol in 1764, refined in 1875 and further developed by Marshall in 1886, Patterson in 1890, and Wood-Jones in 1908 [9–17]. Other significant contributions to understanding the role of the spinal ligaments [10–19] were Mitsichelli, 1709; Porfur du Petit, 1710; Huber, 1739; Rolando, 1809 (substantia gelatinosa); and Stilling, 1824 (microtome). Experimental studies of the spinal segments were also reported by Burdach (1826), Truck (1849), Clark (1851), Lissauer (1855), Goll (1860), Fleshing (1876), Gowers (1880), Bastian (1890), and Flatau (1894).

1.6 Contribution of Hans Karl Barkow

Hans Karl Barkow (1798–1873), a German anatomist and physiologist, was born on August 4, 1798, and educated in Berlin (Geifswald and Friedrich Wilhelm Universities) [11–19]. He obtained his doctorate in 1821 at Greifswald and was appointed professor of anatomy at the same university from 1826 to 1835. He was a professor at Breslau between 1835 and 1873. He was also the director of the Anatomical Institute from 1845 [11–19]. In addition to the two major ligaments at the craniocervical junction (CCJ) (the alar and transverse ligaments), he described Barkow's ligament, a rare accessory ligament located anterosuperior to the dens. The alar ligament is a horizontal band attached to the occipital condyles [16–22]. The width, length, and thickness of Barkow's ligament are 4 mm, 2.5 cm, and 3.5 mm, respectively. Anatomically, its action is to resist extension of the atlanto-occipital joint, a function synergic with the anterior atlanto-occipital membrane [16–22].

1.7 Contributions of Sir Henry Morris, Wenzel Gruber, and Friedrich Arnold

Sir Henry Morris (7 January 1844 to 14 June 1926), anatomist and surgeon, was born in Petworth, Sussex, UK in 1844 (Fig. 1.8) and educated at Epsom and University College, London. In 1861, he worked in Guy's Hospital. He also worked in the urological surgery and cancer wards of Middlesex Hospital in 1870. In 1879, he published his "Anatomy of the Joints," a study of the morphological parts (ligaments, joints, etc.) where the head joins the spinal column, the CCJ region [11, 14–20].

Wenzel Gruber (1814–1890), anatomist, was born on 24 September 1814 in the small village of Krukanice near Pilsen, now in the Czech Republic [11, 16–22]. He studied at the University of Prague and then in St. Petersburg, Russia, and moved back to Austria in 1888. In Lang's textbook, "Gruber's ligament" denoted a ligament extending from the transverse occipital ligament posteriorly to the apical ligament anteriorly. Gruber served as the scientific director of practical and applied anatomy for over 30 years. He died from a stroke in Vienna on September 30, 1890 [16–22].

Philipp Friedrich Arnold (8 January 1803 to 5 July 1890), anatomist and physiologist, was born in Edenkoben (Rheinpfalz), Germany (Fig. 1.9) and studied at the University of Heidelberg. His name became associated with several anatomical structures, such as nerve, ganglion, and canal [16–21]. Anatomically, external fibers belonging to the accessory atlanto-axial ligament (AAAL), called the "lateral occipito-axial ligament," oblique fibrous bundles inserting the lateral surface of the foramen magnum over the posterior surface of the axis, are called "Arnold's ligament." These fibers insert on the lateral of the atlas, reinforcing the atlanto-axial capsule; some have used the eponym for the entire AAAL [16–22].

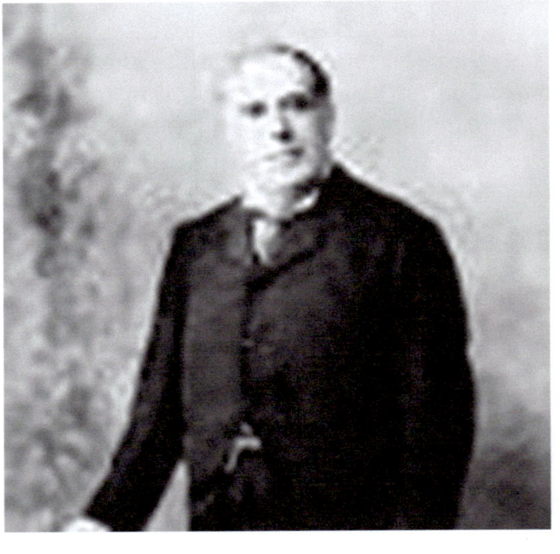

Fig. 1.8 Henry Morris (1844–1926)

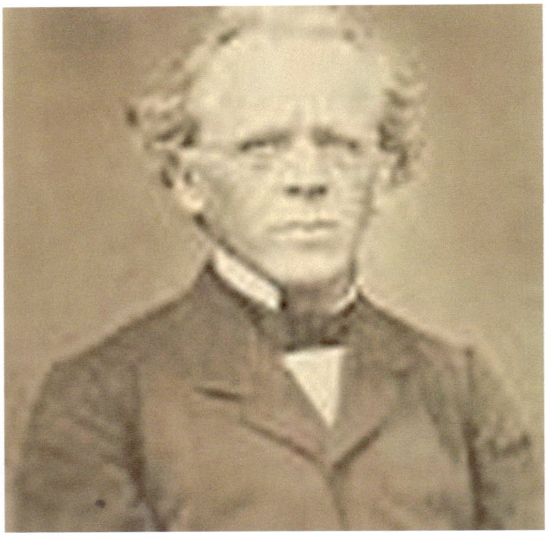

Fig. 1.9 Philipp Friedrich Arnold (1803–1890)

1.8 Modern Era Studies

In 1838, Key documented a case report involving ossification of the posterior longitudinal ligament (PLL) in the cervical spine. Wood-Jones in 1913 performed a specific anatomical analysis of all the spinal elements, including the course of the spinal ligaments [8–14]. In 1942, 100 years after Key, Oppenheimer reported a total of eighteen cases of calcification or ossification of the anterior longitudinal ligament and the PLL. Even then, its clinical importance was not widely recognized. In 1960, Tsukimoto reported a case of PLL ossification in the cervical spine. Only in Japan was ossification of the PLLs indexed as an official disease in 1975, and the first guideline was published in 2005, with an additional directive published in 2019 [11–18]. Taylor, in 1929, used cervical tractions, and Crutchfield, in 1933, incorporated modern, innovative elements (Edmonton Extension Tongs) into his tractions to achieve better clinical results. Gardner in 1972 improved the Crutchfield cervical system (Gardner Wells Tongs) [11–18]. The halo system was successfully presented by Perry and Nickel in 1959, and Harrington developed an innovative rod and hook system in 1962 [19–26].

In 1962, Sir Frank Hodsworth (22 September 1904 to December 1969) proposed the two-column spine model. He was an orthopedic surgeon from England, UK, recognized as a pioneer in the fields of rehabilitation, spinal injuries, and spinal segments. In 1983, Francis Denis from the USA (1946) described a novel, very comprehensive and useful classification system, the so-called Dennis Classification, to facilitate scientific communication and medical dialogue regarding these fractures and their treatments [19–24].

The continuing evolution of neuroradiology through X-ray, three-dimensional (3D) X-ray, computed tomography (CT), 3D CT and especially magnetic resonance imaging (MRI) and functional MRI has provided a better understanding of the anatomy, the kinematics, and the biomechanics of the spinal column and the spinal ligaments [27–34]. Accurate imaging is a crucial aspect of the armamentarium of neurosurgeons and spine surgeons worldwide, facilitating better treatment of spinal diseases and spinal trauma to improve the Quality of Life (QOL) of patients, particularly their Health-related Quality of Life (HRQL) [28–34].

1.9 Conclusion

Throughout the ages, considerable scientific effort has been invested in enhancing the anatomical, physiological, morphological, and structural understanding of the spinal ligaments. All of these contributions demonstrate the need for reciprocal interactions to develop more successful and safer neuro-anatomical, morphological, neurosurgical, and spinal procedures and approaches for the human nervous system, thereby achieving optimal results. The modern era provides the tools (diagnostics, radiological, imaging, physiological, etc.) to achieve better results and improve understanding of the complexity and importance of the spinal ligaments in the marvelous and complex entity that is the human body.

References

1. Castiglioni A. Storia della Medicina. A Mondadori; 1936.
2. Castiglioni A. Storia della Medicina. A Mondadori; 1948.
3. Castiglioni A. La medicina ai tempi e nell'opera di Dante Roma, Leonardo da Vinci, 1922 Trieste, Biblioteca dei Civici Musei di Storia ed Arte, inv. CMA 9839.
4. Syrmos N, Ampatzidis G, Fachantidou A, Mouratidis I, Syrmos C. Historical back training in most important points of neurosurgery. Ann General Psychiatry. 2010;9(Suppl 1):S89.
5. Syrmos NC, Giannouli V, Kottas S, Turgut M. History of cranial subdural hematoma. In: Subdural Hematoma: Past to Present to Future Management; 2021. p. 33–43.
6. Syrmos NC, Giannouli V, Turgut M. The sutures of the skull: a historical perspective the sutures of the skull: anatomy, Embryology, Imaging, and Surgery, 2021, pp. 7–18.
7. Goodrich JT. How to get in and out of the skull: from tumi to "hammer and chisel" to the Gigli saw and the osteoplastic flap. Neurosurg Focus. 2014;36(4):E6.

8. Sakai K, Yoshii T, Furuya T, Machino M. Research history, pathology and epidemiology of ossification of the posterior longitudinal ligament and ligamentum flavum. J Clin Med. 2022;11(18):5386.
9. Naderi S, Türe U, Pait TG. History of the spinal cord localization. Neurosurg Focus. 2004;16(1):E15.
10. Matsunaga S, Sakou T. Ossification of the posterior longitudinal ligament of the cervical spine: etiology and natural history. Spine (Phila Pa 1976). 2012;37(5):E309–14.
11. Sanan A, Rengachary SS. The history of spinal biomechanics. Neurosurgery. 1996;39(4):657–68.
12. Heary RF, Madhavan K. The history of spinal deformity. Neurosurgery. 2008;63(3 Suppl):5–15.
13. Hardy TA. Spinal cord anatomy and localization. Continuum (Minneap Minn). 2021;27(1):12–29.
14. Pearce JM. The development of spinal cord anatomy. Eur Neurol. 2008;59(6):286–91.
15. Schiller MD, Mobbs RJ. The historical evolution of the management of spinal cord injury. J Clin Neurosci. 2012;19(10):1348–53.
16. Rai R, Tubbs RS. Barkow's ligament. In: Tubbs RS, Iwanaga J, Loukas M, Oskouian RJ, editors. Clinical anatomy of the ligaments of the Craniocervical junction. UK: Cambridge Scholars Publishing; 2019. p. 213–9.
17. Naderi S, Andalkar N, Benzel EC. History of spine biomechanics: part II--from the Renaissance to the 20th century. Neurosurgery. 2007;60(2):392–403.
18. Tubbs RS. Miscellaneous ligaments of the craniocervicl junction including Arnold's, Gruber's, and Gerber's ligaments. In: Tubbs RS, Iwanaga J, Loukas M, Oskouian RJ, editors. Clinical anatomy of the ligaments of the Craniocervical junction. UK: Cambridge Scholars Publishing; 2019. p. 233–41.
19. Tubbs RS. The ligaments and joints connecting the head with the spinal column from Morris' the anatomy of the joints. In: Tubbs RS, Iwanaga J, Loukas M, Oskouian RJ, editors. Clinical anatomy of the ligaments of the Craniocervical junction. UK: Cambridge Scholars Publishing; 2019. p. 25–50.
20. Lang J. Clinical anatomy of the cervical spine. New York: Thieme Medical Publishers; 1993.
21. Naňka O. Wáclav Leopold Gruber (1814-1890) [Wenzel Leopold Gruber (1814-1890)]. Cas Lek Cesk. 2015;154(2):95–7.
22. Ashby N, Squiers J. A historical perspective on the development of modern concepts of tissue perfusion: prehistory to the twentieth century. Crit Care Nurs Clin North Am. 2014;26(3):297–309.
23. Kotani Y, Takahata M, Abumi K, Ito M, Sudo H, Minami A. Cervical myelopathy resulting from combined ossification of the ligamentum flavum and posterior longitudinal ligament: report of two cases and literature review. Spine J. 2013;13(1):e1–6.
24. Koike Y, Takahata M, Nakajima M, Otomo N, Suetsugu H, Liu X, Endo T, Imagama S, Kobayashi K, Kaito T, Kato S, Kawaguchi Y, Kanayama M, Sakai H, Tsuji T, Miyamoto T, Inose H, Yoshii T, Kashii M, Nakashima H, Ando K, Taniguchi Y, Takeuchi K, Ito S, Tomizuka K, Hikino K, Iwasaki Y, Kamatani Y, Maeda S, Nakajima H, Mori K, Seichi A, Fujibayashi S, Kanchiku T, Watanabe K, Tanaka T, Kida K, Kobayashi S, Takahashi M, Yamada K, Takuwa H, Lu HF, Niida S, Ozaki K, Momozawa Y, Genetic Study Group of Investigation Committee on Ossification of the Spinal Ligaments, Yamazaki M, Okawa A, Matsumoto M, Iwasaki N, Terao C, Ikegawa S. Genetic insights into ossification of the posterior longitudinal ligament of the spine. Elife. 2023;12:e86514.
25. Ohara Y. Ossification of the ligaments in the cervical spine, including ossification of the anterior longitudinal ligament, ossification of the posterior longitudinal ligament, and ossification of the ligamentum flavum. Neurosurg Clin N Am. 2018;29(1):63–8.
26. Swanson LW. Neuroanatomical Terminology. Oxford: Oxford University Press; 2015. p. 296–9.
27. Brambilla GA. Storia delle scoperte fisico-medico-anatomico-chirurgiche fatte dagli uomini illustri italiani. Tom 2. Giulio Cesare Aranzio. Milano: Nel Imperial Monistero di s. Ambrogio Maggiore; 1781. p. 188–98.
28. Kobayashi S, Matsushima T, Sakai T, Matsushima K, Bertalanffy H, Rutka JT. Evolution of microneurosurgical anatomy with special reference to the history of anatomy, surgical anatomy, and microsurgery: historical overview. Neurosurg Rev. 2022;45(1):253–61.
29. Fiester P, Rao D, Soule E, Orallo P, Rahmathulla G. Anatomic, functional, and radiographic review of the ligaments of the craniocervical junction. J Craniovertebr Junction Spine. 2021;12(1):4–9.
30. Fiester P, Soule E, Patel J, Jenson M, Rao D. Interrelationship between craniocervical dissociation spectrum injuries and atlantoaxial instability on trauma cervical MRI examinations. Cureus. 2022;14(11):e31238.
31. Peters B, Parizel PM, Van Goethem JW. Age-related changes to the craniocervical ligaments in asymptomatic subjects: a prospective MR study. Eur Spine J. 2020;29(5):1029–35.
32. Baumert B, Wörtler K, Steffinger D, Schmidt GP, Reiser MF, Baur-Melnyk A. Assessment of the internal craniocervical ligaments with a new magnetic resonance imaging sequence: three-dimensional turbo spin echo with variable flip-angle distribution (SPACE). Magn Reson Imaging. 2009;27(7):954–60.
33. Sakai T. Historical evolution of anatomical terminology from ancient to modern. Anat Sci Int. 2007;82(2):65–81.
34. Syrmos NC. The seven miracles of neurosurgery. J Neurosurg Sci. 2020;64(4):407.

Development of the Spinal Ligaments

2

Natalia Molik and R. Shane Tubbs

2.1 Introduction

The embryonic period, encompassing the first 8 weeks post-fertilization, marks a critical time in forming the body's foundational structures. It begins with the formation of the morula, which migrates through the fallopian tube and transforms into a blastocyst by the end of the first week [1]. This blastocyst features a cavity, the blastocele, and gives rise to a bilaminar structure composed of epiblast and hypoblast layers [1]. By the second week, a primitive streak appears within the epiblast, and gastrulation begins, during which the three primary germ layers—definitive endoderm, ectoderm, and mesoderm—are formed [1].

The mesoderm, situated between the ectoderm and endoderm, plays a critical role in the development of connective tissues throughout the body [1]. It comprises four distinct regions: axial mesoderm (which includes the prechordal plate and notochord), paraxial mesoderm (presomitic), intermediate mesoderm, and lateral plate mesoderm [1]. The notochord, a hollow structure derived from the axial mesoderm, serves as a precursor to the vertebral column and plays a crucial role in the induction of the neural plate.

N. Molik · R. S. Tubbs (✉)
Tulane University School of Medicine,
New Orleans, LA, USA
e-mail: rtubbs@tulane.edu

Connective tissues, including cartilage, bone, blood, and specific organs, originate from the mesoderm, mesenchyme acting as a vital precursor [2]. Mesenchyme has a loose composition, consisting primarily of ground substance and sparse collagen fibers, providing the foundational matrix from which various connective tissues develop [2].

As development progresses, somites form from the paraxial mesoderm adjacent to the neural tube. These segmental structures differentiate to generate the sclerotome, which is essential for forming the spine and its associated structures, including the spinal ligaments [1]. By the fourth week of embryogenesis, sclerotome cells migrate around the notochord and neural tube, merging to form vertebral precursors [1]. This process is accompanied by the formation of intervertebral discs; the sclerotome contributes to the anulus fibrosus, while remnants of the notochord develop into the nucleus pulposus.

Ligaments are essential for stabilizing the spine, supporting its structure, and facilitating movement [2]. Composed of dense connective tissue, primarily made of collagen, ligaments serve as strong yet flexible bands or sheets connecting various skeletal system components [2]. Some ligaments, particularly elastic ligaments along the vertebral column, contain parallel bundles of elastic fibers alongside the collagen fibers, enhancing their flexibility [2]. The formation of spinal ligaments is closely linked to the growth

M. Turgut et al. (eds.), *Ligaments of the Vertebral Column*,
https://doi.org/10.1007/978-3-032-09070-6_2

and differentiation of surrounding structures, including vertebrae and intervertebral discs.

Ultimately, the intricate relationship between the mesoderm, mesenchyme, and the development of spinal ligaments underscores the complexity of connective tissue formation in the body [2]. As these structures mature, they provide the support and stability essential for a functional musculoskeletal system. Understanding the origins and maturation of spinal ligaments provides valuable insights into their roles in spinal health, injury prevention, and the biomechanical challenges the spine faces throughout life.

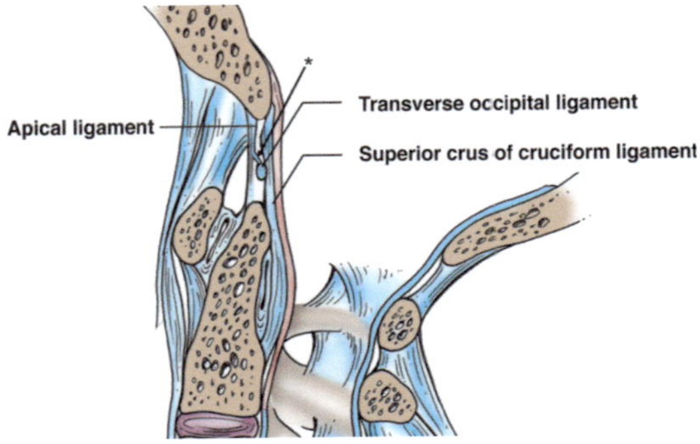

Fig. 2.1 Sagittal view noting the ligaments of the craniocervical junction. Note the anterior atlantooccipital membrane just anterior to the apical ligament. Gruber's ligament is seen at the *

2.2 Craniocervical Ligaments

2.2.1 Atlantooccipital Ligaments

2.2.1.1 Function

The atlantooccipital ligaments are essential for stabilizing the connection between the atlas (C1) and the occipital bone at the craniocervical junction [3]. They prevent excessive movement and maintain proper alignment, supporting the head's weight and aiding in posture [3]. In addition to their stabilizing function, they allow for a degree of flexibility and movement, facilitating flexion, extension, and some lateral motion of the head. The primary components of these ligaments are the anterior atlantooccipital membrane, the posterior atlantooccipital membrane, and the lateral atlantooccipital ligament [3].

2.2.1.2 Origin and Composition

The anterior atlantooccipital membrane (Fig. 2.1) is a thin, dense sheet of fibrous connective tissue comprising densely woven fibers that extend between the anterior margin of the foramen magnum and the upper border of the anterior arch of the atlas (C1) [4].

The posterior atlantooccipital membrane (Fig. 2.2) is also a sheet of dense fibrous connective tissue; it connects the posterior border of the foramen magnum to the posterior arch of the atlas [4]. Several studies have established a connection between the posterior atlantooccipital membrane, the rectus capitis posterior minor muscle, and the spinal dura mater [4].

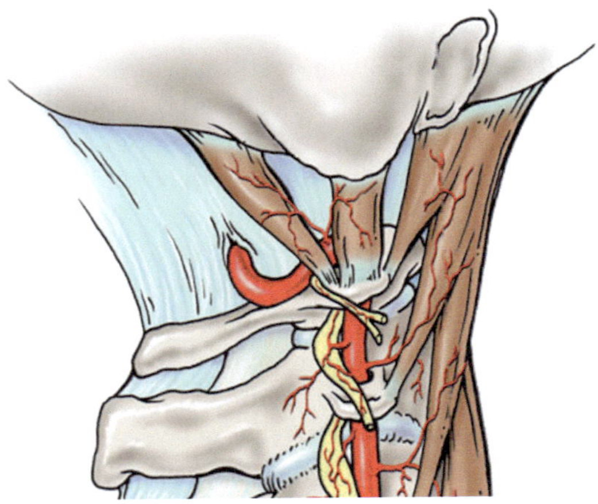

Fig. 2.2 Lateral view of the craniocervical junction noting the right vertebral artery piercing the posterior atlantooccipital membrane

The lateral atlantooccipital ligament, composed of dense connective tissue, connects to the anterolateral side of the transverse process of the atlas and inserts into the jugular process of the occipital bone. It runs laterally to the anterior atlantooccipital membrane, its fibers oriented in a direction opposite to those of the rectus capitis lateralis muscle [4].

While there is limited literature on the specific origins of the atlantooccipital membranes and ligaments, it is known that the craniocervical junction (CCJ) is of mesodermal origin and begins to form during the third gestational week [3], when the mesoderm divides into segmental clusters called somites. Once mature, these somites differentiate into ventromedial sclerotomes and dorsolateral dermomyotomes [3]. The sclerotomes ultimately develop into the vertebral bodies, neural arches, ligaments, and membranes.

2.2.1.3 Pathology

Atlantooccipital dissociation represents the most common cervical spine injury following a motor vehicle collision and is usually highly unstable with significant neurological morbidity [3].

2.2.2 Barkow's Ligament

2.2.2.1 Function

Barkow's ligament (Fig. 2.3) is positioned horizontally between the occipital condyles, located behind the alar ligaments and the apex of the odontoid process [5]. Its primary function, in conjunction with the anterior atlantooccipital membrane, is to prevent extension of the atlanto-occipital joint [5]. It also reinforces the stabilizing effect of the transverse ligament at the median atlantoaxial joint, contributing to overall stability in this critical region [6].

2.2.2.2 Origin and Composition

Barkow's ligament has been observed in fetuses aged 28–38 weeks of intrauterine life [5]. Its fibers run anterior to the alar ligaments, positioned just in front of the superior aspect of the dens, though they do not attach to those structures. The anatomical location and characteristics of Barkow's ligament have led researchers to question whether it is a distinct structure or simply a deeper component of the anterior atlantooccipital membrane [5].

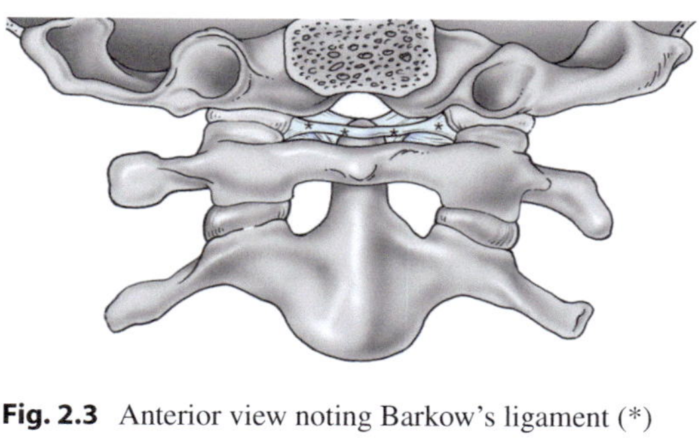

Fig. 2.3 Anterior view noting Barkow's ligament (*)

2.2.2.3 Pathology

Barkow's ligament contributes to the stability of the craniocervical junction (CCJ). Various clinical conditions can compromise the stability of this joint owing to ligamentous and biomechanical changes [5]. For example, Down syndrome, IVA mucopolysaccharidosis, Klippel-Feil syndrome, osteogenesis imperfecta, and Chiari type I malformations are associated with ligament laxity, which can increase the risk of neurological injury [5].

The CCJ is inherently less stable in children, making them more vulnerable to injury and subsequent neurological morbidity if there is trauma at this joint [5].

2.2.3 Apical Ligament

2.2.3.1 Function

The apical ligament (Figs. 2.1 and 2.4) stretches from the tip of the odontoid process (dens) to the basion, situated between the anterior occipital membrane and the cruciform ligament [3]. It extends from the tip of the dens to the anterior edge of the foramen magnum [3]. Despite its ana-

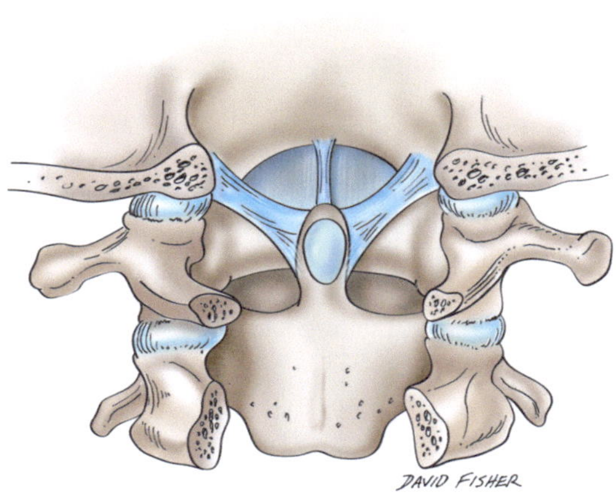

Fig. 2.4 Posterior view demonstrating the apical ligament connecting the tip of the odontoid process to the basion. Also note the laterally positioned alar ligaments

tomical presence, the apical ligament makes only a minimal contribution to the stability of the CCJ.

2.2.3.2 Origin and Composition

This ligament was once thought to be a derivative of the notochord, but histological studies have cast doubt on this, at least in adults.

2.2.3.3 Pathology

This ligament is absent in up to 20% of cadaveric dissections [3].

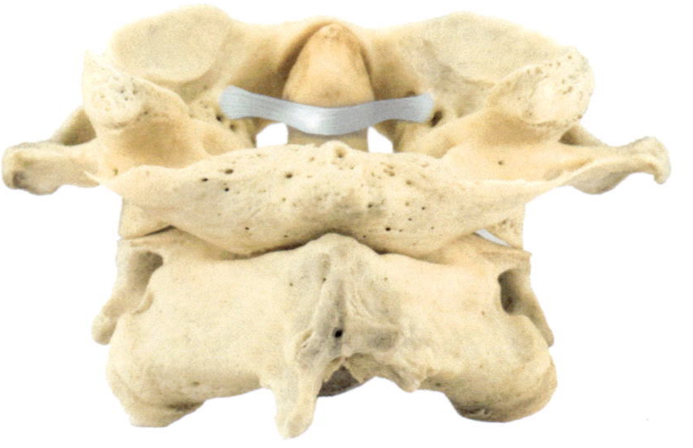

Fig. 2.5 The transverse ligament of the atlas

2.2.4 Transverse Occipital Ligament

2.2.4.1 Function

The transverse occipital ligament (TOL) (Fig. 2.1) is a minor accessory ligament of the CCJ. It is posterosuperior to the odontoid process and the alar ligament [4]. It crosses the foramen magnum horizontally, connecting the inner surfaces of the occipital condyles, positioned posterior to the alar ligament and superior to the transverse ligament [4]. Its primary function is to aid in stabilizing the CCJ during lateral bending, flexion, and axial rotation [7].

2.2.4.2 Origin and Composition

The TOL consists of dense, regular connective tissue rich in collagen fibers, interspersed with fibroblasts [7]. It has been observed in fetuses as early as 8–9 weeks of gestation and is believed to originate from the axial component of the first cervical sclerotome [7].

2.2.4.3 Pathology

The TOL is present in only about 10% of the population, although there is considerable discrepancy among researchers regarding its prevalence [4]. Its appearance is very similar to that of the alar ligament, making it challenging to distinguish the two [4].

2.2.5 Transverse Ligament of the Atlas

2.2.5.1 Function

The transverse ligament of the atlas (Fig. 2.5) is an essential component of the cruciform ligament and is the primary stabilizing ligament at the atlantoaxial joint. It could be considered the most important ligament in the body [8]. It is the strongest and thickest ligament in the craniocervical region [9]. Its main role is stabilizing the CCJ by securely anchoring the odontoid process (dens) to the posterior aspect of the anterior arch of the atlas (C1). The transverse ligament facilitates rotational movement in the neck [9].

2.2.5.2 Origin and Composition

The transverse ligament starts to develop around 6 weeks of gestation. It forms alongside the alar ligament from a shared mesenchymal condensation at the pro-atlas segment, emerging slightly earlier than the alar ligament [10]. Both ligaments arise from the first cervical sclerotome, along with the basal dental segments [11]. By 14–15 weeks of gestation, the transverse ligament can be identified as a relatively thin band connecting the lateral masses of the atlas (C1). At the same time, joint cavitation around the odontoid process is still incomplete, except for the mid-anterior portion [10]. At this developmental stage, a network of collagen fibers and a thin layer of articular cartilage have not yet formed [10]. The transverse ligament also lacks a weaker longitudinal band extending to the posterior surface of the axis, which is part of the cruciform ligament. Instead, it features a ring-like sheath that encircles the tip of the odontoid process, leaving it exposed to the primitive epidural space [10].

2.2.5.3 Pathology

If the transverse ligament is disrupted by trauma, the atlantoaxial joints become poorly equipped to tolerate axial rotation [10]. Specific individuals also suffer congenital abnormalities in the structure or thickness of the transverse ligament, which can make them more susceptible to instability [10]. Those born with conditions such as Down syndrome frequently have lax connective tissues, contributing to instability in the atlanto-axial joint [10].

2.2.6 Alar Ligament

2.2.6.1 Function

The alar ligament (Fig. 2.4), together with the transverse ligament, forms the cruciform ligament, which anchors the axis to the base of the skull [10]. These paired ligaments originate from the posterior surface of the upper dens and extend either caudocranially or horizontally [10].

The primary function of the alar ligaments is to limit axial rotation and lateral flexion of the head, helping to prevent anterior displacement of the atlas (C1) if the transverse ligament is ruptured [10]. This stabilizing role is crucial for maintaining the integrity of the CCJ.

2.2.6.2 Origin and Composition

The alar ligament can be observed in fetal specimens as early as 6–7 weeks of gestation and originates from a common mesenchymal condensation at the pro-atlas segment, similar to the transverse ligament [10]. It develops from the axial component of the first cervical sclerotome. By 14–15 weeks of gestation, the alar ligament is identifiable and consists of a broad band connecting the odontoid process to the occipital condyle [11]. It attaches to the posterior aspect of the odontoid process at the upper level and the lateral aspects at the lower level [11].

The fibers of this ligament are composed exclusively of collagen and are generally oriented horizontally, upward, or downward, their orientation being strongly influenced by the position of the occipital bone [12].

2.2.6.3 Pathology

Rarely do nodular calcifications or ossifications occur in the alar ligament. These can mimic a type III fracture of the occipital condyle or a type I fracture of the odontoid process [12].

Failure of the alar ligament can lead to excessive axial rotation, potentially resulting in compression or dissection injuries to the vertebral artery and damage to the spinal accessory nerves [12]. This instability underscores the significance of the alar ligament in preserving the integrity of the CCJ and safeguarding surrounding structures [12].

2.2.7 Accessory Atlantoaxial Ligament

The accessory atlantoaxial ligament (Fig. 2.6) inserts medially into the posterior surface of the axis and extends laterally and superiorly to attach to the lateral mass of the atlas (C1), located posterior to the transverse ligament. It can also send an extension more cranially to attach onto the occipital bone. This ligament is thought to enhance craniocervical stability [4].

Although limited research exists on the embryological origin of the accessory atlantoaxial ligament, sclerotomes are known to form the vertebrae and their associated ligaments [3]. The ligament develops as part of the maturation of structures that stabilize the atlantoaxial joint.

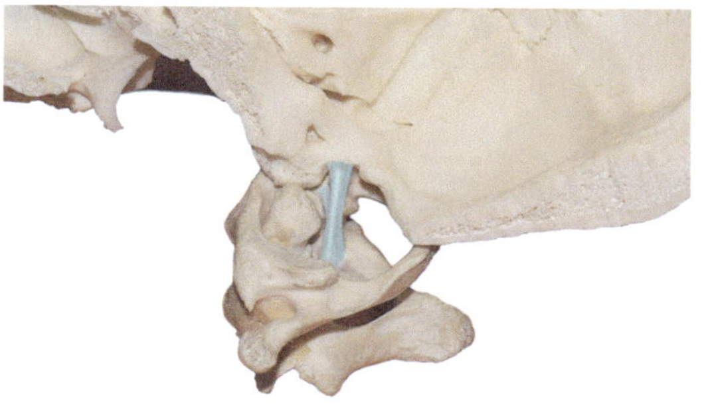

Fig. 2.6 The right accessory atlanto-axial ligament

2.3 Thoracic Ligaments

2.3.1 Facet Capsular Ligament

2.3.1.1 Function

The facet capsular ligament encases the facet joint by linking the posterolateral articular facet joints of adjacent vertebrae [13]. It functions with other accessory ligaments of the vertebral column, which help stabilize the column and its joints [8].

2.3.1.2 Origin and Composition

The facet capsular ligament has a collagen-rich exterior and an elastin-rich interior, which provides both strength and flexibility [13]. The details of its formation in the embryo are not fully understood, but it is known to originate from the mesoderm and sclerotomes of the developing vertebral column. As adjacent sclerotomes form vertebrae, the facet capsular ligaments develop to stabilize the zygapophysial joints, ensuring proper spinal function [13]. Further research is needed to clarify the specific developmental processes involved.

2.3.1.3 Pathology

Injury to the facet capsular ligament is commonly associated with whiplash resulting from sudden neck movements [8]. There are also reports of ossification in these ligaments, leading to reduced flexibility and increased stiffness, which can cause pain and restricted movement [8]. This underscores the crucial role of the capsular ligament in spinal health and function.

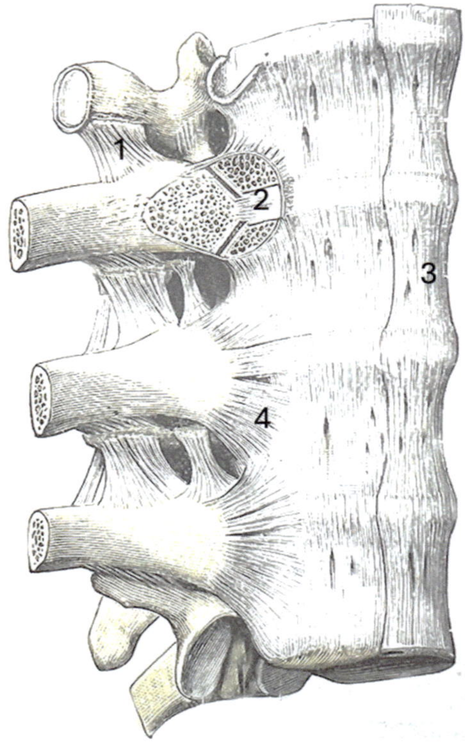

Fig. 2.7 The superior costotransverse ligament (1), intra-articular ligament of the head of the rib (2), anterior longitudinal ligament (3) and radiate ligament (4). (After Testut)

2.3.2 Radiate Ligament of the Costovertebral Joint

2.3.2.1 Function

The radiate ligament (Fig. 2.7) of the costovertebral joint connects the head of the rib to the adjacent vertebral body, facilitating only minimal gliding movements at the facets [8]. This ligament stabilizes the costovertebral joint, allowing for controlled motion while ensuring the rib remains securely attached to the spine during respiration [14]. Its structural integrity is essential for maintaining proper thoracic function and facilitating effective breathing mechanics [14].

2.3.2.2 Origin and Composition

The radiate ligament of the costovertebral joint consists of dense, regular connective tissue and can be identified as early as 8 weeks of gestation [15]. Although the specifics of its development in the embryo remain largely unclear, the costovertebral joints are known to originate from the central sclerotome and arthrotome of a single somite; this process occurs without resegmentation [15].

2.3.3 Intra-Articular Ligament of the Head of the Rib

2.3.3.1 Function

The intra-articular ligament of the head of the rib (Fig. 2.7) is a small yet significant structure that connects the two articular surfaces of the rib's head to the corresponding vertebral body [8]. Its primary function is to provide additional support to the costovertebral joint during movement. This ligament is crucial for maintaining proper alignment between the ribs and vertebrae, especially during respiratory movements [8]. By stabilizing the joint, the intra-articular ligament ensures smooth and coordinated rib motion, essential for effective breathing mechanics [8].

2.3.3.2 Origin and Composition

Similar to the radiate ligament of the costovertebral joint, the intra-articular ligament develops as an integral component of this joint's formation [15]. It typically appears around the same time as the costovertebral joints, approximately 8 weeks of gestation [15].

2.3.4 Superior Costotransverse Ligament

2.3.4.1 Function

The superior costotransverse ligament (Fig. 2.7) stabilizes the costotransverse joint by linking the neck of the rib to the transverse process of the vertebra. It is also essential for controlling the extent of rotation and lateral flexion of the ribcage during respiratory movements [8].

2.3.4.2 Origin and Composition

Like other ligaments related to the costovertebral joint, the superior costotransverse ligament originates from mesodermal tissue surrounding the developing vertebrae and ribs [15]. It usually becomes identifiable around 8 weeks of gestation [15].

2.3.4.3 Pathology

Injury or absence of the costovertebral ligaments can lead to increased rib movement in relation to the vertebrae during breathing [8]. This instability compromises the function of the ribcage as a protective "box" for the thoracic organs, rendering them more vulnerable to injury from external impacts or excessive stress [8]. Preserving the integrity of these ligaments is crucial for providing structural support and safeguarding essential thoracic structures [8].

2.3.5 Costotransverse Ligament

2.3.5.1 Function

The costotransverse ligament limits rib movement at the costotransverse joint during respiration, thereby promoting optimal expansion of the thoracic cavity [8]. It also reinforces the front part of the costotransverse joint, contributing to overall stability during breathing [8].

2.3.5.2 Origin and Composition

This ligament consists of short fibers that stretch from the back of the rib's neck to the front of the neighboring transverse process [8]. From an embryological perspective, the development of the costotransverse ligament is associated with the formation of the costovertebral and costotransverse joints, which typically begin to develop around 8 weeks of gestation [15].

2.3.5.3 Pathology

In the 11th and 12th ribs, the costotransverse ligament is rudimentary or absent [8].

2.3.6 Lateral Costotransverse Ligament

2.3.6.1 Function

The lateral costotransverse ligament strengthens the posterior aspect of the costotransverse joint [8]. It stabilizes the connection between the rib and the transverse process of the vertebra, preventing excessive movement.

2.3.6.2 Origin and Composition

Embryologically, the development of the lateral costotransverse ligament aligns with the formation of the costovertebral and costotransverse joints, which occur around 8 weeks of gestation [15].

2.4 Lumbar Ligaments

2.4.1 Anterior Longitudinal Ligament

2.4.1.1 Function

The anterior longitudinal ligament (ALL) is a crucial stabilizer of the spine (Fig. 2.7). It is the strongest and largest among the spinal ligaments, essential for limiting the movement of spinal segments during extension [8]. At its uppermost end, the ALL is anchored to the basilar occipital bone and extends downward to the anterior tubercle of the atlas (C1) and the anterior surface of the axis (C2) [8]. Moving further downward, it continues to the anterior surface of the sacrum, so it spans the entire length of the anterior aspect of the vertebral column [8]. It attaches to the anterior aspect of each vertebral body and the front of the anulus fibrosus, providing critical support and stability throughout the spinal column [8].

2.4.1.2 Origin and Composition

The ALL consists of numerous densely packed collagen fibers intertwined with a few elastic fibers and is organized into three layers: superficial, intermediate, and deep [8]. The superficial layers attach to the intervertebral discs and the anterior edges of the vertebral bodies, creating flexible, secondary connections to their midsections. This configuration helps to fill the concave areas and contributes to a smoother, more flattened appearance of the anterior vertebral column [8]. The intermediate fibers connect 2–3 vertebrae; the deep fibers establish direct links between adjacent vertebral bodies.

The ALL can be identified in human fetuses as early as 8 weeks of gestation. Between the seventh and eighth weeks of fetal development, it forms from an interstitial matrix surrounding the cartilaginous vertebrae [2]. During this period, a strong attachment to the anterior surface of the centra is also established [2]. Its fibers generally blend with the external surface of the anulus fibrosus, leading to different interpretations of its anatomical origins.

The ALL has been shown to contribute to the ossification of the fetal vertebral body during development [16]. Its attachments are primarily associated with cortical bone, as the ALL is highly connected to the anterior cortical wall via fiber bundles, reflecting the typical progression of ligament formation [8, 16]. By 30 weeks of gestation, the anterior cortical wall is attached and incorporated into the ALL [16]. In contrast, the anulus fibrosus is anchored to the vertebral end plate, and the fibers of the adult anulus that connect to bone are integrated into the ring apophysis, which is classified as non-cortical [8]. This developmental divergence suggests that the short, deep fibers of the ALL should not be considered part of the anulus fibrosus associated with vertebral cartilage [8].

2.4.1.3 Pathology

The ALL is unique among spinal ligaments. It is the only structure that limits the extension of the vertebral column, making it particularly important in assessing and diagnosing cervical acceleration-deceleration injuries, commonly known as whiplash [8].

The ALL can also be linked to diffuse idiopathic skeletal hyperostosis (DISH) or Forestier disease. This rare condition is characterized by excessive calcification or thickening of the ligament in the cervical region [8]. This pathological alteration can result in complications such as difficulties swallowing due to the calcified ligament compressing the esophagus [8]. It can also lead to radiculomyelopathy due to the narrowing of the cervical spine [8].

2.4.2 Posterior Longitudinal Ligament

2.4.2.1 Function

The Posterior Longitudinal Ligament (PLL) (Fig. 2.8) plays a vital role in stabilizing the spine, primarily functioning to resist hyperflexion of the vertebral column by preventing the

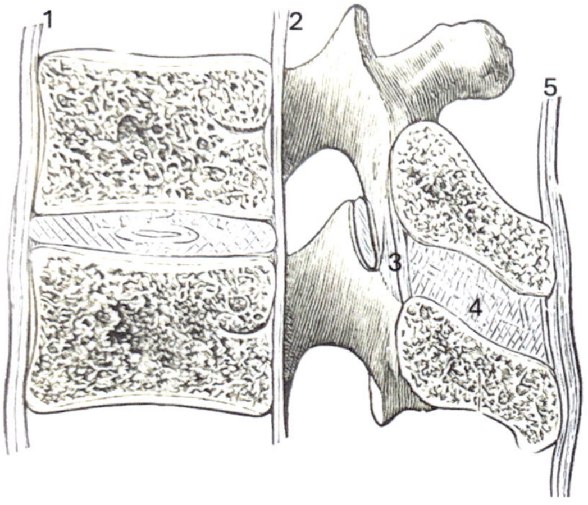

Fig. 2.8 The anterior longitudinal ligament (1), posterior longitudinal ligament (2), ligamentum flavum (3), interspinous ligament (4) and supraspinous ligament (5). (After Testut)

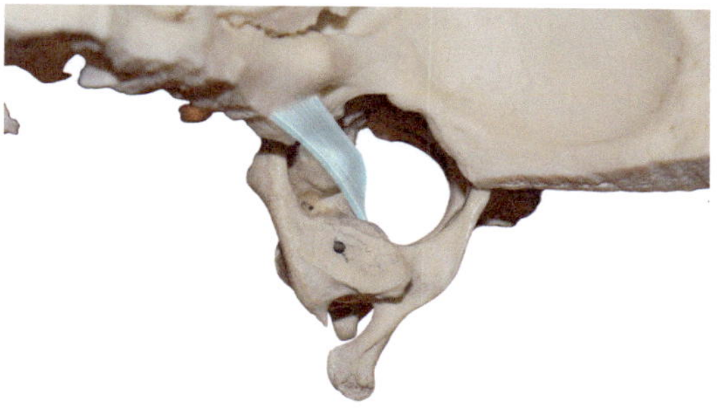

Fig. 2.9 The tectorial membrane

posterior ends of the vertebral bodies from separating [8]. It consists of a band of longitudinal fibers that extend along the entire length of the vertebral canal on the posterior surfaces of the vertebrae, connecting them to the posterior aspect of the anulus fibrosus [8]. This anatomical arrangement helps to prevent posterior herniation of the nucleus pulposus [8]. At its rostral end, the PLL connects C2 to the intracranial aspect of the base of the skull, known as the tectorial membrane (Fig. 2.9), which provides structural support and stability to the upper cervical spine [8].

2.4.2.2 Origin and Composition

The PLL consists mainly of collagen fibers, but it features more elastic fibers than the ALL, enhancing its flexibility. The arrangement of collagenous and elastin fibers follows a cephalocaudal orientation and is denser and more compact than that of the ALL [8]. The PLL is structured into two layers: a thick, deep layer firmly attached to the posterior surface of each vertebra and a thinner, superficial layer extending from the tectorial membrane [1].

Hamid et al. (2002) demonstrated that the PLL can be identified in fetuses as early as 13 weeks of gestation [17]. At this developmental stage, its anterior aspect connects to the posterior surface of the vertebral body, giving it a double-layered appearance near the basivertebral vein [17]. At the intervertebral disc level, the PLL attaches to the posterior edge of the anulus fibrosus. At the same time, the anterior portion of the dura mater links to the back of the PLL via connective tissue.

By 15 weeks, the PLL's deep and superficial layers are recognizable. At the vertebral body, it takes on a triangular shape, with the deep fibers oriented longitudinally and the superficial fibers positioned horizontally [17]. Although the PLL continues to attach to the anulus fibrosus at the intervertebral disc level, its triangular contour is no longer apparent [17]. The dura mater remains connected to the back of the PLL through fibrous tissue, anchoring it to the vertebral discs.

At 21 weeks, the attachment between the dura mater and PLL appears more ligament-like at the level of the vertebral body, with the anterior dura also connecting to its superficial layer [17]. However, a gap forms between the dura and the PLL at the intervertebral disc level, where the PLL still adheres to the anulus fibrosus [17]. The connections between the dura mater and PLL weaken, reducing to a few strands of connective tissue.

By 32 weeks, the PLL regains its triangular shape and remains connected to the dura mater at the level of the vertebral body [17]. The dura mater adheres to the PLL at the intervertebral disc, its fibers oriented across the intervertebral foramen.

At 39 weeks, the deep layer of the PLL anchors firmly to the fibrous tissue of the vertebral body, while the anterior dura connects to the superficial layer only through fibrous formations [17]. At the intervertebral disc level, the PLL's superficial layer remains attached to the anulus fibrosus.

Importantly, studies have indicated that the tectorial membrane is absent in specimens between 14 and 15 weeks of gestation, suggesting that this structure develops later as it fuses with the cranial dura mater and is separated from the transverse ligament by a thin layer of areolar tissue [10].

2.4.2.3 Pathology

The PLL has a limited capacity to resist hyperflexion of the vertebral column, which helps prevent and redirect posterior herniation of the nucleus pulposus [8]. It is densely populated with nerve endings, meaning that injuries to it, such as those from whiplash or acute spinal trauma, can lead to localized pain [8]. This discomfort arises as the nucleus pulposus exerts pressure on the nerve endings within the PLL [8].

The PLL can become ossified in older adults, contributing to radiculomyelopathy [8].

2.4.3 Ligamentum Flavum

2.4.3.1 Function

The ligamentum flavum (LF) (Fig. 2.8) comprises a series of ligaments that interconnect the laminae of neighboring vertebrae, forming alternating sections of the posterior wall of the vertebral canal [8]. It is present bilaterally within each vertebral canal and converges at the midline. Each LF spans from the posterior surface of the lamina of the vertebra below to the anterior surface of the lamina of the vertebra above [8]. Extending from the base of the skull to the pelvis, it is positioned anteriorly and centrally between the laminae, thereby contributing to the posterior aspect of the vertebral canal [8].

The LF is crucial for counteracting the separation of the vertebral laminae during spinal flexion [8]. It achieves this by restricting abrupt flexion movements and aiding in the return of the vertebral column to an upright posture [8]. This function helps maintain the spine's natural curvature and protects the intervertebral discs from potential injury.

2.4.3.2 Origin and Composition

The yellow coloration of the ligamentum flavum (LF) is primarily attributable to its rich content of elastic fibers; it comprises approximately 80% elastic fibers and 20% collagen fibers. The elastic fibers are arranged parallel to the longitudinal axis of the ligament [8]. Two types are present: elastic fibers and elaunin fibers [8]. The elastic fibers predominate in the central region of the ligament. In contrast, the elaunin fibers, composed of scattered elastin deposits interspersed with microtubules, are more concentrated near the ligament's bony attachments [18].

The LF is a bilateral structure that can be detected as early as 12 weeks of gestation [2]. As fetal development progresses, the right and left portions of the LF either fuse at the midline or partially unite with gaps that allow venous connections to be made to the vertebral venous plexuses [19]. The formation of the LF is intricately connected to the development of the laminae [10]. Its origin can be traced back to a hypercellular layer located on the anterior side of the laminar cartilage. By 15 weeks of gestation, it has thickened; however, the embryonic LF has a lower density of elastic fibers than its adult counterpart [2].

The components of elastogenesis crucial for forming the LF have been researched. Elastogenesis involves several proteins, including tropoelastin (the soluble precursor of elastin), fibrillin-1 (Fib-1), lysyl oxidase (LOX), and fibulin-4 (Fbln-4) [19]. Fib-1 is a key component of microfibrils, which serve as scaffolding on which tropoelastin is deposited, while LOX facilitates the cross-linking of properly aligned tropoelastin monomers into mature elastin. Fbln-4 is believed to aid in tropoelastin deposition and/or cross-linking [19].

One study showed that elastic fibers within the LF first appear on postnatal day seven, initially presenting as thin and disorganized [19]. By postnatal day 14, these fibers become more organized, aligning longitudinally and adopting a wavy or crimped shape. Between postnatal days 14 and 35, they straighten, and by postnatal day 56, while there is no change in diameter or orientation, they appear denser [19]. At 2 years of age, the elastin fibers show fragmentation in various tissue areas.

Markers for elastin synthesis in the LF indicate that staining for tropoelastin peaks from postnatal day seven to postnatal day 35, followed by a significant reduction in staining after postnatal day 56 up to 2 years [19]. Fibrillin-1 demonstrates the most intense staining from embryonic week 16 to postnatal day 0, while fibulin-4 shows the strongest staining at postnatal day 14 [19]. In contrast, lysyl oxidase stains most intensely between postnatal days seven and 21.

2.4.3.3 Pathology

Anatomical variations in the midline gaps of the LF depend on the vertebral level. Yoon et al. (2014) showed that the prevalence of these midline gaps is greater in the cervical and thoracic regions than at lumbar levels; they are particularly notable at C5-C6 and T10-T11, with lower frequencies at T4-T5 and below T2 [19].

The LF is absent along the anterior half of the anterior laminar surface, a detail that holds practical significance for surgeons aiming to prevent incidental durotomy during laminectomy procedures [20]. This ligament comprises two distinct layers with a "gliding" space between them; notably, the outer layer is discontinuous at the midline. This anatomical characteristic can provide a strategic entry point for safely dividing the ligament without harming the dura mater below [20].

Hematoma formation within the LF is a rare source of radiculopathy, typically resulting from a partial tear in a previously degenerated ligament. This injury leads to intrafilamentary bleeding, manifesting as mild, non-neurological symptoms [20]. Subsequent fibrinolysis and hemolysis can significantly increase the volume of the LF mass, exacerbating symptoms and potentially causing considerable neural compression.

During hyperextension, the LF can protrude into the spinal canal, risking compression of the spinal cord, particularly in conditions such as spinal stenosis, ossification of the posterior longitudinal ligament (PLL), or ossification of the LF itself [8].

2.4.4 Supraspinous Ligament

2.4.4.1 Function

The supraspinous ligament (SSL) (Fig. 2.8) is crucial for restricting spinal flexion. This strong, fibrous structure stretches from the apex of each spinous process, linking vertebra C7 down to the sacrum [18]. Superior to C7, the SSL transitions into the ligamentum nuchae, displaying distinctive structural features. As it descends toward the lumbar area, it becomes thicker and broader, ultimately integrating with the adjacent fascia.

2.4.4.2 Origin and Composition

The SSL comprises three layers—superficial, middle, and deep—each characterized by parallel-aligned tendinous fibers that define its appearance [18]. The superficial layer consists of longitudinally-arranged collagen fibers that span across 3–4 spinous processes. The middle layer extends over 2–3 spinous processes and incorporates fibers from the posterior layer of the thoracolumbar fascia and the aponeurosis of the longissimus thoracis muscle [1]. The deep layer connects adjacent spinous processes and is formed from strong tendinous fibers originating from the aponeurosis of the longissimus thoracis [8].

Notably, the rostral portion of the SSL, known as the ligamentum nuchae, is primarily composed of the aponeuroses of the trapezius, splenius capitis, rhomboids, and the posterior serratus muscles [21]. Studies of bovine specimens indicate that isolated elastic fibers within the ligamentum nuchae begin to emerge around the midpoint of gestation [21]. Initially, these fibers form bundles of microfibrils, identifiable around gestational day 280, with small elastin cores developing by embryonic day 135 [21]. Throughout the remainder of gestation, the prevalence of these core-sheath complexes increases. They eventually fuse laterally, which enhances the elastin content and results in thicker fibers.

2.4.4.3 Pathology

The absence of the SSL at the lumbosacral junction can heighten spinal mobility in this region. This deficiency may also contribute to the onset of low back pain and various musculoskeletal disorders frequently associated with the lumbosacral area [8]. Moreover, the SSL is subjected to the greatest load during spinal flexion, rendering it vulnerable to injury during acute spinal trauma, as in whiplash [8].

2.4.5 Interspinous Ligament

2.4.5.1 Function

The interspinous ligament (ISL) (Fig. 2.8) is a slender, membrane-like structure that connects neighboring vertebral spinous processes [1]. Its fibers run from the base to the tip of each spinous process, where they interact with the supraspinous ligament (SSL) on the posterior side and the ligamentum flavum (LF) on the anterior side. The ISL exhibits varying degrees of development across the spine: it is relatively underdeveloped in the cervical region, elongated and narrow in the thoracic area, and thicker and broader in the lumbar region [8]. Its primary roles include providing minimal resistance during flexion and preventing the separation of the spinous processes.

2.4.5.2 Origin and Composition

The ISL comprises three layers, each consisting of collagenous tissue, characterized by cells organized in rows interspersed among bundles of type I collagen fibers [8]. These layers are categorized as anterior, middle, and posterior. The anterior layer is a posterior extension of the LF. It contains fibers that orient posterocranially, extending from the LF to the anterior portion of the lower border of the spinous process above [8]. This layer also incorporates elastic fibers, the density of which increases as the ISL integrates with the LF [8].

The middle layer consists entirely of collagen fibers originating from the anterior portion of the upper border of the spinous process above. In contrast, the posterior layer comprises collagenous fibers that attach to the posterior half of the upper border of the spinous process below. This layer extends behind the posterior edge of the upper spinous process, connecting with either the SSL or the medial tendons of the erector spinae muscle [8].

Interestingly, the ISL has a higher concentration of cells than the LF, with fibroblasts arranged in linear formations within its central region and chondrocytes located near its bony attachments. The specific origins of this ligament in the embryo remain largely unclear.

2.4.5.3 Pathology

Pathological issues involving the ISL are frequently linked to degenerative alterations in the spinal column, which can lead to spinal instability [18]. Such instability has the potential to cause a herniated nucleus pulposus (NP), which can, in turn, lead to radiculopathy and various other painful spinal conditions [18].

2.4.6 Iliolumbar Ligament

2.4.6.1 Function

The iliolumbar ligament (Fig. 2.10) is symmetrically anchored to the tip of the anteroinferior portion of the L5 transverse process, and in certain instances, it also attaches to the L4 transverse process. It projects laterally to form a connection with the pelvis [8]. It is essential for restricting excessive motion and ensuring stability at the lumbosacral junction, effectively preventing anterior displacement of the L5 vertebra over the sacrum.

2.4.6.2 Origin and Composition

The iliolumbar ligament is reliably present by gestational age 11–15 weeks [22]. The anterior portion originates from the tip of the L5 transverse process and attaches to the anterior aspect of the iliac wing [22]. The posterior portion also arises from the tip of the L5 transverse process but extends in a more oblique, cranial direction toward the ilium's crest [22]. In neonates, the iliolumbar ligament initially shows muscular characteristics, lacking collagen fibers and standard ligamentous properties [8]. It begins to develop by the end of the first decade of life, becoming fully collagenous by the conclusion of the second decade. By the third decade, it is dis-

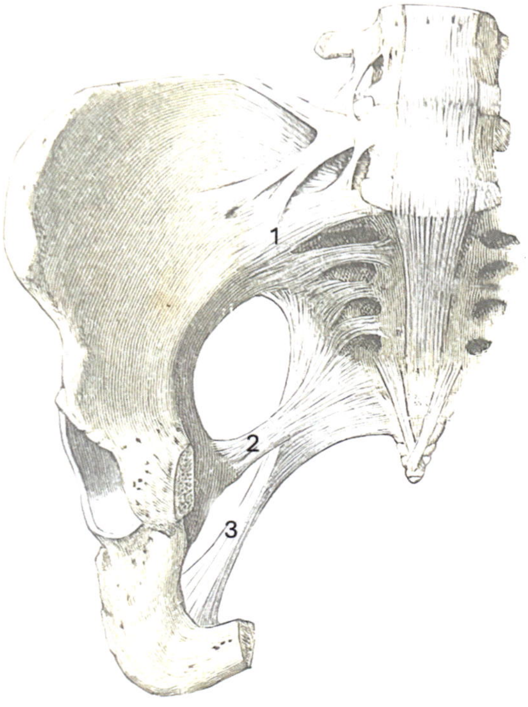

Fig. 2.10 The anterior sacroiliac ligament (1), sacrospinous ligament (2), and sacrotuberous ligament (3). Also, note the more proximal iliolumbar ligament, which is not labeled

tinctly recognizable as a ligament and contains numerous collagen fibers [18]. During the fifth decade, signs of hyaline degeneration begin to appear, and by the sixth decade, fatty infiltration and hyalinization are accompanied by calcification throughout the ligament.

2.4.6.3 Pathology

The human iliolumbar ligament has anatomical variations. Typically, it comprises a single band connecting the tip of the costal process of L5 to the iliac crest [23]. The most frequent variation features two bands: the anterior band is oval, while the posterior band has a rectangular or fan-like configuration [23].

This ligament stabilizes the sacroiliac joint by restricting excessive movement, which can help mitigate the risk of low back pain [8]. A loss of stability in this joint significantly contributes to the development of non-specific low back pain [8].

2.5 Sacroiliac Ligaments

2.5.1 Anterior Sacroiliac Ligament

2.5.1.1 Function

The anterior sacroiliac ligament (Fig. 2.10) is an anterior-inferior thickening of the fibrous capsule, characterized by a less distinct structure than other sacroiliac ligaments. It comprises elongated, transversely aligned ligamentous fibers stretching from the ala and the sacrum's anterior aspect to the ilium's anterior surface [8]. Its main role is to inhibit dislocation of the sacroiliac joint [8].

2.5.1.2 Origin and Composition

The anterior sacroiliac ligament is formed from dense connective tissue. Although details of its development remain somewhat unclear, it is associated with the broader development of the sacroiliac joint, which takes place around 8–12 weeks of gestation [24]. At this point, a well-defined articular joint can be recognized, and its stability is ensured by the posterior ligamentous framework.

During fetal development, the joint surfaces are smooth, and by roughly 5 months of gestation, a delicate fibrous septum begins to connect the surfaces. By 37 weeks of gestation, the joint capsule is lined by a synovial membrane [24]. The sacroiliac joint features two types of cartilage: thicker fibrocartilage on the sacral side and hyaline cartilage on the iliac side. The joint capsule and ligamentous structures mature into a robust, fibrous configuration throughout the first decade of life.

2.5.1.3 Pathology

Throughout pregnancy, loosening of the sacroiliac ligaments reduces the interlocking function of the sacroiliac joint, allowing for greater pelvic rotation [18]. This change contributes significantly to the lordotic posture often observed in pregnant individuals. Moreover, as this ligamentous relaxation extends beyond the pelvis during the later stages of pregnancy, the risk of S1 joint dislocation increases [8].

The anterior sacroiliac ligament is thin and particularly vulnerable to injury, making it a common source of pain.

2.5.2 Posterior Sacroiliac Ligament

2.5.2.1 Function

The posterior sacroiliac ligament is robust, linking the posterior superior iliac spine (PSIS) and the iliac crest to the third and fourth segments of the sacrum [24]. It ultimately merges with the sacrotuberous ligament. Its primary role is to inhibit anterior and inferior displacement of the sacrum, thereby ensuring stability in the pelvic region.

2.5.2.2 Origin and Composition

Like the anterior sacroiliac ligament, details of the development of the posterior sacroiliac ligament have not been well elucidated [24]. Nonetheless, it is closely linked to the formation of the sacroiliac joint, as previously mentioned.

2.5.2.3 Pathology

Injury to the posterior sacroiliac ligament can result in heightened counternutation or backward tilting of the sacrum in relation to the ilium [8]. Furthermore, edema or swelling of this ligament can exert pressure on the S1, S2, and/or S3 nerves, causing zones of ischemia due to impaired microvascular circulation, which may lead to low back pain [25].

2.5.3 Sacrotuberous Ligament

2.5.3.1 Function

The sacrotuberous ligament (Fig. 2.10) links the sacrum, ilium, and coccyx to the ischial tuberosity [8]. It is a fan-shaped fibrous band of connective tissue that provides stability to the posterior pelvis [26]. Its posterior portion originates cranially at the sacrum and inserts caudally at the ischial tuberosity. At the same time, its anterior section begins caudally at the sacrum and inserts cranially at the ischial tuberosity [8]. This ligament contains various muscle fibers that are continuous with it. The superficial fibers are interconnected with the tendon of the biceps femoris, while the fibers on the posterior surface attach to the lowest fibers of the gluteus maximus [8]. This anatomical configuration enhances pelvic stability and contributes to the movements of the lower limb [8]. The primary function of this ligament is to prevent upward tilting of the lower end of the sacrum.

2.5.3.2 Origin and Composition

Although details of the development of this ligament are not established, it is thought to be linked to the formation of the sacroiliac joint, which becomes recognizable around 12 weeks of gestation.

2.5.3.3 Pathology

The lateral branch of the S1 nerve extends deep into the long posterior sacroiliac ligament. Swelling or pressure in this structure can lead to compression of the S1 nerve, along with the adjacent S2 and S3 nerves. This compression can result in diminished blood flow, contributing to the development of ischemic zones [8].

2.5.4 Sacrospinous Ligament

2.5.4.1 Function

The sacrospinous ligament (Fig. 2.10) is a triangular band of connective tissue located on the pelvic side of the sacrotuberous ligament. It originates from the lower sacrum and upper coccyx, extending laterally to attach to the ischial spine, which helps to prevent excessive movement and maintain the integrity of the pelvis [26]. It also effectively divides the greater sciatic notch into the greater sciatic foramen and the lesser sciatic notch into the lesser sciatic foramen [26].

2.5.4.2 Origin and Composition

Similar to the sacrotuberous ligament, the development of this ligament is not well understood, but it is linked to the development of the sacroiliac joint.

2.5.4.3 Pathology

As in the sacrotuberous ligament (above).

2.5.5 Anterior Sacrococcygeal Ligament

2.5.5.1 Function

The anterior sacrococcygeal ligament (Fig. 2.10) consists of irregular fibers that extend onto the pelvic surfaces of both the sacrum and coccyx, anchoring to the ALL [8]. Its primary function is to collaborate with the posterior sacrococcygeal ligament to enhance the stability of the sacroiliac joint.

2.5.5.2 Origin and Composition

There is little information in the literature regarding the origin of the anterior sacrococcygeal ligament. However, it develops from mesodermal tissue in the lateral plate mesoderm, which contributes to the development of the pelvis and associated structures [27].

2.5.6 Superficial Posterior Sacrococcygeal Ligament

The superficial posterior sacrococcygeal ligament is a flat structure that extends from the margin of the sacral hiatus to the posterior surface of the coccyx, effectively covering the lower sacral canal [8]. While little is known about its origin in the embryo, its development is believed to resemble that of the anterior sacrococcygeal ligament, which emerges from mesodermal tissue as the sacral and coccygeal regions are forming [27]. This ligament helps to stabilize the sacrococcygeal junction [8].

2.5.7 Deep Posterior Sacrococcygeal Ligament

The deep posterior sacrococcygeal ligament extends from the posterior aspect of the fifth sacral vertebral body to the dorsum of the coccyx, corresponding to the PLL [27]. Its origin is thought to be similar to that of the anterior and superficial posterior sacrococcygeal ligaments, emerging from mesodermal tissue during the development of the sacral and coccygeal regions [26]. It is crucial for stabilizing the sacrococcygeal junction.

2.5.8 Lateral Sacrococcygeal Ligament

The lateral sacrococcygeal ligament is on either side of the deep posterior sacrococcygeal ligament [8]. It connects the transverse process of the coccyx to the inferolateral angle of the sacrum, effectively completing the foramen through which the S5 nerve traverses [8]. This ligament is important for stabilizing the sacrococcygeal junction and enhancing the overall integrity of the pelvic region [27]. Its origin in the embryo remains poorly understood.

2.5.9 Intercornual Sacrococcygeal Ligament

The intercornual sacrococcygeal ligament links the cornua of the sacrum and coccyx on either side [8]. Its origin parallels that of the other sacrococcygeal ligaments, emerging from mesodermal tissue during the formation of the sacrum and coccyx [27]. It is essential for stabilizing the junction between these anatomical structures.

2.6 Conclusions

The ligaments of the spine have a complex arrangement and development. Knowledge of this embryology can help better understand congenital malformations and pathological findings.

References

1. Pesenti S, Philip N, Bollini G. Embryology of the vertebral column. In: Spinal anatomy: modern concepts. Cham: Springer International Publishing; 2019. p. 19–24.

2. Mescher AL. Junqueira's basic histology: text and atlas. 7th ed. McGraw-Hill Education LLC; 2023.
3. Offiah CE, Day E. The craniocervical junction: embryology, anatomy, biomechanics and imaging in blunt trauma. Insights Imaging. 2016;8(1):29–47. https://doi.org/10.1007/s13244-016-0530-5.
4. Alvi MA, Moghaddamjou A, Fehlings MG. Anatomy and physiology of cervical spine and cervical spinal cord. In: Degenerative cervical myelopathy. Academic; 2023. p. 11–33.
5. Moraes P, Baptista S. The ligament of barkow is a solid structure in human fetuses. Coluna/Columna. 2023;22(4) https://doi.org/10.1590/s1808-185120222204272760.
6. Tubbs RS, Dixon J, Loukas M, Shoja MM, Cohen-Gadol AA. Ligament of Barkow of the craniocervical junction: its anatomy and potential clinical and functional significance. J Neurosurg Spine. 2010;12(6):619–22. https://doi.org/10.3171/2009.12.spine09671.
7. Lenz R, Moore GD, Panchani PN, DiLandro AC, Battaglia F, Tubbs RS, Shoja MM, Loukas M, Kozlowski PB, D'Antoni AV. The transverse occipital ligament: an anatomic, histologic, and radiographic study. Spine J. 2012;12(7):596–602. https://doi.org/10.1016/j.spinee.2012.07.005.
8. Asma Mian Butt, Gill C, Amin Demerdash, Watanabe K, Loukas M, Rozzelle CJ, R. Shane Tubbs. A comprehensive review of the sub-axial ligaments of the vertebral column: part II histology and embryology. Childs Nerv Syst. 2015;31(7):1061–6. https://doi.org/10.1007/s00381-015-2730-6.
9. Tubbs RS, Hallock JD, Radcliff V, Naftel RP, Mortazavi M, Shoja MM, Loukas M, Cohen-Gadol AA. Ligaments of the craniocervical junction: a review. J Neurosurg Spine. 2011;14(6):697–709.
10. Abe H, Ishizawa A, Cho KH, Suzuki R, Fujimiya M, Rodríguez-Vázquez JF, Murakami G. Fetal development of the transverse Atlantis and alar ligaments at the craniovertebral junction. Clin Anat. 2011;25(6):714–21. https://doi.org/10.1002/ca.22020.
11. Pang D, Thompson DNP. Embryology and bony malformations of the craniovertebral junction. Childs Nerv Syst. 2010;27(4):523–64. https://doi.org/10.1007/s00381-010-1358-9.
12. Debernardi A, D'Aliberti G, Talamonti G, Villa F, Piparo M, Collice M. The Craniovertebral junction area and the role of the ligaments and membranes. Neurosurgery. 2011;68(2):291–301. https://doi.org/10.1227/NEU.0b013e3182011262.
13. Nikpasand M, Abbott RE, Kage CC, Singh S, Winkelstein BA, Barocas VH, Ellingson AM. Cervical facet capsular ligament mechanics: estimations based on subject-specific anatomy and kinematics. JOR Spine. 2023;6(3) https://doi.org/10.1002/jsp2.1269.
14. Saker E, Graham RA, Nicholas R, D'Antoni AV, Loukas M, Oskouian RJ, Tubbs RS. Ligaments of the costovertebral joints including biomechanics, innervations, and clinical applications: a comprehensive review with application to approaches to the thoracic spine. Cureus. 2016;8(11) https://doi.org/10.7759/cureus.874.
15. Scaal M. Early development of the vertebral column. Semin Cell Dev Biol. 2016;49:83–91. https://doi.org/10.1016/j.semcdb.2015.11.003.
16. Jin ZW, Song KJ, Lee NH, Nakamura T, Fujimiya M, Murakami G, Cho BH. Contribution of the anterior longitudinal ligament to ossification and growth of the vertebral body: an immunohistochemical study using the human fetal lumbar vertebrae. Surg Radiol Anat. 2010;33(1):11–8. https://doi.org/10.1007/s00276-010-0725-2.
17. Hamid M, Fallet-Bianco C, Delmas V, et al. The human lumbar anterior epidural space: morphological comparison in adult and fetal specimens. Surg Radiol Anat. 2002;24(3–4):194–200. https://doi.org/10.1007/s00276-002-0041-6.
18. Asma Mian Butt, Gill C, Amin Demerdash, Watanabe K, Loukas M, Rozzelle CJ, R. Shane Tubbs. A comprehensive review of the sub-axial ligaments of the vertebral column: part I anatomy and function. Childs Nerv Syst. 2015;31(7):1037–59. https://doi.org/10.1007/s00381-015-2729-z.
19. Yoon SP, Kim HJ, Choi YS. Anatomic variations of cervical and high thoracic Ligamentum Flavum. Korean J Pain. 2014;27(4):321–5. https://doi.org/10.3344/kjp.2014.27.4.321.
20. Chang U, Lee MC, Kim DH. Posterior approach to the Midcervical spine. In: Surgical anatomy & techniques to the spine. WB Saunders; 2006. p. 57–64. https://doi.org/10.1016/b978-1-4160-0313-7.50011-1.
21. Brown JP, Lind RM, Burzesi AF, Kuo CK. Elastogenic protein expression of a highly elastic murine spinal ligament: the Ligamentum Flavum. PLoS One. 2012;7(6):e38475. https://doi.org/10.1371/journal.pone.0038475.
22. Uhthoff HK. Prenatal development of the iliolumbar ligament. J Bone Joint Surg. 1993;75(1):93–5. https://doi.org/10.1302/0301-620x.75b1.8421046.
23. Dąbrowski K, Ciszek B. Anatomy and morphology of iliolumbar ligament. Surg Radiol Anat. 2023;45(2):169–73. https://doi.org/10.1007/s00276-022-03070-y.
24. Misawa H, Ohtsuka K, Nakata K, Kinoshita H. Embryological study of the spinal ligaments in human fetuses. J Spinal Disord. 1994;7(6):495–598.
25. Dydyk AM, Forro SD, Hanna A. Sacroiliac joint injury. PubMed; StatPearls Publishing; 2020. https://www.ncbi.nlm.nih.gov/books/NBK557881/
26. Chaudhry SR, Chaudhry K. Anatomy, abdomen and pelvis, ligaments. PubMed; StatPearls Publishing; 2020. https://www.ncbi.nlm.nih.gov/books/NBK493215/
27. Lee SH, Yang M, Won H, Kim Y-D. Coccydynia: anatomic origin and considerations regarding the effectiveness of injections for pain management. Korean J Pain. 2023;36(3):272–80. https://doi.org/10.3344/kjp.23175.

Histogenesis of the Spinal Ligaments (Light and Electron Microscopy)

3

Aylin Gökhan, Ebru Eroğlu, Okan Derin, Servet Çelik, and Yiğit Uyanıkgil

3.1 Introduction

The vertebral column, a main axis of the human musculoskeletal system, provides both structural support and protection for the spinal cord and associated neural elements. This architecture is supported by the spinal ligaments, specialized connective tissues that confer stability, flexibility, and mechanical resilience to the spine. They include the anterior longitudinal ligament (ALL), posterior longitudinal ligament (PLL), ligamentum flavum (LF), interspinous ligament (ISL), and supraspinous ligament (SSL), all specifically adapted to their biomechanical roles, balancing tensile strength with elasticity to accommodate dynamic spinal movements.

Developing the spinal ligaments is a complex, tightly regulated process that integrates embryological, molecular, cellular, and biomechanical factors. Mesenchymal condensations of the paraxial mesoderm differentiate into highly specialized extracellular matrix (ECM) components under genetic, environmental, and mechanical stimuli. This histogenic process ensures that the properties of the ligaments are aligned with their distinct functional roles—stabilizing vertebral segments, resisting hyperextension, or supporting flexion and recoil during motion.

Understanding the development, structure, and function of spinal ligaments is crucial for diagnosing and managing ligament-related pathologies, which are associated with a wide range of spinal disorders. Conditions such as ossification of the posterior longitudinal ligament (OPLL), ligament hypertrophy, and diffuse idiopathic skeletal hyperostosis (DISH) entail structural and functional disruptions that compromise spinal stability and neural integrity. Advances in imaging technologies, molecular biology, and regenerative medicine have improved the diagnosis and treatment of these pathologies, offering novel therapeutic approaches to restore ligament function and improve patient outcomes.

A. Gökhan · E. Eroğlu
Department of Histology and Embryology, Ege University Faculty of Medicine, Bornova, İzmir, Türkiye

O. Derin
Department of Anatomy, Ege University Faculty of Medicine, Bornova, İzmir, Türkiye

S. Çelik
Department of Anatomy, Ege University Faculty of Medicine, Bornova, İzmir, Türkiye

Interventional Anatomy and Plastination Research Center, Ege University, Bornova, İzmir, Türkiye

Y. Uyanıkgil (✉)
Department of Histology and Embryology, Ege University Faculty of Medicine, Bornova, İzmir, Türkiye

Interventional Anatomy and Plastination Research Center, Ege University, Bornova, İzmir, Türkiye
e-mail: yigituyanikgil@gmail.com

M. Turgut et al. (eds.), *Ligaments of the Vertebral Column*,
https://doi.org/10.1007/978-3-032-09070-6_3

This chapter examines the histogenesis, structural composition, and functional biomechanics of the spinal ligaments, with an emphasis on their developmental origins and physiological roles. It also explores diagnostic and therapeutic innovations, including advances in regenerative medicine, tissue engineering, and surgical interventions. By integrating foundational research with clinical applications, this work highlights the importance of interdisciplinary approaches for advancing spinal healthcare and addressing ligament-related disorders.

3.2 Embryonic Origin of the Major Spinal Ligaments

The vertebral column is a biomechanical axis and a protective framework for the human body. Spinal ligaments are vital for preserving vertebral column stability, flexibility, and functional integrity. They originate during embryogenesis from mesenchymal cells derived from the paraxial mesoderm. This process begins with aggregating mesenchymal progenitors into somites, which segment along the cranio-caudal axis of the developing embryo. Each somite differentiates into distinct compartments: the sclerotome, dermatome, and myotome. The sclerotome, in particular, contributes to the formation of vertebrae, ribs, and ligamentous structures in the axial skeleton [1, 2].

The embryonic development of spinal ligaments is a highly regulated process involving cellular differentiation, molecular signaling, and extracellular matrix organization. Mesenchymal cells within the sclerotome differentiate into fibroblasts and other connective tissue cells, which synthesize and organize the extracellular matrix components necessary for ligament formation. Key molecular pathways, including Sonic Hedgehog (Shh), Transforming Growth Factor Beta (TGF-β), and Bone Morphogenetic Proteins (BMPs), orchestrate these processes, ensuring the proper alignment and mechanical properties of the ligaments.

The structural and functional specialization of each ligament is shaped not only by genetic and molecular factors but also by mechanical forces. Fetal movements are critical for aligning collagen fibers and enhancing the tensile strength of the developing ligaments, optimizing their resilience and functionality throughout life.

Disruption of these tightly regulated developmental processes can result in congenital anomalies or predispose individuals to ligament pathologies such as ossification or degeneration. A comprehensive understanding of the embryonic origins and mechanisms of development of the spinal ligaments provides a foundation for diagnosing and treating such conditions, offering critical insights for both basic research and clinical practice.

3.2.1 Major Ligaments of the Vertebral Column

The structural arrangement of the spinal ligaments reflects their critical biomechanical roles in stabilizing the vertebral column while allowing flexibility. Their distinct anatomical positions and specialized functions are crucial for maintaining spinal health and optimal movement.

3.2.1.1 Anterior Longitudinal Ligament (ALL)

The anterior longitudinal ligament (ALL) is the most anteriorly positioned spinal ligament, running along the length of the vertebral bodies and intervertebral discs. Its primary role is to prevent hyperextension, thereby maintaining spinal alignment across a wide range of movements. It is also critical for distributing loads by transmitting significant compressive forces during spinal activities [3, 4]. Its structural integrity is vital for preserving spinal stability, particularly under axial loading and bending forces.

3.2.1.2 Posterior Longitudinal Ligament (PLL)

Situated along the posterior surfaces of the vertebral bodies within the vertebral canal, the posterior longitudinal ligament (PLL) restricts hyperflexion. It contributes to spinal stabilization, especially in the lumbar region, where flexion movements are more pronounced. Its primary function is to prevent excessive forward bending and to preserve spinal alignment, making it indispensable for mitigating degenerative complications such as spondylolisthesis and spinal canal stenosis [5–7].

3.2.1.3 Ligamentum Flavum (LF)

The ligamentum flavum (LF), located posterior to the PLL, connects the laminae of adjacent vertebrae. This ligament is distinguished by its high elastin content, which confers exceptional elasticity and recoil, enabling it to accommodate natural spinal movements. As a dynamic stabilizer, the LF ensures stability during flexion and extension, absorbs mechanical forces, and safeguards neural structures against injury [8, 9]. Its distinctive biomechanical properties are critical for maintaining the spine's functional resilience.

3.2.1.4 Interspinous Ligament (ISL)

Positioned between the spinous processes of adjacent vertebrae, the interspinous ligament (ISL) stabilizes the spine during flexion by preventing excessive separation of those processes. Collaborating with the supraspinous ligament (SSL), it provides posterior stabilization and limits flexion-induced motion. Preserving the ISL during spinal surgeries has been shown to improve postoperative outcomes and minimize the risk of instability [10, 11]. Its stabilizing function is especially crucial during dynamic spinal movements.

3.2.1.5 Supraspinous Ligament (SSL)

The supraspinous ligament (SSL) extends along the tips of the spinous processes from the seventh cervical vertebra (C7) to the sacrum. It resists excessive flexion and enhances posterior spinal stability. It is essential for preserving spinal alignment and preventing excessive motion. Injury to this ligament has been associated with conditions such as proximal junctional kyphosis and increased spinal instability [12, 13]. Maintaining the integrity of the SSL is particularly important in patients with degenerative spinal diseases, as it supports the functional capacity of the vertebral column [14].

The sequential organization of these ligaments from anterior to posterior ensures a functional balance between spinal stability and mobility. The ALL resists hyperextension, the PLL restricts hyperflexion, the LF contributes dynamic stabilization through its elasticity, the ISL maintains alignment during flexion, and the SSL reinforces posterior stability. Understanding these ligaments is crucial for optimizing clinical outcomes in spinal surgery and rehabilitation.

3.2.2 Molecular and Cellular Mechanisms of Ligamentogenesis

The embryogenesis of spinal ligaments is a multifaceted process governed by differentiating mesenchymal cells into ligament-forming fibroblasts. This process is tightly regulated by transcriptional programs, signaling pathways, and ECM dynamics, all of which collectively establish the structural and functional characteristics of the spinal ligaments.

The cellular microenvironment plays a crucial role in ligamentogenesis. Experimental evidence highlights the involvement of growth factors such as PDGF and TGF-β, which mediate mesenchymal cell migration and differentiation. PDGF facilitates the migration of mesenchymal cells adjacent to sclerotome-derived cartilage via a PI3K-dependent mechanism [15]. Mechanical forces are also critical; cyclic tensile strain enhances osteogenic gene expression, which is regulated by BMP signaling [16].

Epigenetic modifications such as DNA methylation also influence ligamentogenesis. Studies indicate reduced methylation in the promoter regions of Wnt pathway genes is associated with increased osteogenic potential, particularly when spinal ligaments are ossified [17]. Mechanical stress also drives mesenchymal differentiation, stimulating osteoblast migration and new bone formation in response to external physical stimuli.

Transcriptional regulation is central to ligament development, beginning with mesenchymal aggregation in the sclerotome. Key transcription factors, including Pax1 and Pax9, guide mesenchymal progenitors toward ligament-forming and chondrogenic lineages [18, 19]. Scleraxis (Scx) is pivotal in fibroblast specification and collagen synthesis, while Mohawk (Mkx) facilitates tenogenic differentiation, further underscoring the role of transcriptional networks in ligamentogenesis [20, 21].

Signaling pathways, such as the Wnt/β-catenin, Sonic Hedgehog (Shh), and BMP pathways, are integral to ligament development. Canonical Wnt signaling regulates mesenchymal cell fate, while Shh signaling patterns the sclerotome and promotes ligament formation. BMPs, particularly BMP2, stimulate ECM production and ossification of ligamentous structures [22–26]. Fibroblasts contribute to ECM assembly by synthesizing types I and III collagen, which provide tensile strength, and elastin, which confers elasticity. Proteoglycans and glycosaminoglycans maintain ECM hydration and viscoelasticity, ensuring biomechanical functionality [27–29].

The interplay of transcription factors, signaling pathways, and epigenetic regulation forms a complex network governing ligament development. Cooperative activities, such as those between noggin and gremlin 1, are critical for axial skeleton development, while retinoic acid modulates the differentiation of intervertebral ligament cells [30, 31]. Key transcription factors such as STAT3 and RUNX2 further enhance ligamentogenesis, promoting osteogenic differentiation and regulating ossification through BMP signaling [32, 33]. These regulatory mechanisms ensure the formation of ligaments and their integration into the vertebral column.

3.2.3 Spatiotemporal Dynamics of Ligament Formation

Ligaments develop through distinct spatial and temporal phases tailored to meet the biomechanical demands of specific spinal regions. During the early fetal period, mesenchymal cells rapidly proliferate and differentiate, producing an ECM enriched with proteoglycans and collagen. These components establish the foundational architecture of the spinal ligaments. By the second trimester, fibroblasts are actively synthesizing dense collagen fibers, particularly in ligaments such as the ALL and PLL, which require tensile strength to resist forces of hyperextension and hyperflexion [34]. Elastogenesis begins concurrently in the ligamentum flavum, where elastin fibers integrate into the ECM to support dynamic movements [35–37].

The interspinous and supraspinous ligaments mature later, and collagen organization aligns to meet the mechanical demands of fetal activity. Fibroblasts drive this process, enhancing the structural integrity of these ligaments [38, 39]. Regional adaptations emerge across the spine, the cervical region developing higher elastin-to-collagen ratios to enhance flexibility, while the ligaments in the lumbar spine thicken to withstand greater axial loads [40, 41]. These region-specific specializations reflect the precise molecular signaling and mechanical forces shaping spinal ligament development.

3.2.4 Embryonic Environment and External Influences

The embryonic environment has a significant influence on ligamentogenesis, regulating oxygen levels, mechanical forces, and biochemical signals. Hypoxia is a critical regulator, enhancing ligament-specific gene expression and stimulating ECM synthesis. Fibroblasts respond to low oxygen tension by producing collagen and proteoglycans, which contribute to the structure and hydration of ligaments. Mechanical forces generated by fetal movements have a complementary effect, aligning collagen fibers and promoting the organization and strength of ligaments. These forces are essential for developing tensile and viscoelastic properties in response to the mechanical demands of the musculoskeletal system [42–45].

Environmental stimuli also activate key biochemical signaling pathways, such as the Wnt/β--catenin and MAPK pathways. These pathways regulate fibroblast differentiation, ECM remodeling, and ligament maturation, ensuring the formation of mechanically robust ligaments [46,

47]. Disruptions of oxygen regulation, mechanical loading, or signaling pathways during development can result in structural anomalies or predispose individuals to degenerative ligamentous conditions later in life [48].

Experimental studies provide significant insights into these regulatory mechanisms, revealing the complex interplay among genetic, epigenetic, and environmental factors. Table 3.1 provides a detailed summary of the developmen-

Table 3.1 Developmental origins, molecular regulation, and functional attributes of spinal ligaments

SLs	Developmental origin	Key signaling pathways	Key transcription factors	ECM contributions	Histological and regulatory features
ALL	Derived from mesenchymal cells in the sclerotome.	Wnt/β-catenin regulates mesenchymal fate; BMP promotes osteogenic processes in pathological states.	Pax1, Pax9 direct differentiation; RUNX2 contributes to ossification in pathological states.	Dense type I collagen provides tensile strength; type III collagen supports flexibility and repair.	Histology shows dense regular connective tissue with parallel collagen fibers; influenced by TGF-β for matrix remodeling and mechanical stress for structural alignment.
PLL	Arises from mesenchymal condensations around the neural tube and notochord.	Wnt and BMP interact with Shh to regulate ligament formation; Shh critical for vertebral patterning.	Pax1, Pax9 guide sclerotomal development; RUNX2 implicated in ossification; STAT3 supports osteogenesis.	Type I collagen provides tensile strength; ECM contains elastin for limited elasticity.	Histologically denser than the ALL, with fibrocartilage regions near vertebral bodies. Excessive BMP/Wnt linked to OPLL, altering histology with calcifications.
LF	Derived from mesenchymal cells in the sclerotome; specialized for elasticity.	BMP and TGF-β pathways regulate elastin synthesis and ECM remodeling.	Scleraxis drives fibroblast differentiation; Mohawk regulates tenogenic lineage commitment.	Elastin dominates ECM (up to 80%), providing stretch and recoil; type I and III collagen maintain structural integrity.	Histology reveals an elastin-rich matrix interspersed with collagen fibers. Mechanical stress enhances elastin fiber differentiation and alignment.
ISL	Develops from mesenchymal condensations between adjacent spinous processes.	Shh and BMP signaling regulate fibroblast differentiation.	Pax1 supports early mesenchymal development; Scleraxis promotes fibroblast ECM production.	Type I collagen ensures tensile strength; moderate elastin supports flexibility under mechanical strain.	Histologically characterized by interwoven collagen bundles arranged to resist tensile forces during flexion. Cyclic mechanical strain enhances fibroblast activity and ECM organization.
SSL	Arises from mesenchymal condensations above spinous processes.	TGF-β promotes fibrous differentiation; BMP directs osteoblast lineage commitment.	Mohawk regulates fibroblast differentiation; RUNX2 influences ossification processes.	Predominantly type I collagen for strength; minor elastin content contributes to flexibility.	Histology highlights a dense collagenous structure with longitudinal fiber alignment. Limited vascularity contributes to slow healing responses.

This table outlines the developmental origins, key molecular signaling pathways, transcription factors, extracellular matrix (ECM) contributions, and regulatory mechanisms involved in the formation and specialization of the major spinal ligaments (SLs). These include the anterior longitudinal ligament (ALL), posterior longitudinal ligament (PLL), ligamentum flavum (LF), interspinous ligament (ISL), and supraspinous ligament (SSL). By summarizing histogenetic processes, it emphasizes the interplay of genetic regulation, ECM composition, and mechanical influences on ligamentogenesis. References are drawn from foundational research on signaling pathways [22, 29, 49], transcription factors [18, 20, 21], ECM roles [1, 27], and regulatory influences [15–17] tal origins, signaling pathways, transcription factors, and extracellular matrix (ECM) contributions involved in forming the five major spinal ligaments. These findings highlight the integration of the regulatory systems underlying ligamentogenesis, offering a comprehensive understanding of the histogenesis and biomechanical functions of the spinal ligaments.

3.3 Cellular Components and Extracellular Matrix Composition

The structural and functional properties of spinal ligaments are governed by the intricate interplay between their cellular components and ECM architecture. This finely tuned system ensures that the ligaments provide biomechanical stability and adaptability, enabling the vertebral column to withstand diverse mechanical forces while maintaining its structural integrity. A deeper understanding of the cellular and ECM composition of spinal ligaments reveals insights into their role in maintaining spinal health and adaptability and also provides a foundation for developing regenerative therapies for ligament injuries and degenerative conditions.

3.3.1 Cellular Components

The cellular architecture of the spinal ligaments is primarily composed of fibroblasts, the principal mediators of ECM synthesis, organization, and remodeling. These spindle-shaped cells align longitudinally with collagen fibers, highlighting their crucial role in maintaining the structural integrity of the extracellular matrix (ECM) [50, 51]. Although fibroblasts are relatively sparse within ligament tissues, they exhibit dynamic metabolic activity, responding to biomechanical stimuli to regulate ECM turnover and facilitate repair. This adaptability is essential for preserving ligament function under normal physiological conditions and during high-impact mechanical stress [52].

In fibrocartilaginous regions, such as the ligamentum flavum, chondrocyte-like cells complement fibroblasts by synthesizing proteoglycans and other extracellular matrix (ECM) components. These molecules enhance the tissue's capacity to resist compressive forces, contributing to its biomechanical resilience [53]. Under mechanical stress, fibroblasts upregulate their metabolic activity, producing new ECM) components to counteract ligament fatigue and microinjury. This dynamic response is crucial for ensuring the functional integrity of the spinal ligaments, even when they are subjected to sustained mechanical loads [54].

The ECM functions as a structural scaffold and a dynamic signaling interface, mediating bioactive interactions that regulate cellular behavior. This dual role is particularly evident in fibroblast-ECM interactions, which maintain the delicate balance between ECM synthesis and degradation. Such equilibrium is essential for ligament health, enabling spinal ligaments to adapt to mechanical stimuli while preserving their biomechanical properties [50]. The ECM's composition, dominated by collagen and elastin, provides the tensile strength and flexibility necessary for ligaments to withstand various mechanical loads. Collagen confers tensile strength, while elastin confers elasticity, ensuring the resilience of these structures under stress [51].

3.3.2 Collagen and Elastin: Fundamental Extracellular Matrix Components

Collagen is the most abundant ECM protein in spinal ligaments. It is the primary determinant of the tensile strength necessary to counteract the mechanical forces generated during spinal motion. Type I collagen predominates in load-bearing ligaments such as the ALL and PLL, forming densely packed fibrils oriented along the primary axes of tensile stress. This structural alignment is critical for resisting deformation under stretching forces during flexion and extension of the spine, contributing significantly to vertebral stability [51, 55, 56]. The biomechanical properties of these ligaments are further enhanced by collagen fibril cross-linking, which confers additional resilience and enhances the capacity to endure repetitive or high-impact mechanical loads [57, 58].

In addition to the predominant type I collagen, type III collagen, though less abundant, is an essential supporting component, conferring flexibility and enabling adaptive tissue repair during ECM remodeling. This collagen subtype is particularly important in maintaining ligament integrity when mechanical conditions vary, ensuring that the ligament retains functional stability while accommodating microstructural adjustments [51, 59]. The dynamic regulation of collagen synthesis and degradation is pivotal for the spinal ligaments; it facilitates the adaptive response to mechanical demands, preserving their functional and structural integrity over time [59, 60].

Elastin, although present in lower concentrations than collagen, is integral to ligaments that require elasticity and recoil. In the ligamentum flavum, elastin constitutes up to 80% of the ECM, conferring the ability to stretch and recover its original conformation during repetitive spinal movements. This elasticity is critical for mitigating encroachment of the spinal canal during dynamic motion, thereby protecting neural elements and preserving functional mobility [51, 61]. In contrast, stabilizing ligaments such as the ALL and PLL have minimal elastin content, reflecting their primary biomechanical role in resisting tensile forces rather than accommodating elastic deformation. This compositional difference highlights the biomechanical specializations of spinal ligaments, elastin-dominant regions supporting dynamic movements, and collagen-rich regions ensuring structural stability and resistance to deformation [51, 61].

3.3.3 Proteoglycans and Glycosaminoglycans: Hydration and Viscoelasticity

Proteoglycans and their associated glycosaminoglycans (GAGs) are integral ECM components that regulate ligament hydration and viscoelasticity. They comprise a protein core with covalently attached GAG chains such as chondroitin sulfate and hyaluronic acid, which attract water to maintain ECM hydration. This hydration is critical for ligaments subject to compressive forces, such as the ligamentum flavum. Proteoglycans also enhance the viscoelastic properties of ligaments, facilitating energy absorption and dissipation during mechanical loading [62].

The distribution of proteoglycans varies among spinal ligaments, reflecting their biomechanical roles. The ligamentum flavum, for example, has a higher proteoglycan content, consistent with its fibrocartilaginous nature and its need to accommodate compression. In contrast, the ISL and SSL have moderate proteoglycan levels, contributing to their ability to distribute loads across the spinal column [62, 63].

3.3.4 Extracellular Matrix Dynamics in Ligament Health and Repair

The ECM exhibits dynamic properties that facilitate ligament adaptation, repair, and regeneration. Fibroblasts coordinate those processes by synthesizing and remodeling ECM components such as collagen, elastin, and proteoglycans. This synergy between cellular and matrix components enables ligaments to respond to mechanical stimuli, ensuring their resilience and functionality [50]. For instance, mechanical loading induces fibroblasts to increase collagen synthesis, reinforcing ligament structure and preventing fatigue-related failure [64].

ECM remodeling becomes critical in cases of ligament injury or degeneration. Dysregulated ECM turnover, often seen in degenerative conditions, can compromise ligament integrity and function [65]. A detailed understanding of ECM dynamics provides a basis for developing therapeutic strategies to enhance ligament repair and regeneration. Emerging approaches, including the use of growth factors, biomimetic scaffolds, and cell-based therapies, leverage insights into ECM biology to restore ligament function [64].

The intricate balance between cellular activity and ECM composition highlights the biological and mechanical sophistication of the spinal ligaments. These insights underpin efforts to maintain ligament health and flexibility throughout life, addressing acute injuries and chronic degenerative conditions [66].

3.4 Histogenesis and Histology of Major Spinal Ligaments

The histogenesis of individual spinal ligaments is a highly specialized process, reflecting the structural and functional requirements of the vertebral column. Each ligament undergoes a distinct developmental pathway, leading to an ECM composition and biomechanical properties tailored to its specific role. For instance, the ligamentum flavum is characterized by a high elastin content, providing the elasticity required for its function. In contrast, the ALL predominantly consists of dense collagen fibers to resist tensile forces during hyperextension. Similarly, the PLL, ISL, and SSL are specifically structured to stabilize and maintain vertebral alignment under varying mechanical stresses. These adaptations stem from their embryonic origins, cellular differentiation processes, and ECM specialization.

Table 3.2 provides a comparative summary of the structural and functional properties of the five principal spinal ligaments. It highlights their dominant ECM components, distinctive structural features, primary functional roles, and regional variations, offering a comprehensive perspective on their biomechanical adaptations and physiological significance.

3.4.1 Anterior Longitudinal Ligament: Development, Structure, and Functional Significance

The anterior longitudinal ligament (ALL), also known as the ligamentum longitudinale anterius, is a crucial component of the vertebral column, serving both mechanical and protective functions. From the occipital bone to the sacrum, the ALL runs along the anterior aspect of the vertebral bodies and intervertebral discs, forming a continuous band of fibrous connective tissue. Its primary biomechanical function is to restrict hyperextension of the spine, thereby preserving

Table 3.2 Structural and functional comparison of spinal ligaments

SLs	Dominant ECM component	Unique structural features	Primary function	Regional variations
ALL	Predominantly type I collagen	High tensile strength; resists excessive extension	Maintains vertebral column integrity; prevents hyperextension	Thickest in lumbar region
PLL	Collagen and elastin (balanced)	Combines tensile strength and moderate elasticity	Stabilizes the spine; prevents excessive flexion or extension	Ossification in cervical spine
LF	60–70% elastin; type I collagen	High elasticity and resilience, enabling stretch and recoil	Accommodates spinal movements; protects spinal cord and nerve roots	Thicker in lumbar spine
ISL	Predominantly type III collagen; moderate elastin	Moderate tensile strength and elasticity; absorbs and dissipates forces	Supports spinous processes; stabilizes spine during dynamic movements	Robust in lumbar spine
SSL	Predominantly type I collagen; moderate elastin	High tensile strength; moderate elasticity for force distribution	Maintains posterior stability; resists flexion during spinal movements	Thickest in lumbar spine

This table provides a comparative overview of the extracellular matrix (ECM) composition, unique structural features, primary functions, and regional variations of the spinal ligaments (SLs), including the anterior longitudinal ligament (ALL), posterior longitudinal ligament (PLL), ligamentum flavum (LF), interspinous ligament (ISL), and supraspinous ligament (SSL). It highlights their adaptations to the biomechanical demands of different spinal regions [25, 38, 39, 60, 67–74] the structural alignment of the vertebral column and preventing excessive anterior translation of vertebral segments. In addition to its stabilizing role, the ALL protects adjacent spinal structures, including the intervertebral discs, spinal cord, and nerve roots, by dissipating tensile forces that arise during dynamic spinal movements [69, 75].

The multifunctional significance of this ligament extends to its involvement in spinal pathologies and surgical procedures. Given its location and biomechanical responsibilities, any disruption to the ALL—whether through trauma, degeneration, or ossification—can profoundly affect spinal stability, mobility, and overall function. Thus, understanding its development, structure, biomechanical properties, and pathological susceptibilities is crucial for advancing spinal health research and improving clinical outcomes (Fig. 3.1).

3.4.1.1 Developmental Origins

The development of the ALL begins during embryogenesis and follows a highly coordinated process involving molecular, genetic, and mechanical factors. During the early stages of embryonic development, mesenchymal cells condense along the anterior surface of the notochord, forming the precursor to the ALL. These cells

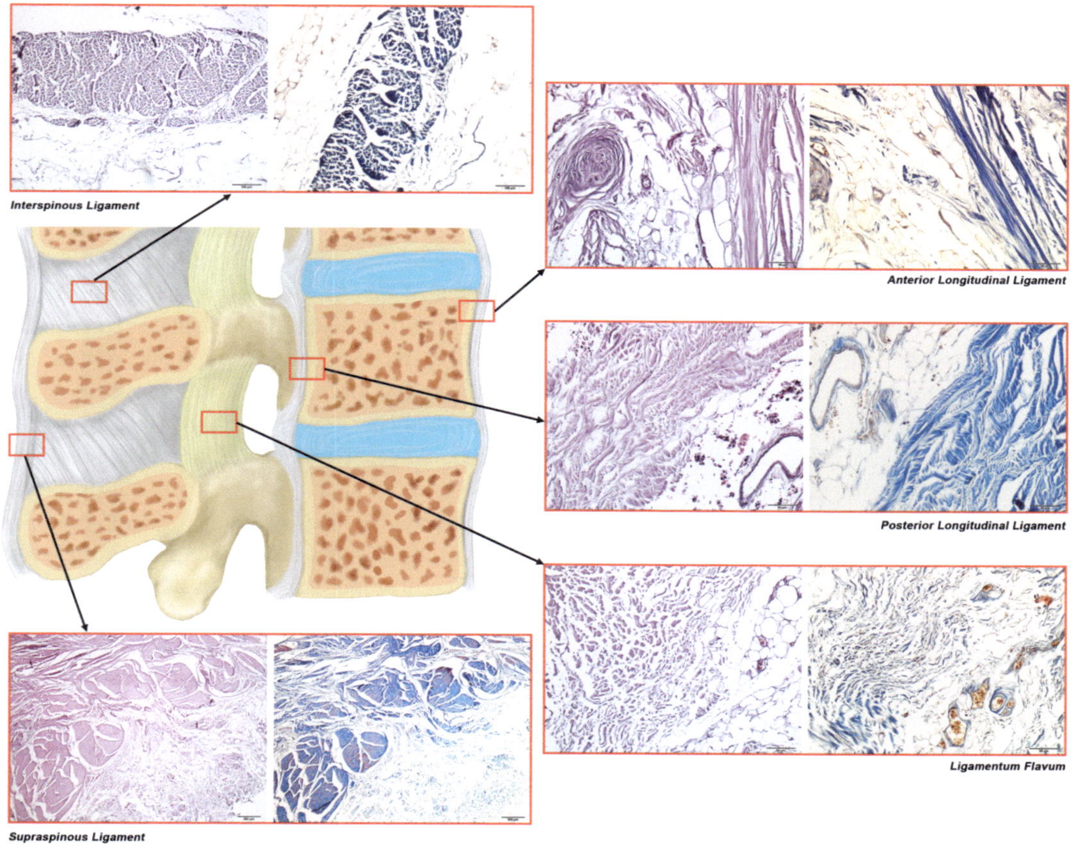

Fig. 3.1 Anatomical localization and histological architecture of the spinal ligaments. The schematic drawing was originally created by the authors. Tissue samples indicated within the red boxes were dissected from adult human cadavers with appropriate institutional permission. Following standard histological procedures, sections were stained with hematoxylin and eosin (H&E) and Masson's trichrome. Images were examined under light microscopy at ×10 magnification

differentiate into fibroblasts, synthesizing type I collagen and other ECM proteins. This differentiation marks the transformation of the ALL into a dense, fibrous structure by the end of the first trimester, enabling it to meet the biomechanical demands of fetal movements. These mechanical stresses are crucial for establishing the tensile properties of the ligament, preparing it to withstand postnatal loads, and supporting spinal stability [76, 77].

The coordination of the development of the ALL with adjacent spinal structures such as vertebrae and intervertebral discs ensures its integration into the overall spinal architecture. This synchronization is vital, allowing the ligament to maintain alignment and integrity within the vertebral column. The biomechanical resilience of the ALL, largely attributable to its collagen composition, is heavily influenced by molecular signaling pathways, including those mediated by TGF-β and FGF. These pathways regulate fibroblast activity, collagen synthesis, and ECM organization. TGF-β, in particular, has been shown to upregulate collagen gene expression, contributing to the tensile strength and mechanical functionality of the ALL [77, 78].

Mechanical loading during fetal development further reinforces the structural integrity of the ALL. Fetal movements exert tensile forces on the developing ligament, stimulating fibroblasts to produce and organize ECM components. This mechanical environment is indispensable for the alignment and orientation of collagen fibers, which confer the strength and elasticity required for the ligament's postnatal role. The dynamic interplay between mechanical stimuli and molecular signaling highlights the importance of biomechanical forces in shaping ligament development [79, 80].

The genetic regulation of ALL development is also crucial. Genes such as DLX5 are involved in fibroblast differentiation and ECM production within spinal ligaments. Dysregulation of these genes has been implicated in developmental anomalies such as DISH and ligament ossification, which can lead to clinical complications. Furthermore, environmental factors such as mechanical stress and injury can modulate the development and maturation of the ALL, potentially resulting in structural adaptations or pathologies [76, 81, 82].

3.4.1.2 Structural Composition

The ALL is a dense, fibrous connective tissue, predominantly composed of type I collagen, which provides high tensile strength and resistance to extension forces. Histologically, ALL is classified as dense, regular connective tissue with minimal elastin content. This composition reflects its primary function as a stabilizing structure rather than requiring flexibility. Proteoglycans within the ECM enhance the ligament's hydration and ability to distribute compressive loads, further supporting its stabilizing role. The balance between collagen and proteoglycan content is critical for maintaining biomechanical integrity. Dysregulation of this balance, for example, by excessive collagen deposition or proteoglycan depletion, has been associated with pathological conditions such as ossification of the ALL, which can result in spinal rigidity and reduced mobility [80, 81, 83–85].

Regional variations in the thickness and composition of the ALL correspond to the differing mechanical demands among spinal segments. For instance, the lumbar region, which bears the greatest axial loads, haincreaser and more robust ALL than the cervical rextracellular matrix (egion, where mobility takes precedence over load-bearing capacity. This regional specialization highlights the ligament's adaptability in meeting the distinct biomechanical requirements of different spinal segments [69].

The layered anatomical organization of the ALL enhances its mechanical function. Its outer layer integrates with the periosteum of the vertebral bodies, providing firm attachment and stability. The inner layer interacts with the anterior anulus fibrosus of the intervertebral discs, reinforcing the intervertebral joints and preventing anterior displacement of the discs. This dual-layered structure enables the ALL to resist hyperextension forces effectively and contribute to overall spinal stability during static postures and dynamic movements [75].

3.4.1.3 Biomechanical Properties and Functional Roles

The ALL is a critical tension band along the anterior spine, counteracting hyperextension forces and ensuring stability during spinal movements. Its dense collagen network allows it to absorb and distribute tensile forces evenly across the vertebral column, reducing the risk of structural injury. Its biomechanical importance is particularly pronounced in the cervical region, where spinal mobility is highest, and the lumbar region, where the risk of hyperextension-related injuries is greatest [69].

Beyond static support, the ALL contributes actively to the dynamic stability of the spine. Limiting anterior vertebral motion helps protect the intervertebral discs and vertebral bodies during rapid or extreme movements, such as those associated with athletic activities or trauma. The ALL also synergizes with posterior spinal elements such as the PLL and ligamentum flavum to maintain the structural and functional alignment of the spinal column [75].

3.4.1.4 Pathological Changes

Ossification: Ossification of the ALL is a pathological condition often associated with DISH. It involves the formation of ectopic bone along the anterior aspect of the vertebral column, reducing ligament flexibility and increasing spinal stiffness. Severe ossification can lead to significant functional impairments such as reduced spinal mobility and compression of adjacent structures. For example, an ossified ALL can compress the esophagus or trachea, resulting in dysphagia or respiratory complications [86, 87].

Degeneration and Trauma: Degenerative changes in the ALL, including thinning and fibrosis, compromise its mechanical integrity and increase the risk of spinal instability. These changes are commonly associated with degenerative disc disease, as reduced intervertebral disc height places additional strain on the ligament. Traumatic injuries such as those resulting from hyperextension forces can cause partial or complete ligament rupture, leading to profound instability and the potential for neurological compromise [75].

3.4.1.5 Clinical and Functional Implications

The ALL is critically important in spinal surgeries, particularly in procedures addressing hyperextension-related injuries or degenerative conditions. Surgical interventions such as anterior cervical decompression or lumbar fusion often require resection of the ALL to access the underlying vertebral bodies or intervertebral discs. However, careful management of the ligament is necessary to preserve spinal stability and prevent complications such as adjacent segment disease [69].

Preoperative imaging, including magnetic resonance imaging (MRI) and computed tomography (CT), is essential for assessing ALL integrity and identifying pathological changes such as ossification or ligament disruption. Advances in minimally invasive surgical techniques have significantly improved outcomes, reducing postoperative complications and shortening recovery times. These innovations emphasize the importance of preserving ligament function and integrity during surgical interventions [75].

3.4.2 Posterior Longitudinal Ligament: Development, Structure, and Functional Significance

The posterior longitudinal ligament (PLL) is a critical connective tissue structure within the vertebral canal. It extends along the posterior surfaces of the vertebral bodies and intervertebral discs, spanning from the axis (C2) to the sacrum. Functionally, it is pivotal in stabilizing the vertebral column by limiting excessive spinal flexion and maintaining the alignment of the vertebrae. It also forms a protective barrier for the spinal canal by reinforcing the posterior annulus fibrosus of the intervertebral discs, thereby reducing the risk of posterior disc herniation into the spinal canal, a potentially deleterious event that can compress the spinal cord or nerve roots. Structurally, the PLL is notable for its distinctive composition, combining dense collagen fibers and fibrocartilage. This combination confers tensile strength and adaptability, enabling the ligament to accommodate the spine's curvatures and biomechanical demands [37] (Fig. 3.1).

3.4.2.1 Developmental Origins

The development of the PLL is a complex multifactorial process that starts during embryogenesis, beginning with mesenchymal condensation along the posterior aspect of the developing vertebral column. Mesenchymal cells differentiate into fibroblasts and chondrocyte-like cells, which have distinct but complementary roles in ligament formation. Fibroblasts synthesize type I collagen, a structural protein critical for tensile strength. At the same time, chondrocyte-like cells produce type II collagen, which provides the elasticity and compressive resistance necessary for the functional versatility of the PLL [88, 89].

During the second trimester of fetal development, the PLL matures significantly. This stage is marked by increased fibrocartilage deposition, matrix organization, and collagen alignment, which are closely related to the mechanical forces exerted by fetal spinal movements. These mechanical stimuli are crucial for guiding the development of the structural properties of the PLL, enabling it to adapt to the biomechanical demands of postnatal life [90–92].

Investigations have highlighted the critical role of fibrocartilage within the PLL in counteracting compressive stresses. This fibrocartilage comprises a matrix enriched in type I and type II collagen, each contributing distinctively to its biomechanical properties. Type I collagen confers tensile strength, enabling the PLL to withstand mechanical forces, while type II collagen confers resilience and elasticity, essential for its adaptive response to dynamic loads [25, 93]. The equilibrium between these collagen types is modulated by mechanical loading, which influences the gene expression pathways involved in collagen synthesis and degradation [63, 76]. Notably, mechanical loading has been shown to upregulate collagen gene expression, enhancing the tensile strength of the PLL and improving its structural integrity [76, 94].

3.4.2.2 Structural Composition

The PLL is histologically and functionally unique, with a complex, stratified structure that supports its dual role in stabilizing the spine and facilitating controlled movement. Its outer layer consists of mainly of dense regular connective tissue rich in type I collagen, which provides tensile strength and resists elongation during spinal flexion. In contrast, its inner layer contains fibrocartilage interspersed with type II collagen, contributing to elasticity and resistance to compressive forces. This layered architecture allows the PLL to distribute mechanical loads effectively while adapting to the dynamic and regionally distinct demands of the vertebral column [91].

The ECM of the PLL incorporates not only collagen but also elastin and proteoglycans, which collectively optimize its biomechanical properties. Elastin fibers contribute to the ligament's flexibility, enabling it to conform to the natural curves of the spine, particularly in the cervical and thoracic regions. Proteoglycans enhance hydration and compressive strength, thereby facilitating the ligament's ability to absorb and distribute dynamic loads. This interplay of structural components ensures that the PLL maintains vertebral alignment and mitigates excessive motion, thereby preserving spinal stability and reducing the risk of injury [70, 95].

The PLL varies in composition and thickness among regions, reflecting its functional specialization. In the cervical and thoracic regions, it is relatively elastic, allowing for greater flexibility to accommodate spinal curvature and mobility. In the lumbar region, where mechanical loads are higher owing to weight-bearing activities, it is thicker and more collagen-rich, providing enhanced tensile strength to support axial loading. These regional adaptations highlight the crucial role of the PLL in maintaining spinal biomechanics across various segments of the vertebral column [91, 95].

3.4.2.3 Biomechanical Properties and Functional Roles

The PLL, located along the posterior vertebral bodies, adapts to tensile and compressive stresses, ensuring spinal stability under mechanical loads. Its viscoelastic nature allows it to accommodate dynamic and static forces, a critical function in conditions such as degenerative intervertebral disc disease, where loading patterns are altered. Age-related changes and degeneration can impair its stabilizing role [4, 82, 96].

The ALL, positioned anteriorly on the vertebral bodies, has high tensile strength, which is essential for preventing hyperextension and excessive posterior motion. It maintains spinal alignment and reduces hyperextension injuries, particularly in athletes, while its distinctive biomechanical properties reinforce spinal stabilization [97, 98].

The ligamentum flavum (LF), interspinous ligament (ISL), and supraspinous ligament (SSL) contribute further to spinal stability. The LF supports dynamic movements by absorbing and dissipating forces, protecting the spinal cord during bending and twisting. However, its hypertrophic response to stress can exacerbate spinal stenosis. The ISL and SSL, though less tensile, stabilize the spine by limiting flexion and preserving posterior column integrity [4, 82, 96] [11, 99]. Together, these ligaments enhance the spine's capacity to withstand mechanical stresses, ensuring the preservation of functional integrity.

Aging, injuries, and systemic conditions such as ankylosing spondylitis influence ligament biomechanics, altering mechanical properties and increasing the risk of instability. Comprehensive insights into these interactions are crucial for advancing therapies for spinal disorders [4, 82]. Conditions such as ankylosing spondylitis can also significantly alter the biomechanical behavior of these ligaments, resulting in increased stiffness and reduced flexibility [100]. A comprehensive understanding of these complex interactions is therefore imperative for developing therapeutic strategies aimed at spinal disorders.

Table 3.3 outlines the tensile properties, elasticity, and functional roles of the spinal ligaments (SLs), emphasizing the resistance of the ALL and PLL to hyperextension and the contributions of the LF, ISL, and SSL to shock absorption, flexion control, and structural alignment. This synthesis highlights their integrated roles in ensuring spinal stability, flexibility, and neural protection [4, 11, 38, 39, 60, 68–70, 74, 77, 81, 82, 101–106].

3.4.2.4 Pathological Changes

The PLL is prone to pathological changes that can compromise its structural and functional integrity. OPLL is characterized by ectopic bone formation within the ligament. This condition, which is more prevalent in East Asian populations, leads to progressive spinal canal stenosis and potentially spinal cord compression. Molecular pathways involving Bone Morphogenetic Protein-2 (BMP-2), Transforming Growth Factor Beta (TGF-β), and RUNX2 are central to the pathogenesis of OPLL, driving osteoblast differentiation and disrupting the flexibility of the ligament [65, 107].

Degenerative changes, including fibrosis, elastin depletion, and proteoglycan loss, are also common in the PLL. These changes result in increased stiffness, reduced elasticity, and a diminished capacity to absorb compressive forces. Such alterations exacerbate conditions such as spinal stenosis and disc herniation, further compromising spinal stability and function [70, 95].

Histological studies of diseased PLL tissue often reveal disorganized collagen fibers, calcification, and fibrosis. Advanced pathologies such as severe OPLL can lead to myelopathy and neurological deficits, necessitating timely clinical intervention [108].

3.4.2.5 Clinical and Functional Implications

The PLL is a critical consideration in spinal surgeries, particularly for conditions such as cervical myelopathy, OPLL, and severe disc herniations. Surgical interventions, including anterior cervical decompression, corpectomy, and laminoplasty, often involve resection of the PLL to relieve spinal canal compression. However, such procedures must account for potential complications, including cerebrospinal fluid leakage and injury to adjacent dura mater, necessitating precise surgical planning and technique [9, 65, 99, 109–112].

Table 3.3 Functional roles of spinal ligaments

SLs	Tensile strength	Elasticity	Primary functional role
ALL	High	Low	Prevents hyperextension; maintains stability during extension
PLL	Moderate	Moderate	Resists flexion; adapts to tensile and compressive forces
LF	Moderate	High	Facilitates dynamic movement; absorbs shock
ISL	Low	Low	Limits flexion; enhances spinal stability
SSL	Low	Low	Provides tensile support; maintains alignment

Consolidated from multiple sources, this table summarizes the tensile strength, elasticity, and functional roles of the spinal ligaments (SLs), including the anterior longitudinal ligament (ALL), posterior longitudinal ligament (PLL), ligamentum flavum (LF), interspinous ligament (ISL), and supraspinous ligament (SSL). The ALL and PLL are emphasized for their roles in stability, while the LF, ISL, and SSL contribute through shock absorption, flexion limitation, and structural alignment [4, 11, 37, 44, 47, 58, 63, 70, 76, 82, 87, 91, 94–99]

Preoperative imaging using MRI and CT is crucial for evaluating PLL pathology and informing surgical strategies. Advances in minimally invasive approaches and neuroprotective techniques have improved outcomes, reducing the incidence of complications and enhancing recovery times [9, 99, 109–111].

The contributions of the PLL to spinal biomechanics and its interaction with adjacent structures underscore its importance in both health and disease. A comprehensive understanding of its structural and functional properties provides critical insights into managing spinal disorders.

3.4.3 The Ligamentum Flavum: Development, Structure, and Functional Significance

The LF is a critical component of the spinal column, contributing to its flexibility, stability, and overall biomechanical integrity. This ligament, which connects the laminae of adjacent vertebrae, is distinguished by its high elastic fiber content, allowing it to stretch and recoil during spinal movements. Extending from the axis (C2) to the sacrum, the LF is vital in maintaining the alignment of the vertebrae, protecting the spinal cord, and meeting the dynamic demands of the vertebral column. According to current scientific knowledge, this section examines the ligament's developmental origins, structural composition, biomechanical properties, and clinical significance (Fig. 3.1).

3.4.3.1 Developmental Origins

The LF develops from mesenchymal tissue during embryogenesis, specifically from the cells surrounding the posterior vertebral arch. By the second trimester of fetal development, mesenchymal cells differentiate into fibroblasts and elastin-secreting cells. These cells synthesize the ECM proteins that give the ligament its characteristic properties. Types I and III collagen dominate the early stages of development, providing the tensile strength necessary for structural support, while elastin production increases during later stages to accommodate the dynamic requirements of fetal movement [34, 113].

The differentiation of these cells is regulated by molecular signaling pathways such as TGF-β and FGF, which influence cell proliferation, matrix synthesis, and tissue organization. These pathways are crucial for the maturation of the LF into a dense, elastic structure that can endure mechanical stress and maintain spinal flexibility. During the final trimester, it thickens and is organized into its layered structure, preparing it for the mechanical demands of postnatal life ([37, 114].

3.4.3.2 Structural Composition

The LF is histologically distinct among spinal ligaments owing to its high elastic fiber content, constituting approximately 60–80% of its structure, depending on the region and physiological conditions. These elastic fibers are densely packed and organized into parallel bundles, interwoven with collagen fibers, primarily types I and III, forming a highly resilient extracellular matrix (ECM). The remaining composition includes fibroblasts, which actively maintain the ECM by synthesizing elastin, collagen, and proteoglycans, as well as sparse vascular networks that supply nutrients to the tissue. This distinctive elastin-collagen matrix provides the LF with remarkable elasticity and tensile strength, enabling it to stretch and recoil during spinal movements without permanent deformation [60, 114, 115].

In addition to its elastic components, the LF contains proteoglycans and glycoproteins within its ECM, contributing to its viscoelastic properties. These molecules are essential for the hydration and structural integrity of the ligament, allowing it to dissipate mechanical loads effectively. The fibroblast population of the LF demonstrates region-specific activity, with elastin synthesis being greater in areas subjected to higher dynamic stresses, such as the lumbar region. This adaptation is essential for the ligament's stabilizing and protective structure [73, 101].

Structural variations along the spinal column further reflect the biomechanical demands placed on the LF. The lumbar spine is thicker and denser, with a lower elastin-to-collagen ratio than the cervical region. This adaptation provides enhanced mechanical support to counteract the greater compressive forces experienced in the lower spine. In contrast, the cervical LF has a higher proportion of elastic fibers, providing the greater flexibility required for the mobility of the upper spinal segments. These regional differences highlight the ligament's ability to balance tensile strength and elasticity according to functional requirements [73, 101].

Pathological changes in the LF often involve remodeling of its histological components, which can impair its biomechanical properties. Conditions such as lumbar spinal stenosis are associated with increased collagen deposition and decreased elastin content, leading to a loss of elasticity and hypertrophy of the ligament. These changes are primarily driven by alterations in cellular activity and ECM turnover. Transforming growth factor-beta (TGF-β) has been implicated in promoting collagen synthesis and inhibiting elastin production, while matrix metalloproteinases (MMPs) degrade elastin, further contributing to the imbalance [116–120].

Histopathological examinations of hypertrophic LF tissue reveal increased fibrosis, disorganized collagen bundles, and reduced elastin fiber density. In advanced cases, the ECM is mineralized, and inflammatory cells are infiltrated. These changes lead to significant stiffening of the ligament, restricting its ability to accommodate spinal movements and resulting in compression of the spinal canal and neural elements. Such pathological remodeling underscores the critical role of maintaining the ligament's histological integrity for normal spinal function and highlights its involvement in degenerative spinal disorders [60, 116, 119, 120].

3.4.3.3 Biomechanical Properties and Functional Roles

The LF is crucial for spinal biomechanics, maintaining tension between adjacent vertebrae and contributing to spinal stability. Its elastic properties enable it to stretch during spinal flexion and recoil during extension, reducing the potential for vertebral misalignment and preserving the integrity of the spinal canal. This function is particularly important in minimizing stress on the intervertebral discs and facet joints, which are prone to degeneration under repetitive loading [121, 122].

The ligament also acts as a dynamic stabilizer, absorbing and dissipating forces during spinal movement. This protective function is critical in transitional zones of the spine, such as the thoracolumbar and lumbosacral junctions, where mechanical loads are greatest. By preventing excessive separation of vertebrae during flexion, the LF contributes to the overall resilience of the vertebral column and protects the spinal cord and nerve roots from mechanical stress [69, 75].

3.4.3.4 Pathological Changes

Degenerative changes in the LF, often associated with aging and chronic mechanical stress, can compromise its structural and functional integrity. These changes include hypertrophy, fibrosis, and ossification, all contributing to a loss of elasticity and increased stiffness. LF hypertrophy is a leading cause of lumbar spinal stenosis, in which thickened ligament tissue encroaches on the spinal canal, compressing neural structures and causing symptoms such as pain, numbness, and motor weakness [123, 124].

Ossification of the ligamentum flavum (OLF) is another significant pathological condition, particularly prevalent in East Asian populations. It is characterized by ectopic bone formation within the ligament, leading to severe spinal canal stenosis and neurological deficits. Molecular studies have implicated BMP-2 and TGF-β signaling pathways in the ossification process, providing potential targets for therapeutic intervention. OLF typically affects the thoracic spine, where the ligament is relatively less elastic, further exacerbating the effects of ossification [107, 125].

3.4.3.5 Clinical and Functional Implications

Pathological changes in the LF are a common indication for surgical intervention, particularly in severe lumbar stenosis or OLF. Surgical decompression, involving partial or complete resection of the LF, is often necessary to relieve spinal cord or nerve root compression. Advances in minimally invasive surgical techniques, such as endoscopic or microscopic decompression, have improved outcomes by preserving surrounding structures and minimizing postoperative complications [108].

Preoperative imaging, including MRI and CT, is essential for assessing the extent of ligament hypertrophy or ossification and planning surgical strategies. These imaging modalities provide detailed assessments of the ligament's thickness, elasticity, and anatomical relationships with adjacent structures, enabling surgical approaches to be tailored to optimize patient outcomes [75, 109].

3.4.4 Interspinous Ligament: Development, Structure, and Functional Significance

The interspinous ligament (ligamentum interspinale) (ISL) is a critical connective tissue structure located between the spinous processes of adjacent vertebrae. It serves structural and functional roles, contributing to spinal stability, biomechanical integrity, and proprioception. Its development, structural composition, and functional significance underscore its importance in maintaining the dynamic balance of the vertebral column. This section provides a comprehensive analysis of the ISL, highlighting its embryological origins, anatomical features, biomechanical properties, and clinical relevance (Fig. 3.1).

3.4.4.1 Developmental Origins

The ISL develops during the embryonic and fetal stages from mesenchymal tissue derived from the paraxial mesoderm. By the fourth week of embryogenesis, mesenchymal cells in the posterior sclerotome condense and differentiate into fibroblasts, which produce the ECM proteins necessary for ligament formation. This matrix predominantly comprises collagen types I and III, providing the tensile strength required for the ligament's stabilizing function.

During fetal development, the ISL undergoes significant remodeling influenced by mechanical forces from increasing fetal movements. These forces stimulate fibroblast activity, promoting the organization and maturation of collagen fibers into thick, parallel bundles. By the third trimester, the ISL has a well-defined structure characterized by dense collagen fibers interspersed with a sparse population of fibrocytes [12, 38].

3.4.4.2 Structural Composition

The ISL, located between the spinous processes of adjacent vertebrae, is mainly composed of dense connective tissue, with type III collagen predominating; the elastin content is moderate. This composition provides tensile strength while allowing limited flexibility. The collagen fibers are arranged in an interwoven, S-shaped configuration, which enhances flexibility and stabilizes the spinous processes during spinal movements. These structural features enable the ligament to resist mechanical forces effectively while accommodating minor adjustments during dynamic activities [38, 126].

Regional variations in ISL structure reflect its adaptation to local biomechanical demands. In the cervical spine, the ligament is thinner and has a higher elastin-to-collagen ratio, supporting the greater flexibility required in this area. In contrast, the lumbar spine exhibits a thicker, more collagen-dense ligament, better suited to withstanding the substantial tensile and compressive forces associated with weight-bearing and movement. These regional differences demonstrate the ligament's functional versatility and ability to provide targeted stability where mechanical demands are highest [73, 101].

The ISL balances tensile strength and elasticity, allowing it to support spinal stability while absorbing and dissipating forces. This property is particularly important during dynamic movements such as twisting or bending, in which the ligament helps distribute mechanical loads and reduces stress on the underlying structures. Its composition, combining type III collagen for tensile strength and elastin for flexibility, makes it well-suited to its stabilizing role in maintaining spinal alignment during complex movements [70].

By adapting to varying mechanical demands and providing critical support during spinal movements, the ISL is pivotal in maintaining the overall stability and functionality of the spine. Understanding its histological and biomechanical characteristics is essential for appreciating its contributions to spinal health and addressing pathologies that can compromise its function.

3.4.4.3 Biomechanical Properties and Functional Roles

The ISL is a fundamental component of the spinal column, particularly important in maintaining stability during flexion movements. Resisting excessive separation of adjacent spinous processes is crucial for preserving vertebral alignment and ensuring the structural integrity of the spine. During flexion, it undergoes tensile strain, which it counteracts through its collagen-rich extracellular matrix. This matrix imparts significant tensile strength while allowing for the necessary elasticity to accommodate dynamic mechanical loads [12]. These biomechanical properties are crucial for the ligament's ability to maintain spinal stability and functionality under various physiological and pathological conditions [38, 80, 82].

In addition to its structural role, the ISL is densely supplied with mechanoreceptors and nociceptors, which facilitate its proprioceptive function. These sensory elements provide essential feedback about spinal position and movement, contributing significantly to postural control and reflexive stabilization of the spine. During activities that require rapid adjustments, such as those involving sudden or complex motions, the proprioceptive input from the ISL enables precise neuromuscular coordination, thereby mitigating the risk of injury. Integrating this sensory information with motor responses is indispensable for maintaining spinal stability, particularly in dynamic contexts where the spine must adapt to changing mechanical demands [77, 82, 102].

The ISL also operates synergistically with other spinal ligaments, including the SSL and the LF, forming a cohesive network that supports and stabilizes the vertebral column. This ligamentous collaboration is essential for distributing mechanical loads evenly across the spine, thereby reducing localized stress and mitigating the risk of injury to individual spinal components. Such cooperative interactions are particularly critical in countering flexion and torsional forces, which impose significant mechanical demands on the spinal column. The interconnected nature of these ligaments amplifies the biomechanical efficiency of the spine, ensuring both stability and adaptability during weight-bearing and dynamic movements [68, 74].

An in-depth understanding of the ISL's biomechanical properties, proprioceptive contributions, and functional interactions with surrounding structures is essential for advancing clinical strategies to manage spinal disorders and injuries. Conditions such as ligamentous sprains, degenerative pathologies, and postural dysfunction often disrupt the ligament's mechanical or sensory functions, compromising spinal stability. Therapeutic interventions, including targeted rehabilitation programs, regenerative therapies, and surgical procedures, are frequently aimed at restoring or augmenting these ligamentous functions. Thus, a thorough exploration of the ISL's multifaceted role in spinal biomechanics is critical for optimizing outcomes in managing spinal health [77, 82, 102].

3.4.4.4 Pathological Changes

The ISL is susceptible to injuries and degenerative changes that can compromise its function. Acute trauma, repetitive microtrauma, and age-related degeneration can lead to structural weakening, inflammation, or calcification of the ligament. These conditions often result in pain, reduced spinal stability, and functional impairment.

Repetitive flexion and extension, particularly in athletes and individuals engaged in physically demanding occupations, place significant stress on the ISL. This can result in partial tears or microtrauma at its attachment sites, leading to localized inflammation and pain. Chronic overuse can also cause fibrosis and reduced ligament elasticity, exacerbating the risk of further injury [12, 127].

Baastrup's disease, also known as "kissing spine syndrome," is a degenerative condition characterized by the abnormal approximation of adjacent spinous processes, often leading to inflammation, hypertrophy of the ISL, and painful pseudoarticulations. Most commonly affecting the lumbar spine, particularly at the L4-L5 level, it arises from age-related degeneration or repetitive mechanical stress, which is exacerbated by contact between the spinous processes due to reduced intervertebral disc height. Clinical symptoms include localized lumbar pain, often worsened by spinal extension and relieved by flexion, with significant functional impairment in severe cases. Imaging modalities such as MRI and CT are crucial for diagnosing interspinous narrowing, sclerosis, and pseudoarticulations. Treatment focuses on conservative approaches, including physical therapy and anti-inflammatory medications, though refractory cases can require corticosteroid injections or surgical intervention to relieve symptoms and restore mobility [128–131].

Calcification of the ISL is a clinically significant condition that can arise from degenerative changes or systemic disorders, including vitamin D-resistant rickets. This condition leads to reduced flexibility of the ligament, which can result in spinal stiffness and pain. The ISL is crucial for stabilizing the spine, particularly during surgical procedures involving the posterior elements of the vertebral column. Preservation of this ligament during surgeries such as laminectomy or interspinous process device implantation is essential to minimize the risk of postoperative complications, including axial pain and instability [132].

Research indicates that the ISL can be calcified through various etiologies, including genetic predispositions and systemic conditions such as vitamin D-resistant rickets. For instance, hereditary vitamin D-resistant rickets (HVDRR) is characterized by mutations in the vitamin D receptor (VDR) gene, leading to skeletal deformities and impaired mineralization [133, 134]. This condition can manifest in various ways, including calcification of ligaments, which can contribute to the overall stiffness and pain experienced by patients [135]. The presence of nociceptors in the ISL suggests that abnormal calcification can lead to significant pain, further complicating the clinical picture [132].

3.4.4.5 Clinical and Functional Implications

The ISL is a critical consideration in spinal surgeries, particularly in procedures involving the posterior elements of the vertebral column. Its preservation is essential for maintaining spinal stability, especially during laminectomy or interspinous process device implantation. Research indicates that preserving the ligament reduces the risk of postoperative complications such as axial pain and instability, emphasizing its biomechanical importance [136].

However, in conditions where the ligament contributes to pathology, such as Baastrup's disease or extensive calcification, surgical resection can be required. Minimally invasive techniques have been developed to target these conditions while minimizing disruption to surrounding structures, thereby preserving overall spinal function [136].

The ISL's functional role extends beyond mechanical support, contributing to the intricate balance of forces that maintain spinal alignment and enable dynamic movement. Its sensory and proprioceptive properties are crucial for maintaining postural control and preventing injury. Understanding the biomechanical and clinical implications of the ISL is essential for managing conditions that affect spinal stability and mobility.

Advances in imaging techniques, such as MRI and high-resolution ultrasound, have made it easier to assess the ligament's integrity and detect pathological changes. These diagnostic tools are invaluable in guiding therapeutic interventions, whether conservative or surgical, to optimize outcomes and restore function.

3.4.5 Supraspinous Ligament: Development, Structure, and Functional Significance

The supraspinous ligament (SSL) is an essential component of the spinal column, spanning the tips of the spinous processes from the seventh cervical vertebra (C7) to the sacrum. Functionally, it is integral to maintaining spinal stability by limiting forward flexion and protecting the vertebral column under mechanical stress. This section explores the embryological development, structural composition, biomechanical roles, and clinical significance of the SSL, highlighting its importance in spinal health and its implications in pathological conditions (Fig. 3.1).

3.4.5.1 Developmental Origins

The SSL development begins during embryogenesis and arises from mesenchymal tissue derived from the paraxial mesoderm. By the fourth week of development, the somites segment along the embryonic axis, and their sclerotome components contribute to the formation of the vertebrae and associated connective tissues, including ligaments. There is mesenchymal condensation along the posterior midline, initiating the differentiation of fibroblasts that synthesize ECM components, predominantly collagen type I. These fibers form the foundational framework of the ligament, providing the tensile strength necessary to resist mechanical forces [10, 137].

During the fetal period, progressive collagen deposition and organization characterize the maturation of the SSL. Fetal movements significantly stimulate this process, and mechanical loading promotes fibroblast activity and ECM alignment. By the third trimester, the ligament achieves a highly organized, longitudinal structure that can accommodate the mechanical demands of the postnatal spine. This structural organization is crucial for the ligament's role in spinal stability, as it interacts with other components of the posterior ligamentous complex, including the ISL and LF, which collectively contribute to the spine's stability during various movements [77].

3.4.5.2 Structural Composition

The SSL, extending along the tips of the spinous processes from the cervical to the sacral regions, primarily comprises dense, parallel-aligned collagen fibers arranged longitudinally. This structural organization gives the ligament significant tensile strength, enabling it to resist stretching forces during spinal flexion. Fibroblasts, the predominant cellular component, are dispersed within the ECM, actively maintaining and repairing the ligament's structural integrity. The ligament contains minimal elastin fibers, emphasizing its role as a rigid stabilizer rather than a highly elastic structure [61, 138].

Regional adaptations in the SSL reflect the biomechanical demands of different spinal segments. In the lumbar region, it is thicker and broader to accommodate the greater tensile forces associated with weight-bearing activities. The cervical region features a thinner SSL, which allows for enhanced flexibility to support the increased range of motion required in the upper spine. These variations highlight the ligament's ability to balance mechanical stability and flexibility in response to regional functional demands [74].

While predominantly collagenous, the SSL contains some elastin fibers, which contribute modestly to its elasticity. This balance of collagen and elastin enables the ligament to absorb and dissipate forces during spinal movements, particularly during dynamic activities such as twisting or bending. The SSL's ability to distribute mechanical loads protects underlying spinal structures from injury and contributes to the overall stability of the vertebral column. These properties make the SSL particularly critical in maintaining the posterior stability of the spine under dynamic loading conditions [70, 126].

The SSL works synergistically with the ISL to form a cohesive stabilizing network for the vertebral column. While the ISL has a higher type III collagen content for tensile resilience, the SSL, with its higher proportion of type I collagen, provides longitudinal tensile strength. Together, these ligaments are essential for ensuring spinal stability and adaptability during motion. Understanding their structural composition and biomechanical roles is necessary for evaluating their contributions to spinal health and managing conditions that could compromise their integrity [10, 70].

The SSL is also enveloped by paravertebral fascia, which enhances its stability and integrates it into the broader connective tissue network of the spine. Limited vascularity is characteristic of the ligament; its blood supply is primarily derived from adjacent musculature and periosteal vessels. This vascular limitation contributes to its relatively slow healing following injury [61, 132, 138].

3.4.5.3 Biomechanical Properties and Functional Roles

The SSL contributes to the stability of the spine in several ways, both static and dynamic. It acts as a mechanical restraint during spinal flexion, limiting the separation of spinous processes and preventing hyperflexion. This function reduces strain on intervertebral discs and adjacent soft tissues, safeguarding the vertebral column against injury [102]. Together with the ISL, the SSL forms a cohesive network that stabilizes the posterior elements of the spine. This interaction is particularly significant during activities involving dynamic loads, such as lifting or bending, in which it prevents excessive vertebral motion and maintains alignment [10].

The SSL contains mechanoreceptors that relay information about spinal position and movement to the central nervous system. This sensory feedback is vital for maintaining posture and coordinating movement, underscoring the ligament's role beyond structural support [5, 139]. The ligament's tensile properties contribute to the distribution of mechanical forces across the vertebral column, reducing the risk of localized stress concentrations that could lead to injury or degeneration [137].

3.4.5.4 Pathological Changes

The SSL is susceptible to degenerative changes associated with aging and chronic mechanical stress. These changes often manifest as fibrosis, calcification, or ligament thinning, leading to reduced flexibility and tensile strength. Such degeneration can contribute to spinal stiffness and heighten the risk of injury under mechanical load.

The SSL is implicated in several pathological conditions. Ankylosing spondylitis, an inflammatory process affecting the SSL, can lead to fibrosis and ossification, contributing to spinal rigidity and an increased risk of fractures. Disruption of the SSL in trauma, such as whiplash injuries, can compromise the stability of the posterior column and exacerbate neurological deficits [74, 139].

Traumatic injuries to the SSL, including sprains or tears, typically result from hyperflexion forces. These injuries can destabilize the posterior ligamentous complex, increasing the risk of vertebral displacement and intervertebral disc herniation. Prompt diagnosis and management prevent long-term instability and pain [103, 140].

3.4.5.5 Clinical and Functional Implications

The SSL is a critical consideration in spinal surgeries, particularly those involving posterior decompression or stabilization. Preservation of the SSL during procedures such as laminectomy or spinal fusion helps maintain postoperative stability and reduces the risk of complications such as axial pain or kyphosis. Surgical techniques that spare the ligament have been shown to enhance recovery outcomes and maintain biomechanical integrity [8].

In cases of severe pathology, such as tumor invasion or extensive ossification, resection of the SSL can be necessary. In such scenarios, careful surgical planning and robust postoperative rehabilitation are essential to minimize functional deficits and ensure optimal recovery [141].

3.5 Collaborative Multidisciplinary Care

Managing spinal ligament pathologies effectively requires a multidisciplinary approach that combines advances in diagnostic imaging, biomechanical principles, surgical techniques, and regenerative medicine. This integrated framework bridges foundational scientific research with clinical applications, addressing the complexities of ligament disorders while fostering innovation and improving patient outcomes.

3.5.1 Basic Science in Diagnosis: Integrated Diagnostic Approaches

Advances in diagnostic imaging have been pivotal in transforming the detection and evaluation of spinal ligament injuries. MRI, with its superior ability to visualize soft tissues, is invaluable for diagnosing conditions such as OPLL and other ligament pathologies. MRI provides detailed insights into such pathologies, including myelomalacia and ossification, and aids in tailoring surgical interventions, such as laminoplasty, for cervical spondylotic myelopathy [25, 40]. CT complements MRI by providing high-resolution imaging of calcifications and bony structures, which are crucial for preoperative planning.

Incorporating biomechanical insights into surgical planning enhances the precision and efficacy of interventions. Understanding the tensile strength, elasticity, and load-bearing capacities of the spinal ligaments allows for customized surgical approaches tailored to the unique biomechanical profile of each patient. This personalized strategy ensures optimal outcomes by aligning surgical techniques with patient-specific needs, emphasizing the role of biomechanics in achieving spinal stability and functionality [70, 75].

Regenerative medicine has emerged as a transformative avenue for treating spinal ligament pathologies. Biological therapies, including mesenchymal stem cell applications and growth factor-based treatments, hold promise for ligament repair and regeneration. Growth factors, such as TGF-β and BMPs, have shown potential in promoting ECM synthesis and ligament healing, as well as modulating pathological processes like ossification. Biomimetic scaffolds incorporating BMPs are being developed to enhance ligament repair, leveraging the body's intrinsic regenerative capacities [142, 143].

The synergy between disciplines is critical for advancing spinal healthcare. Collaboration between basic scientists and clinicians fosters a holistic understanding of spinal ligament pathologies. Genetic research on diffuse idiopathic skeletal hyperostosis provides valuable insights for early screening and preventive strategies in high-risk populations. Furthermore, emerging technologies, such as machine learning algorithms, are revolutionizing the predictive modeling of clinical outcomes, including recovery trajectories in spinal cord injuries, highlighting the importance of interdisciplinary collaboration in improving patient care [25, 144].

3.5.2 Basic Science in Treatment: Comprehensive Therapeutic Strategies

Advancing the understanding of cellular and molecular mechanisms underlying ligament development and pathology has opened avenues for innovative therapeutic interventions to improve ligament repair, regeneration, and functionality. These approaches capitalize on the intricate signaling pathways and biomechanical properties that govern ligament integrity, offering potential for both clinical and experimental applications.

3.5.2.1 Regenerative Therapies

Regenerative therapies harness the body's natural healing processes to restore ligament function. Using BMPs in conjunction with biomimetic scaffolds represents a significant advance in ligament repair. BMPs, particularly BMP-2 and BMP-7, play a pivotal role in promoting mesenchymal stem cell differentiation into ligament-forming fibroblasts and enhancing extracellular matrix (ECM) production, which is critical for maintaining tensile strength and resilience. Biomimetic scaffolds, designed to mimic the native ligament environment, provide a structural framework that supports cell attachment, proliferation, and matrix deposition. These scaffolds can be augmented with bioactive molecules to accelerate healing and improve the mechanical properties of repaired ligaments [41, 142].

3.5.2.2 Engineered Ligaments

Advances in tissue engineering have led to the development of engineered ligaments designed to simulate the mechanical and functional characteristics of native ligaments. Modulating TGF-β signaling is a promising strategy in this context. TGF-β not only regulates collagen synthesis but is also essential for ligament organization and remodeling. By fine-tuning TGF-β activity, it is possible to enhance the structural integrity and mechanical performance of engineered ligaments, making them suitable for surgical implantation and load-bearing applications. Moreover, integrating these ligaments with bone-to-bone attachments, facilitated by BMP-4 and other osteogenic factors, further enhances their applicability in reconstructive surgeries [40, 143].

3.5.2.3 Targeted Therapies

Targeted therapies using FGFs offer solutions for restoring elasticity and resilience in ligaments affected by degenerative conditions. FGFs, particularly FGF-2, stimulate fibroblast proliferation and elastin synthesis, addressing the loss of elasticity in conditions such as ligament hypertrophy or fibrosis. These therapies can also mitigate the progression of ossification in ligaments, as FGFs counteract excessive collagen deposition and preserve the biomechanical flexibility of affected tissues. Delivery systems, such as nanoparticle-based carriers, are being explored to enhance the precision and efficacy of FGF-based treatments, thereby minimizing systemic side effects and maximizing local therapeutic benefits [142, 143].

3.5.2.4 Emerging Approaches

Advances in regenerative medicine, particularly in gene editing and cell-based therapies, are redefining the management of ligament pathologies through highly targeted and effective interventions. Among these, CRISPR/Cas9 gene-editing technology represents a transformative breakthrough, enabling precise genomic modifications to address the molecular underpinnings of ligament disorders. This approach is particularly relevant for conditions such as OPLL, a debilitating pathology characterized by ectopic bone formation within spinal ligaments. CRISPR/Cas9 facilitates the correction of pathogenic mutations associated with OPLL, offering the potential to mitigate risk factors, halt disease progression, and manage ligament pathologies at their genetic origins. By addressing disease mechanisms at the molecular level, this technology holds promise for revolutionizing the treatment landscape for genetically predisposed ligament conditions [64, 145].

In parallel, mesenchymal stem cell therapies have emerged as a powerful avenue for ligament regeneration, particularly when combined with bioactive molecules such as TGF-β and BMPs. MSCs have multipotent differentiation capabilities, enabling them to transform into ligament-relevant cell types, including fibroblasts and chondrocytes. Bioactive agents, such as BMP-2 and TGF-β1, significantly enhance the osteogenic and chondrogenic differentiation of ligament-derived stem cells, thereby facilitating tissue repair and regeneration. These agents also stimulate ECM production, repair microstructural injury, and improve the biomechanical properties of ligament tissues. TGF-β1 is pivotal in regulating collagen synthesis, a process essential for the repair and regeneration of ligament tissue. At the same time, BMP-2 plays a crucial role in facilitating ECM organization and structural remodeling, both of which are essential for restoring ligament functionality [64].

A particularly innovative strategy for enhancing the efficacy of these regenerative therapies involves integrating mechanobiological stimuli, such as cyclic tensile loading, which replicates the physiological mechanical environment of native ligaments. Mechanobiological interventions are increasingly recognized for their capacity to guide stem cell differentiation, enhance extracellular matrix (ECM) production, and promote collagen fiber alignment. Mechanical loading has been shown to regulate the expression of critical signaling molecules, including TGF-β and BMP, thereby accelerating tissue healing and improving structural integrity. For instance, cyclic tensile loading not only facilitates ECM alignment but also enhances cell proliferation and differentiation, enabling ligament tissues to form with biomechanical properties similar to those of their healthy counterparts [146, 147].

These emerging approaches highlight the critical interplay among genetic, cellular, and mechanical factors in ligament healing and regeneration. By combining advanced gene-editing tools, MSC-based therapies, and mechanobiological interventions, regenerative medicine provides a multidimensional approach to addressing structural and functional deficits associated with ligament pathologies. Future research should prioritize the optimization of these therapies by leveraging patient-specific models and precision medicine techniques to improve treatment outcomes. Continuing innovation in these areas will significantly expand their clinical applicability, offering new hope for patients suffering from ligament-related disorders.

3.5.2.5 Future Directions

Integrating advanced regenerative therapies with cutting-edge imaging modalities and computational modeling is paving the way for precision medicine in treating ligament pathologies. Emerging predictive models, powered by machine learning, offer the ability to analyze patient-specific biomechanical and molecular profiles, enabling the development of tailored therapeutic strategies. This is particularly critical for ligament injuries, where individual variability in healing responses can significantly influence treatment efficacy. By incorporating large datasets, machine learning algorithms can predict the effectiveness of gene-editing technologies, MSC-based therapies, and mechanobiological interventions, facilitating personalized treatment plans to enhance safety and efficacy [148].

Advances in bioprinting technologies are poised to transform personalized regenerative medicine by enabling the creation of ligament constructs with region-specific extracellular matrix (ECM) compositions and mechanical gradients. These constructs are engineered to replicate the native structure and biomechanical characteristics of ligaments, addressing the specific functional demands of various spinal regions. For instance, bioprinted constructs can be optimized to withstand the tensile forces prevalent in the lumbar spine or to support the flexibility required in the cervical spine. Such precise customization enhances the mechanical integration of regenerated ligaments while promoting critical cellular processes, including ECM remodeling and collagen fiber alignment, which are essential for achieving durable and functional recovery [149].

The convergence of computational modeling, predictive analytics, and advanced biomaterials engineering constitutes a paradigm shift in ligament regeneration. By integrating these technologies into clinical workflows, clinicians can develop more precise and effective treatment protocols. Key research priorities include the development of scalable bioprinting platforms, refining machine learning algorithms to incorporate diverse patient datasets, and validating patient-specific models for clinical application. These interdisciplinary advances will significantly enhance the ability of regenerative medicine to deliver truly personalized and effective therapies for ligament injuries and degenerative conditions, ultimately improving patient outcomes and quality of life.

3.6 Conclusion

Spinal ligaments play a crucial role in maintaining the stability, mobility, and resilience of the vertebral column. Their histogenesis, originating from mesenchymal condensations of the paraxial mesoderm, exemplifies a highly orchestrated process involving cellular, molecular, and biomechanical mechanisms. These ligaments differentiate into specialized ECM components that confer essential tensile strength, elasticity, and adaptability, aligning with their distinct functional roles in facilitating controlled motion, stabilizing vertebral segments, and accommodating physiological mechanical stresses.

The intricate interplay between cellular activity and mechanical forces during ligament development optimizes their structural and functional properties. Fetal movements, for instance, are essential for collagen alignment and ligament maturation, ensuring mechanical resilience throughout life. Disruptions of these developmental processes or degenerative changes highlight the need for comprehensive insights into ligament biomechanics and histogenesis to inform diagnostic and therapeutic advances.

Recent advancements in molecular biology, imaging technologies, and regenerative medicine have significantly enhanced our understanding of spinal ligament physiology and pathology. Innovations such as biomimetic scaffolds, mesenchymal stem cell therapies, and bioactive molecules, including TGF-β and BMPs, hold substantial promise for ligament repair and regeneration. Mechanobiological interventions, including cyclic tensile loading, replicate the physiological environment necessary for ECM organization, further enhancing ligament healing and functional recovery. Concurrently, minimally invasive surgical techniques that integrate biomechanical insights improve outcomes for ligament-related pathologies while preserving structural integrity.

Future research should prioritize the integration of mechanobiological, molecular, and genetic insights to elucidate the complex dynamics of ligament development and repair. Investigations into the role of mechanical forces in histogenesis and regeneration have significant implications for optimizing rehabilitation protocols and improving tissue engineering methods. Furthermore, identifying genetic predispositions to ligament pathologies such as OPLL could enable precision medicine approaches to be tailored to individual biomechanical profiles and susceptibility.

In conclusion, the histogenesis and functional specialization of spinal ligaments are crucial to the stability and mobility of the vertebral column. Disruptions of these processes are closely tied to significant spinal pathologies, underscoring the need to bridge fundamental research to clinical practice. Interdisciplinary collaborations that incorporate molecular, biomechanical, and regenerative perspectives hold immense potential for revolutionizing the prevention, treatment, and management of ligament-related disorders, ultimately enhancing spinal healthcare and improving patient outcomes.

References

1. Williams S, Alkhatib B, Serra R. Development of the axial skeleton and intervertebral disc. Curr Top Dev Biol. 2019;133:49–90. https://doi.org/10.1016/bs.ctdb.2018.11.018.
2. Ikeda Y, Nakajima A, Aiba A, Koda M, Okawa A, Takahashi K, Yamazaki M. Association between serum leptin and bone metabolic markers, and the development of heterotopic ossification of the spinal ligament in female patients with ossification of the posterior longitudinal ligament. Eur Spine J. 2011;20:1450–8. https://doi.org/10.1007/s00586-011-1688-7.
3. Marchi L, Abdala N, Oliveira L, Amaral R, Coutinho E, Pimenta L. Stand-alone lateral interbody fusion for the treatment of low-grade degenerative spondylolisthesis. Sci World J. 2012;2012 https://doi.org/10.1100/2012/456346.
4. Cornaz F, Widmer J, Farshad-Amacker NA, Spirig JM, Snedeker JG, Farshad M. Biomechanical contributions of spinal structures with different degrees of disc degeneration. Spine (Phila Pa 1976). 2021;46:E869–77. https://doi.org/10.1097/BRS.0000000000003883.
5. Pizones J, Izquierdo E, Sánchez-Mariscal F, Zúñiga L, Álvarez P, Gómez-Rice A. Sequential damage assessment of the different components of the posterior ligamentous complex after magnetic resonance imaging interpretation: prospective study 74 traumatic fractures. Spine (Phila Pa 1976). 2012;37 https://doi.org/10.1097/BRS.0b013e3182422b2b.

6. Takagi Y, Yamada H, Ebara H, Hayashi H, Iwanaga T, Shimozaki K, Kitano Y, Kagechika K, Tsuchiya H. Thoracic spondylolisthesis and spinal cord compression in diffuse idiopathic skeletal hyperostosis: a case report. J Med Case Rep. 2017;11 https://doi.org/10.1186/s13256-017-1252-0.
7. Mehta G, Shetty UC, Meena D, Tiwari AK, Nama KG, Aseri D. Evaluation of diagnostic accuracy of magnetic resonance imaging in posterior Ligamentum complex injury of thoracolumbar spine. Asian Spine J. 2021;15:333–9. https://doi.org/10.31616/ASJ.2020.0027.
8. Kim JS, Cheung ZB, Arvind V, Caridi J, Cho SK-WW. Role of posterior ligamentous reinforcement in proximal junctional kyphosis: a cadaveric biomechanical study. Asian Spine J. 2019;13:68–76. https://doi.org/10.31616/ASJ.2018.0102.
9. Mori K, Yoshii T, Hirai T, Iwanami A, Takeuchi K, Yamada T, Seki S, Tsuji T, Fujiyoshi K, Furukawa M, Nishimura S, Wada K, Koda M, Furuya T, Matsuyama Y, Hasegawa T, Takeshita K, Kimura A, Abematsu M, Haro H, Ohba T, Watanabe M, Katoh H, Watanabe K, Ozawa H, Kanno H, Imagama S, Ito Z, Fujibayashi S, Yamazaki M, Matsumoto M, Nakamura M, Okawa A, Kawaguchi Y. Prevalence and distribution of ossification of the supra/interspinous ligaments in symptomatic patients with cervical ossification of the posterior longitudinal ligament of the spine: a CT-based multicenter cross-sectional study. BMC Musculoskelet Disord. 2016;17:1–7. https://doi.org/10.1186/s12891-016-1350-y.
10. Kaulhausen T, Zarghooni K, Stein G, Knifka J, Eysel P, Koebke J, Sobottke R. The interspinous spacer: a clinicoanatomical investigation using plastination. Minim Invasive Surg. 2012;2012:538697. https://doi.org/10.1155/2012/538697.
11. Widmer J, Cornaz F, Scheibler G, Spirig JM, Snedeker JG, Farshad M. Biomechanical contribution of spinal structures to stability of the lumbar spine – novel biomechanical insights. Spine J. 2020;20:1705–16. https://doi.org/10.1016/j.spinee.2020.05.541.
12. Kulkarni R, Ramyashree R. Interspinous ligament as a pain generator. J Recent Adv Pain. 2016;2:54–5. https://doi.org/10.5005/jp-journals-10046-0040.
13. Hedman TP, Ohnmeiss DD, Leasure J, Raji OR, Hochschuler SH. Interspinous-Interbody fusion via a strictly lateral surgical approach: a biomechanical stabilization comparison to constructs requiring both lateral and posterior approaches. Cureus. 2023; https://doi.org/10.7759/cureus.41918.
14. Ploumis A, Christodoulou P, Kapoutsis D, Gelalis I, Vraggalas V, Beris A. Surgical treatment of lumbar spinal stenosis with microdecompression and interspinous distraction device insertion. A case series. J Orthop Surg Res. 2012;7 https://doi.org/10.1186/1749-799X-7-35.
15. Wang Y, Serra R. PDGF mediates TGFβ-induced migration during development of the spinous process. Dev Biol. 2012;365:110–7. https://doi.org/10.1016/j.ydbio.2012.02.013.
16. Sugita D, Nakajima H, Kokubo Y, Takeura N, Yayama T, Matsumine A. Cyclic tensile strain facilitates ossification of the cervical posterior longitudinal ligament via increased Indian hedgehog signaling. Sci Rep. 2020;10 https://doi.org/10.1038/s41598-020-64304-w.
17. Chiba N, Furukawa KI, Takayama S, Asari T, Chin S, Harada Y, Kumagai G, Wada K, Tanaka T, Ono A, Motomura S, Murakami M, Ishibashi Y. Decreased DNA methylation in the promoter region of the WNT5A and GDNF genes may promote the osteogenicity of mesenchymal stem cells from patients with ossified spinal ligaments. J Pharmacol Sci. 2015;127:467–73. https://doi.org/10.1016/j.jphs.2015.03.008.
18. Takahashi Y, Wakabayashi R, Kitajima S, Uchiyama H. Epichordal vertebral column formation in Xenopus laevis. J Morphol. 2024;285 https://doi.org/10.1002/jmor.21664.
19. Sánchez RS, Sánchez SS. Characterization of pax1, pax9, and uncx sclerotomal genes during Xenopus laevis embryogenesis. Dev Dyn. 2013;242:572–9. https://doi.org/10.1002/dvdy.23945.
20. Alberton P, Popov C, Prägert M, Kohler J, Shukunami C, Schieker M, Docheva D. Conversion of human bone marrow-derived mesenchymal stem cells into tendon progenitor cells by ectopic expression of scleraxis. Stem Cells Dev. 2012;21:846–58. https://doi.org/10.1089/scd.2011.0150.
21. Otabe K, Nakahara H, Hasegawa A, Matsukawa T, Ayabe F, Onizuka N, Inui M, Takada S, Ito Y, Sekiya I, Muneta T, Lotz M, Asahara H. Transcription factor Mohawk controls tenogenic differentiation of bone marrow mesenchymal stem cells in vitro and in vivo. J Orthop Res. 2015;33:1–8. https://doi.org/10.1002/jor.22750.
22. Topol L, Jiang X, Choi H, Garrett-Beal L, Carolan PJ, Yang Y. Wnt-5a inhibits the canonical Wnt pathway by promoting GSK-3-independent β-catenin degradation. J Cell Biol. 2003;162:899–908. https://doi.org/10.1083/jcb.200303158.
23. Choi KS, Lee C, Harfe BD. Sonic hedgehog in the notochord is sufficient for patterning of the intervertebral discs. Mech Dev. 2012;129:255–62. https://doi.org/10.1016/j.mod.2012.07.003.
24. Choi KS, Harfe BD. Hedgehog signaling is required for formation of the notochord sheath and patterning of nuclei pulposi within the intervertebral discs. Proc Natl Acad Sci USA. 2011;108:9484–9. https://doi.org/10.1073/pnas.1007566108.
25. Dong J, Xu X, Zhang Q, Yuan Z, Tan B. Dkk1 acts as a negative regulator in the osteogenic differentiation of the posterior longitudinal ligament cells. Cell Biol Int. 2020;44:2450–8. https://doi.org/10.1002/cbin.11452.
26. Mukherjee A, Rotwein P. Akt promotes BMP2-mediated osteoblast differentiation and bone devel-

opment. J Cell Sci. 2009;122:716–26. https://doi.org/10.1242/jcs.042770.
27. Cox MK, Appelboom BL, Ban GI, Serra R. Erg cooperates with TGF-β to control mesenchymal differentiation. Exp Cell Res. 2014;328:410–8. https://doi.org/10.1016/j.yexcr.2014.08.015.
28. Haddad-Weber M, Prager P, Kunz M, Seefried L, Jakob F, Murray MM, Evans CH, Nöth U, Steinert AF. BMP12 and BMP13 gene transfer induce ligamentogenic differentiation in mesenchymal progenitor and anterior cruciate ligament cells. Cytotherapy. 2010;12:505–13. https://doi.org/10.3109/14653241003709652.
29. Ban GI, Williams S, Serra R. Antagonism of BMP signaling is insufficient to induce fibrous differentiation in primary sclerotome. Exp Cell Res. 2019;378:11–20. https://doi.org/10.1016/j.yexcr.2019.01.026.
30. Stafford DA, Brunet LJ, Khokha MK, Economides AN, Harland RM. Cooperative activity of noggin and gremlin 1 in axial skeleton development. Development. 2011;138:1005–14. https://doi.org/10.1242/dev.051938.
31. Wu X, Chen Q, Washio Y, Yokoi H, Suzuki T. Excess retinoic acid induces fusion of Centra by degenerating intervertebral ligament cells in Japanese flounder, Paralichthys olivaceus. J Exp Zool B Mol Dev Evol. 2016;326:464–73. https://doi.org/10.1002/jez.b.22717.
32. Fan D, Chen Z, Chen Y, Shang Y. Mechanistic roles of leptin in osteogenic stimulation in thoracic ligament flavum cells. J Biol Chem. 2007;282:29958–66. https://doi.org/10.1074/jbc.M611779200.
33. Iwasaki K, Furukawa KI, Tanno M, Kusumi T, Ueyama K, Tanaka M, Kudo H, Toh S, Harata S, Motomura S. Uni-axial cyclic stretch induces Cbfa1 expression in spinal ligament cells derived from patients with ossification of the posterior longitudinal ligament. Calcif Tissue Int. 2004;74:448–57. https://doi.org/10.1007/s00223-002-0021-1.
34. Taha H, Bareksei Y, Albanna W, Schirmer M. Ligamentum flavum cyst in the lumbar spine: a case report and review of the literature. J Orthop Traumatol. 2010;11:117–22. https://doi.org/10.1007/s10195-010-0094-y.
35. Krymchenko R, Coşar Kutluoğlu G, van Hout N, Manikowski D, Doberenz C, van Kuppevelt TH, Daamen WF. Elastogenesis in focus: navigating elastic fibers synthesis for advanced dermal biomaterial formulation. Adv Healthc Mater. 2024;13:2400484. https://doi.org/10.1002/adhm.202400484.
36. Bennasroune A, Romier-Crouzet B, Blaise S, Laffargue M, Efremov RG, Martiny L, Maurice P, Duca L. Elastic fibers and elastin receptor complex: Neuraminidase-1 takes the center stage. Matrix Biol. 2019;84:57–67. https://doi.org/10.1016/j.matbio.2019.06.007.
37. Uchida K, Yayama T, Cai HX, Nakajima H, Sugita D, Guerrero AR, Kobayashi S, Yoshida A, Chen KB, Baba H. Ossification process involving the human thoracic ligamentum flavum: role of transcription factors. Arthritis Res Ther. 2011;13 https://doi.org/10.1186/ar3458.
38. Scapinelli R, Stecco C, Pozzuoli A, Porzionato A, Macchi V, De Caro R. The lumbar interspinous ligaments in humans: anatomical study and review of the literature. Cells Tissues Organs. 2006;183:1–11. https://doi.org/10.1159/000094901.
39. Zhang Y, Xu H, Hu X, Zhang C, Chu T, Zhou Y. Histopathological changes in supraspinous ligaments, ligamentum flava and paraspinal muscle tissues of patients with ankylosing spondylitis. Int J Rheum Dis. 2016;19:420–9. https://doi.org/10.1111/1756-185X.12305.
40. Hyun SY, Lee JH, Kang KJ, Jang YJ. Effect of FGF-2, TGF-β-1, and BMPs on Teno/ligamentogenesis and osteo/cementogenesis of human periodontal ligament stem cells. Mol Cells. 2017;40:550–7. https://doi.org/10.14348/molcells.2017.0019.
41. Fuchigami S, Nakamura T, Furue K, Sena K, Shinohara Y, Noguchi K. Recombinant human bone morphogenetic protein-9 potently induces osteogenic differentiation of human periodontal ligament fibroblasts. Eur J Oral Sci. 2016;124:151–7. https://doi.org/10.1111/eos.12249.
42. Zelzer E, Blitz E, Killian ML, Thomopoulos S. Tendon-to-bone attachment: from development to maturity. Birth Defects Res C Embryo Today. 2014;102:101–12. https://doi.org/10.1002/bdrc.21056.
43. Bobzin L, Roberts RR, Chen HJ, Crump JG, Merrill AE. Development and maintenance of tendons and ligaments. Development (Cambridge). 2021;148 https://doi.org/10.1242/dev.186916.
44. Quinn KP, Winkelstein BA. Preconditioning is correlated with altered collagen fiber alignment in ligament. J Biomech Eng. 2011;133 https://doi.org/10.1115/1.4004205.
45. Ichioka H, Yamamoto T, Yamamoto K, Honjo K, et al. Biomechanical force induces the growth factor production in human periodontal ligament-derived cells. Odontology. 2016;104:27–34. https://doi.org/10.1007/s10266-015-0206-5.
46. Li M, Zhang C, Yang Y. Effects of mechanical forces on osteogenesis and osteoclastogenesis in human periodontal ligament fibroblasts: a systematic review of in vitro studies. Bone Joint Res. 2021;8:19–31. https://doi.org/10.1302/2046-3758.81.BJR-2018-0060.R1.
47. Huang H, Yang R, Zhou Y. Mechanobiology of periodontal ligament stem cells in orthodontic tooth movement. Stem Cells Int. 2018;2018 https://doi.org/10.1155/2018/6531216.
48. Hanhan S, Ejzenberg A, Goren K, Saba F, Suki Y, Sharon S, Shilo D, Waxman J, Spitzer E, Shahar R, Atkins A, Liebergall M, Blumenfeld A, Deutsch D, Haze A. Skeletal ligament healing using the recombinant human amelogenin protein. J Cell Mol Med. 2016;20:815–24. https://doi.org/10.1111/jcmm.12762.

49. Alvarez-Medina R, Cayuso J, Okubo T, Takada S, Martí E. Wnt canonical pathway restricts graded Shh/Gli patterning activity through the regulation of Gli3 expression. Development. 2008;135:237–47. https://doi.org/10.1242/dev.012054.
50. Ham SM, Song MJ, Yoon H-S, Lee DH, Chung JH, Lee S-T. SPARC is highly expressed in young skin and promotes extracellular matrix integrity in fibroblasts via the TGF-β signaling pathway. Int J Mol Sci. 2023;24:12179. https://doi.org/10.3390/ijms241512179.
51. Naya Y, Takanari H. Elastin is responsible for the rigidity of the ligament under shear and rotational stress: a mathematical simulation study. J Orthop Surg Res. 2023;18 https://doi.org/10.1186/s13018-023-03794-6.
52. Zhang Q, Liu C, Hong S, Min J, Yang Q, Hu M, Zhao Y, Hong L. Excess mechanical stress and hydrogen peroxide remodel extracellular matrix of cultured human uterosacral ligament fibroblasts by disturbing the balance of MMPs/TIMPs via the regulation of TGF-β1 signaling pathway. Mol Med Rep. 2017;15:423–30. https://doi.org/10.3892/mmr.2016.5994.
53. Dai C, Guo L, Yang L, Wu Y, Gou J, Li B. Regional fibrocartilage variations in human anterior cruciate ligament tibial insertion: a histological three-dimensional reconstruction. Connect Tissue Res. 2015;56:18–24. https://doi.org/10.3109/03008207.2014.970183.
54. Yang X, Sun C, Meng X, Chen G, Fan T, Zhang C, Chen Z. LGR5 regulates osteogenic differentiation of human thoracic ligamentum flavum cells by Wnt signalling pathway. J Cell Mol Med. 2022;26:3862–72. https://doi.org/10.1111/jcmm.17420.
55. Tseng HW, Pitt ME, Glant TT, McRae AF, Kenna TJ, Brown MA, Pettit AR, Thomas GP. Inflammation-driven bone formation in a mouse model of ankylosing spondylitis: sequential not parallel processes. Arthritis Res Ther. 2016;18:35. https://doi.org/10.1186/s13075-015-0805-0.
56. Zhao Q, Yang Y, Wu P, Huang C, Zhang R, Li Q, Shi B. Biomechanical study of the C5–C8 cervical extraforaminal ligaments. J Orthop Surg Res. 2020;15 https://doi.org/10.1186/s13018-020-02006-9.
57. Reese SP, Underwood CJ, Weiss JA. Effects of decorin proteoglycan on fibrillogenesis, ultrastructure, and mechanics of type I collagen gels. Matrix Biol. 2013;32:414–23. https://doi.org/10.1016/j.matbio.2013.04.004.
58. Stender CJ, Rust E, Martin PT, Neumann EE, Brown RJ, Lujan TJ. Modeling the effect of collagen fibril alignment on ligament mechanical behavior. Biomech Model Mechanobiol. 2018;17:543–57. https://doi.org/10.1007/s10237-017-0977-4.
59. Min J, Li B, Liu C, Guo W, Hong S, Tang J, Hong L. Extracellular matrix metabolism disorder induced by mechanical strain on human parametrial ligament fibroblasts. Mol Med Rep. 2017;15:3278–84. https://doi.org/10.3892/mmr.2017.6372.
60. Chen MH, Hu CK, Chen PR, Chen YS, Sun JS, Chen MH. Dose-dependent regulation of cell proliferation and collagen degradation by estradiol on ligamentum flavum. BMC Musculoskelet Disord. 2014;15 https://doi.org/10.1186/1471-2474-15-238.
61. Iorio JA, Jakoi AM, Singla A. Biomechanics of degenerative spinal disorders. Asian Spine J. 2016;10:377–84. https://doi.org/10.4184/asj.2016.10.2.377.
62. Hillgärtner M, Linka K, Itskov M. Failure of adhesive bonds between proteoglycans causes viscoelasticity of soft tissues. Pamm. 2016;16:87–8. https://doi.org/10.1002/pamm.201610032.
63. Zhang B, Chen G, Yang X, Fan T, Chen X, Chen Z. Dysregulation of MicroRNAs in hypertrophy and ossification of Ligamentum Flavum: new advances, challenges, and potential directions. Front Genet. 2021;12 https://doi.org/10.3389/fgene.2021.641575.
64. Wei B, Li Z, Lin Y, Hu X, Xu L, Wang S, Ji M, Lu J. BMP-2/TGF-β1 gene insertion into ligament-derived stem cells sheet promotes tendon–bone healing in a mouse. Biotechnol J. 2023;18 https://doi.org/10.1002/biot.202200470.
65. Antikievicz DEP, Rossi GB, Maldaun MVC, Gripp D, et al. Analysis of Myelomalacia and posterior longitudinal ligament ossification as prognostic factors in patients with cervical Spondylotic myelopathy submitted to Laminoplasty. Arquivos Brasileiros de Neurocirurgia: Braz Neurosur. 2022;41:e102–7. https://doi.org/10.1055/s-0042-1742298.
66. Zhandarov K, Blinova E, Ogarev E, Sheptulin D, Terekhina E, Telpukhov V, et al. Intervertebral canals and Intracanal ligaments as new terms in Terminologia anatomica. Diagnostics. 2023;13 https://doi.org/10.3390/diagnostics13172809.
67. Losiniecki AJ, Serrone JC, Keller JT, Bohinski RJ. Lumbar ligamentum flavum: spatial relationships to surrounding anatomical structures and technical description of en bloc resection. J Neurol Surg A Cent Eur Neurosurg. 2013;74:388–92. https://doi.org/10.1055/s-0033-1348350.
68. Iwanaga J, Ishak B, Saga T, Singla A, Impastato D, Chapman JR, Oskouian RJ, David G, Porzionato A, Reina MA, Macchi V, de Caro R, Tubbs RS. The lumbar Ligamentum Flavum does not have two layers and is confluent with the Interspinous ligament: anatomical study with application to surgical and interventional pain procedures. Clin Anat. 2020;33:34–40. https://doi.org/10.1002/ca.23437.
69. Becker CA, Kuhlein T, Walter S, Kistler M, Bruder J, Rubenbauer B, Greiner A, Böcker W, Kubmaul AC. Novel tape suture osteosynthesis for hyperextension injuries of the subaxial cervical spine: a biomechanical study. Vivo (Brooklyn). 2023;37:124–31. https://doi.org/10.21873/invivo.13061.
70. Qu X, Chen Z, Fan D, Sun C, Zeng Y, Guo Z, Qi Q, Li W. MiR-199b-5p inhibits osteogenic differentiation in ligamentum flavum cells by targeting

JAG1 and modulating the Notch signalling pathway. J Cell Mol Med. 2017;21:1159–70. https://doi.org/10.1111/jcmm.13047.
71. Kosuri KC, Venumadhav N, Siddaraju KS. Ossified ligamentum longitudinale anterius in adult human dry vertebrae. J Clin Diagn Res. 2014;8:AC04-6. https://doi.org/10.7860/JCDR/2014/8691.4702.
72. Harada Y, Furukawa KI, Asari T, Chin S, Ono A, Tanaka T, Mizukami H, Murakami M, Yagihashi S, Motomura S, Ishibashi Y. Osteogenic lineage commitment of mesenchymal stem cells from patients with ossification of the posterior longitudinal ligament. Biochem Biophys Res Commun. 2014;443:1014–20. https://doi.org/10.1016/j.bbrc.2013.12.080.
73. Nihei A, Hagiwara K, Kikuchi M, Yashiro T, Hoshino Y. Histological investigation of rabbit ligamentum flavum with special reference to differences in spinal levels. Anat Sci Int. 2003;78:162–7. https://doi.org/10.1046/j.0022-7722.2003.00050.x.
74. Merter A, Karaca MO, Yazar T. Biomechanical effects of sequential resection of the posterior ligamentous complex on intradiscal pressure and resistance to compression forces. Acta Orthop Traumatol Turc. 2019;53:502–6. https://doi.org/10.1016/j.aott.2019.08.016.
75. Holzgreve F, Maurer-Grubinger C, Isaak J, Kokott P, Mörl-Kreitschmann M, Polte L, Solimann A, Wessler L, Filmann N, van Mark A, Maltry L, Groneberg DA, Ohlendorf D. The acute effect in performing common range of motion tests in healthy young adults: a prospective study. Sci Rep. 2020;10 https://doi.org/10.1038/s41598-020-78846-6.
76. Tang T, Zhu Z, He Z, Wang F, Chen H, Liu SS, Zhan M, Wang J, Tian W, Chen D, Wu X, Liu X, Zhou Z, Liu SS. DLX5 regulates the osteogenic differentiation of spinal ligaments cells derived from ossification of the posterior longitudinal ligament patients via NOTCH signaling. JOR Spine. 2023;6 https://doi.org/10.1002/jsp2.1247.
77. Anderson B, Shahidi B. The impact of spine pathology on posterior ligamentous complex structure and function. Curr Rev Musculoskelet Med. 2023;16:616–26. https://doi.org/10.1007/s12178-023-09873-9.
78. Kato H, Braddock DT, Ito N. Genetics of diffuse idiopathic skeletal hyperostosis and ossification of the spinal ligaments. Curr Osteoporos Rep. 2023;21:552–66. https://doi.org/10.1007/s11914-023-00814-6.
79. Sim O, Ryu D, Lee J, Lee C. Stress distribution on spinal cord according to type of laminectomy for large focal cervical ossification of posterior longitudinal ligament based on finite element method. Bioengineering. 2022;9 https://doi.org/10.3390/bioengineering9100519.
80. Akinci SZ, Karabulut D, Doğru SC, Sürmen HK, Yaman O, Arslan YZ. Effect of a pedicle screw fixation system on lumbar spinal segments: a finite element study. Turkiye Klinikleri J Med Sci. 2023;43:372–81. https://doi.org/10.5336/MEDSCI.2023-99005.
81. Zhai J, Guo S, Li J, Chen B, Zhao Y. Progression of spinal ligament ossification in patients with thoracic myelopathy. Orthop Surg. 2022;14:1958–63. https://doi.org/10.1111/os.13291.
82. Cornaz F, Widmer J, Farshad-Amacker NA, Spirig JM, Snedeker JG, Farshad M. Intervertebral disc degeneration relates to biomechanical changes of spinal ligaments. Spine J. 2021;21:1399–407. https://doi.org/10.1016/j.spinee.2021.04.016.
83. Alsoof D, Anderson G, Disilvestro KJ, McDonald CL, Kuris EO, Daniels AH. Diffuse spinal hyperostosis causing severe spinal stenosis and thoracic myelopathy. Orthop Rev (Pavia). 2022;14 https://doi.org/10.52965/001C.37832.
84. Beauséjour MH, Wagnac E, et al. Numerical investigation of spinal cord injury after flexion-distraction injuries at the cervical spine. J Biomech Eng. 2022;144 https://doi.org/10.1115/1.4052003.
85. Ünal M, Sezgin AB. Dura mater: anatomy and clinical implication. J Behav Brain Sci. 2021;11:239–47. https://doi.org/10.4236/jbbs.2021.1110019.
86. Mizuno J, Nakagawa H, Song J. Symptomatic ossification of the anterior longitudinal ligament with stenosis of the cervical spine. J Bone Joint Surg Seri B. 2005;87:1375–9. https://doi.org/10.1302/0301-620X.87B10.16742.
87. Ohlerth S, Steiner G, Geissbühler U, Flückiger M. Diffuse idiopathic skeletal hyperostosis in the dog (DISH): a review. Schweiz Arch Tierheilkd. 2016;158:331–9. https://doi.org/10.17236/sat00061.
88. Watanabe K, Mochida J, Nomura T, Okuma M, Sakabe K, Seiki K. Effect of reinsertion of activated nucleus pulposus on disc degeneration: an experimental study on various types of collagen in degenerative discs. Connect Tissue Res. 2003;44:104–8. https://doi.org/10.1080/03008200390200247.
89. Wang X, Sun J, Tan J, Fang P, Chen J, Yuan W, Chen H, Liu Y. Effect of sIL-13Rα2-Fc on the progression of rat tail intervertebral disc degeneration. J Orthop Surg Res. 2019;14 https://doi.org/10.1186/s13018-019-1361-0.
90. Yu CC, Hao DJ, Ma YL, Huang DG, Li HK, Feng H, Hou Q. The role of posterior longitudinal ligament in cervical disc replacement: an ovine cadaveric biomechanical analysis. Med Sci Monit. 2016;22:1843–9. https://doi.org/10.12659/MSM.899138.
91. Sato R, Uchida K, Kobayashi S, Yayama T, Kokubo Y, Nakajima H, Takamura T, Bangirana A, Itoh H, Baba H. Ossification of the posterior longitudinal ligament of the cervical spine: histopathological findings around the calcification and ossification front. J Neurosurg Spine. 2007;7:174–83. https://doi.org/10.3171/SPI-07/08/174.
92. Inoue T, Nakamura T, Ikeda T, Takagi K. Effect of extracellular matrix protein on the rate of proteoglycan synthesis in rabbit intervertebral disc cells. J Spinal Disord Tech. 2005;18:52–7. https://doi.org/10.1097/01.bsd.0000128056.03461.6b.

93. Sun N, Liang Y, Hu B, Feng J, Lin G, Chen X, Rui G. circSKIL promotes the ossification of cervical posterior longitudinal ligament by activating the JNK/STAT3 pathway. Exp Ther Med. 2021;22 https://doi.org/10.3892/etm.2021.10193.
94. Mine T, Ihara K, Kawamura H, Date R, Umehara K. Collagen expression in various degenerative meniscal changes: an immunohistological study. J Orthop Surg (Hong Kong). 2013;21:216–20. https://doi.org/10.1177/230949901302100221.
95. Ji L, Huang P, Wang Q, Li X, Li Y. Modulation of the biological network of lumbar spinal stenosis by Tongdu Huoxue decoction based on clinical metabolomics. Front Mol Biosci. 2023;10:1074500. https://doi.org/10.3389/fmolb.2023.1074500.
96. Aleksić V, Ilić R, Milićević M, Milisavljević F, Joković M. Ligamentum flavum hypertrophy in a patient with pott's disease. Srp Arh Celok Lek. 2020;148:757–60. https://doi.org/10.2298/SARH191201077A.
97. Blais M, Shahidi B, Anderson B, O'Brien E, Moltzen C, Iannacone T, Eastlack RK, Mundis GM. The influence of ligament biomechanics on proximal junctional kyphosis and failure in patients with adult spinal deformity. JOR Spine. 2023;6 https://doi.org/10.1002/jsp2.1277.
98. Getgood A, Brown C, Lording T, Amis A, Claes S, Geeslin A, Musahl V, Amis A, Brown C, Cavaignac E, Claes S, Daggett M, Dejour D, Engebretsen L, Feng H, Fleming B, Fu F, Geeslin A, Getgood A, Guenther D, Helito CP, Herbst E, Inderhaug E, Karlsson J, Kittl C, Kuroda R, LaPrade R, Landreau P, Lording T, Mueller W, Musahl V, Neyret P, Noyes F, Pearle A, Saithna A, Smigielski R, Sonnery-Cottet B, Spalding T, Van Dyck P, Verdonk P, Williams A, Wilson A, Zaffagnini S. The anterolateral complex of the knee: results from the international ALC consensus group meeting. Knee Surg Sports Traumatol Arthrosc. 2019;27:166–76. https://doi.org/10.1007/s00167-018-5072-6.
99. Lerchl T, El Husseini M, Bayat A, Sekuboyina A, Hermann L, Nispel K, Baum T, Löffler MT, Senner V, Kirschke JS. Validation of a patient-specific musculoskeletal model for lumbar load estimation generated by an automated pipeline from whole body CT. Front Bioeng Biotechnol. 2022;10 https://doi.org/10.3389/fbioe.2022.862804.
100. Abilash Kumar AK, Mohd QMQ, Ahmad ZAH, Towil B. Fracture-dislocation at C6-C7 level with quadriplegia after traditional massage in a patient with ankylosing spondylitis: a case report. Malays Orthop J. 2017;11:75–7. https://doi.org/10.5704/MOJ.1707.013.
101. Iwanaga J, Simonds E, Yilmaz E, Schumacher M, Patel M, Tubbs R. Anatomical and biomechanical study of the lumbar interspinous ligament. Asian J Neurosurg. 2019;14:1203–6. https://doi.org/10.4103/ajns.ajns_87_19.
102. Li Y, Shen Z, Huang M, Wang X. Stepwise resection of the posterior ligamentous complex for stability of a thoracolumbar compression fracture. Medicine. 2017;96 https://doi.org/10.1097/MD.0000000000007873.
103. Huang Y, Wang W, Zhang L, Teng Y, Zhan Z, Yang H, Yang P. The relationship between MRI findings of posterior ligamentous complex and lumbar instability in degenerative spondylolisthesis. Int J Gen Med. 2024;17:2279–87. https://doi.org/10.2147/ijgm.s452735.
104. Edwards CR, Liou CJ, Ahmed S, Wong TT, Ahmad ZY. A case-based review of spine ligamentous anatomy and pathology. Contemp Diagn Radiol. 2024;47:8–8. https://doi.org/10.1097/01.CDR.0001027108.12301.bf.
105. Johnson GM, Zhang M. Regional differences within the human supraspinous and interspinous ligaments: a sheet plastination study. Eur Spine J. 2002;11:382–8. https://doi.org/10.1007/s00586-001-0378-2.
106. Zhao Y, Xiang Q, Jiang S, Lin J, Li W. Revealing the novel metabolism-related genes in the ossification of the ligamentum flavum based on whole transcriptomic data. JOR Spine. 2024;7 https://doi.org/10.1002/jsp2.1357.
107. Kawaguchi Y, Nakano M, Yasuda T, Seki S, Suzuki K, Yahara Y, Makino H, Kitajima I, Kimura T. Serum biomarkers in patients with ossification of the posterior longitudinal ligament (OPLL): inflammation in OPLL. PLoS One. 2017;12 https://doi.org/10.1371/JOURNAL.PONE.0174881.
108. Chen Y, Liu X, Chen D, Wang X, Yuan W. Surgical strategy for ossification of the posterior longitudinal ligament in the cervical spine. Orthopedics. 2012;35 https://doi.org/10.3928/01477447-20120725-25.
109. Tamburrelli FC, Meluzio MC, Burrofato A, Perna A, Proietti L. Minimally invasive surgery procedure in isthmic spondylolisthesis. Eur Spine J. 2018;27:237–43. https://doi.org/10.1007/s00586-018-5627-8.
110. Salzmann SN, Okano I, Jones C, Zhu J, Lu S, Onyekwere I, Balaji V, Reisener MJ, Chiapparelli E, Shue J, Carrino JA, Girardi FP, Cammisa FP, Sama AA, Hughes AP. Preoperative MRI-based vertebral bone quality (VBQ) score assessment in patients undergoing lumbar spinal fusion. Spine Journal. 2022;22:1301–8. https://doi.org/10.1016/j.spinee.2022.03.006.
111. Hirai T, Yoshii T, Nagoshi N, Takeuchi K, Mori K, Ushio S, Iwanami A, Yamada T, Seki S, Tsuji T, Fujiyoshi K, Furukawa M, Nishimura S, Wada K, Furuya T, Matsuyama Y, Hasegawa T, Takeshita K, Kimura A, Abematsu M, Haro H, Ohba T, Watanabe M, Katoh H, Watanabe K, Ozawa H, Kanno H, Imagama S, Ando K, Fujibayashi S, Koda M, Yamazaki M, Matsumoto M, Nakamura M, Okawa A, Kawaguchi Y. Distribution of ossified spinal lesions in patients with severe ossification of the posterior longitudinal ligament and prediction of ossification at each segment based on the cervical OP index classification: a multicenter study (JOSL CT

study). BMC Musculoskelet Disord. 2018;19 https://doi.org/10.1186/s12891-018-2009-7.
112. Yang H, Sun J, Shi J, Guo Y, Zheng B, Wang Y, Xu X, Shi G. Anterior controllable antedisplacement fusion as a choice for 28 patients of cervical ossification of the posterior longitudinal ligament with dura ossification: the risk of cerebrospinal fluid leakage compared with anterior cervical corpectomy and fusion. Eur Spine J. 2019;28:370–9. https://doi.org/10.1007/s00586-018-5813-8.
113. Jain S, Jindal P, Girdhar P, Bharti B, Verma R. Ligamentum Flavum cyst-a rare cause of Lumbar Canal stenosis: a case report with review of literature. J Minimall Invasive Spine Surg Tech. 2021;6:57–60. https://doi.org/10.21182/jmisst.2020.00234.
114. Desai AA, Trivedi A, Chandraker BL, Kadam R. Report of a rare case: Ligamentum Flavum cyst. MGM J Med Sci. 2015;2:208–12. https://doi.org/10.5005/jp-journals-10036-1075.
115. Nizamani WM. Ligamentum flavum cyst: an uncommon but recognizable and surgically correctable category of juxtafacet cyst. Radiol Case Rep. 2018;13:302–4. https://doi.org/10.1016/j.radcr.2017.09.009.
116. Park JB, Kong CG, Suhl KH, Chang ED, Riew KD. The increased expression of matrix metalloproteinases associated with elastin degradation and fibrosis of the ligamentum flavum in patients with lumbar spinal stenosis. Clin Orthop Surg. 2009;1:81–9. https://doi.org/10.4055/cios.2009.1.2.81.
117. Yabe Y, Hagiwara Y, Tsuchiya M, Honda M, Hatori K, Sonofuchi K, Kanazawa K, Koide M, Sekiguchi T, Itaya N, Itoi E. Decreased elastic fibers and increased proteoglycans in the ligamentum flavum of patients with lumbar spinal canal stenosis. J Orthop Res. 2016;34:1241–7. https://doi.org/10.1002/jor.23130.
118. Sobański D, Bogdał P, Staszkiewicz R, Sobańska M, Filipowicz M, Czepko RA, Strojny D, Grabarek BO. Evaluation of differences in expression pattern of three isoforms of the transforming growth factor beta in patients with lumbosacral stenosis. Cell Cycle. 2024;23:555–72. https://doi.org/10.1080/15384101.2024.2345484.
119. Sun C, Zhang H, Wang X, Liu X. Ligamentum flavum fibrosis and hypertrophy: molecular pathways, cellular mechanisms, and future directions. FASEB J. 2020;34:9854–68. https://doi.org/10.1096/fj.202000635R.
120. Sun X, Sun X, Sun X, Chen Z, Sun S, Wang W, Wang W, Zhang T, Zhang T, Zhang T, Kong C, Kong C, Lu S, Lu S. Dynamic stabilization adjacent to fusion versus posterior lumbar Interbody fusion for the treatment of lumbar degenerative disease: a meta-analysis. Biomed Res Int. 2020;2020 https://doi.org/10.1155/2020/9309134.
121. Li X, Guan Z, Chen X, Chen B, Kong L, Han J, Zhang W. Modified minimally invasive technique for decompression and reduction of thoracolumbar burst fracture with neurological symptoms: technical note. J Orthop Surg Res. 2021;16 https://doi.org/10.1186/s13018-021-02783-x.
122. Okuda T, Baba I, Fujimoto Y, Tanaka N, Sumida T, Manabe H, Hayashi Y, Ochi M. The pathology of ligamentum flavum in degenerative lumbar disease. Spine (Phila Pa 1976). 2004;29:1689–97. https://doi.org/10.1097/01.BRS.0000132510.25378.8C.
123. Wang Y, Yang L, Lei T, Lin YS, Qi XB, Wang ZH, Cao JM. Benefits and risks of subsection laminectomy with pedicle screw fixation for ossification of the ligamentum flavum of the thoracic spine: a retrospective study of 30 patients. Med Sci Monit. 2019;25:6341–50. https://doi.org/10.12659/MSM.915318.
124. Wildi LM, Kurrer MO, Benini A, Weishaupt D, Michel BA, Brühlmann P. Pseudocystic degeneration of the lumbar ligamentum flavum: a little known entity. J Spinal Disord Tech. 2004;17:395–400. https://doi.org/10.1097/01.bsd.0000109837.59382.0e.
125. Yokosuka K, Park JS, Jimbo K, Yoshida T, Yamada K, Sato K, Takeuchi M, Yamagishi SI, Nagata K. Immunohistochemical demonstration of advanced glycation end products and the effects of advanced glycation end products in ossified ligament tissues in vitro. Spine (Phila Pa 1976). 2007;32 https://doi.org/10.1097/01.brs.0000263417.17526.35.
126. Chao YH, Tsuang YH, Sun JS, Sun MG, Chen MH. Centrifugal force induces human ligamentum flavum fibroblasts inflammation through activation of JNK and p38 pathways. Connect Tissue Res. 2012;53:422–9. https://doi.org/10.3109/03008207.2012.685132.
127. Simpson S, Krabak BJ. Interspinous ligament calcification in a collegiate gymnast. PM and R. 2014;6:742–5. https://doi.org/10.1016/j.pmrj.2014.01.007.
128. Okada K, Ohtori S, Inoue G, Orita S, Eguchi Y, Nakamura J, Aoki Y, Ishikawa T, Miyagi M, Kamoda H, Suzuki M, Kubota G, Sakuma Y, Oikawa Y, Inage K, Sainoh T, Toyone T, Yamauchi K, Takahashi K. Interspinous ligament lidocaine and steroid injections for the management of Baastrup's disease: a case series. Asian Spine J. 2014;8:260–6. https://doi.org/10.4184/asj.2014.8.3.260.
129. Clark KEN, Jawad ASM. Clinical vignette: impingement of the lumbar spinous processes causing lumbar back pain. J R College Physicians Edinburgh. 2023;53:288–9. https://doi.org/10.1177/14782715231211018.
130. Baastrup CI. On the spinous processes of the lumbar vertebrae and the soft tissues between them, and on pathological changes in that region. Acta Radiol. 1933;14:52–5. https://doi.org/10.3109/00016923309132353.
131. Spirollari E, Feldstein E, Ng C, Vazquez S, Kinon MD, Gandhi C, Tyagi R. Correction of sagittal balance with resection of kissing spines. Cureus. 2021; https://doi.org/10.7759/cureus.16874.

132. Richardson AM, Gernsback JE, Kolcun JPG, Vanni S. Treatment of posttraumatic lumbar interspinous ligament calcification with partial resection of spinous processes and calcified interspinous ligaments: case report. J Neurosurg Spine. 2019;30:362–6. https://doi.org/10.3171/2018.9.SPINE18401.
133. Casey G, Mcpherson T, Kini U, Ryan F, Taibjee SM, Moss C, Burge S. Hereditary vitamin D-resistant rickets presenting as alopecia. Pediatr Dermatol. 2014;31:519–20. https://doi.org/10.1111/pde.12327.
134. Faiyaz-Ul-Haque M, Aldhalaan W, Alashwal A, Bin-Abbas BS, Alsagheir A, Alotaiby M, Rafiq Z, Zaidi SHE. Hereditary 1,25-dihydroxyvitamin D-resistant rickets (HVDRR): clinical heterogeneity and long-term efficacious management of eight patients from four unrelated Arab families with a loss of function VDR mutation. J Pediatr Endocrinol Metab. 2018;31:861–8. https://doi.org/10.1515/jpem-2017-0312.
135. Ali RS, Abdulhussein R, Esrick M, Sen M. A rare presentation of rickets mimicking Sacroiliitis: a case report and literature review. Cureus. 2022; https://doi.org/10.7759/cureus.26033.
136. Hamdy H, Abotakia T, Allam A. Mini open spinous process splitting laminectomy in the management of cervical Spondylotic myelopathy. Egyp Spine J. 2017;23:6–12. https://doi.org/10.21608/esj.2017.6753.
137. Tai CL, Hsieh PH, Chen WP, Chen LH, Chen WJ, Lai PL. Biomechanical comparison of lumbar spine instability between laminectomy and bilateral laminotomy for spinal stenosis syndrome – an experimental study in porcine model. BMC Musculoskelet Disord. 2008;9 https://doi.org/10.1186/1471-2474-9-84.
138. Robertson D, Willardson R, Parajuli D, Cannon A, Bowdenn AE. The lumbar supraspinous ligament demonstrates increased material stiffness and strength on its ventral aspect. J Mech Behav Biomed Mater. 2013;17:34–43. https://doi.org/10.1016/j.jmbbm.2012.07.009.
139. Pizones J, Zúniga L, Sánchez-Mariscal F, Lvarez PA, Gómez-Rice A, Izquierdo E. MRI study of post-traumatic incompetence of posterior ligamentous complex: importance of the supraspinous ligament. Prospective study of 74 traumatic fractures. Eur Spine J. 2012;21:2222–31. https://doi.org/10.1007/s00586-012-2403-z.
140. Tsukamoto M, Morimoto T, Kobayashi T, Muranaka K, Yoshihara T, Maeda K, Sonohata M, Kasai Y, Otani K, Mawatari M. The relationship between traction spurs, Modic change, vacuum phenomenon, and segmental instability of the lumbar spine. Sci Rep. 2022;12 https://doi.org/10.1038/s41598-022-14244-4.
141. Paolo P, Roberto S, Emanuele C, Gabriele R, Massimo M, Giacomo E, Marco S, Maria F, Riccardo B, Mearini M, Bergomi R, Panciani PP, Stefini R, Esposito G, Sicuri GM, Costi E, Ronchetti G, Fontanella M. Dorsal paddle leads implant for spinal cord stimulation through laminotomy with midline structures preservation. Surg Neurol Int. 2012;3:164. https://doi.org/10.4103/2152-7806.105275.
142. Jin SK, Lee JH, Hong JH, Park JK, Seo YK, Kwon SY. Enhancement of osseointegration of artificial ligament by nano-hydroxyapatite and bone morphogenic protein-2 into the rabbit femur. Tissue Eng Regen Med. 2016;13:284–96. https://doi.org/10.1007/s13770-016-9051-z.
143. Lee-Barthel A, Lee CA, Vidal MA, Baar K. Localized BMP-4 release improves the enthesis of engineered bone-to-bone ligaments. Transl Sports Med. 2018;1:60–72. https://doi.org/10.1002/tsm2.9.
144. Nam DC, Lee HJ, Lee CJ, Hwang SC. Molecular pathophysiology of ossification of the posteriolongitudinal ligament (OPLL). Biomol Ther (Seoul). 2019;27:342–8. https://doi.org/10.4062/biomolther.2019.043.
145. McMillan A, Nguyen MK, Gonzalez-Fernandez T, Ge P, Yu X, Murphy WL, Kelly DJ, Alsberg E. Dual non-viral gene delivery from microparticles within 3D high-density stem cell constructs for enhanced bone tissue engineering. Biomaterials. 2018;161:240–55. https://doi.org/10.1016/j.biomaterials.2018.01.006.
146. Shah TA, Rogers MB. Unanswered questions regarding sex and BMP/TGF-β signaling. J Dev Biol. 2018;6 https://doi.org/10.3390/JDB6020014.
147. Cao Y. Opposing roles of BMP and TGF-β signaling pathways in pancreatitis: mechanisms and therapeutic implication. Adv Res Gastroenterol Hepatol. 2019;13 https://doi.org/10.19080/argh.2019.13.555871.
148. Zhang QZ, Chen C, Chang MB, Shanti RM, Cannady SB, O'Malley BW, Shi S, Le AD. Oral rehabilitation of patients sustaining orofacial injuries: the UPenn initiative. Adv Dent Res. 2019;30:50–6. https://doi.org/10.1177/0022034519877400.
149. Abdelhamid MAA, Khalifa HO, Ki MR, Pack SP. Nanoengineered silica-based biomaterials for regenerative medicine. Int J Mol Sci. 2024;25 https://doi.org/10.3390/ijms25116125.

Morphologic Anatomy of the Spinal Ligaments

4

Mirwais Alizada, Pengfei Li, Zeyuan Zhang, Yuanzhi Xu, and Yilin Liu

4.1 Introduction

Spinal ligaments are categorized into vertebral body ligaments and vertebral arch ligaments. Vertebral body ligaments are mainly composed of anterior longitudinal ligament, posterior longitudinal ligament. Vertebral Arch Ligaments are made up of ligamentum flavum, lumbar interspinous ligaments, supraspinous ligament, intertransverse ligaments, nuchal ligament, iliolumbar ligament, capsular ligaments, midline interlaminar ligament respectively. Present chapter focuses on the morphology and anatomy of above spinal ligaments.

4.1.1 Vertebral Body Ligaments

4.1.1.1 Anterior Longitudinal Ligament (ALL)

The anterior longitudinal ligament (ALL) is a strong and wide ligament that runs along the front of the vertebral bodies, from the occipital bone to the sacrum [1, 2]. It starts at the base of the occipital bone and attaches to the front of the atlas (C1) and the axis (C2). Then, it continues down to the upper sacrum (Fig. 4.1) [3, 4]. The ligament changes in size as it moves down, becoming wider and thicker in the thoracic spine compared to the cervical and lumbar areas. This is because the lower spine carries more weight. ALL is thicker and narrower over the vertebral bodies than it is over the intervertebral discs (IVDs) [1, 2].

The ligament is strongly attached to the outer layer of the vertebral bodies and the annulus fibrosus of the intervertebral discs, with stronger attachments at the discs than at the vertebral bodies [5]. ALL is mostly made of dense, longitudinal collagen fibers with some elastic fibers, giving it strength and flexibility needed for spine stability [6–10].

ALL has three layers: superficial, intermediate, and deep. Each layer has different fiber directions and attachment points. The deep layer has short fibers that connect individual intervertebral joints, extending over the discs and attaching to the edges of the vertebral bodies (Fig. 4.2). These fibers attach directly to the bone or the covering of the vertebrae [1, 2].

The superficial layers, which cover the deeper fibers, have longer collagen fibers that connect several intervertebral segments. Like the deep fibers, the superficial fibers attach to the top and bottom vertebral endplates, helping to provide stability across multiple segments [1, 2].

ALL works biomechanically through its different layers. The superficial fibers connect several vertebrae, providing wide mechanical

M. Alizada · P. Li · Z. Zhang · Y. Xu · Y. Liu (✉)
Department of Orthopaedic Surgery, The First Affiliated Hospital of Zhengzhou University, Zhengzhou, China
e-mail: liu212381@126.com

M. Turgut et al. (eds.), *Ligaments of the Vertebral Column*,
https://doi.org/10.1007/978-3-032-09070-6_4

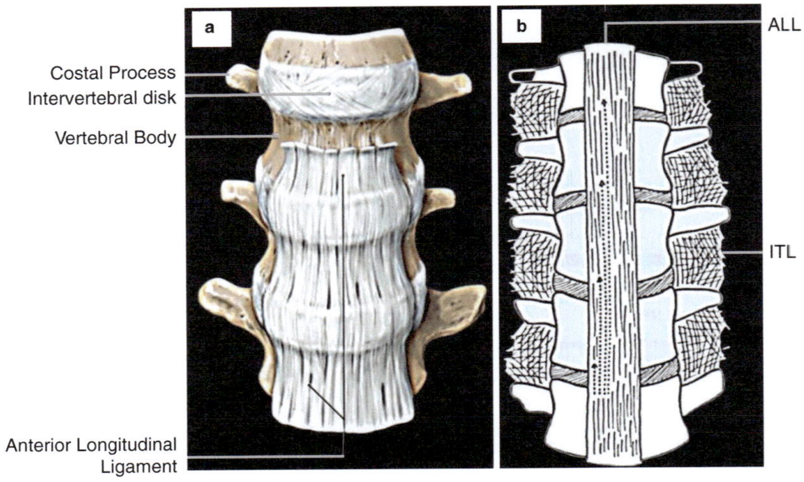

Fig. 4.1 Anterior longitudinal ligament. (**a**) Anterior view. (**b**) Classic descriptions of ALL and the intertransverse ligaments (ITL). The arrows indicate the span of various fibers in the anterior longitudinal ligament stemming from the L5 vertebra. (Source: (**a**) Schünke M, Schulte E, Schumacher U, Ross LM, Lamperti ED. Thieme atlas of anatomy: general anatomy and musculoskeletal system. Thieme Medical Publishers, Incorporated; Copyright 2014. (**b**). After Bogduk N 2012 Clinical Anatomy of the Lumbar Spine and Sacrum, fourth ed. Edinburgh: Churchill Livingstone)

support, while the shorter, deeper fibers help maintain stability in specific segments. The deeper fibers are strongly attached to the vertebral bodies and discs, improving stability and controlling movement [2, 6].

In the lumbar spine, ALL mainly attaches to the front edges of the vertebral bodies, but it also has secondary connections to the curved front surfaces of the vertebrae. The main part of the ligament stretches across this curve, with some deep fibers blending with the covering of the vertebrae. The space between the ligament and the vertebrae contains loose connective tissue, blood vessels, and nerves [8]. Over the intervertebral discs, ALL is loosely connected to the front part of the annulus fibrosus by loose connective tissue, rather than being firmly attached [1].

The structure of ALL allows it to be an important stabilizer along the spine, especially in the lumbar and cervical regions where stress is highest. It provides strong, continuous support in the front to keep the vertebrae aligned, prevent hyperextension, and protect the front parts of the spine from injury [9–11].

4.1.1.2 Posterior Longitudinal Ligament (PLL)

PLL lies on the posterior surfaces of the vertebral bodies in the vertebral canal, attached between the body of axis (C2) and the sacrum, and continuous with the membrane tectoria above (Fig. 4.3) [1, 2].

PLL consists of superficial and deep connective tissue layers, typically differentiated by their morphology and fiber arrangement. The superficial layer is positioned further posterior compared to the deeper layer. Distinguishing PLL from the dura mater is often challenging. The superficial fibers span across three to four vertebrae, while the deeper fibers connect adjacent vertebrae, functioning as peri-vertebral ligaments that are closely associated with—and, in adults, fused to—the annulus fibrosus of the intervertebral discs [12].

The ligament is broad at the cervical and upper thoracic levels and maintains a consistent width. However, in the lower thoracic and lumbar regions, it becomes denticulated, appearing narrow over the vertebral bodies and broadening over the intervertebral discs [13].

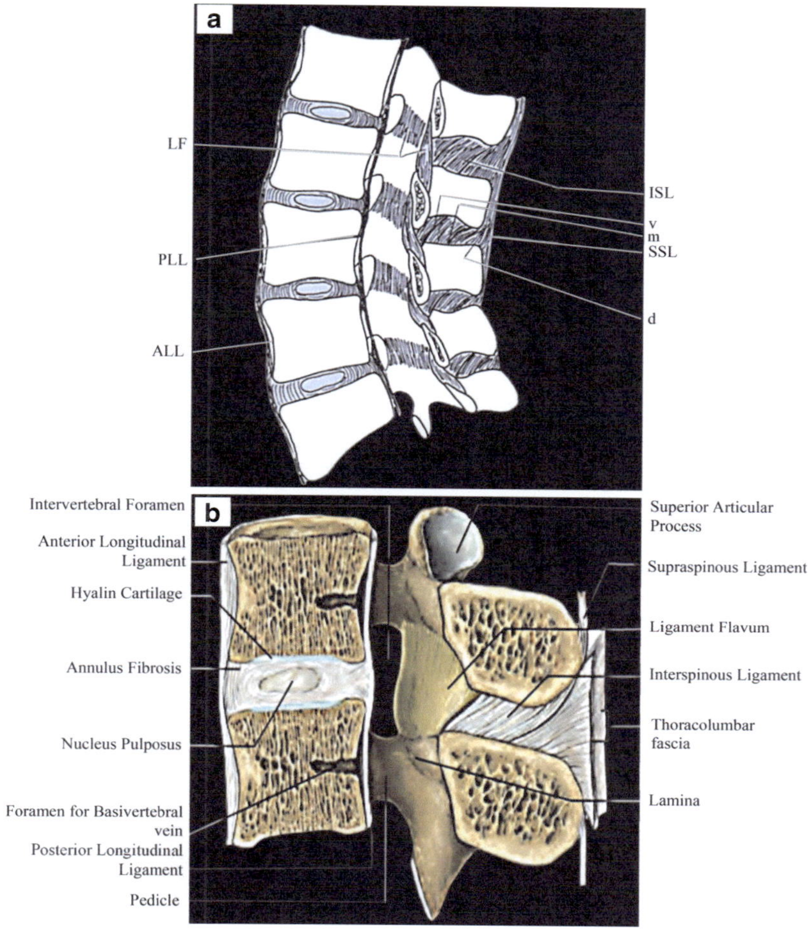

Fig. 4.2 Anterior longitudinal ligament. (**a**) A median sagittal section of the lumbar spine to show its various ligaments. ALL, anterior longitudinal ligament; ISL, interspinous ligament: v, ventral part; m, middle part; d, dorsal part; PLL, posterior longitudinal ligament; SSL, supraspinous ligament. LF, ligamentum flavum, viewed from within the vertebral canal, and in sagittal section at the midline. (**b**) A median sagittal section through the upper lumbar vertebral column showing discs and ligaments. (Source: (**a**) Bogduk N 2012 Clinical Anatomy of the Lumbar Spine and Sacrum, fourth ed. Edinburgh: Churchill Livingstone. (**b**) Standring S, Gray's Anatomy, The Anatomical Basis of Clinical Practice 41st ed. Edinburgh: Churchill Livingstone. Copyright 2020)

PLL features a central band of fibers, approximately 8 to 10 mm wide, extending across multiple vertebral segments. Its broad attachment to the intervertebral discs creates a "fanlike" appearance, giving the ligament a denticulate structure over each vertebral body. This denticulate appearance is more pronounced in the lower thoracic and lumbar regions, where the superficial layer maintains a more uniform width [2, 14].

Despite this general pattern, significant morphological variation exists within the lumbar region, where both the central fibers and the "fan-like" portion tend to decrease in width from L1 to L5. The deep layer, which adheres to the superficial layer along the midline, maintains a more consistent diameter throughout its length, measuring 2 to 3 mm at its narrowest point. PLL overall also exhibits a denticulate appearance [2, 15].

In the cervical region, PLL presents as a broad, band-like structure, maintaining a similar width over both the intervertebral discs and verte-

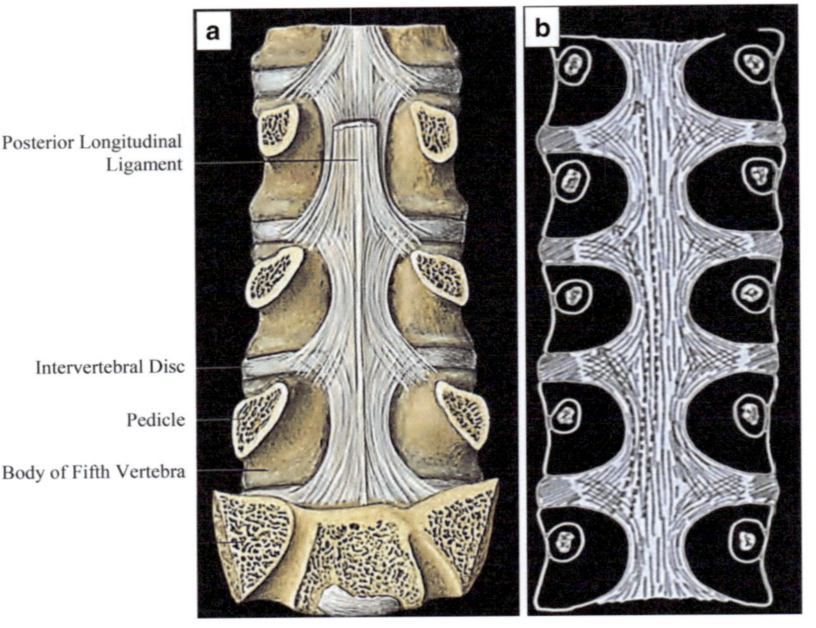

Fig. 4.3 The posterior longitudinal ligament. (**a**) The dotted lines indicate the span of some of the constituent fibers of the ligament arising from the L5 vertebra. (**b**) The posterior longitudinal ligament in the lumbar region. (Source: (**a**) Bogduk N 2012 Clinical Anatomy of the Lumbar Spine and Sacrum, fourth ed. Edinburgh: Churchill Livingstone. (**b**) Standring S, Gray's Anatomy, The Anatomical Basis of Clinical Practice 41st ed. Edinburgh: Churchill Livingstone. Copyright 2020)

bral bodies. Moving inferiorly, the ligament becomes progressively more denticulate, with its widest portion over the intervertebral disc (IVD). While distinguishing between the superficial and deep fibers at the level of the IVD is challenging, their attachment to the margins of the vertebral bodies and the intervening annulus fibrosus remains distinct [16].

The fibers of both layers appear to converge, forming a shared attachment. The superficial and deep layers are both anchored to a midline bony septum on the posterior surface of the vertebral body, extending between the superior and inferior margins. However, this attachment is not always continuous due to deficiencies in the septum within the central third of the vertebral body. The fiber orientation in the PLL is consistent across all levels, with the central fibers of the superficial layer being more vertically aligned compared to the "fanlike" portion. Although the deep layer is visible through the superficial layer, its exact fiber orientation may be difficult to determine [16, 17].

4.2 Vertebral Arch Ligaments

4.2.1 Ligament Flavum

The ligamentum flavum (plural: ligamenta flava) consists of paired elastic ligaments that connect the laminae of neighboring vertebrae at the back of the vertebral canal, from the axis (C2) to the first sacral vertebra (Fig. 4.2) [1, 2]. These ligaments meet at the midline, forming an angle with an opening at the front. Each ligament is shaped like a quadrilateral and runs diagonally from top to bottom and side to side. This diagonal orientation increases as you go down the spine. At the midline, the left and right ligaments join at a 90° angle, open in the front (Fig. 4.4). The ligament attaches to the lower border of the lamina above and measures 14–22 mm in height, 11–23 mm in width at the lower part, and 3.5–6 mm in thickness [18, 19].

Under magnification with an operating microscope, the ligamentum flavum is seen to have two separate layers. The superficial layer has fiber

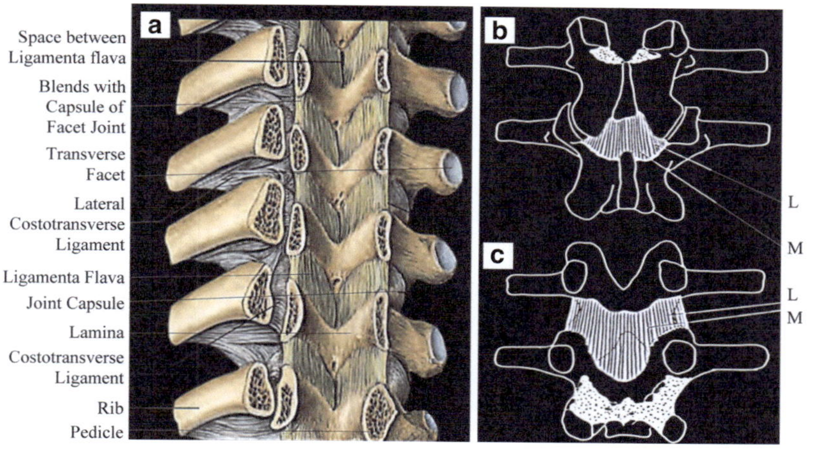

Fig. 4.4 The ligamentum flavum at the L2–3 level. (**a**) The ligamenta flava and costotransverse ligaments, ventral aspect. (**b**) Posterior view. (**c**) Anterior view (from within the vertebral canal). The medial (M) and lateral (Ll divisions) of the ligament are labelled. The shaded areas depict the sites of attachment of the ligamentum flavum at the levels above and below 12–3. In (**b**) the silhouettes of the laminae and inferior articular processes behind the ligament are indicated by the dotted lines. (Source: (**a**) After Bogduk N 2012 Clinical Anatomy of the Lumbar Spine and Sacrum, fourth ed. Edinburgh: Churchill Livingstone. (**b** and **c**) Standring S, Gray's Anatomy, The Anatomical Basis of Clinical Practice 41st ed. Edinburgh: Churchill Livingstone. Copyright 2020)

bundles that are aligned in the frontal plane, curving upward and extending from one lamina to the next. This layer merges with the joint capsule and stays evenly thin [20]. The deeper layer is more structured, with fibers running parallel to the sagittal plane, getting thicker from the sides toward the center. It also strengthens the joint capsule but can sometimes be free at the outer edge [21]. Between these two layers is a "gliding space," most noticeable in the lumbar spine, without any important blood vessels or nerves. At the midline, a vertical "split" separates the left and right superficial layers, while the deeper layers stay connected. The ligamentum flavum touches the erector spinae muscles at the back [18–20].

The yellow color of the ligamentum flavum comes from its high content of elastic fibers, which makes it different from other spinal ligaments that are mostly made of collagen [20]. Histologically, the ligamentum flavum is 80% elastin and 20% collagen. The elastic fibers are spread throughout the ligament, but at the ends, there are modified fibers called elaunin, which are made of elastin and microtubules [20, 22].

The front surface of the ligament is covered by a smooth, thin membrane. The ligament is thin, wide, and long in the cervical region, thicker in the thoracic region, and thickest in the lumbar region [23].

4.2.2 Interspinous Ligaments

The lumbar interspinous ligaments (ISLs) are made of thin, short fibers that connect the edges of neighboring spinous processes [1, 2]. These ligaments come from three places: the ligamenta flava, the vertebral laminae, and the lower surface of the spinous processes (Fig. 4.2). In the lumbar region, ISLs are thicker and shaped like a rhombus or quadrilateral, often found in pairs [24]. They extend forward toward the ligamentum flavum and backward toward the supraspinous ligament, when it is present [25].

The structure of ISLs differs in the thoracic, lumbar, and cervical regions. In the thoracic region, ISLs are narrow and long, while in the lumbar region, they are thicker, quadrilateral, and usually appear as pairs, separated by a narrow gap. In the lumbar region, collagen fibers run diagonally downward and forward, with only the deepest fibers forming true ligaments [24, 26]. The more dorsal fibers come from the tendons of the longissimus thoracis muscle, which extend into the interspinous space and attach to the top edge of the spinous process, not the tip. In contrast, in the cervical region, there are no distinct interspinous ligaments [27]. Instead, the median septum of the ligamentum nuchae passes between the cervical spinous processes [24, 27].

4.2.3 Supraspinous Ligament

The supraspinous ligament is a strong, fibrous cord that connects the tips of the spinous processes from vertebrae C7 to L4 or L5 (Fig. 4.2) [1, 2]. Below its lower end, the fibers of the right and left lumbodorsal fascia cross at the midline. This ligament is often incomplete or missing in some areas [26].

The supraspinous ligament has three layers: superficial, central, and deep. In children, all layers are made of tendinous tissue. However, by the early twenties, the central and deep layers start to change into fibrocartilage, and this change becomes more noticeable by middle age. The superficial fibers cover three to four vertebrae, the central fibers span two to three, and the deepest fibers connect neighboring spinous processes, continuing into the interspinous ligament [2, 27].

In the thoracic and lumbar regions, the supraspinous ligament mainly acts as a tendinous seam formed by the dorsal muscles, rather than as a separate ligament structure [6, 9–11, 23, 28, 29].

Most of the supraspinous ligament is made up of tendons from muscles with attachments along the back midline, like the semispinalis, longissimus, trapezius, and latissimus dorsi. Only the outermost fibers are not connected to any muscle. Below L4 or L5, the ligament is replaced by the crossing fibers of the latissimus dorsi [2, 27].

4.3 Intertransverse Ligaments

The intertransverse ligaments have a complex structure and can be understood in different ways. They are made of connective tissue sheets that stretch from the upper edge of one transverse process to the lower edge of the next transverse process above (Fig. 4.1) [1, 2]. Unlike typical ligaments, the intertransverse ligaments do not have clear inner or outer edges, and their collagen fibers are less tightly packed and not as well organized as true ligaments. Instead, they look more like membranes, which is why they are often called "false ligaments" [2, 30].

The medial and lateral extensions of these membranes suggest that, instead of being true ligaments, they are part of a larger fascial system that separates or defines certain paravertebral compartments. The only true ligament in this area is the ligament of Bourgery, which connects the base of a transverse process to the mamillary process below [31].

In the intertransverse spaces, these ligaments form a septum that separates the front muscles of the lumbar spine from the back muscles. On the side, the intertransverse ligaments have two layers: the anterior layer (also called the anterior layer of the thoracolumbar fascia), which covers the front of the quadratus lumborum muscle, and the posterior layer, which joins with the transversus abdominis aponeurosis to form the middle layer of the thoracolumbar fascia [31, 32].

Medially, the intertransverse ligament splits into two layers. The dorsal layer attaches to the side of the vertebral lamina across from the intertransverse space and blends with the joint capsule below. The ventral layer curves forward, covering the side of the vertebral bodies, and eventually joins with the anterior longitudinal ligament (Fig. 4.5). This part forms a membrane that encloses the outer end of the intervertebral foramen, with two openings. The upper opening allows nerve branches to pass to the psoas muscle, while the lower opening allows the ventral ramus of the spinal nerve and the spinal branches of the lumbar arteries and veins to pass through [2, 31, 32].

Between the ventral and dorsal layers of the intertransverse ligament is a wedge-shaped space called the superior articular recess, which allows for movement of the zygapophysial joint below [2, 23].

In the cervical region, these ligaments have a few irregular fibers and are mostly replaced by intertransverse muscles. In the thoracic region,

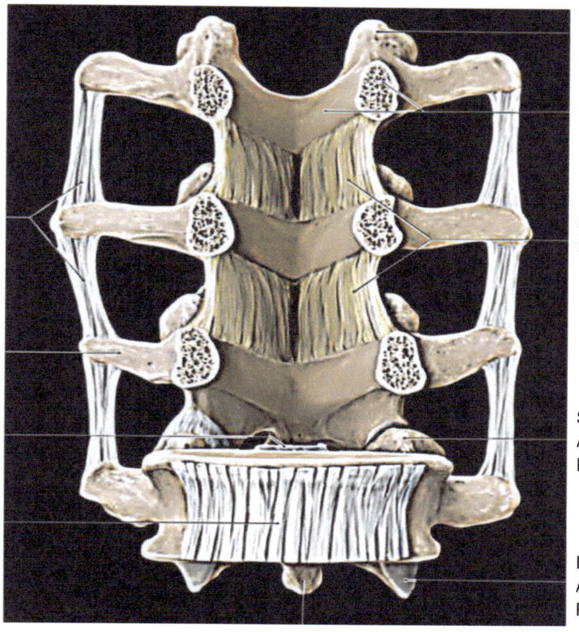

Fig. 4.5 Ligamenta flava and intertransverse ligaments, anterior view (after removal of the L2–L4 vertebral bodies). (The other vertebral arch ligaments are not visible in this view.) (Source: S, Gray's Anatomy, The Anatomical Basis of Clinical Practice 41st ed. Edinburgh: Churchill Livingstone. Copyright 2020)

they are cord-like and closely linked to nearby muscles, while in the lumbar region, they are thin and membranous [32].

4.3.1 Nuchal Ligament (Ligamentum Nuchae)

The nuchal ligament is a triangular fibroelastic structure between the paired muscles of the back of the neck. It is wide at its base, where it attaches to the cervical vertebrae, and becomes narrower as it rises toward the skull (Fig. 4.6) [33]. At the top, it attaches to the external occipital protuberance and the medial nuchal line of the occipital bone. At the bottom, it extends to the spinous processes of all cervical vertebrae, from C1 (atlas) to C7 [33, 34].

The nuchal ligament has two parts: (1) the lamellar portion, which is the front double-layered section with fatty tissue between the layers, and (2) the funicular portion, a fibrous structure at the back formed by the fusion of the lamellar layers [33].

The nuchal ligament is located in the center of the neck, separating paired structures and serving as an attachment point for midline neck muscles like the trapezius, rhomboids, and splenius capitis [35]. In a side view, it appears triangular, with the back edge of the triangle formed by the funicular portion, stretching from the spinous process of C7 to the external occipital protuberance [33, 34].

The second border of the nuchal ligament is at the front, where the lamellar portion attaches to the spinous processes of the cervical vertebrae and the posterior arch of C1. The third border is at the top, where the lamellar portion attaches along the median occipital protuberance, extending from the back of the foramen magnum to the external occipital protuberance [33].

The two layers of the nuchal ligament come together to form the funicular portion at the back [23]. At the occipital bone, the lamellar portion merges with the periosteum on the sides. In the middle, the lamellar portion in the suboccipital region serves as the attachment point for the medial edge of the rectus capitis posterior minor muscle [34, 36].

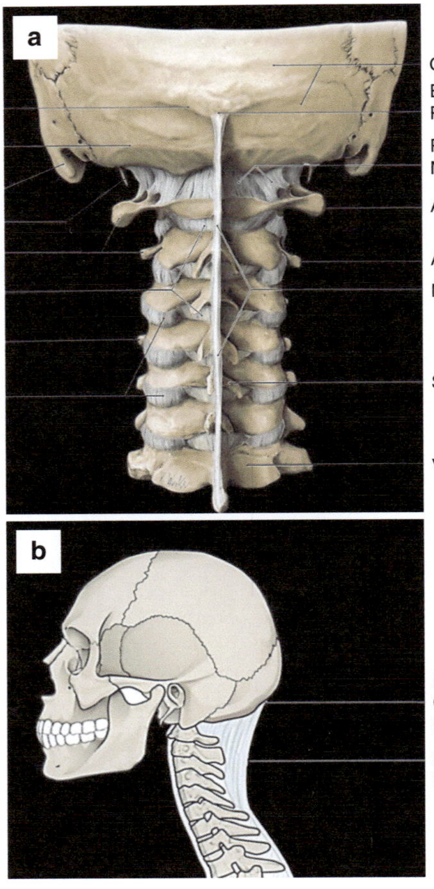

Fig. 4.6 Nuchael ligament. (**a**) lateral view. (**b**) Posterior view. (Source: (**a**) Schünke M, Schulte E, Schumacher U, Ross LM, Lamperti ED. Thieme atlas of anatomy: general anatomy and musculoskeletal system. Thieme Medical Publishers, Incorporated; Copyright 2014. (**b**) Base-Line Healing © Copyright L. S. Blyth 2017–2024)

4.3.2 Iliolumbar Ligament

The iliolumbar ligament is an important stabilizer in the lumbar spine, connecting the transverse process of the fifth lumbar vertebra (L5) to the ilium on both sides [2, 37]. It stretches from the tip of the L5 transverse process to the inner surface of the ilium and the inner edge of the iliac crest. However, its shape and even its existence are debated [37].

Early anatomical descriptions identified five distinct parts of the iliolumbar ligament: the anterior, superior, posterior, inferior, and vertical iliolumbar ligaments (Fig. 4.7) [38]. Recent studies confirm the presence of anterior and posterior parts of the iliolumbar ligament but question the existence of a superior part, without discussing the inferior or vertical portions. These differences in findings may be clarified with further research [39].

The superior iliolumbar ligament is likely overstated, as it is actually the anterior fascia of the quadratus lumborum and lacks the characteristics of a true ligament, such as properly aligned collagen fibers connecting two bones. The vertical and inferior iliolumbar ligaments are often confused with the ventral sacroiliac ligament, but they attach to the lumbar vertebrae and ilium, not the sacrum. Therefore, they should still be called "iliolumbar ligaments."

Another study confirmed the presence and attachment of the anterior, dorsal, and inferior parts of the iliolumbar ligament, and also found an additional part called the "sacroiliac part." This section has fibers that connect between the sacrum and ilium, below the L5 transverse pro-

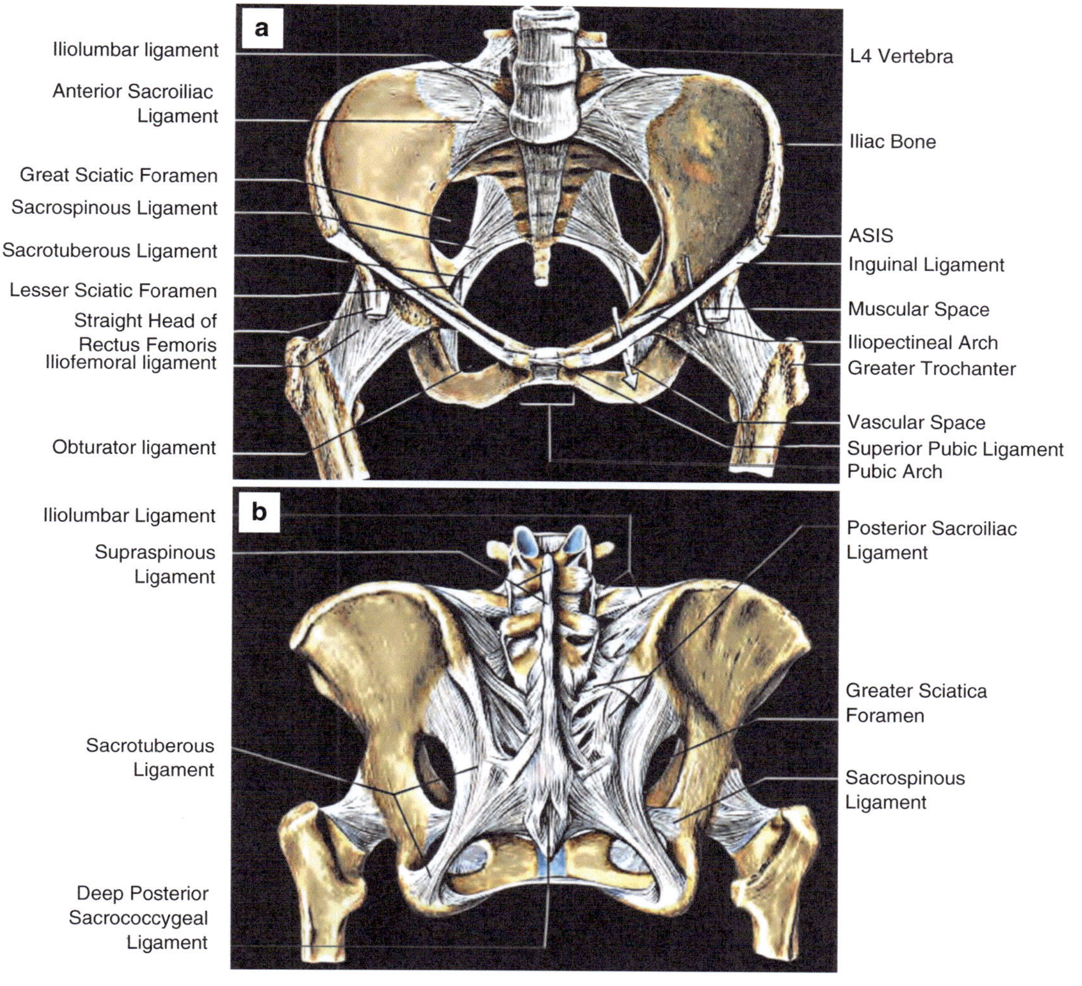

Fig. 4.7 The iliolumbar ligament. (**a**) Anterior aspect, ASIS, anterior superior iliac spine. (**b**) Posterior aspect. (Source: Standring S, Gray's Anatomy, The Anatomical Basis of Clinical Practice 41st ed. Edinburgh: Churchill Livingstone. Copyright 2020)

cess, and merge with the lowest fibers of the anterior band [40].

Despite identifying its parts, the existence of the iliolumbar ligament has been questioned. One study found it only in adults, while in neonates and children, it appears as muscle tissue. The suggestion is that this muscle gradually transforms into ligament tissue over time.

In contrast, another study strongly rejected the idea that the iliolumbar ligament is absent in fetuses, showing that it is present as early as 11.5 weeks of gestation [40].

The iliolumbar ligament is made of dense, fibrous connective tissue, mostly composed of collagen fibers that provide strength and resistance to stretching, crucial for stabilizing the lumbar spine and pelvis. It is a thick, flat band with a somewhat triangular or fan-like shape, widening as it extends from the lumbar vertebrae to its attachment on the ilium [2, 37].

The fibers of the iliolumbar ligament run diagonally from the lumbar transverse processes to the ilium. This alignment helps the ligament resist lateral and rotational forces, stabilizing the connection between the lumbar spine and the pelvis [2, 37–39].

4.3.3 Capsular Ligaments

The capsular ligaments, or articular capsules, are ligaments that surround and stabilize the synovial joints of the spine. They enclose the facet (zygapophyseal) joints between the articular processes of adjacent vertebrae and are essential for maintaining the stability and function of the spinal column (Fig. 4.8) [2, 34, 41, 42].

The capsular ligaments are made of dense fibrous connective tissue, mainly consisting of collagen fibers arranged at right angles. They also contain some elastic fibers and many fibroblasts. Unlike elastic ligaments, these ligaments have limited elasticity and primarily provide stability. The capsular ligaments form a thin, fibrous capsule around the facet joints, blending with surrounding tissues and reinforcing the joint as continuous structures [42]. The thickness and width of the capsular ligaments vary in different parts of the spine. In the cervical region, they are thinner to allow more mobility and flexibility. In the thoracic spine, they are slightly thicker, providing more stability. In the lumbar region, the capsular ligaments are much thicker and stronger to support the increased demand for stability in this weight-bearing area [41, 42].

The capsular ligaments attach to the edges of the facet joints, covering the articular surfaces of the superior and inferior articular processes of adjacent vertebrae, forming a capsule around each joint. The fibers encircle the joint to limit movement and ensure stability. Inside the capsule, a synovial membrane lines the surface and produces synovial fluid, which lubricates the joints and reduces friction. The outer layer is made of dense connective tissue, providing support and preventing excessive movement [42, 43].

The capsular ligament in the spine undergoes one of the greatest amounts of stretch in the lumbar region, either the most or second most. This high degree of stretch highlights its important role in maintaining stability while allowing controlled movement in the lumbar spine [11, 28, 43].

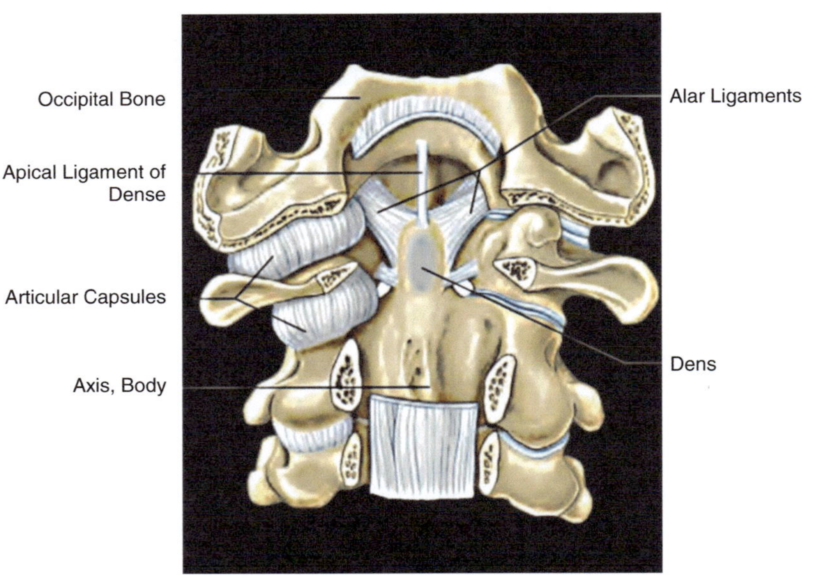

Fig. 4.8 Capsular ligament. (Source: Standring S, Gray's Anatomy, The Anatomical Basis of Clinical Practice 41st ed. Edinburgh: Churchill Livingstone. Copyright 2020)

4.3.4 Midline Interlaminar Ligament

The midline interlaminar ligament (MIL) is a thin, vertical ligament located in the middle between the right and left ligamenta flava (LF), but it remains separate from them (Fig. 4.9) [44]. MIL averages 9.03 ± 4.29 mm in length (ranging from 1.60 to 18.73 mm) and 4.94 ± 1.56 mm in width (ranging from 2.61 to 9.68 mm). It is loose during spinal flexion and tightens during extension, remaining relatively loose during lateral flexion [44, 45]. The MIL has fewer elastic fibers than the ligamentum flavum but contains more nerve fibers. Its dimensions do not vary significantly across different lumbar levels, and it is present in 90% of people [44, 45].

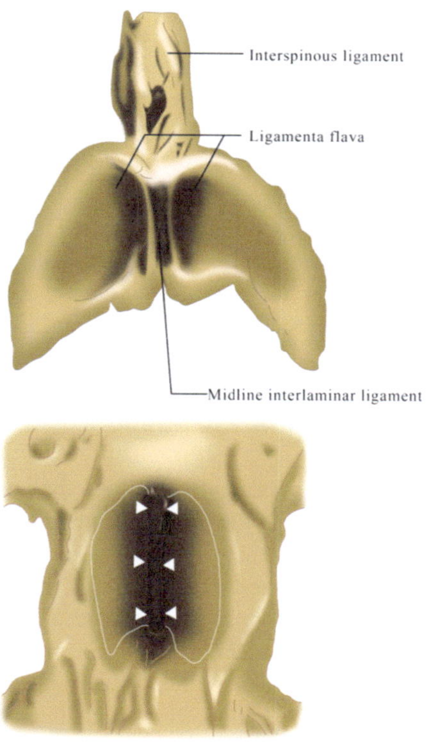

Fig. 4.9 Midline interlaminar ligament

4.4 Conclusion

Through an in-depth literature review, we uncovered critical insights into the morphology of spinal ligaments. Here is a summary of our findings:

4.4.1 Anterior Longitudinal Ligament (ALL)

It is a strong ligament along the front of the spine, stretching from the occipital bone to the sacrum. It is thicker in the thoracic region to handle heavier loads and attaches firmly to both the vertebral bodies and discs.

ALL has three layers—superficial, intermediate, and deep—that provide stability across different spine segments. Its dense collagen fibers help stabilize the spine, keep vertebrae aligned, prevent excessive backward bending, and protect the front of the spine, especially in high-stress areas like the lower back and neck.

4.4.2 Posterior Longitudinal Ligament (PLL)

The posterior longitudinal ligament (PLL) runs along the back of the spine from C2 to the sacrum. It has two layers: the outer layer spans several vertebrae, while the inner layer connects nearby vertebrae and attaches to the intervertebral discs. The PLL is wide in the neck, but it narrows and looks "fan-shaped" in the lower spine, especially over the discs. Its fibers come together at a central point on each vertebra, helping to keep the spine stable, with some changes in width in the lower back.

4.4.3 Ligament Flavum

It connects the laminae of adjacent vertebrae from C2 to the sacrum. Each ligament is elastic, quadrilateral-shaped, and meets at a 90° angle at the midline. It has two layers—a thin superficial layer and a structured deeper layer, separated by a "gliding space." Composed mainly of elastic fibers, the ligament's yellow color distinguishes it from other spinal ligaments. It varies in thickness, being thinnest in the cervical region and thickest in the lumbar region.

4.4.4 Interspinous Ligament

The lumbar interspinous ligaments (ISLs) connect adjacent spinous processes, forming thick, rhombus-shaped pairs in the lumbar spine. They attach forward to the ligamentum flavum and backward to the supraspinous ligament. ISL structure differs by region: narrow in the thoracic spine, thicker in the lumbar, and absent in the cervical, where the ligamentum nuchae's median septum serves a similar role.

4.4.5 Supraspinous Ligament

It is a fibrous cord connecting the tips of spinous processes from C7 to L4 or L5, which merges with the lumbodorsal fascia. It has three layers that change from tendons in children to fibrocartilage by adulthood. In the thoracic and lumbar spine, it mainly acts as a tendinous seam for back muscles. It consists mostly of muscle tendons, with only the outer fibers not attached to muscles.

4.4.6 Intertransverse Ligament

The intertransverse ligaments are thin connective tissue sheets connecting adjacent transverse processes. Unlike true ligaments, they lack organized collagen and resemble membranes, often called "false ligaments." They contribute to a fascial system defining paravertebral compartments, with only the ligament of Bourgery being a true ligament in this area. In the lumbar region, they form a septum separating front and back muscles, with two layers: an anterior layer covering the quadratus lumborum muscle and a posterior layer merging with the thoracolumbar fascia. Medially, the ligament splits to form a membrane around the intervertebral foramen, allowing passage of nerves and blood vessels. Regionally, the ligaments are mostly muscle in the cervical area, cord-like in the thoracic region, and membranous in the lumbar area.

4.4.7 Nuchal Ligament

The nuchal ligament is a triangular, fibroelastic structure between the neck muscles, broad at its base along the cervical vertebrae and narrowing toward the skull. It attaches from the external occipital protuberance to the spinous processes from C1 to C7. The ligament has two parts: the lamellar portion (a front, double-layered section) and the funicular portion (a fused, fibrous back section). It serves as an attachment for neck muscles like the trapezius and rhomboids. The lamellar portion also anchors the rectus capitis posterior minor in the suboccipital region and connects to the occipital bone.

4.4.8 Iliolumbar Ligament

The iliolumbar ligament stabilizes the lumbar spine by connecting the transverse process of L5 to the ilium. Its structure, debated in anatomy, has traditionally been described with five parts (anterior, superior, posterior, inferior, and vertical). Recent studies confirm anterior and posterior parts, while the "superior" is often just fascia from the quadratus lumborum, and the inferior and vertical parts resemble the ventral sacroiliac ligament. The ligament is dense with collagen, creating a strong, fan-shaped band that helps resist lateral and rotational forces, supporting lumbar and pelvic stability. Its development appears to transition from muscle in infancy to ligament in adulthood.

4.4.9 Capsular Ligament

Capsular ligaments, or articular capsules, surround and stabilize the spine's synovial facet joints. Made mostly of collagen fibers with limited elasticity, they form a thin capsule around each joint, adapting in thickness by region: thinner in the cervical spine for flexibility, thicker in the thoracic for stability, and thickest in the lumbar area to support weight-bearing demands. These ligaments attach around the facet joint edges, limiting movement and ensuring stability. A synovial membrane inside produces fluid for lubrication. Capsular ligaments experience a significant stretch in the lumbar region, balancing stability with controlled movement.

4.4.10 Midline Interlaminar Ligament (MIL)

It is a thin vertical ligament situated between, but separate from, the right and left ligamenta flava. It measures around 9 mm in length and 5 mm in width, loosening during spinal flexion and tightening during extension. The MIL has fewer elastic fibers but more nerve fibers than the ligamentum flavum and is present in 90% of people, with consistent dimensions across lumbar levels.

In conclusion, the spine's supporting ligaments contribute to stability, flexibility, and protection across various regions. The Anterior Longitudinal Ligament (ALL) and Posterior Longitudinal Ligament (PLL) provide front and back support, preventing excessive movements. Depending on the spine region, the Ligamentum Flavum and Interspinous Ligaments (ISL) connect vertebrae with varying elasticity and thickness. The Supraspinous Ligament links spinous tips, adapting with age, while Intertransverse Ligaments act as "false ligaments" supporting paravertebral compartments. The Nuchal Ligament supports neck muscles, and the Iliolumbar Ligament stabilizes the lumbar spine. Capsular Ligaments surround facet joints, and the Midline Interlaminar Ligament (MIL) supports movement control, adapting to spinal motion.

References

1. Standring S. Gray's anatomy international edition: the anatomical basis of clinical practice. Elsevier Health Sciences. 2020;(21):731–2.
2. Bogduk N. Clinical anatomy of the lumbar spine and sacrum. Elsevier Health Sciences 2005 (01); 39–48.
3. Gray's Anatomy. 39th edition: the anatomical basis of clinical practice. AJNR Am J Neuroradiol. 2005;26(10):2703–4.
4. Drake R, Vogl A, Mitchell A. Gray's anatomy for students. Elsevier Health Sciences. 2009 (04); 21–23.
5. François RJ. Ligament insertions into the human lumbar vertebral body. Acta Anat (Basel). 1975;91(3):467–80.
6. White AA, Punjabi MM. Clinical biomechanics of the spine. 2nd ed. Lippincott Williams & Wilkins; 1990. p. 18–9.
7. Behrsin JF, Briggs CA. Ligaments of the lumbar spine: a review. Surg Radiol Anat. 1988;10(3):211–9.
8. Standring S, Gray's Anatomy DS. The anatomical basis of clinical practice. 40th ed. Churchill Livingstone Elseveir; 2008. p. 1163–1177, 1185–6.
9. Benzel EC. Biomechanics of Spine Stabilization. 3rd ed. Georg Thieme Verlag; 2017. (7); 8–9, 55, 63, 97, 98, 114, 120–122, 176, 188, 273, 304.
10. Banton RA, CMPT A, Bending L. Biomechanics of the spine. J Spinal Res Found. 2012;7(2):12–20.
11. Pintar FA, Yoganandan N, Myers T, Elhagediab A, Sances A. Biomechanical properties of human lumbar spine ligaments. J Biomech. 1992;25(11):1351–6.
12. Loughenbury PR, Wadhwani S, Soames RW. The posterior longitudinal ligament and peridural (epidural) membrane. Clin Anat. 2006;19(6):487–92.
13. Aryal V, Black AC, Jimenez A. Anatomy, back, posterior longitudinal ligament. In: StatPearls [Internet]. Treasure Island (FL): StatPearls Publishing; 2024.
14. Tubbs RS, Loukas M, Phantana-Angkool A, Shoja MM, Ardalan MR, Shokouhi G, Oakes WJ. Posterior distraction forces of the posterior longitudinal ligament stratified according to vertebral level. Surg Radiol Anat. 2007;29(8):667–70.
15. Drake R, Vogl A, Mitchell A. Gray's anatomy for students. Philadelphia, PA: E Churchill Livingstone/Elsevier; 2015. p. 51–2.
16. Salaud C, Ploteau S, Hamel O, Armstrong O, Hamel A. Morphometric study of the posterior longitudinal ligament at the lumbar spine. Surg Radiol Anat Springer-Verlag France. 2018;40(5):563–9.
17. Matsunaga S, Sakou T. Ossification of the posterior longitudinal ligament of the cervical spine: etiology and natural history. Spine (Phila Pa 1976) 2012 Mar 1;37(5):E309–E314.
18. Viejo-Fuertes D, Liguoro D, Rivel J, Midy D, Guerin J. Morphologic and histologic study of the ligamentum flavum in the thoraco-lumbar region. Surg Radiol Anat. Springer Nature, Surg Radiol Anat. 1998;20(3):171–6.

19. Abdel-Meguid EM. An anatomical study of the human lumbar ligamentum flavum. Neurosciences (Riyadh). 2008;13(1):11–6.
20. Nihei A, Hagiwara K, Kikuchi M, Yashiro T, Hoshino Y. Histological investigation of rabbit ligamentum flavum with special reference to differences in spinal levels. Anat Sci Int Blackwell Publishing. 2003;78(3):162–7.
21. Willard FH, Vleeming A, Schuenke MD, Danneels L, Schleip R. The thoracolumbar fascia: Anatomy, function and clinical considerations. J Anat. 2012;221(6):507–36.
22. Wiltse LL. Anatomy of the extradural compartments of the lumbar spinal canal. Peridural membrane and circumneural sheath. Radiol Clin North Am. 2000;38(6):1177–206.
23. Bogduk N, Mercer S. Biomechanics of the cervical spine. I: Normal kinematics. Clin Biomech (Bristol, Avon). 2000;15(9):633–48.
24. Iwanaga J, Simonds E, Yilmaz E, Schumacher M, Patel M, Tubbs RS. Anatomical and biomechanical study of the lumbar Interspinous ligament. Asian J Neurosurg. 2019;14(4):1203–6.
25. Scapinelli R, Stecco C, Pozzuoli A, Porzionato A, Macchi V, De Caro R. The lumbar interspinous ligaments in humans: anatomical study and review of the literature. Cells Tissues Organs. 2006;183(1):1–11.
26. Heylings DJ. Supraspinous and interspinous ligaments of the human lumbar spine. J Anat. 1978;125(Pt 1):127–31.
27. Rissanen PM. The surgical anatomy and pathology of the supraspinous and interspinous ligaments of the lumbar spine with special reference to ligament ruptures. Acta Orthop Scand Suppl. 1960;46:1–100.
28. White AA, Punjabi MM. Clinical biomechanics of the spine. 1st ed. Lippincott Williams & Wilkins; 1985. p. 20–5.
29. Biomechanics of Spine Stabilization. AJNR Am J Neuroradiol. 2002;23(7):1261.
30. Parson SH. Clinically oriented Anatomy, 6th edn. J Anat. 2009;215(4):474.
31. Charpy A, Nicolas A, Poirier PJ. Traité d'anatomie humaine. Masson et cie; 1984.
32. Lewin T, Moffett B, Vidik A. The morphology of the lumbar synovial interveertebral joints. Acta Morphol Neerl Scand. 1962;4:299–319.
33. Kadri PA, Al-Mefty O. Anatomy of the nuchal ligament and its surgical applications. Neurosurgery 2007 61(5 Suppl 2):301–304; discussion 304.
34. Dean NA, Mitchell BS. Anatomic relation between the nuchal ligament (ligamentum nuchae) and the spinal dura mater in the craniocervical region. Clin Anat. 2002;15(3):182–5.
35. Mercer S, Bogduk N. The ligaments and annulus fibrosus of human adult cervical intervertebral discs. Spine (Phila Pa 1976). 1999;24(7):619–26. discussion 627-8
36. Takeshita K, Peterson ET, Bylski-Austrow D, Crawford AH, Nakamura K. The nuchal ligament restrains cervical spine flexion. Spine (Phila Pa 1976). 2004;29(18):E388–93.
37. Fujiwara A, Tamai K, Yoshida H, Kurihashi A, Saotome K, An HS, Lim TH. Anatomy of the iliolumbar ligament. Clin Orthop Relat Res. 2000;380:167–72.
38. Hanson P, Sonesson B. The anatomy of the iliolumbar ligament. Arch Phys Med Rehabil. 1994;75(11):1245–6.
39. Luk KDK, Ho HC, Leong JCY. The iliolumbar ligament. A study of its anatomy, development and clinical significance. J Bone Joint Sur – Series B. 1986;68(2):197–200.
40. Rucco V, Basadonna PT, Gasparini D. Anatomy of the iliolumbar ligament: a review of its anatomy and a magnetic resonance study. Am J Phys Med Rehabil. 1996;75(6):451–5.
41. Przybyla AS, Skrzypiec D, Pollintine P, Dolan P, Adams MA. Strength of the cervical spine in compression and bending. Spine (Phila Pa 1976). 2007;32(15):1612–20.
42. Yahia LH, Garzon S. Structure on the capsular ligaments of the facet joints. Ann Anat. 1993;175(2):185–8.
43. Singh S, Winkelstein BA. Characterization of the L4/L5 rat facet capsular ligament macromechanical and microstructural responses to tensile failure loading. J Biomech Elsevier Ltd. 2023;157. PMID: 37523884.
44. Simonds E, Iwanaga J, Ishak B, Reina MA, Oskouian RJ, Tubbs RS. Discovery of a new ligament of the lumbar spine: the midline interlaminar ligament. Spine J. 2020;20(7):1134–7.
45. Millhuff A, Haddad H, Draper MS, Motzko M, Glueck E, Holland B, Wright B. The midline interlaminar ligament of the spine: An anatomical study. Clin Anat John Wiley and Sons Inc; 2023 36(4):618–623.

5 Biochemical Characterization of the Spinal Ligaments

Ayça Tuzcu and Kenan Yörük

5.1 Introduction

5.1.1 Importance of Spinal Ligaments in Biomechanical and Biochemical Context

The spinal ligaments are specialized connective tissue structures that play a critical role in maintaining spinal stability and controlling segmental motion. Their mechanical performance is largely determined by the composition and organization of extracellular matrix (ECM) components, particularly type I and III collagen, elastin, and glycosaminoglycans. For example, the ligamentum flavum physiologically contains a high elastin to collagen ratio, reaching up to 75% elastin in fetal tissue. However, with advancing age, elastin content decreases while type I collagen increases, leading to changes in the tissue's mechanical properties and a reduction in elasticity [1]. These structures are not static; they undergo continuous remodeling in response to various biological and mechanical stimuli throughout life. Aging, repetitive mechanical stress, and microinjury contribute to the progressive loss of elastic fibers and accumulation of collagen, particularly in the ligamentum flavum. As a result, the ligament gradually loses its elastic properties, becomes fibrotic, and undergoes functional deterioration [2].

5.1.2 Focus on Ligamentum Flavum

The ligamentum flavum (LF) is a connective tissue structure located between the vertebral arches, characterized by a higher elastin content compared to other spinal ligaments. This elasticity allows it to accommodate the physiological movements of the spinal canal. However, with advancing age, chronic mechanical loading, and inflammatory processes, elastin content decreases and is progressively replaced by type I collagen. This structural transition reduces tissue flexibility and predisposes the LF to hypertrophy and fibrosis [1, 2].

In particular, mineral deposits observed in the LF, such as hydroxyapatite and calcium pyrophosphate dihydrate, may contribute to the development of lumbar spinal stenosis by promoting tissue rigidity and mass effect on the spinal canal [3].

5.1.3 Biochemical Disruption as a Basis for Pathology

The disruption in the balance of structural proteins in ligament tissue (e.g., loss of elastin, increase in collagen) leads to loss of

A. Tuzcu (✉) · K. Yörük
Department of Biochemistry, Aydın Adnan Menderes University Faculty of Medicine, Efeler, Aydın, Türkiye
e-mail: aycaurhan@gmail.com

M. Turgut et al. (eds.), *Ligaments of the Vertebral Column*,
https://doi.org/10.1007/978-3-032-09070-6_5

biomechanical properties and transformation of the tissue into fibrotic and mineralized structures. Microdamage in collagen fibrils may serve as nucleation sites for mineral deposition. These biochemical processes have a crucial function in the development of spinal canal narrowing, nerve compression, and the resulting clinical symptoms [4].

5.2 Biochemical Components of Spinal Ligaments

The spinal ligaments possess a rich ECM structure, primarily composed of elastin, type I and type III collagen, proteoglycans, and glycosaminoglycans. These components form the biochemical foundation that ensures both the mechanical strength and flexibility of the spine [5].

5.2.1 Structural Proteins: Collagens and Elastin

The primary structural protein of spinal ligaments is type I collagen, which provides resistance against tensile forces. Type III collagen is present in smaller amounts and contributes to tissue elasticity, playing a role in the repair process. For example, in the ligamentum flavum, approximately 85% of the collagen is type I and 15% is type III, reflecting its strong tensile capacity with limited elasticity. This collagen ratio may vary depending on the type of ligament and can change significantly in response to aging, trauma, or chronic mechanical loading. Elastin is abundantly found in structures requiring high elasticity, such as the ligamentum flavum. However, with aging, elastin fibers degrade and are replaced by collagen, leading to reduced tissue elasticity and subsequent fibrosis and thickening [1, 2].

5.2.2 Proteoglycans and Glycosaminoglycans

The main proteoglycans found in spinal ligaments are decorin and biglycan. These molecules interact with collagen fibrils to regulate the process of fibrillogenesis, help maintain the water content of the ECM, and contribute to the tissue's resistance to compressive forces. They also play a crucial role in tissue degradation and remodeling by interacting with enzymes such as matrix metalloproteinases (MMPs) [6, 7].

In the ligamentum flavum, proteoglycans—particularly chondroitin-6-sulfate and dermatan sulfate—play a fundamental role in maintaining tissue hydration and viscoelasticity due to their hydrophilic nature. These molecules act as shock absorbers, supporting the biomechanical function of the spinal ligaments. A study by Okada et al. demonstrated age-related changes in glycosaminoglycan composition, including an increase in dermatan sulfate and chondroitin-6-sulfate content in elderly specimens. Such alterations may impair ligament hydration and elasticity, contributing to degenerative processes in the spinal column [8].

5.2.3 Cellular Components and ECM Turnover

The structural integrity of spinal ligaments depends not only on ECM components but also on resident fibroblasts, which are responsible for synthesizing key proteins such as collagen, elastin, and proteoglycans. Mechanical stress activates these cells, initiating ECM remodeling. This process is regulated by matrix MMPs and tissue inhibitors of metalloproteinases (TIMPs), which together maintain the balance between ECM synthesis and degradation. Chronic loading, aging, and inflammatory signaling disrupt this balance, leading to fibrosis, loss of elastic fibers, and progressive mineralization in the ligamentum flavum [9].

5.2.4 Age-Related and Mechanical Adaptations

Spinal ligaments undergo significant biochemical and structural changes with aging. Alterations such as a decrease in elastin fibers, an increase in type I collagen, and a loss of glycosaminoglycans lead to ligaments becoming more rigid and less elastic. This condition is particularly characterized by thickening (hypertrophy) and loss of flexibility in the ligamentum flavum [10].

Mechanical stress, including compression and repetitive flexion-extension, plays a central role in the pathophysiology of the ligamentum flavum. It activates fibroblasts and induces the expression of cytokines such as transforming growth factor beta-1 (TGF-β) and interleukin-6 (IL-6). These factors stimulate the production of extracellular matrix components, including collagen, and promote tissue remodeling. While initially compensatory, sustained signaling under chronic mechanical loading can lead to excessive matrix accumulation, fibrosis, and progressive calcification [9].

5.3 Mechanisms Underlying Ligament Degeneration

Ligament degeneration is a complex process that disrupts spinal biomechanics and often leads to clinical symptoms. This process results from the combined effects of multiple factors, including aging, repetitive mechanical stress, inflammation, oxidative damage, and genetic predisposition. Degenerative changes—particularly in the ligamentum flavum—can result in altered collagen/elastin ratios, loss of proteoglycans, fibrosis, and even ossification. These biochemical disruptions lay the groundwork for clinical outcomes such as spinal canal narrowing, nerve root compression, and spinal instability.

5.3.1 Degenerative Disc Disease and Ligament Interactions

Reduction in disc height during degenerative disc disease shifts axial loading to the posterior elements of the spine, particularly the ligamentum flavum. This results in mechanical stretching and fibroblast activation, promoting ECM remodeling and hypertrophy. Physical stress induces the upregulation of type I collagen and TGF-β1, leading to fibrosis and a loss of tissue elasticity [11]. In addition to mechanical stress, the degenerated disc microenvironment is rich in inflammatory cytokines such as interleukin-1β (IL-1β) and tumor necrosis factor-α (TNF-α). These cytokines stimulate fibroblasts within the ligamentum flavum to increase the expression of MMP-2 and MMP-9, which degrade structural ECM proteins like collagen and elastin [12]. Moreover, oxidative stress plays a synergistic role in accelerating the degeneration of the ligamentum flavum. Chuang et al. showed that age-related increases in reactive oxygen species (ROS) activate the Akt and mitogen-activated protein kinase (MAPK) pathways, further promoting inflammation, fibroblast senescence, and apoptosis within the ligamentum flavum [13]. These molecular alterations diminish tissue elasticity and enhance LF thickening, thereby contributing to spinal canal narrowing and neurogenic symptoms.

5.3.2 Osteoarthritis-Linked Ligament Remodeling

Osteoarthritis (OA) is a common musculoskeletal disorder characterized by the progressive degeneration of articular cartilage. However, this process is not limited to cartilage damage alone; it represents a widespread tissue remodeling that affects all components of the joint, including the subchondral bone, synovium, meniscus, and spinal ligaments [14]. Structural changes observed in spinal ligaments, including collagen accumulation, elastin degradation, and fibrosis, particularly in the ligamentum flavum, contribute to reduced spinal flexibility and limited range of motion, which are key factors in the clinical presentation of degenerative spine conditions [13]. The remodeling process observed in spinal ligaments due to OA is triggered by both increased mechanical stress and a chronically inflamed microenvironment. Simultaneously, pro-inflammatory cytokines abundantly present in OA tissues, including IL-6, IL-1β, and TNF-α, contribute to increased oxidative stress and ECM degradation in ligament cells [15]. Among the primary enzymes involved in this process, MMP-9 plays a critical role by degrading ECM components such as collagen and elastin, thereby compromising ligament integrity. In contrast, the compensatory increase in TIMPs is insufficient, preventing adequate control of matrix degradation [16]. Studies have demonstrated that hypertrophic ligamentum flavum tissue exhibits increased expression of α-smooth muscle actin, indicating a phenotypic transition of resident fibroblasts into myofibroblasts. This cellular transformation is associated with enhanced type I collagen synthesis and remodeling of the fibrotic extracellular matrix [17]. Furthermore, hyperactivation of the TGF-β1/Smad signaling pathway has been identified as a central mechanism in this fibrotic transformation [18]. Histopathological analyses have demonstrated that ligamentum flavum tissues from OA patients exhibit increased type I and III collagen, decreased elastin, and marked accumulation of glycosaminoglycans [1]. Such structural remodeling not only reduces intersegmental mobility but also contributes to spinal canal narrowing, thereby promoting neurological symptoms. In recent years, epigenetic modifications have also been implicated in ligament remodeling. Specifically, alterations in DNA methylation and microRNA expression affect fibroblast proliferation and ECM production, contributing to the pathogenesis of OA [19]. These findings collectively suggest that OA cannot be explained solely by mechanical wear and tear; instead, it represents a multifactorial disorder involving complex biochemical and cellular mechanisms.

5.3.3 Hypertrophy and Fibrosis of the Ligamentum Flavum

LF is an elastic connective tissue located between the laminae of the vertebrae that supports the structural integrity of the spinal canal and regulates tension during flexion-extension movements. Under physiological conditions, LF is rich in elastin, providing the spine with its necessary flexibility. However, with aging, mechanical loading, and degenerative diseases, the tissue undergoes hypertrophy and fibrosis, particularly in the lumbar region, which constitutes a significant cause of spinal stenosis [14]. The primary mechanism of LF hypertrophy involves degeneration of elastic fibers and their replacement with disorganized type I collagen, resulting in fibrotic remodeling [20]. This not only leads to physical thickening of the ligament but also to a significant loss of its elastic properties. Histopathological analyses of hypertrophied LF have shown marked fibroblast proliferation, neovascularization, and chronic inflammatory cell infiltration [2]. At the molecular level, growth factors, including TGF-β1, connective tissue growth factor, and vascular endothelial growth factor, are upregulated in hypertrophic LF tissue. These mediators promote the transdifferentiation of fibroblasts into a myofibroblast phenotype, thereby enhancing ECM deposition [11]. Additionally, this fibrotic response is reinforced through signaling cascades involving Smad2/3 and MAPK pathways [2]. Another hallmark of LF fibrosis is the phenotypic shift of ligament cells through a process resembling epithelial-mesenchymal transition, which increases cellular plasticity and further exacerbates fibrotic progression [21]. Environmental stressors, including oxidative stress, mitochondrial dysfunction, and tissue hypoxia, have also been implicated in upregulating fibrosis-associated gene expression in LF cells [13]. Recently, several studies have focused on the role of immune cell infiltration and the formation of a fibroinflammatory microenvironment in LF hypertrophy. In particular, M1 macrophages and mast cells have been shown to initiate and sustain fibrotic remodeling in the ligament tissue [2]. These findings suggest that LF hypertrophy is not merely a consequence of mechanical stress but also involves a distinct immune-inflammatory disease process.

5.3.4 Ossification Mechanisms

Ossification processes occurring in spinal ligaments, particularly in structures such as the ligamentum flavum and the posterior longitudinal ligament, represent severe pathological conditions that can result in compression of the spinal cord or nerve roots. This condition is commonly referred to as ossified posterior longitudinal ligament (OPLL), which is notably more prevalent among Asian populations [22]. The ossification process in spinal ligaments, such as the posterior longitudinal ligament and ligamentum flavum, involves the reprogramming of native ligament fibroblasts into chondrocyte-like cells that deposit a calcified extracellular matrix, recapitulating endochondral bone formation and leading to spinal canal narrowing and potential myelopathy [22]. From a molecular perspective, dysregulation of the Wnt/β-catenin signaling pathway plays a central role in OPLL development, as activation of Wnt signaling promotes osteoblastic differentiation of ligament cells through increased expression of Wnt3a, LRP5/6, and β-catenin [23]. Epigenetic regulation has recently emerged as a significant factor in the mechanisms of ligament ossification. Studies of ligament tissues from OPLL patients have demonstrated the downregulation of specific microRNAs, such as miR-10a and miR-140, accompanied by the activation of genes involved in osteogenesis [24]. These epigenetic alterations may contribute to ossification both in genetically predisposed individuals and in spinal segments subjected to chronic mechanical stress. Furthermore, recent findings indicate that chronic inflammation and oxidative stress-mediated through IL-6, TNF-α, and the accumulation of ROS also contribute to osteogenic transformation [25]. Collectively, these data suggest that OPLL is a multifactorial pathological process influenced not only by genetic and mechanical factors but also by systemic and environmental components.

5.3.5 Inflammatory Diseases

The structural integrity of spinal ligaments may be compromised during inflammatory diseases due to both direct inflammatory cell infiltration and secondary tissue remodeling. In particular, chronic inflammatory rheumatic disorders can affect connective tissue components, leading to ligament thickening, fibrosis, or ossification.

Ankylosing spondylitis is a prototypical axial spondyloarthritis that initiates at the entheses and is characterized by aberrant bone formation along the spinal ligaments. Mechanical stress and microdamage at entheseal sites activate local antigen-presenting cells, inducing the secretion of IL-23, which drives the differentiation of IL-17-producing T cells. This cytokine milieu promotes both tissue inflammation and new bone formation via osteoblast activation, particularly affecting the ligamentum flavum, anterior longitudinal ligament, and interspinous ligaments [19, 26, 27].

Rheumatoid arthritis often involves the cervical spine, where chronic synovitis can extend to adjacent ligamentous structures. Inflammatory infiltration of the transverse and alar ligaments, especially between C1 and C2, may lead to instability and atlantoaxial subluxation. MRI-based studies and histological analyses have confirmed ligamentous thickening and pannus invasion in these regions. Moreover, elevated levels of MMP-1, MMP-9, and TNF-α, along with reduced TIMP expression, contribute to matrix degradation. NF-κB and JAK/STAT signaling cascades further amplify these processes through enhanced fibroblast activation and cytokine production [28–31].

Psoriatic arthritis is another seronegative spondyloarthropathy frequently involving spinal entheses. Microscopic enthesitis initiates a pathological cascade involving IL-23, IL-17, and IL-22, leading to chronic inflammation, fibrocartilage metaplasia, and subsequent ossification at ligamentous attachment sites. Enthesophyte formation along the vertebral column has been confirmed in both imaging and histopathologic studies, underscoring the active role of cytokine-mediated bone remodeling [32–34].

Spinal ligaments may also be indirectly affected in connective tissue disorders such as Systemic Lupus Erythematosus and Mixed Connective Tissue Disease. These conditions can compromise the structural integrity of connective tissues, leading to reduced elasticity and progressive fibrosis. Dysregulation of cytokine signaling disturbs the balance between the synthesis and degradation of connective tissue components [35].

Inflammatory processes in spinal ligaments activate various enzymes, particularly MMP-2 and MMP-9, which degrade type I and type III collagen, thereby impairing tissue architecture. Moreover, the imbalance in TIMP-1 and TIMP-2 accelerates ECM degradation [21]. Alongside fibroblast activation, there is altered expression of ECM proteins such as fibronectin, tenascin-C, and decorin. These alterations contribute not only to the deterioration of mechanical properties but also to the progression of chronic fibrotic remodeling [7]. Signaling pathways such as NF-κB and JAK/STAT also play critical roles in the activation of inflammatory cells and cytokine secretion. These cascades promote the infiltration of immune cells into ligament tissue and upregulate the expression of pro-inflammatory genes. In ligament cells exposed to chronic inflammation, markers of oxidative stress, including ROS and inducible nitric oxide synthase, are upregulated, thereby exacerbating cellular damage [13].

5.3.6 Genetic Influences on the Structural Integrity of Spinal Ligaments

The structural integrity and biomechanical properties of spinal ligaments are significantly influenced by genetic factors. In particular, hereditary syndromes associated with connective tissue disorders alter ligament elasticity, tensile strength, and cellular composition, thereby predisposing to degenerative or structurally unstable changes.

One such condition is Ehlers-Danlos syndrome, which is primarily characterized by ligamentous hyperlaxity and mechanical weakness due to mutations in genes responsible for type V collagen synthesis. These alterations are frequently associated with spinal instability, scoliosis, and intervertebral disc degeneration. In individuals with Ehlers-Danlos syndrome, fibroblasts derived from ligament tissue exhibit impaired synthesis of extracellular matrix proteins and disrupted fibrillar organization [36]. Marfan syndrome is a heritable connective tissue disorder primarily caused by mutations in the FBN1 gene, which encodes fibrillin-1, a critical glycoprotein involved in the formation of elastic fibers. Impairment in fibrillin-1 synthesis results in a defective elastic fiber architecture, compromising the structural and biomechanical integrity of spinal ligaments. As a result, individuals with Marfan syndrome frequently present with ligamentous laxity, kyphoscoliosis, and postural abnormalities, reflecting the systemic weakness of connective tissue [37, 38].

Among genetically mediated ossifying disorders, one of the most well-characterized conditions is OPLL. This disorder, which is particularly prevalent in East Asian populations, has been associated with genetic variants in *ENPP1*, *COL11A2*, *BMP2*, and *TGF-β1*. These genes are involved in regulating bone formation, ECM protein synthesis, and osteoblast differentiation [39].

5.4 Biochemical Markers and Mechanisms

The pathophysiology of spinal ligament degeneration, particularly ligamentum flavum hypertrophy and fibrosis, extends far beyond mechanical stress and structural alterations. In recent years, a growing body of evidence has underscored the pivotal role of biochemical markers and molecular pathways in mediating these pathological transformations. These mechanisms not only reflect the biological response of ligamentous tissue to chronic strain and aging but also actively drive the progression of fibrotic remodeling, inflammation, and ossification.

Among the most studied biochemical mediators are TGF-β1, a key regulator of fibroblast-to-myofibroblast transition; MMPs and their TIMPs, which orchestrate extracellular matrix turnover; ROS, which mediate oxidative stress responses; and proinflammatory cytokines such as IL-6, TNF-α, and interleukin-17 (IL-17), which establish a chronic inflammatory microenvironment [2]. These molecular players do not act in isolation. Instead, they participate in interconnected signaling cascades—such as the TGF-β/SMAD, NF-κB, and MAPK pathways—that regulate fibroblast activity, ECM composition, and immune cell infiltration. The dysregulation of

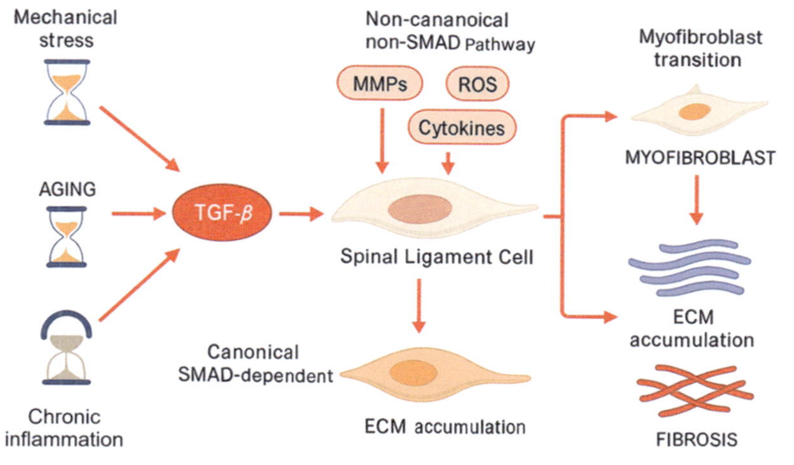

Fig. 5.1 Molecular mechanisms contributing to spinal ligament degeneration. The diagram illustrates the interplay among key biochemical mediators, including TGF-β1, ROS, MMPs/TIMPs, and proinflammatory cytokines (IL-6, TNF-α, and IL-17). These factors act through signaling cascades including TGF-β/SMAD, NF-κB, and MAPK pathways, collectively promoting fibroblast act

these pathways results in altered biomechanical properties of the spinal ligaments, contributing to clinical manifestations such as lumbar spinal stenosis, ligament ossification, and axial rigidity [40].

Understanding these biochemical mechanisms is essential not only for elucidating the molecular basis of ligament degeneration but also for identifying potential biomarkers for early diagnosis and novel therapeutic targets. In this section, we outline the major molecular pathways and marker molecules involved in spinal ligament pathology, offering an integrated view of how biochemical signals influence the degenerative process.

An integrated illustration of these interconnected molecular pathways, including TGF-β1, MMPs/TIMPs, ROS, and proinflammatory cytokines, is seen in Fig. 5.1, providing a conceptual framework for the biochemical basis of spinal ligament degeneration.

5.4.1 TGF-β1, SMAD Pathway, and Myofibroblast Transition

TGF-β1 is a central cytokine involved in tissue remodeling and fibrosis across various organs, and it plays a pivotal role in the pathogenesis of ligamentum flavum hypertrophy (LFH). In the context of spinal ligament biochemistry, TGF-β1 mediates fibroblast-to-myofibroblast differentiation, a phenotypic switch that underlies excessive ECM deposition and tissue thickening. TGF-β1 initiates its biological effects by binding to the TGF-β type II receptor (TβRII), which subsequently recruits and phosphorylates the TGF-β type I receptor (TβRI). The activated receptor complex phosphorylates receptor-regulated SMADs (R-SMADs), particularly SMAD2 and SMAD3. These R-SMADs form a complex with the common mediator SMAD4 and translocate into the nucleus, where they regulate the transcription of genes responsible for ECM production, such as COL1A1, fibronectin, and α-smooth muscle actin. This gene activation leads to the differentiation of fibroblasts into myofibroblasts, cells that exhibit contractile properties and contribute to fibrosis by secreting large amounts of collagen and other ECM components [2]. Recent studies using human ligamentum flavum tissue samples have demonstrated that TGF-β1 expression is significantly elevated in hypertrophied specimens compared to normal tissue. Moreover, nuclear localization of phosphorylated SMAD2/3 is positively correlated with both α-smooth muscle actin expression and ligament thickness, supporting a direct link between TGF-β1/SMAD signaling and LFH pathogenesis [41]. Importantly, mechanical stress and chronic inflammation—both prevalent in degenerative spinal conditions—are known to stimulate local TGF-β1 secretion by resident cells and infiltrating macrophages. In vitro experiments have confirmed that cyclic mechanical strain can upregulate TGF-β1 mRNA and protein expression in human ligament fibroblasts, thereby promoting fibrotic gene transcription via SMAD-dependent pathways [42]. In addition to canonical SMAD signaling, non-SMAD pathways, such as MAPK (ERK, JNK, p38) and PI3K/AKT, also modulate TGF-β1-induced fibrosis; however, their role in spinal ligament pathology remains less well-defined. However, some evidence suggests that these alternative pathways may synergize with SMADs to enhance myofibroblast persistence and ECM stiffness, creating a self-amplifying fibrotic loop [43]. Given its central role, the TGF-β1/SMAD axis has emerged as a potential therapeutic target. Pharmacologic inhibition of TGF-β1 signaling using small molecules or neutralizing antibodies has shown efficacy in reducing ECM accumulation and myofibroblast activation in preclinical models. However, due to the pleiotropic roles of TGF-β1 in tissue homeostasis and immune regulation, systemic inhibition carries potential risks, and localized or targeted delivery strategies are under investigation [44].

5.4.2 Matrix Metalloproteinases and Tissue Inhibitors of Metalloproteinases

MMPs are a family of zinc-dependent endopeptidases responsible for the degradation of ECM components such as collagen, elastin, laminin, and proteoglycans. In spinal ligaments, particularly the ligamentum flavum, MMPs play a critical role in maintaining ECM homeostasis and mediating pathological remodeling during hypertrophy and fibrosis. Among the MMP family, MMP-2 (gelatinase A) and MMP-9 (gelatinase B) have been most consistently implicated in ligamentum flavum degeneration and fibrosis. These enzymes degrade denatured collagens (gelatins) and basement membrane components, and their activity is tightly regulated at the transcriptional level and by activation of latent proenzymes. Additionally, MMP-13 (collagenase 3), which targets fibrillar collagens such as type I and III, has also been detected in hypertrophied ligament tissue, especially in areas undergoing active remodeling [45].

MMP activity is counterbalanced by TIMPs, a family of four endogenous inhibitors (TIMP-1 to TIMP-4) that bind MMPs in a 1:1 stoichiometry. TIMP-1 primarily inhibits MMP-9, while TIMP-2 is more selective for MMP-2. In healthy ligament tissue, the balance between MMPs and TIMPs is essential for maintaining structural integrity and preventing pathological degradation or over-deposition of ECM components. However, in ligamentum flavum hypertrophy, this balance is often disrupted.

Recent immunohistochemical and transcriptomic analyses of human hypertrophied ligamentum flavum samples have shown elevated expression of MMP-2 and MMP-9, often accompanied by a relative reduction or mislocalization of TIMP-1 and TIMP-2. This imbalance promotes an environment of excessive ECM turnover, which paradoxically leads to both matrix destruction and aberrant fibrotic reconstruction [46]. Furthermore, pro-inflammatory cytokines such as IL-1β, TNF-α, and IL-17, commonly elevated in degenerative spine disease, can upregulate MMP expression in fibroblasts and macrophages via the NF-κB and MAPK pathways. These signaling cascades also suppress TIMP production, further aggravating the proteolytic environment. Interestingly, studies have also revealed that mechanical stress and oxidative injury contribute to increased MMP activity, linking biomechanical factors with biochemical degradation [47]. In addition to their degradative roles, certain MMPs are involved in non-ECM functions, such as modulating cytokine availability, cleaving cell surface receptors, and influencing cell migration. Thus, their dysregulation in spinal ligaments may have far-reaching consequences beyond matrix turnover alone. Targeting the MMP/TIMP axis is an area of therapeutic interest. Inhibiting MMPs pharmacologically or restoring TIMP levels through gene therapy has shown promise in preclinical models of tissue fibrosis. However, due to the complex roles of MMPs in both degradation and regeneration, therapeutic modulation must be precisely timed and tissue-specific to avoid adverse outcomes [48].

5.4.3 Reactive Oxygen Species and Oxidative Stress

ROS, including superoxide anions (O_2^-), hydrogen peroxide (H_2O_2), and hydroxyl radicals (•OH), are natural byproducts of cellular metabolism, primarily originating from mitochondrial oxidative phosphorylation and enzymatic reactions involving NADPH oxidases (NOX). While physiological levels of ROS act as signaling molecules in processes such as cell proliferation and differentiation, excessive or unbalanced ROS production, termed oxidative stress, is detrimental to tissue integrity and function.

In the context of spinal ligaments, particularly the ligamentum flavum, oxidative stress has emerged as a key mediator of fibrotic remodeling and degenerative changes. Several studies have reported elevated levels of oxidative damage markers, such as 8-hydroxy-2′-deoxyguanosine (8-OHdG) and malondialdehyde (MDA), in hypertrophied ligament tissues, indicating persistent oxidative injury. ROS influence ligament pathology through multiple mechanisms. Firstly, they activate pro-fibrotic signaling pathways, notably TGF-β1/SMAD, by enhancing the transcription and release of TGF-β1 from fibroblasts and macrophages. This creates a feedback loop wherein ROS potentiate fibrosis, and fibrotic cells generate further ROS. Secondly, ROS modulate the activity of MMPs, promoting ECM degradation and turnover. Oxidative stress also suppresses the expression of antioxidant enzymes, such as superoxide dismutase (SOD), glutathione peroxidase (GPx), and catalase, thereby further exacerbating the redox imbalance [13]. Recent transcriptomic and immunohistochemical analyses of degenerative ligamentum flavum tissues have identified the overexpression of NOX4, an isoform of NADPH oxidase associated with chronic ROS generation. NOX4-mediated ROS production is associated with increased fibroblast proliferation, myofibroblast differentiation, and expression of fibrosis-related genes including ACTA2, COL1A1, and FN1 [49]. Moreover, mechanical loading, often altered in degenerative spine conditions, has been shown to increase mitochondrial ROS production in ligament cells. This biomechanical-oxidative interface likely contributes to ligament degeneration through mechanotransduction pathways involving p38 MAPK and NF-κB, which are redox-sensitive transcription factors that regulate inflammatory and fibrotic gene expression [13]. Therapeutically, antioxidants have been explored as modulators of spinal ligament pathology. Compounds such as N-acetylcysteine (NAC), resveratrol, and melatonin have demonstrated efficacy in vitro in reducing ROS levels, inhibiting myofibroblast activation, and restoring ECM balance. However, clinical translation remains limited due to challenges in tissue-specific delivery and sustained bioavailability [50].

5.4.4 Cytokines: IL-6, TNF-α, and IL-17

Proinflammatory cytokines are central mediators of tissue remodeling, immune cell recruitment, and fibrotic transformation in various musculoskeletal pathologies, including degenerative changes in spinal ligaments. Among these, IL-6, TNF-α, and IL-17 have been identified as key drivers in inflammation-induced fibrosis and hypertrophy in the ligamentum flavum and other spinal ligament structures.

5.4.4.1 IL-6 and Fibroinflammatory Signaling

IL-6 is a pleiotropic cytokine that signals through both classical (membrane-bound IL-6R) and trans-signaling (soluble IL-6R) pathways, the latter being more relevant in chronic inflammation. In spinal ligament tissue, IL-6 levels are significantly elevated in hypertrophied samples, particularly in patients with lumbar spinal stenosis (LSS) [51]. IL-6 promotes the expression of fibrogenic genes such as COL1A1, ACTA2, and TGF-β1, while also stimulating STAT3 phosphorylation, which supports fibroblast proliferation and myofibroblast transition. In vitro studies using human ligament fibroblasts have shown that IL-6 stimulation enhances ECM protein secretion and increases the expression of MMPs thus contributing to a dual phenotype of degradation and fibrosis. Moreover, IL-6 amplifies oxidative stress responses, often acting synergistically with ROS to drive chronic tissue injury [45].

5.4.4.2 TNF-α and ECM Disruption

TNF-α is another potent proinflammatory cytokine implicated in ligamentum flavum degeneration. It exerts its effects through the activation of NF-κB and MAPK pathways, leading to the transcription of genes involved in inflammation, cell survival, and ECM remodeling. Elevated levels of TNF-α have been detected in ligamentum flavum tissues from patients with spinal stenosis and disc degeneration and are associated with increased fibronectin and collagen type III expression [13]. TNF-α also facilitates macrophage infiltration and polarization toward an M1 phenotype, which sustains the local inflammatory milieu. Additionally, TNF-α can enhance the production of IL-6 and IL-1β, establishing a pro-inflammatory cytokine loop that further exacerbates ligament thickening and fibrosis.

5.4.4.3 IL-17 and Autoimmune-Linked Fibrosis

In spinal ligament pathology, it is plausible, based on studies in other fibrotic tissues, that IL-17A may activate fibroblasts, augment TGF-β1 expression, and enhance MMP/NOX4-mediated oxidation [2]. However, direct experimental validation in ligamentum flavum cell models is currently lacking. IL-17 also potentiates the effects of TNF-α and IL-6 through synergistic interactions, leading to sustained inflammation and ECM dysregulation. In ligaments from patients with axial spondyloarthritis, increased IL-17 expression correlates with early fibrosis and ossification, suggesting its role in both fibrotic and osteogenic transformation.

5.4.4.4 Therapeutic Considerations

Given the central role of these cytokines in ligament pathology, targeting IL-6 (e.g., tocilizumab), TNF-α (e.g., etanercept, infliximab), or IL-17 (e.g., secukinumab) has therapeutic potential not only in systemic diseases, such as axial spondyloarthritis, but also in localized spinal fibrosis. However, translation of these biologics into degenerative spinal conditions remains under investigation, particularly with regard to delivery, safety, and tissue-specific efficacy [52–54].

5.5 Conclusion and Future Perspectives

Spinal ligament degeneration is a multifactorial process involving biochemical, mechanical, and immunological components, with the ligamentum flavum serving as a principal model for studying these pathologies [14]. The interplay between ECM components, such as type I/III collagen, elastin, proteoglycans, and glycosaminoglycans, and cellular signaling pathways (e.g., TGF-β/SMAD, MAPK, and NF-κB) mediates the transition between adaptive and maladaptive remodeling [2]. Recent histopathological and molecular studies have confirmed that fibroblast-to-myofibroblast transition and oxidative stress–driven matrix disruption are central events in fibrosis and hypertrophy [13]. Furthermore, chronic mechanical strain accelerates ECM turnover and inflammatory cytokine expression, which over time contributes to ligament stiffening and spinal canal narrowing [2].

5.5.1 Diagnostic and Prognostic Biomarker Potential

Emerging evidence has suggested the utility of molecular markers, such as MMP-2, MMP-9, TIMP-1, IL-6, and TGF-β1, as early indicators of spinal ligament degeneration [7, 45, 51]. Proteomic and transcriptomic profiling of hypertrophic ligamentum flavum tissues has identified candidate markers like fibronectin, tenascin-C, and NOX4, which correlate with both fibrosis severity and clinical symptoms [21]. Future studies should aim to validate such biomarkers in large cohorts and integrate them with advanced imaging tools to improve diagnostic precision.

5.5.2 Translational and Therapeutic Pathways

Therapeutic strategies targeting fibrosis-related pathways are under development, with preclinical studies demonstrating the efficacy of TGF-β1 inhibitors, antioxidant agents, and MMP blockers in reducing ECM accumulation and inflammatory cell infiltration. However, due to the pleiotropic effects of these pathways in tissue repair and immune regulation, systemic blockade may carry risks such as impaired wound healing or immunosuppression [55]. Localized drug delivery systems, including hydrogels, nanoparticles, and scaffold-based therapeutics, are being investigated to enhance site-specific efficacy while minimizing systemic toxicity [56]. Immunomodulatory approaches, particularly the neutralization of IL-17 and TNF-α, have shown potential in inflammatory ligament pathologies, especially those associated with ankylosing spondylitis [26].

5.5.3 Future Research Directions

Future investigations should adopt integrative methodologies, such as single-cell RNA sequencing, metabolomics, and spatial transcriptomics, to unravel cellular heterogeneity and niche-specific responses within ligament tissues [19]. Animal models that recapitulate the fibrotic and ossific phenotypes observed in humans are critically needed to test disease-modifying therapies [57]. Furthermore, epigenetic regulation—through microRNAs, histone modifications, and DNA methylation—offers a novel dimension to explore pathogenesis and reversibility in ligament remodeling [24]. Finally, interdisciplinary collaborations between spine surgeons, bioengineers, and molecular biologists will be essential to translate these findings into clinical interventions that preserve ligament function and spinal mobility [39].

References

1. Voelker A, Schroeter F, Steinke H, Heyde CE. Degeneration of the lumbar spine and its relation to the expression of collagen and elastin in facet joint capsules and ligament flavum. Acta Orthop Traumatol Turc. 2022;56(3):210–6. https://doi.org/10.5152/j.aott.2022.21314. PMID: 35703510; PMCID: PMC9612638.
2. Silwal P, Nguyen-Thai AM, Alexander PG, Sowa GA, Vo NV, Lee JY. Cellular and molecular mechanisms of hypertrophy of Ligamentum Flavum. Biomolecules. 2024;14(10):1277. https://doi.org/10.3390/biom14101277. PMID: 39456209; PMCID: PMC11506588.
3. Seki S, Kawaguchi Y, Ishihara H, Oya T, Kimura T. Lumbar spinal stenosis due to a large calcified mass in the ligamentum flavum. Asian Spine J. 2013;7(3):236–41. https://doi.org/10.4184/asj.2013.7.3.236. Epub 2013 Sep 4. PMID: 24066222; PMCID: PMC3779778
4. Orzechowska S, Świsłocka R, Lewandowski W. Model of pathological collagen mineralization based on spine ligament calcification. Materials (Basel). 2020;13(9):2130. https://doi.org/10.3390/ma13092130. PMID: 32375359; PMCID: PMC7254246
5. Rifai NH, Andrea Rita, Wittwer CT. Tietz fundamentals of clinical chemistry and molecular diagnostics. 9th ed. St. Louis: Elsevier; 2023.
6. Salimi H, Suzuki A, Habibi H, Orita K, Hori Y, Yabu A, Terai H, Tamai K, Nakamura H. Biglycan expression and its function in human ligamentum flavum. Sci Rep. 2021;11(1):4867. https://doi.org/10.1038/s41598-021-84363-x. PMID: 33649499; PMCID: PMC7921587.
7. Wang S, Qu Y, Fang X, Ding Q, Zhao H, Yu X, Xu T, Lu R, Jing S, Liu C, Wu H, Liu Y. Decorin: a potential therapeutic candidate for ligamentum flavum hypertrophy by antagonizing TGF-β1. Exp Mol Med. 2023;55(7):1413–23. https://doi.org/10.1038/s12276-023-01023-y. Epub 2023 Jul 3. PMID: 37394592; PMCID: PMC10394053.
8. Okada A, Harata S, Takeda Y, Nakamura T, Takagaki K, Endo M. Age-related changes in proteoglycans of human ligamentum flavum. Spine (Phila Pa 1976). 1993;18(15):2261–6. https://doi.org/10.1097/00007632-199311000-00020.
9. Ma Q, Feng X, Chen Y, Zhang J, Sun C. Mechanical stress contributes to ligamentum flavum hypertrophy by inducing local inflammation and myofibroblast transition in the innovative surgical rabbit model. Front Immunol. 2025;16:1541577. https://doi.org/10.3389/fimmu.2025.1541577. PMID: 40303410; PMCID: PMC12037363.

10. Hayashi K, Ishidou Y, Yonemori K, Nagamine T, Origuchi N, Maeda S, Imamura T, Kato M, Yoshida H, Sampath TK, ten Dijke P, Sakou T. Expression and localization of bone morphogenetic proteins (BMPs) and BMP receptors in ossification of the ligamentum flavum. Bone. 1997;21(1):23–30. https://doi.org/10.1016/s8756-3282(97)00080-x.
11. Cao YL, Duan Y, Zhu LX, Zhan YN, Min SX, Jin AM. TGF-β1, in association with the increased expression of connective tissue growth factor, induce the hypertrophy of the ligamentum flavum through the p38 MAPK pathway. Int J Mol Med. 2016;38(2):391–8. https://doi.org/10.3892/ijmm.2016.2631. Epub 2016 Jun 8. PMID: 27279555; PMCID: PMC4935458.
12. Chen X, Wang Z, Deng R, Yan H, Liu X, Kang R. Intervertebral disc degeneration and inflammatory microenvironment: expression, pathology, and therapeutic strategies. Inflamm Res. 2023;72(9):1811–28. https://doi.org/10.1007/s00011-023-01784-2. Epub 2023 Sep 4
13. Chuang HC, Tsai KL, Tsai KJ, Tu TY, Shyong YJ, Jou IM, Hsu CC, Shih SS, Liu YF, Lin CL. Oxidative stress mediates age-related hypertrophy of ligamentum flavum by inducing inflammation, fibrosis, and apoptosis through activating Akt and MAPK pathways. Aging (Albany NY). 2020;12(23):24168–83. https://doi.org/10.18632/aging.104105. Epub 2020 Nov 20. PMID: 33223505; PMCID: PMC7762458.
14. Sairyo K, Biyani A, Goel V, Leaman D, Booth R Jr, Thomas J, Gehling D, Vishnubhotla L, Long R, Ebraheim N. Pathomechanism of ligamentum flavum hypertrophy: a multidisciplinary investigation based on clinical, biomechanical, histologic, and biologic assessments. Spine (Phila Pa 1976). 2005;30(23):2649–56. https://doi.org/10.1097/01.brs.0000188117.77657.ee.
15. Miller RE, Miller RJ, Malfait AM. Osteoarthritis joint pain: the cytokine connection. Cytokine. 2014;70(2):185–93. https://doi.org/10.1016/j.cyto.2014.06.019. Epub 2014 Jul 24. PMID: 25066335; PMCID: PMC4254338.
16. Wang C, Wei Z, Yu T, Zhang L. Dysregulation of metalloproteinases in spinal ligament degeneration. Connect Tissue Res. 2023;64(4):310–22. https://doi.org/10.1080/03008207.2022.2160327. Epub 2023 Jan 4
17. Hur JW, Bae T, Ye S, Kim JH, Lee S, Kim K, Lee SH, Kim JS, Lee JB, Cho TH, Park JY, Hur JK. Myofibroblast in the ligamentum flavum hypertrophic activity. Eur Spine J. 2017;26(8):2021–30. https://doi.org/10.1007/s00586-017-4981-2. Epub 2017 Feb 8
18. Shen J, Li S, Chen D. TGF-β signaling and the development of osteoarthritis. Bone Res. 2014;2:14002. https://doi.org/10.1038/boneres.2014.2. PMID: 25541594; PMCID: PMC4274935.
19. Kiełbowski K, Herian M, Bakinowska E, Banach B, Sroczyński T, Pawlik A. The role of genetics and epigenetic regulation in the pathogenesis of osteoarthritis. Int J Mol Sci. 2023;24(14):11655. https://doi.org/10.3390/ijms241411655. PMID: 37511413; PMCID: PMC10381003.
20. Shafaq N, Suzuki A, Terai H, Nakamura H, Takaoka K. Histopathological analysis of hypertrophic ligamentum flavum in degenerative lumbar canal stenosis focus on the expression of bmps signaling components. In: Spine: Affiliated Society Meeting Abstracts, vol. 58; 2010. p. 58.
21. Sun C, Zhang H, Wang X, Liu X. Ligamentum flavum fibrosis and hypertrophy: molecular pathways, cellular mechanisms, and future directions. FASEB J. 2020;34(8):9854–68. https://doi.org/10.1096/fj.202000635R. Epub 2020 Jul 1
22. Yan L, Gao R, Liu Y, He B, Lv S, Hao D. The pathogenesis of ossification of the posterior longitudinal ligament. Aging Dis. 2017;8(5):570–82. https://doi.org/10.14336/AD.2017.0201. PMID: 28966802; PMCID: PMC5614322.
23. Yayama T, Mori K, Okumura N, Nishizawa K, Kumagai K, Nakamura A, Imai S. Wnt signaling pathway correlates with ossification of the spinal ligament: a microRNA array and immunohistochemical study. J Orthop Sci. 2018;23(1):26–31. https://doi.org/10.1016/j.jos.2017.09.024. Epub 2017 Oct 26
24. Zhang B, Chen G, Yang X, Fan T, Chen X, Chen Z. Dysregulation of MicroRNAs in hypertrophy and ossification of Ligamentum Flavum: new advances, challenges, and potential directions. Front Genet. 2021;12:641575. https://doi.org/10.3389/fgene.2021.641575. PMID: 33912216; PMCID: PMC8075056.
25. Nam DC, Lee HJ, Lee CJ, Hwang SC. Molecular pathophysiology of ossification of the posterior longitudinal ligament (OPLL). Biomol Ther (Seoul). 2019;27(4):342–8. https://doi.org/10.4062/biomolther.2019.043. PMID: 31042677; PMCID: PMC6609106.
26. Sieper J, Poddubnyy D, Miossec P. The IL-23-IL-17 pathway as a therapeutic target in axial spondyloarthritis. Nat Rev Rheumatol. 2019;15(12):747–57. https://doi.org/10.1038/s41584-019-0294-7. Epub 2019 Sep 24
27. Kim SH, Lee SH. Updates on ankylosing spondylitis: pathogenesis and therapeutic agents. J Rheum Dis. 2023;30(4):220–33. https://doi.org/10.4078/jrd.2023.0041. Epub 2023 Sep 6. PMID: 37736590; PMCID: PMC10509639.
28. Di Muzio C, Conforti A, Bruno F, Currado D, Berardicurti O, Navarini L, Pavlych V, Di Cola I, Biaggi A, Di Donato S, Marino A, Lorusso S, Ursini F, Barile A, Masciocchi C, Cipriani P, Giacomelli R, Ruscitti P. The assessment of atlantoaxial joint involvement in patients with rheumatoid arthritis, results from an observational "real-life" study. Sci Rep. 2023;13(1):20146. https://doi.org/10.1038/s41598-023-46069-0. PMID: 37978246; PMCID: PMC10656509.
29. Chen Q, Wang H, Zhang M, Chen F, Guo X, Lu X, Ni B, Guo Q. Open reduction for potentially reducible atlantoaxial dislocation secondary to transverse

ligament laxity in patients with rheumatoid arthritis. World Neurosurg. 2022;167:e789–94. https://doi.org/10.1016/j.wneu.2022.08.097. Epub 2022 Aug 28
30. Pulik Ł, Łęgosz P, Motyl G. Matrix metalloproteinases in rheumatoid arthritis and osteoarthritis: a state of the art review. Reumatologia. 2023;61(3):191–201. https://doi.org/10.5114/reum/168503. Epub 2023 Jul 2. PMID: 37522140; PMCID: PMC10373173.
31. Ding Q, Hu W, Wang R, Yang Q, Zhu M, Li M, Cai J, Rose P, Mao J, Zhu YZ. Signaling pathways in rheumatoid arthritis: implications for targeted therapy. Signal Transduct Target Ther. 2023;8(1):68. https://doi.org/10.1038/s41392-023-01331-9. PMID: 36797236; PMCID: PMC9935929.
32. Araujo EG, Schett G. Enthesitis in psoriatic arthritis (part 1): pathophysiology. Rheumatology (Oxford). 2020;59(Suppl 1):i10–4. https://doi.org/10.1093/rheumatology/keaa039. PMID: 32159793; PMCID: PMC7065460.
33. Azuaga AB, Ramírez J, Cañete JD. Psoriatic arthritis: pathogenesis and targeted therapies. Int J Mol Sci. 2023;24(5):4901. https://doi.org/10.3390/ijms24054901. PMID: 36902329; PMCID: PMC10003101.
34. Pignon C, Bibas N, Lopez-Medina C, Fautrel B, Gossec L. Clinical enthesitis in patient with psoriatic arthritis, a systematic literature review with metaanalysis. Joint Bone Spine. 2025;92(2):105807. https://doi.org/10.1016/j.jbspin.2024.105807. Epub 2024 Oct 30
35. Martin JC, Baeten DL, Josien R. Emerging role of IL-17 and Th17 cells in systemic lupus erythematosus. Clin Immunol. 2014;154(1):1–12. https://doi.org/10.1016/j.clim.2014.05.004. Epub 2014 May 23
36. Malfait F, Francomano C, Byers P, Belmont J, Berglund B, Black J, Bloom L, Bowen JM, Brady AF, Burrows NP, Castori M, Cohen H, Colombi M, Demirdas S, De Backer J, De Paepe A, Fournel-Gigleux S, Frank M, Ghali N, Giunta C, Grahame R, Hakim A, Jeunemaitre X, Johnson D, Juul-Kristensen B, Kapferer-Seebacher I, Kazkaz H, Kosho T, Lavallee ME, Levy H, Mendoza-Londono R, Pepin M, Pope FM, Reinstein E, Robert L, Rohrbach M, Sanders L, Sobey GJ, Van Damme T, Vandersteen A, van Mourik C, Voermans N, Wheeldon N, Zschocke J, Tinkle B. The 2017 international classification of the Ehlers-Danlos syndromes. Am J Med Genet C Semin Med Genet. 2017;175(1):8–26. https://doi.org/10.1002/ajmg.c.31552.
37. Judge DP, Dietz HC. Marfan's syndrome. Lancet. 2005;366(9501):1965–76. https://doi.org/10.1016/S0140-6736(05)67789-6. PMID: 16325700; PMCID: PMC1513064.
38. Ramirez F, Dietz HC. Marfan syndrome: from molecular pathogenesis to clinical treatment. Curr Opin Genet Dev. 2007;17(3):252–8. https://doi.org/10.1016/j.gde.2007.04.006. Epub 2007 Apr 27. Erratum in: Curr Opin Genet Dev. 2007 Aug;17(4):367.
39. Nakajima M, Takahashi A, Tsuji T, Karasugi T, Baba H, Uchida K, Kawabata S, Okawa A, Shindo S, Takeuchi K, Taniguchi Y, Maeda S, Kashii M, Seichi A, Nakajima H, Kawaguchi Y, Fujibayashi S, Takahata M, Tanaka T, Watanabe K, Kida K, Kanchiku T, Ito Z, Mori K, Kaito T, Kobayashi S, Yamada K, Takahashi M, Chiba K, Matsumoto M, Furukawa K, Kubo M, Toyama Y; Genetic Study Group of Investigation Committee on Ossification of the Spinal Ligaments; Ikegawa S. A genome-wide association study identifies susceptibility loci for ossification of the posterior longitudinal ligament of the spine. Nat Genet. 2014 46(9):1012-1016. doi: https://doi.org/10.1038/ng.3045. Epub 2014 Jul 27.
40. Luo K. Signaling cross talk between TGF-β/Smad and other signaling pathways. Cold Spring Harb Perspect Biol. 2017;9(1):a022137. https://doi.org/10.1101/cshperspect.a022137. PMID: 27836834; PMCID: PMC5204325.
41. Wang L, Chang M, Tian Y, Yan J, Xu W, Yuan S, Zhang K, Liu X. The role of Smad2 in transforming growth factor β_1-induced hypertrophy of Ligamentum Flavum. World Neurosurg. 2021;151:e128–36. https://doi.org/10.1016/j.wneu.2021.03.147. Epub 2021 Apr 5
42. Han F, Wang J, Ding L, Hu Y, Li W, Yuan Z, Guo Q, Zhu C, Yu L, Wang H, Zhao Z, Jia L, Li J, Yu Y, Zhang W, Chu G, Chen S, Li B. Tissue engineering and regenerative medicine: achievements, future, and sustainability in Asia. Front Bioeng Biotechnol. 2020;8:83. https://doi.org/10.3389/fbioe.2020.00083. PMID: 32266221; PMCID: PMC7105900.
43. Finnson KW, Almadani Y, Philip A. Non-canonical (non-SMAD2/3) TGF-β signaling in fibrosis: mechanisms and targets. Semin Cell Dev Biol. 2020;101:115–22. https://doi.org/10.1016/j.semcdb.2019.11.013. Epub 2019 Dec 26
44. Porte J, Jenkins G, Tatler AL. Myofibroblast TGF-β activation measurement in vitro. Methods Mol Biol. 2021;2299:99–108. https://doi.org/10.1007/978-1-0716-1382-5_6.
45. Sugimoto K, Nakamura T, Tokunaga T, Uehara Y, Okada T, Taniwaki T, Fujimoto T, Mizuta H. Matrix metalloproteinase promotes elastic fiber degradation in ligamentum flavum degeneration. PLoS One. 2018;13(8):e0200872. https://doi.org/10.1371/journal.pone.0200872. PMID: 30067795; PMCID: PMC6070248.
46. Torun YM, Delen E, Doğanlar O, Doğanlar ZB, Delen Ö, Orakdöğen M. Effects of Expression of Matrix Metalloproteinases and Discoidin Domain Receptors in Ligamentum Flavum Fibrosis in Patients with Degenerative Lumbar Canal Stenosis. Asian Spine J. 2023;17(1):194–202. https://doi.org/10.31616/asj.2021.0380. Epub 2022 Sep 27. PMID: 36163678; PMCID: PMC9977973.
47. Kwon WK, Ham CH, Choi H, Baek SM, Lee JW, Park YK, Moon HJ, Park WB, Kim JH. Elucidating the effect of mechanical stretch stress on the mechanism of ligamentum flavum hypertrophy: development of a novel in vitro multi-torsional stretch loading device. PLoS One. 2022;17(10):e0275239. https://

doi.org/10.1371/journal.pone.0275239. PMID: 36269774; PMCID: PMC9586365.
48. Charzewski Ł, Krzyśko KA, Lesyng B. Structural characterisation of inhibitory and non-inhibitory MMP-9-TIMP-1 complexes and implications for regulatory mechanisms of MMP-9. Sci Rep. 2021;11(1):13376. https://doi.org/10.1038/s41598-021-92881-x. PMID: 34183752; PMCID: PMC8238946.
49. Duan Y, Ni S, Zhao K, Qian J, Hu X. Immune cell infiltration and the genes associated with ligamentum flavum hypertrophy: identification and validation. Front Cell Dev Biol. 2022;10:914781. https://doi.org/10.3389/fcell.2022.914781. PMID: 36036007; PMCID: PMC9400804.
50. Hsu YC, Chuang HC, Tsai KL, Tu TY, Shyong YJ, Kuo CH, Liu YF, Shih SS, Lin CL. Administration of N-Acetylcysteine to regress the Fibrogenic and Proinflammatory effects of oxidative stress in hypertrophic Ligamentum Flavum cells. Oxidative Med Cell Longev. 2022;2022:1380353. https://doi.org/10.1155/2022/1380353. PMID: 36338342; PMCID: PMC9629932.
51. Nakamura T, Okada T, Endo M, Nakamura T, Oike Y, Mizuta H. Angiopoietin-like protein 2 promotes inflammatory conditions in the ligamentum flavum in the pathogenesis of lumbar spinal canal stenosis by activating interleukin-6 expression. Eur Spine J. 2015;24(9):2001–9. https://doi.org/10.1007/s00586-015-3835-z. Epub 2015 Mar 4
52. Mualem W, Liu J, Balu A, Chesney K, Nair MN. Biomarkers related to hypertrophy of the ligamentum flavum: a systematic review of the literature. J Neurosurg Spine. 2024;41(1):33–45. https://doi.org/10.3171/2024.2.SPINE23991.
53. Braun J, Kiltz U, Bühring B, Baraliakos X. Secukinumab in axial spondyloarthritis: a narrative review of clinical evidence. Ther Adv Musculoskelet Dis. 2021;13:1759720X211041854. https://doi.org/10.1177/1759720X211041854. PMID: 34471428; PMCID: PMC8404628.
54. Dougados M, van der Heijde D, Sieper J, Braun J, Citera G, Lenaerts J, van den Bosch F, Wei JC, Pedersen R, Bonin R, Jones H, Marshall L, Logeart I, Vlahos B, Bukowski JF, Maksymowych WP. Effects of Long-term Etanercept treatment on clinical outcomes and objective signs of inflammation in early nonradiographic axial Spondyloarthritis: 104-week results from a randomized, Placebo-Controlled Study. Arthritis Care Res (Hoboken). 2017;69(10):1590–8. https://doi.org/10.1002/acr.23276. Epub 2017 Aug 31.
55. Kim KK, Sheppard D, Chapman HA. TGF-β1 signaling and tissue fibrosis. Cold Spring Harb Perspect Biol. 2018;10(4):a022293. https://doi.org/10.1101/cshperspect.a022293. PMID: 28432134; PMCID: PMC5880172.
56. Dewi NM, Meiliana A, Defi IR, Amalia R, Sartika CR, Wijaya A, Barliana MI. Targeted therapy for skeletal muscle fibrosis: regulation of Myostatin, TGF-β, MMP, and TIMP to maintain extracellular matrix homeostasis. Biologics. 2025;19:213–29. https://doi.org/10.2147/BTT.S508221. PMID: 40260056; PMCID: PMC12011048.
57. Wang B, Gao C, Zhang P, Sun W, Zhang J, Gao J. The increased motion of lumbar induces ligamentum flavum hypertrophy in a rat model. BMC Musculoskelet Disord. 2021;22(1):334. https://doi.org/10.1186/s12891-021-04203-x. PMID: 33823825; PMCID: PMC8025532.

Biomechanical Properties of the Spinal Ligaments

6

Joe Iwanaga and R. Shane Tubbs

6.1 Introduction

The sub-axial ligaments of the spinal column help stabilize the vertebral column joints. The three main joints in the vertebral column stabilized by the sub-axial ligaments are the vertebral joints, costovertebral joints, and the sacroiliac joints. The vertebral joints consist of the intervertebral synovial and cartilaginous joints, both of which are the major components in forming a functional spinal unit. The costovertebral joints, only associated with the thoracic vertebrae, are a vital component in allowing adequate movement of the ribcage necessary for ventilation, yet can provide a sturdy encasement for the protection of the thoracic organs. The sacroiliac joints attach the sacrum to the left and right ilium.

In particular, the sub-axial ligaments allow the vertebrae significant mobility within a predetermined range while providing the structural integrity necessary to safely house the spinal cord in the vertebral canal. There are two classifications of spinal sub-axial ligaments: the intrasegmental and intersegmental systems. The intrasegmental system consists of ligaments that hold individual adjacent vertebrae together and include such ligaments as the ligamentum flavum, the interspinous ligament, and the intertransverse ligament. Meanwhile, the intersegmental system is responsible for holding together multiple vertebrae using a single ligament, but its ligaments are much longer than those of the intrasegmental system. The intersegmental system comprises ligaments, including the anterior and posterior longitudinal ligaments, as well as the supraspinous ligament. Several ligaments of the subaxial spine are well known among the medical community due to the pathology associated with their rupture, calcification, and other conditions. These ligaments include the anterior longitudinal ligament, known for its involvement in the diagnosis of cervical acceleration-deceleration injury, i.e., whiplash, as well as the ligamentum flavum.

6.2 Functional Spinal Unit

The functional spinal unit, i.e., the spinal motion segment, is the smallest physiological motion unit of the spine to exhibit the biomechanical characteristics applicable to the entire spine. It consists of two adjacent vertebral bodies held together by the two facet synovial joints known as the zygapophysial joints, formed by each vertebra's articular processes, the intervertebral disc

J. Iwanaga (✉)
Department of Neurosurgery, Tulane Center for Clinical Neurosciences, Tulane University School of Medicine, New Orleans, LA, USA
e-mail: jiwanaga@tulane.edu

R. S. Tubbs
Tulane University School of Medicine, New Orleans, LA, USA

M. Turgut et al. (eds.), *Ligaments of the Vertebral Column*,
https://doi.org/10.1007/978-3-032-09070-6_6

between the two vertebral bodies, and all adjoining ligaments; however, the functional spinal unit excludes any other connective tissues, such as muscles and tendons. These three joints allow for vertebral motion, including flexion, extension, rotation, and lateral bending, at the level of the functional spinal unit.

The zygapophysial joint is a synovial joint between the inferior articular process of the superior vertebrae and the superior articular process of the inferior vertebrae in each functional spinal unit [1]. There are two zygapophysial joints in each functional spinal unit, one on either side of the midline of the vertebrae [1]. A synovial joint is formed by articulating bones coated with articular cartilage united by a joint/articular capsule spanning and enclosing the articular cavity; the capsule is composed of an outer fibrous layer lined by a serous synovial membrane [1]. The synovial joint cavity is a potential space containing a small amount of lubricating synovial fluid, which the synovial membrane secures [1]. Any non-articulating surface of a synovial joint is covered by synovial membrane [1].

The other joint involved in the functional spinal unit is the intervertebral disc between the adjacent vertebral bodies. These discs provide a strong attachment between the vertebral bodies, thus uniting them into a continuous semi-rigid column [1]. These discs account for approximately 20–25% of the height of the vertebral column [1]. The intervertebral disc comprises an outer layer of concentric lamellae of fibrocartilage known as the anulus fibrosus. In contrast, the inner portion of the intervertebral disc, encased by the anulus fibrosus, is the nucleus pulposus [1]. The nucleus pulposus consists mainly of water, giving it a semifluid nature, which permits the disc to have significant compressibility and allows for a wide array of movements [1].

6.3 Biomechanics of the Vertebral Joints

The zygapophysial joints determine the movements permitted and restricted between adjacent regions (cervical, thoracic, or lumbar) [1]. Although movements between adjacent vertebrae are relatively small, the aggregate of all the individual movements gives the vertebral column its extensive range of movement [1].

This diarthrodial facet joint is an important anatomical region of the spine due to its biomechanical role in facilitating the articulation of the vertebrae in the spinal column [2]. Together with the intervertebral disc, the bilateral facet joints transfer loads and guide and constrain motions in the spine due to their geometry and mechanical function [2]. This mechanical behavior ensures the normal health and function of the spine during physiologic loading but can also lead to its dysfunction when the tissues of the facet joint are altered either by injury, degeneration, or as a result of surgical modification of the spine [2]. In general, the inclination angle of the articular surfaces of the facet joint in the sagittal plane ranges from 20° to 78° in the cervical region, 55° to 80° in the thoracic region, and 82° to 86° in the lumbar region [2]. The angle between the articulating surfaces in the axial plane ranges from 70° to 96°, 85° to 120°, and 15° to 70° off of the midline in the cervical, thoracic, and lumbar regions, respectively, with increasing orientation angles moving towards the lower levels in the lumbar spine [2].

Regarding the cervical zygapophysial joints, the superior facets face superoposteriorly while the inferior facets face directly inferoanteriorly [1]. The unique characteristics of the cervical vertebrae and their articulations give this region the greatest range and array of movements amongst all the vertebral regions [1]. Based upon a study done by Onan et al. in 1998 utilizing fresh frozen cervical vertebrae, they determined that isolated cervical facet joints allowed flexion up to 19°, extension up to 14°, lateral bending up to 28°, and rotation up to 17° [3]. However, this study does elaborate that joint movements within the constraints of the facet capsule were less than if the joints were isolated [3].

The thoracic zygapophysial joints have superior facets that face posteriorly and slightly laterally, while the inferior facets face anteriorly and medially [1]. The thoracic vertebrae have the least mobility of the three regions, mainly due to the attachment of the rib cage to the vertebrae, the almost vertical orientation of the facet joint, and the superimposing spinous processes [1]. These attachments limit the amount of flexion, extension, and lateral bending in the thoracic region; however, the most rotation per joint in the vertebral column is seen in the thoracic region [1].

The lumbar zygapophysial joints involve superior facets directed posteromedially with inferior facets directed anterolaterally [1]. This arrangement of facets allows for a joint that permits flexion, extension, and lateral flexion while inhibiting rotation [1]. In 2007, Serhan et al. showed that destabilization of a lumbar facet joint leading to an isolated lumbar zygapophysial joint that allowed for 12.2° of flexion-extension, increased from 8.7° with the joint intact in its capsule [4]. Lateral bending in an isolated lumbar facet joint allows for 10.2°, increased from 9.0° with the intact joint capsule [4]. Axial rotation in an isolated lumbar zygapophysial joint is 7.2°, which decreases to 3.8° in an intact lumbar facet joint [4].

The intervertebral disc is very prominent for its function as a shock absorber due to its resilient deformability; however, it is also a vertebral joint that permits movement between adjacent vertebrae [1]. Due to the fibrogelatinous nucleus pulposus occupying the center of the intervertebral disc, surrounded by the anulus fibrosus, compressive forces on the vertebral column cause the nucleus pulposus to flatten out and the anulus fibrosus to bulge. This allows the shock absorption from the weight-bearing force, such as that exhibited by standing or lifting weights, to be absorbed by the disc rather than the bony portions of the vertebral column [1]. During flexion or extension, the intervertebral disc will bulge anteriorly or posteriorly, respectively, such that the nucleus pulposus acts as a fulcrum [1]. During lateral bending, the nucleus pulposus will cause a lateral bulge towards the side of the movement.

Thus, the overall function of the facet joints is to prevent the two adjacent vertebrae joined by the facet joint from engaging in relative motions that could overload and damage any surrounding spinal structures, such as the intervertebral disc, the nerve roots exiting the spinal column, and the spinal cord itself [2]. The intervertebral disc absorbs approximately 75–97% of the compressive load applied to the lumbar spine, while 3–25% is absorbed by the posterior elements of the vertebral column; this posterior force is also known as the "facet force" [2].

6.4 Anterior Longitudinal Ligament

6.4.1 Anatomy

The anterior longitudinal ligament is composed of a strong band of collagenous fibers that extends along the anterior aspect of the vertebral column [5–8]. The anterior longitudinal ligament is attached to the basilar occipital bone rostrally, extends to the anterior tubercle of the atlas (C1) as well as the front of the body of the axis (C2), and runs caudally to the anterior of the sacrum [5]. The anterior longitudinal ligament is narrower and thicker over the vertebral bodies than when it passes over the intervertebral discs [5, 7]. The anterior longitudinal ligament is also thicker and narrower in the thoracic region than in the cervical and lumbar regions, and broadens as it travels caudally [5]. The average width of the anterior longitudinal ligament in the lumbar spine in 25 cadaveric specimens was measured to be 37.1 mm with a mean cross-sectional area of 32.4 mm^2 with a range from 10.6 to 52.5 mm^2 [9].

The anterior longitudinal ligament consists of numerous collagen fibers that are densely packed and constitute three distinct layers: superficial, intermediate, and deep [5, 6, 8]. The superficial fibers are the longest, spanning three to five vertebrae; the intermediate fibers span two to three vertebrae; and the deep fibers span from one vertebral body to the next, connecting adjacent vertebrae [5, 8]. These longitudinal fibers attach firmly to the intervertebral discs and the anterior margins of the vertebral bodies [5–7]. These fibers form looser, secondary attachments to the mid-portion of the vertebral bodies, filling their concave surfaces and flattening the appearance of the anterior surface of the vertebral column [6].

The deep fibers of the anterior longitudinal ligament blend with the periosteum at this point, while the more superficial fibers bridge the concavity [6]. The fibers from the anterior longitudinal ligament also blend with the external surface of the anulus fibrosus, which has led anatomists to have varying opinions on the origins of these fibers [6]. While some authors believe these fibers to be part of the anulus fibrosus and others feel it constitutes a "disc capsule," Bogduk demonstrated that the deep fibers of the anterior longitudinal ligament should not be considered part of the anulus fibrosus due to differences in the embryological origin of these two structures [6]. Accordingly, the fibers of the anterior longitudinal ligament have attachments to cortical bone, which is always the case with ligaments [6]. In 1997, Bogduk demonstrated that the anulus fibrosus does not attach to cortical bone but to the vertebral end plate [6]. Bogduk also illustrated some key differences in the structure of the anterior longitudinal ligament at various regions of the vertebral column, such as the thoracic region, where the anterior longitudinal ligament was not associated with any of the prevertebral muscles and therefore stood alone [6]. Another distinction was made in the lumbar spine at the point where the crura of the diaphragm attached to the first three lumbar vertebrae [6]. In this region, the tendons of the crura extend caudally beyond the three vertebrae and form much of what is described as the anterior longitudinal ligament in this region [6]. This peculiarity has led Bogduk to suggest that the anterior longitudinal ligament may, to some extent, be a continuation of a tendon attachment in addition to its ligamentous nature [6].

6.4.2 Biomechanics

The anterior longitudinal ligament functions primarily to maintain the stability of the vertebral column by restricting the motion of the spinal segments during extension [1, 6]. While Neumann et al. [10] suggested that the anterior longitudinal ligament functions during extension, lateral bending, and axial rotation, Zander et al. [11] believed that the anterior longitudinal ligament is only loaded during extension and is unloaded during other spinal column movements [10, 11]. The anterior longitudinal ligament is the strongest and largest of the spinal ligaments and is the only one that limits extension; the remaining intervertebral ligaments limit flexion movements [1, 10, 11]. In a study conducted by Neumann et al. in 1992, they found the stiffness of the anterior longitudinal ligament to be significantly greater than that of the posterior spinal ligaments [10]. They also noted that the strength of the anterior longitudinal ligament decreased slightly in subjects aged 21–43 years [10]. In a subsequent study in 1993, Neumann et al. found the mean failure loads of bone-anterior longitudinal ligament-bone complexes to be 802 Newtons (N) [12]. This result differs drastically from other studies, with mean values ranging from 330 to 473 N [12]. Neumann and colleagues explained this difference by the properties of the specimens used in their study, suggesting that the difference is due to the use of specimens from younger, presumably less sedentary subjects, whereas other studies used anterior longitudinal ligament specimens from older subjects [12]. They also found that younger anterior longitudinal ligament specimens were more than twice as strong as older specimens [12]. However, they proposed that bone mineral content is a more accurate predictor of bone-ligament-bone structural properties than is age, as there is a linear increase in ultimate force, stiffness, and energy of this complex with increasing bone density [12]. In 1992, Pintar et al. reported a mean stiffness value for the anterior longitudinal ligament in the lumbar spine to be 33.0 N/mm with a margin of 15.7 N/mm [9]. The highest values of energy to failure were observed for the anterior longitudinal ligament and the supraspinous ligament, with values ranging from 0.82–8.68 joules (J) for the anterior longitudinal ligament and 3.18–11.64 J for the supraspinous ligament [9]. According to Panjabi et al. (1982), this failure is due to the ligaments needing to withstand more force and deformation functionally [13]. Failure stresses were similar between the anterior longitudinal ligament and posterior longitudinal ligament (posterior longitudinal ligament) at 8.2–16.1 MPa and 7.2–28.4 MPa, respectively [9]. The stress and strain at failure values reported by Pintar et al. in 1992 were similar to those reported by Chazal et al. in 1985 [9, 14].

6.5 Posterior Longitudinal Ligament

6.5.1 Anatomy

The posterior longitudinal ligament (posterior longitudinal ligament) is a band of longitudinal fibers that runs within the vertebral canal along the posterior aspect of the vertebral bodies [5–8]. Rostrally, the posterior longitudinal ligament is continuous with the tectorial membrane, a broad and strong band inside the vertebral canal whose superficial and deep laminae are attached to the posterior surface of the axial body with the superficial laminae expanding as it travels rostral to the upper surface of the basilar occipital bone and attaching above the foramen magnum and blending with the cranial dura mater, and attaches to the body of the axis (C2) before extending along the vertebral column to the sacrum [5]. In the cervical and upper thoracic regions, the posterior longitudinal ligament is broad and uniform in width, measuring 10–15 mm in width, but becomes almost saw-toothed in appearance as it reaches the lower thoracic and lumbar regions [5–8]. This is because the ligament narrows as it passes over the vertebral bodies and expands over the intervertebral discs caudally [8]. In 1993, Lang described the changing course of the fibers as they reach the thoracolumbar transition; rather than running in a caudal direction and attaching to the tip of the vertebral body below, the lateral deep fibers at this level take a horizontal path and extend out to the intervertebral foramen, covering the lower half of the anulus fibrosus and attaching at its lateral opening [8]. The average width of the posterior longitudinal ligament in the lumbar spines of 21 cadaveric specimens was 33.3 mm, with a mean cross-section area of 5.2 mm^2 [9].

The fibers of the posterior longitudinal ligament are more compact than those of the anterior longitudinal ligament [7]. Between the ligamentous fibers lay the basivertebral veins and venous rami that drain them into anterior internal vertebral plexuses [5]. Early studies also describe an abundance of free and encapsulated nerve endings within the posterior longitudinal ligament [8]. Similar to the anterior longitudinal ligament, the superficial fibers of the posterior longitudinal ligament can span anywhere from three to five vertebrae, and the deepest fibers between adjacent vertebrae [5, 6]. However, these layers are more pronounced in the immediate postnatal years [5]. Examination of the layers of the posterior longitudinal ligament showed that the superficial fibers measure a length of 0.5–1.0 cm [8]. The fibers of the posterior longitudinal ligament attach more firmly to the intervertebral discs than the vertebral bodies, with deep fibers fused to the anulus fibrosus of the intervertebral disc in the adult spine and the superficial fibers being more easily separable from the deeper fibers when over the vertebral bodies [5, 8]. The deep layer of the posterior longitudinal ligament will form a narrow ligament at the middle of the vertebral body, but, as it travels caudally and approaches the upper edge of the intervertebral space, it will diverge towards the lip of the next lower vertebral body as well as a portion of the pedicle of that next lower vertebral body [8]. As per Bogduk, the deep fibers of the posterior longitudinal ligament fuse with the fibers of the anulus fibrosus but ultimately penetrate through them to attach to the posterior margins of the vertebral bodies [6]. In this way, these deep fibers act much like "paravertebral ligaments" [5].

6.5.2 Biomechanics

The posterior longitudinal ligament functions to resist hyperflexion of the vertebral column by resisting separation of the posterior ends of the vertebral bodies [1, 6]. However, due to the polysegmental nature of this ligament, its force is applied over several inter-body joints as opposed to just one [6]. The posterior longitudinal ligament also functions to prevent posterior herniation of the nucleus pulposus [1]. It contains nociceptive nerve endings and is the source of pain from intervertebral disc herniation as the anulus fibrosus impinges on the ligament [1]. Pintar et al. reported the posterior longitudinal ligament has the smallest cross-sectional area with a mean of 5.2 mm^2, compared to the other lumbar spinal ligaments [9]. This ligament had the lowest value of energy to failure, at a range of 0.07–0.33 J, as well as the least strain at failure, ranging between 11.3% and 16.2% [9]. Failure stresses were found to be similar between the anterior longitudinal ligament and posterior longitudinal ligament at 8.2–16.1 MPa and 7.2–28.4 MPa, respectively [9]. Similar values for stress and strain at failure were reported by Chazal et al. in 1985 [9, 14]. The mean stiffness value for the posterior longitudinal ligament in the lumbar spine was 20.4 ± 11.9 Nmm^{-1} [9].

6.6 Ligamentum Flavum

6.6.1 Anatomy

The ligamenta flava are a series of ligaments that connect the lamina of adjacent vertebrae to form alternating sections of the posterior wall of the vertebral canal [1, 5–7]. The ligamentum flavum are present bilaterally at each vertebral level, converging in the midline [1, 6]. This ligament's perpendicular fibers attach to the anterior surface of the lower edge of the lamina above as well as the inferior aspect of the pedicle, and descend to the posterior surface of the upper edge of the lamina below [1, 5–7, 15]. As this ligament descends inferiorly, it will divide into a medial and lateral portion with the medial portion passing to the back of the next lower lamina to attach to the rough area on the upper quarter of the posterior surface of the lamina and the lateral portion passing in front of the zygapophysial joint formed by two vertebrae that the ligament connects [6]. Inferiorly, the lateral portion of each ligament extends to the midpoint between two pedicles and forms the anterior capsule of the zygapophysial joint as it attaches to the anterior aspects of the inferior and superior articular processes of the zygapophysial joint [5, 6, 15]. In fact, the most lateral fibers will extend along the root of the superior articular process as far as the next lower pedicle to which they are attached [6]. Where the posterior margins of the ligament meet as the ligament's attachments extend from the zygapophysial capsule to where the laminae fuse to form spines, the ligament is only partially united with intervals being left for veins connecting the internal to posterior external posterior vertebral venous plexus [5]. In 1992 Pintar and colleagues measured the lumbar ligamentum flavum in 22 cadaveric specimens and found that on average, the ligamentum flavum measures 15.2 mm in length with a mean cross-sectional area of 84.2 mm^2 [9]. In the cervical region, the ligamentum flavum are thin and broad, thickening as they descend caudally with the thickest ligaments found in the lumbar region [1, 5]. The average thickness of the ligamentum flavum, both at midline and laterally, was noted to be 2–3 mm by Yong-Hing and colleagues in 1976 [15].

6.6.2 Biomechanics

The ligamentum flavum functions to oppose separation of the vertebral laminae during spinal flexion [1, 5–7]. This is accomplished by arresting abrupt flexion and aiding in restoring the vertebral column to an erect posture, thereby preserving the normal curvature of spine and protecting the intervertebral discs from injury [1, 5–7, 16]. The elastic nature of this ligament plays an important role in maintaining this function, as a collagenous ligament would be able to resist separation but would buckle when the laminae are approximated [6]. Buckling is minimal with an elastic ligament, protecting the contents of the spinal canal from damage [6]. The elastic nature of this ligament aids in restoring a flexed lumbar spine to its extended position, while the lateral division of the ligament will prevent the anterior capsule of the zygapophysial joint from being nipped within the joint capsule during movement [6]. The ligamentum flavum exerts a disc pressure of 0.7 kg/cm^2 and serves to pre-stress the intervertebral disc; however, the biological significance of this is unknown [6]. The lateral portion of the ligament prevents injury to the anterior capsule of the zygapophysial joint during movement [6]. While some believe that the ligamentum flavum (ligamentum flavum) assists in extending the spine with the help of the erector spinae muscles, Bogduk questions the importance of this ligament in producing extension movements [6, 15]. Pintar et al. reported the ligamentum flavum exhibited the greatest cross-sectional area compared to the other lumbar spinal ligaments, with a mean area of 84.2 ± 17.9 mm^2, similar to the values reported by Panjabi et al. in 1991 [9, 17]. The ligamentum flavum had the lowest overall failure stresses, ranging from 1.3 to 4.1 MPa, with findings similar to those reported by Nachemson and Evans in 1968 [9, 18]. Similar values for stress and strain at failure were reported by Chazal et al. in 1985 [9, 14]. Panjabi et al. [17] reported ligamentum flavum lengths ranging from 11.6 to 16.0 mm, which is similar to the range (13.0–18.0 mm) reported by Pintar et al. [9, 17]. The mean stiffness value for the ligamentum flavum was 27.2 ± 9.2 Nmm^{-1} [9].

There have been no reported disabilities in patients with the ligamentum flavum excised at single or multiple sites; this is most likely due to the location rather than the function of the ligament, as it lies immediately behind the vertebral canal and is therefore immediately adjacent to nervous structures within the canal [6]. The lateral extensions of the ligamentum flavum had elasticity of the medial and anterior capsule of the posterior joints that balanced the elasticity of the intervertebral disc [15].

6.7 Supraspinous Ligament

6.7.1 Anatomy

The supraspinous ligament is composed of a strong fibrous cord connecting the tips of the spinous processes of the vertebral column [1, 5–7]. Fibrocartilage has been noted to be present where the ligament attaches to the spinous process [7]. There are inconsistencies in the description of the supraspinous ligament among anatomists, with many anatomists describing the supraspinous ligament as beginning at the seventh cervical vertebra, where it merges with the nuchal ligament to extend to the occipital protuberance, and extending in a caudal direction along the length of the vertebral column to the sacrum [1, 5, 7]. As this ligament passes caudally, it will thicken and become broader in the lumbar region, where it will blend intimately with the neighboring fascia [5]. While there is no disagreement about where the ligament begins cranially, Parke, Heylings, and Bogduk all suggest that the supraspinous ligament extends caudally only as far as the fifth lumbar vertebra [5, 6, 19, 20]. According to Bogduk, the supraspinous ligament bridges the L4-L5 interspace in only 5% of individuals [6]. He suggests that the ligament ends at the third lumbar spinous process in 22% of individuals, and at L4 in the remaining 73% [6]. Caudal to L5, the supraspinous ligament is replaced by the medial tendons of the erector spinae muscle [19]. The average length of the supraspinous ligament in the lumbar spine is 25.2 mm with a mean cross-sectional area of 25.2 mm^2 based on a study of 22 cadaveric specimens [9].

The supraspinous ligament consists of three layers: superficial, middle, and deep [6]. Similar to the anterior longitudinal ligament, the superficial fibers are composed of longitudinally oriented collagen fibers and extend over three to four spinous processes [5, 6]. This layer ranges in size from a few thin bundles of fibers to very thick bundles measuring 5–6 mm in width and 3–4 mm in thickness, with the majority falling somewhere between these extremes [6]. Deep to this layer comes the middle layer, which spans two to three spinous processes, has a thickness of 1 mm, and is composed of fibers of the posterior layer of the thoracolumbar fascia and the aponeurosis of the longissimus thoracis muscle [6]. The deepest layer of supraspinous ligament connects adjacent spinous processes and consists of strong tendinous fibers of the aponeurosis of the longissimus thoracis muscle [6]. This layer is reinforced by the tendon of the multifidus muscle [6].

Given the tendinous nature of the middle and deep layers of the supraspinous ligament, Bogduk questions the validity of the supraspinous ligament as a true ligament [6].

6.7.2 Biomechanics

The supraspinous ligament functions to limit flexion, but provides little resistance to the separation of the spinous processes [6, 19]. Heylings suggests that the absence of the supraspinous ligament at the lumbosacral junction may account for the increased mobility of the spine in this region [19]. He also suggests that this absence may play a role in the etiology of low back pain and the musculoskeletal disorders that often affect the lumbosacral junction [19]. In 1999, Gudavalli and Triano used computer modeling to assess the lumbar spinal ligaments and found that the supraspinous ligament carries the greatest load during flexion, followed by the ligamentum flavum, capsular ligament, intertransverse, and interspinous ligaments [21]. They also found that the supraspinous ligament undergoes the most significant increase in length [21]. Hindle and colleagues in 1990 found that the supraspinous and interspinous ligaments carried very little load during the first half of flexion but resisted a much greater load toward the end of flexion [22]. They suggest that while these ligaments are helpful in limiting passive flexion when acting in concert with other support structures, they lack much mechanical function when isolated [22]. Due to its continuous nature, the supraspinous ligament was found to have one of the greatest original lengths, next to the anterior longitudinal ligament and posterior longitudinal ligament, compared to other spinal ligaments [9]. The highest values of energy to failure were observed for the anterior longitudinal ligament and the supraspinous ligament, with values ranging from 0.82 to 8.68 J and 3.18 to 11.64 J, respectively [9]. Pintar et al. also reported the supraspinous ligament with the highest strain at failure (70.6–115.0%) [9]. The mean stiffness value reported for the supraspinous ligament was 23.7 ± 10.9 Nmm [9].

6.8 Interspinous Ligament

6.8.1 Anatomy

The interspinous ligament is a thin and almost membranous ligament connecting adjacent vertebral spinous processes [1, 5–7]. Its attachments extend from the root to the apex of each spinous process, meeting the supraspinous ligament posteriorly and the ligamentum flavum anteriorly [1, 5, 7]. The interspinous ligament is poorly developed in the neck, elongated and narrow in the thoracic region, and thicker and broader in the lumbar region [5, 7]. There are inconsistencies in the description of the fibers of the interspinous ligament [19]. With regard to the cervical bundles, some anatomists describe these bundles of the interspinous ligament as part of the nuchal ligament, while others describe them as distinct interspinous fascicles [5]. Also, major discrepancies exist regarding the lumbar supraspinous and interspinous ligaments in man [19]. Many anatomists describe these fibers as crossing the interspinous space in a posterocaudal direction [5, 20, 23]. However, Heylings, Rissanen, Grant, and Bogduk describe the fibers as traversing in a posterocranial direction, especially in the lumbar spine, where, anteriorly, the interspinous ligament is essentially a paired structure with ligaments on each side split by a midline cavity filled with fat [6, 19, 24, 25]. However, this cavity is not present more posteriorly [6]. Pintar et al. reported the average length in of the interspinous ligament in the lumbar spine of 18 studied specimens as 16 mm with a standard deviation of 3.2, and a mean cross-sectional area of 35.1 mm^2 with a standard deviation of 15.0 [9].

Heylings in 1978 postulated that to allow the ligament to maintain a physiologically desirable degree of tensile control throughout the movement from extension to flexion but to still be stable enough to bring this movement to a halt, the ligaments needed to directed almost radially to the axis of movement as seen in the collateral ligaments of the joints in the limbs [19]. The fibers that cross the interspinous space in a posterocranial direction fulfill these criteria but if the fibers were running in the posterocaudal direction, they would either limit flexion too early if the fibers ran a straight course between their attachments, or they would be so lax in extension that the ligament would be useless in controlling in the spine except in the movement of flexion [19].

6.8.2 Biomechanics

The interspinous ligament functions along with the ligamentum flavum and supraspinous ligament to provide protection and stability to the vertebral joints and store muscular energy during movement [16]. It functions weakly to limit flexion especially in the lumbar spine; the interspinous ligament also serves to resist separation of the spinous processes because the fibers run almost perpendicular to the direction of separation of the spinous processes [6, 19]. Hindle and colleagues found that the supraspinous and interspinous ligaments carried very little load during the first half of flexion but resisted a much greater load towards the end of flexion [22]. They suggest that while these ligaments are helpful in limiting passive flexion when acting in concert with other support structures, they lack much mechanical function when isolated [22]. They also noted that when the supraspinous ligament was removed, the interspinous ligament resisted 75% of the load on its own [22]. The interspinous ligament is the only spinal ligament that is not loaded during lateral bending [11]. When compared to the other lumbar ligaments, this ligament was recorded to exhibit the lowest overall stiffness, at a value of 11.5 +/− 6.6 Nmm^{-1}, with the joint capsule giving the highest stiffness at a value of 33.9 +/− 10.7 Nmm^{-1} as well as the lowest stress value, ranging between 1.8 and 5.9 MPa [9].

6.9 Intertransverse Ligament

6.9.1 Anatomy

The intertransverse ligament is a complex ligament, interpreted in various ways, that consists of sheets of connective tissue extending from the superior border of one transverse process to the inferior border of the transverse process above [1, 5–7]. In the cervical region, this ligament consists of a few irregular and scattered fibers interspersed and within and largely replaced by the intertransverse muscles [1, 5]. The intertransverse ligament is composed of rounded fibrous cords in the thoracic region intimately blended with adjacent muscles, and thin and membranous fibers in the lumbar region [1, 5, 7]. Thus Bogduk stated the intertransverse ligament is not a true ligament but rather a membranous continuation of muscular fibers with the medial and lateral continuations comprising part of a complex fascial system that separates certain paravertebral compartments [6]. In fact, Bogduk states the only true ligament in the intertransverse area is the ligament of Bourgery; this ligament connects the base of the transverse process to the mammillary process below [6].

The intertransverse ligament is not considered a true ligament, as it lacks distinct medial and lateral borders, and its collagen fibers are not as densely packed nor are they as regularly oriented as the fibers of true ligaments [6, 26]. Another reason why this ligament has been questioned as a true ligament is that its fibrous fascicles between the transverse processes of the adjacent vertebral do not directly attach to the upper and lower transverse processes as Jiang et al. described in 1994 using a study of 32 human cadavers [26]. This study suggested that the ligament consisted of tendinous fascicles of the semispinalis thoracis muscle and tendons of the levatore costrarum longi muscle with the former fascicles arising from the transverse process and inserting via tendons into the spinous process and the latter fascicles arising from the ends of the transverse process and passing obliquely downward and laterally until eventually inserting into the outer surface of the rib caudal to the vertebrae from which it originated [26]. This hypothesis was corroborated by the fact that these fasicular fibers thought to be ligamentous fibers were inseparable from the muscular fibers during dissection of the 32 human cadavers [26]. These features suggest that the intertransverse ligament resembles a membrane, rather than a ligament with its ligamentous appearance produced by the interweaving of muscle tendons between adjacent transverse processes [26].

In the lumbar spine, the intertransverse ligament forms a septum dividing the anterior musculature from the posterior musculature in the intertransverse spaces [6]. Laterally, the ligament divides into two layers: an anterior layer of thoracolumbar fascia that covers the front of the quadratus lumborum muscle, and a posterior layer that blends with the transversus abdominis aponeurosis to form the middle layer of the thoracolumbar fascia [6]. Medially, the intertransverse ligament splits into two leaves: posterior and anterior [6]. The posterior leaf extends medially and attaches to the lateral margin of the lamina of the vertebra lying opposite to the intertransverse space while inferiorly blending with the capsule of the adjacent facet joint [6]. Meanwhile, the anterior leaf curves forward and extends over the lateral surface of vertebral bodies and blends with the lateral margins of the anterior longitudinal ligament [6]. By covering the lateral aspect of the vertebral column, the anterior leaf forms a membranous sheet that closes the outer end of the interventricular foramen [6]. As such, this anterior leaf has 2 noted perforations that transmit structures into and out of the intervertebral foramen [6]. Running through the superior opening are nerve branches to the psoas muscle, and running through the inferior opening are the anterior rami of spinal nerves, as well as spinal branches of lumbar arteries and veins [6]. Sandwiched between the posterior and anterior leaves is a wedge-shaped space called the superior articular recess that serves to accommodate movements of the sub-adjacent facet joint [6]. This recess is filled with fat that is continuous with the intra-articular in the joint below via the foramen in the superior capsule [6].

6.9.2 Biomechanics

Similar to most of the other ligaments of the subaxial spine, the intertransverse ligament is loaded during flexion [11]. The intertransverse ligament and anterior longitudinal ligament carry the highest load during lateral bending movements of the vertebral column [11]. However, the intertransverse ligament is the only ligament that is not loaded during torsion. Gudavalli and Triano assessed ligament loads using a computer model. They concluded that the supraspinous ligament undergoes the maximum increase in length during torsion, followed by the interspinous ligament, ligamentum flavum, facet capsular ligament, and finally, the intertransverse ligament [21].

6.10 Facet Capsular Ligament

6.10.1 Anatomy

The facet capsular ligament fully encases the facet joint by covering the joint in a rostral to caudal direction with a non-uniform thickness [2]. The lumbar facet capsule has been reported to be approximately 2.0 mm thick in the posterior region while being as much as 3.2 mm thick in the anterior region [2]. The superior and inferior regions of the capsule have been reported to be approximately 2.4 mm thick [2]. *Gray's Anatomy* identifies three distinct types of intracapsular structures: adipose tissue fat pads (anterosuperior, posteroinferior or a combination of the two), fibroadipose meniscoids (located at the superior or inferior pole or both poles of the capsule), and connective tissue rims (either anterior or posterior or both) [5]. While the fat pads of the facet capsules are similar to those found in many other joint capsules, the connective tissue rims of the zygapophysial joint are representative of the capsular ligament [5]. Each joint is surrounded by a thin, loose capsular ligament, which attaches to the margins of the articular processes of adjacent vertebrae [1, 7]. The average length of the capsular ligament in the lumbar spine in 24 individuals' capsular ligaments was measured to be 16.4 mm (±2.9) and an average cross-sectional area of 43.8 mm^2 (±28.3) [9].

6.10.2 Biomechanics

Together with other accessory ligaments of the vertebral column, the capsular ligaments help stabilize the vertebral column and its joints. In the cervical region, the loose nature of this ligament allows for a wide range of movement [1]. However, in the sacral spine, the capsular ligament functions to prevent the lumbar vertebrae from sliding anteriorly down the incline of the sacrum [1]. This is because the facets on S1 face posteromedially and interlock with the anterolateral-facing inferior facets of the L5 vertebra [1].

Due to the make-up of the facet capsular ligament, it can only provide mechanical resistance when the two adjacent vertebrae articulating in the zygapophysial joint undergo movement relative to one another [2]. The role of the ligament was demonstrated in studies using C3–C7 cadaveric spine segments subjected to 100 N of compression with either 2 nanometer (Nm) of sagittal bending or 5 Nm of axial torsion, before and after graded bilateral removal of the capsular ligament [2]. After removal of 50% of the facet capsule, axial rotation increased by 19% when torsion was applied, while the vertical distance between the C4 and C6 spinous processes increased by 5% under flexion [2]. The extent of axial torsion and posterior displacement increased by 25% and 32%, respectively, after 75% of the facet capsule was removed [2]. The increases in the range of motion observed after capsular transection or removal support the hypothesis that the facet capsular ligament provides a substantial contribution to constraining vertebral motion, particularly flexion and lateral bending/torsion [2].

6.11 Iliolumbar Ligament

6.11.1 Anatomy

The iliolumbar ligament is attached to the tip of the anteroinferior aspect of the L5 transverse process bilaterally, as well as the L4 transverse process in some cases. It radiates laterally to attach to the pelvis [5, 6]. The iliolumbar ligament will begin to radiate as it passes laterally from the transverse process and will split into two bands, upper and lower, to attach to the pelvis [5]. The lower bands (the lumbosacral portion of the iliolumbar ligament) will originate from the inferior aspect of the L5 transverse process and travel to the anterosuperior lateral surface of the sacrum and eventually blend in with the anterior sacroiliac ligament [5]. The upper bands will traverse laterally and attach to the inner lip of the iliac crest just anterior to the sacroiliac articulation, with the superior portion of the upper bands becoming continuous with the thoracolumbar fascia [5, 6]. The psoas major muscle surrounds the iliolumbar ligament anteriorly; the muscles occupying the vertebral groove surround the iliolumbar ligament posteriorly and superiorly by the quadratus lumborum [5].

Early anatomists postulated that the iliolumbar ligament consisted of 5 parts [6]. The anterior part was a well-developed ligamentous band who fibers span the entire anteroinferior border of the L5 transverse process (from the border of L5 vertebral body to the tip of the L5 transverse process) [6]. As the fibers from the medial end of the L5 transverse process pass laterally, they will begin to cover the fibers arising from the lateral end and the tip of the L5 transverse process, such that all the fibers become continuous as they leave the transverse process and pass posterolaterally to attach to the ilium [6]. The upper surface of this anterior bundle of the iliolumbar ligament forms the site of attachment of the ligament to the inferior portion of the quadratus lumborum muscle [6]. The superior bundle of the iliolumbar ligament is thought to be formed from the anterior and posterior thickenings of the fascia that surround the base of the quadratus lumborum muscle; these thickenings will attach to the anterosuperior border of the L5 transverse process near the lateral tip [6]. As this bundle travels laterally, it will separate to pass in front of and behind the quadratus lumborum muscle and ultimately attach to the ilium superiorly and inferiorly blend with the anterior ligament to form a channel from which the quadratus lumborum muscle arise [6]. The posterior bundle of the iliolumbar ligament arises from the tip and posterior border of the L5 transverse process and will insert into the ligamentous area of the ilium behind the origin of the quadratus lumborum; of a unique side note, the deepest fibers of the longissimus lumborum arise from the posterior bundle of the iliolumbar ligament [6]. The fourth part of the iliolumbar ligament is the inferior bundle, which arises from the lower border of the transverse process and the body of L5 vertebra [6]. These fibers will pass downwards and laterally across the surface of the anterior sacroiliac ligament to attach to the superoposterior part of the iliac fossa [6]. To distinguish these fibers from the anterior sacroiliac ligament, one needs to observe the oblique orientation of the inferior bundle of the iliolumbar ligament [6]. The final portion of the iliolumbar ligament is the vertical bundle, which arises from the anteroinferior border of the L5 transverse process and will descend almost vertically to attach to the posterior end of the iliopectineal line of the pelvis [6]. The significance of this bundle is that it forms the lateral margin of the channel through which the L5 anterior ramus enters the pelvis [6].

According to Bogduk, a recent study confirmed the presence of the anterior and posterior parts of the iliolumbar ligament but denied the existence of the superior part, while not commenting on the inferior and vertical parts [6]. This study states that the superior part is actually the anterior fascia of the quadratus lumborum muscle and, as such, lacks the characteristic features of a true ligament, which includes oriented collagen fibers passing directly from one bone to another [6]. The vertical and inferior bundles of the iliolumbar ligament were overlooked as part of the anterior sacroiliac ligament because these bundles attach to the lumbar portion and ilium and not the sacrum and ilium as previously thought; thus these bundles are now thought to deserve the name “iliolumbar ligament” and not “anterior sacroiliac ligament” [6].

In 1998, Hanson et al. found that the mean length of the iliolumbar ligament in Caucasians was approximately 33.2 mm while the length in African Americans was approximately 61.8 mm [27]. These differences were also observed to be true in both sexes, i.e., African American females had iliolumbar ligaments that were longer than those of Caucasian females [27].

Thus, the numerous insertions and fiber directions of the iliolumbar ligament suggest a diversity of biomechanical functions for the iliolumbar ligament [28].

6.11.2 Biomechanics

The iliolumbar ligament is the most important ligament to restraining excess movement and to maintaining stability at the lumbosacral junction [28, 29]. The iliolumbar ligament is composed of two bands, the anterior and posterior bands, both of which serve different functions [29]. While its overall function is multifocal, the iliolumbar ligament as a whole is thought to be a ligament that prevents forward sliding of the L5 vertebrae onto the sacrum [6]. The anterior band of the iliolumbar ligament is thought to be responsible for “squaring” the L5 vertebrae on the sacrum and preventing the tilt of the vertebrae in the coronal plane as well as to prevent lateral bending. In contrast, the posterior band is thought to prevent anterior slipping of the L5 vertebrae over the sacrum during weight-bearing movements, as well as helping to resist forward bending [6, 29, 30]. Together with the strong intervertebral disc, the iliolumbar ligament helps stabilize the lumbosacral junction and may have a significant role in maintaining the lumbosacral stability in patients with lumbosacral pathology [6, 29].

During flexion, the iliolumbar ligament will significantly limit the anterior displacement of the L5 vertebra [30]. When the iliolumbar was divided bilaterally, there was a 77.5% increase noted in anterior flexion of L5, with the posterior bands accounting for the majority, approximately 61.2%, of the increase, and the anterior bands contributing only a small amount to the anterior stability of the L5 [30]. Meanwhile, during extension, a 20.41% increase in flexion of L5 was noted after bilateral division of the ligament; however, in this case, it was the anterior band that contributed to all the stability during extension [30]. Lateral bending with bilateral division of the ligament resulted in a dramatic 141.7% increase in flexion of L5 during contralateral bending, with much of this increase attributed to the anterior bands [30]. During torsion of the L5 vertebrae, division of the iliolumbar ligament did not produce much change in the flexion of L5, but both bands together did restrict torsion by 5.3% [30]. These results by Sims and Moorman suggest that the iliolumbar ligament plays a very insignificant role in limiting the displacement of L5 onto the sacrum during torsion, thus suggesting that other structures are primarily responsible for limiting this displacement during torsion [30].

Yamamoto et al. performed in vitro studies on four fresh cadavers of males aged 25–45 (total of 8 ligament specimens) to evaluate the biomechanical function of the iliolumbar ligament both intact and after transection of the ligament [31]. This study involved applying a load of 10 N-m to the intact iliolumbar ligament, a right transected iliolumbar ligament, and bilateral transected iliolumbar ligaments, with the movements of the vertebral column tested before and after the transaction [31]. Flexion increased by 0.9° or approximately 12% after removal of right iliolumbar ligament and by 1.7° or approximately 23% after bilateral iliolumbar ligament removal [31]. Extension increased by 0.6° (11%) with right iliolumbar ligament transection and by 1.1° (20%) with bilateral iliolumbar ligament transaction [31]. The iliolumbar ligaments significantly restricted the motion of the vertebral column to the contralateral side when subjected to a torsional load [31]. Thus bilateral iliolumbar ligaments will significantly restrict the movements of the lumbosacral junction in the directions of flexion and extension with a slight increase in destabilization seen with unilateral transection and a statistically significant increase in destabilization seen with bilateral transection; however, when comparing all the movements of flexion, extension, right and left lateral bending, and right and left axial rotation, the iliolumbar ligament seems to be most effect in resisting lateral bending of the vertebral column [31].

In addition to stabilizing the lumbosacral junction, the iliolumbar ligament may also play an important role in stabilizing the sacroiliac joint by restraining excess movement and thus possibly helping to prevent the onset of low back pain [28, 32]. In his 2003 study, Pool-Goudzwaard defined stability as the ability of a joint to bear loading forces without allowing for any uncontrolled displacements [32]. He states that the ligaments of this lumbopelvic and sacroiliac region contribute to stability by controlling the relative positions of the joint, thus restricting the joint to only those positions that the joint can handle when loading forces are applied [32]. The existence of the sacroiliac part of the iliolumbar ligament, verified by MRI and cryosectioning of the pelvis in coronal and transverse planes, reinforces the thinking that the iliolumbar ligament has a direct restraining effect on movements in the sacroiliac joints [28]. In 2001, Pool-Goudzwaard et al. studied 12 human specimens and applied incremental moment to the sacroiliac joint to induce rotation in the sagittal plane [28, 32]. The results of this study indicated that the sacroiliac joint mobility in the sagittal plane increased monumentally after the total transection of both iliolumbar ligaments, with most of the increase seen after cutting the anterior band of the ligament [32]. This suggests that the iliolumbar ligaments restrict sacroiliac joint mobility in the sagittal plane, with the anterior band of the iliolumbar ligament contributing to most of this restriction [32]. What seems strange is that the locality of the anterior band of the iliolumbar ligament seems to draw skepticism as to how this band can restrict the sacroiliac joint's mobility in the sagittal plane [32]. However, Pool-Goudzwaard explained in his 2003 study that postulated that this phenomenon could be due to the orientation of the auricular surfaces of the sacroiliac joint with respect to the fiber direction of the anterior band of the iliolumbar ligament [32]. The shape of the sacrum is a wedge, with the anterior aspect of the sacrum being larger than the posterior aspect of the sacrum [32]. With the auricular surfaces of sacroiliac joint being oriented posteromedially and anterolaterally, one would expect most of the restriction from the ligaments during sagittal rotation of the sacroiliac joint to be parallel to this orientation of the auricular surfaces [32]. Since the most anterior fibers of the anterior band of the iliolumbar ligament are arranged more parallel to the auricular surfaces of the sacroiliac joint compared to the fibers of the other components of the iliolumbar ligament, loading of the anterior band of the iliolumbar ligament is likely to be stimulated by sacroiliac rotation in the sagittal plane [32].

While several recent studies of the lumbopelvic region have demonstrated support for the hypothesis that loss of the stability of the sacroiliac joints is crucial in the etiology of non-specific low back pain, it is now believed that a variety of factors in addition to loss of ligamentous support such as decrease in muscle forces and dysfunction of the mechanoreceptors in the ligamentous system of the lumbosacral area that are important for activation of the muscles necessary for posture control all play a role in the development of non-specific low back pain [32].

6.12 Costovertebral/Costotransverse Joint

The costovertebral and costotransverse joints are the articulations that connect the 12 pairs (24 total) of ribs to the thoracic vertebrae. When these ribs attach to the bodies of the thoracic vertebrae, they attach at two separate places on the rib, the head and the tubercle of the rib [1]. Where the head attaches to the thoracic vertebrae, it will attach to two convex facets that are from adjacent vertebrae [1]. The head of the rib will articulate with the superior costal facet of the corresponding vertebrae as well as the inferior costal facet of the vertebrae superior to it [1]. The crest of the head of the rib will articulate with the corresponding intervertebral disc [1]. Due to this bi-vertebral attachment, a synovial (gliding) joint is formed that contributes to the mobility of ribs to allow for expansion and retraction during the process of breathing [1]. However, regarding the heads of ribs 1, 10, 11, and 12, they will only articulate with a single vertebra, T1, T10, T11, and T12, respectively [5].

Meanwhile the tubercle of the rib articulates with facets on the tips of the transverse process of the vertebrae that matches its numbering, i.e., the head of the sixth rib will articulate with the superior costal facet of the T6 vertebral body and inferior costal facet of the T5 vertebral body as well as the intervertebral disc between T5 and T6 vertebral bodies and the tubercle of the sixth rib will articulate with the transverse process of the sixth rib [1]. This joint is referred to as the costotransverse joint and is also a synovial joint [1]. Just as there is an exception for the rib heads articulations, there is such an exception for the tubercles of the ribs, as the 11th and 12th ribs do not articulate with the transverse processes and as a result have freer movements [5].

To inhibit many movements and allow for just slight gliding movements through the costovertebral and costotransverse joints, several strong costotransverse ligaments constrain these joints [1]. The articular surfaces on the tubercles of the superior 6 ribs are convex and will fit into the concavities on the transverse processes, allowing for rotation around a transverse axis [1]. This results in elevation and depression movements of the sternal ends of the ribs and the sternum in the sagittal plane, a dynamic that is known as a pump-handle movement [1]. The gliding movements seen as a result of the articulations of the 7th–tenth ribs' flat tubercles with the transverse processes of T7-T10 allow for elevation and depression of the lateral-most portions of these ribs in the transverse plane, resulting in the so-called bucket-handle movement [1]. These movements in conjunction with one another during inspiration will increase the AP and transverse diameter of the thorax, allowing for expansion of the cavity that will draw air into the lungs [1].

The fibrous capsules of the heads of ribs are composed of short and strong fibers that connect the costal heads to the circumference of articular surfaces formed by interventricular discs and demifacets of adjacent vertebrae [1, 5, 7]. There are 12 fibrous capsules on each side of the body (1 for each rib head), equaling a total of 24 fibrous capsules. The fibrous capsule is the strongest in the anterior section, a site where the fibrous capsule will form a radiate ligament of the head of the rib [1]. However, the capsule is most distinct at the superior and inferior portions of the costal head articulation [7]. The upper fibers will traverse the corresponding intervertebral foramina to blend with the posterior aspects of the intervertebral discs to form a symphysis, also known as an amphiarthrosis, which is a slightly movable joint [5]. Meanwhile, the posterior fibers are continuous with the costotransverse ligaments [5].

6.13 Radiate Ligament of the Costovertebral Joint

6.13.1 Anatomy

The costovertebral radiate ligament fans out from the anterior portion of the head of a rib to connect the rib to the bodies of two adjacent vertebrae as well as the intervertebral disc between the two adjacent vertebral bodies [1, 5, 7]. This ligament consists of three flat fasciculi, which are attached to the anterior part of the head of the rib just beyond the articular surface [5]. The superior fasciculus ascends to the vertebral body above, while the inferior fasciculus ascends to the vertebral body below the articulation [5]. Meanwhile, the intermediate fasciculus has the shortest and least distinct fibers of the three fasciculi, with the fibers running horizontally and attaching to the corresponding intervertebral disc [1].

Some exceptions to this attachment do exist. For example, regarding the first rib, the radiate ligament, which is not divided into the three fasciculi, will attach to the C7 vertebral body and the T1 vertebral body [5]. Regarding the joints of the 10th–12th rib heads, which only articulate with a single vertebral body, the ligament does not have the tri-fascicular arrangement [5]. Instead, the fibers of the ligament will attach to the vertebral body above the corresponding rib, as well as the corresponding rib, i.e., the 11th rib radiate ligament will attach to the T10 vertebral body as well as the 11th rib [5].

The radiate ligaments are located along the spinal column and, as such, have a relationship with neurovascular structures in this area [7]. The radiate ligament is situated anterior to the thoracic ganglia of the sympathetic trunk and the pleura [7]. On the right side of the body, the radiate ligaments are located anterior to the azygos vein [7]. Located posterior to the radiate ligaments at each vertebral level are the inter-articular ligaments and the synovial membranes [7].

6.13.2 Biomechanics

The radiate ligament connects the rib head to the vertebral bodies so closely that only slight gliding movements will occur at the facets [1]. Even with this tight connection, the slightest movement here may produce a relatively large excursion of the distal/sternal/anterior end of a rib [1].

6.14 Intra-articular Ligament of the Head of Rib

6.14.1 Anatomy

The intra-articular (inter-articular in older texts) ligament of the head of the rib is a short and flat ligament that attaches the crest of the head of the rib to the intervertebral disc within the joint capsule [1, 5, 7]. This ligament will attach laterally to the crest of the head of the rib, separating the costal articular facets, and will attach medially to the intervertebral disc; in fact, this ligament will divide the joint space into two synovial cavities [1, 5, 7]. This ligament, however, is not seen in the first rib head's joint capsule as well as the 10th–12th rib head's joint capsule [1, 5, 7]. These ribs' heads will articulate with their corresponding vertebral bodies without the use of an intra-articular ligament [1]. Thus, in these four ribs stated above, there is only one synovial cavity in the joint, as well as only one synovial membrane [7].

6.14.2 Biomechanics

While the main function of the intra-articular ligament of the head of the rib is to divide the joint capsule into two synovial cavities, the intra-articular ligament will act as the axis around which rotation will occur [1]. While the costotransverse ligaments will limit movements of the ribs to slight gliding, the articular surfaces on the tubercles of the superior six ribs are convex and, as such, will fit into the concavities on the transverse processes of the vertebrae [1]. As a result, rotation will occur around a transverse axis that traverses the intra-articular ligament and the head and neck of the rib that results in elevation and depression movements of the sternal ends of the ribs and the sternum in the sagittal plane; this movement is the pump-handle movement responsible for assisting in increasing the anterior-posterior diameter of the chest during inspiration [1].

6.15 Superior Costotransverse Ligament

6.15.1 Anatomy

The superior costotransverse ligament is a broad ligament, with a varied texture ranging from a woven/membrane-like texture to a tendon-like texture, that joins the crest of the neck of the rib to the transverse process superior to the rib [1, 26]. With its fibers oriented superolaterally to inferomedially except for a small bundle that runs inferolaterally, the superior costotransverse ligament connects the transverse process superior to the rib to the costal neck, with the rib already being connected to its corresponding transverse process by two separate joints, the lateral costotransverse ligament, the costotransverse ligament, and the radiate ligament [26]. The superior costotransverse ligament, classified as a true ligament, is sometimes divided by anatomists into a strong "anterior costotransverse ligament" and a weak "posterior costotransverse ligament" between which the levator costae and external intercostal muscles lie [1, 7, 26]. The anterior portion will attach between the crest of the costal neck and the lower aspect of the transverse process above the rib, with its lateral end blending in with the internal intercostal membrane as it is crossed by the intercostal vessels and nerve, and its medial border forming a free edge [5, 26]. While Jiang did not mention the existence of a posterior layer, *Gray's Anatomy* states the posterior layer will attach on the posterior surface of costal neck and ascend posteromedially to the transverse process above, with its lateral end blending in the external intercostal muscles [5, 26]. The aperture bounded by this ligament and the vertebrae permits the passage of the spinal nerve as well as the posterior branch of the intercostal artery [1]. Posterior to this ligament passes the posterior ramus of the thoracic nerve, while the anterior ramus of the intercostal nerve passes anterior to the superior costotransverse ligament [7].

However, on the first rib, no superior costotransverse ligament exists [5] and on the shaft of the 12th rib near its head arises the lumbocostal ligament, which will attach to the base of the 1st lumbar transverse process; this lumbocostal ligament is located in series with the superior costotransverse ligaments [5].

The superior costotransverse ligament is the only spinal ligament that will connect adjacent vertebrae on the lateral aspect of the spine; the lateral costotransverse ligament will only connect the transverse process to its own rib [26]. Jiang found that the average length of the superior costotransverse ligament did not differ with sex but did increase significantly as one moves down the vertebral levels with an average length of 8 +/− 2 mm at T7 vertebral level and an average length of 13 +/− 3 mm at T10 vertebral level [26]. The average cross-sectional area between the levels was found to be 5 +/− 2 mm^2 at T7 level and 8 +/− 5 mm^2 at T10 level [26].

6.15.2 Biomechanics

The superior costotransverse ligament, along with the costotransverse and lateral costotransverse ligament, binds the costotransverse joint, which limits these joints' movements to slight gliding [1]. However, the superior costotransverse ligament was found by Jiang et al. to have the characteristics appropriate for involvement in the active lateral balancing of the spine [26]. The fact that the superior costotransverse ligament is the only ligament that connects adjacent vertebrae on the lateral aspect of the spine further reaffirms its importance in maintaining lateral stability between adjacent vertebrae [26]. In their 1994 study, Jiang et al. provided evidence that the superior costotransverse ligament plays a role in maintaining lateral spine balance, which is only evident in species with a bipedal stance [26]. They tested the spinal ligaments of quadrupeds, including dogs, rats, mice, and hamsters, and found that these species lack superior costotransverse ligaments [26]. They concluded that the spines of quadrupeds do not require the balance laterally that bipedal organisms so require; as such, there may be no need for the superior costotransverse ligament in quadrupeds [26]. Because of the lack of supplementary structure of the lateral aspect of the spine, the costotransverse ligament is susceptible to damage from excessive strain [26].

6.16 Costotransverse Ligament

6.16.1 Anatomy

The costotransverse ligament is a ligament composed of many short fibers that stretch from the rough posterior aspect neck of the rib to the anterior aspect of the adjacent transverse process thus filling the costotransverse foramen [1, 5, 7]. However, as seen with other ribs, some exceptions exist with the costotransverse ligament. In the 11th and 12th ribs, the costotransverse ligament is either rudimentary or completely absent [5].

6.16.2 Biomechanics

The costotransverse ligament will strengthen the anterior aspect of the costotransvserse joint [1].

6.17 Lateral Costotransverse Ligament

6.17.1 Anatomy

The lateral costotransverse ligament is a short but strong, thick ligament that passes obliquely from the posterior apex of the transverse process to the rough non-articular part of the adjacent costal tubercle [1, 5, 7]. Each of these true ligaments, as it travels superiorly and laterally from the transverse process to the rib tubercle, forms an acute angle with the vertical line of the spine [26]. The lateral costotransverse ligament of the upper ribs, which are shorter and more oblique compared to the lateral costotransverse ligament of the lower ribs, will ascend from the transverse processes. In comparison, the lateral costotransverse ligament of the lower ribs will descend from the transverse processes [5].

6.17.2 Biomechanics

The lateral costotransverse ligament will strengthen the posterior aspect of the costotransverse joint. In contrast, the costotransverse ligament will strengthen the anterior aspect of the costotransverse joint, as previously stated in the paper [1]. Because of the connection between the ribs and the transverse processes, these ligaments formed a rigid bond compared to the bond formed by the connection between the upper transverse processes and the lower ribs by the superior costotranverse ligament [26]. Due to this almost rigid connection, the lateral costotranverse ligament does not appear to allow for very much flexibility [26]. However, this ligament did not seem to have the characteristics necessary for significant involvement in the active lateral balancing of the spine [26]. As such, this ligament is unlikely to be strained during lateral bending of the spine [26].

6.18 Accessory Ligament

6.18.1 Anatomy

The accessory ligament, if present, is usually medial to the superior costotransverse ligament [5]. While it is variable in its attachments, the bands of the ligament will usually pass from a depression located on the rib medial to a costal tubercle and span to the inferior articular process immediately above this depression [5]. However, some fibers of the ligament will also pass to the base of the transverse process [5]. To differentiate this ligament from the superior costotransverse ligament, one must look for the posterior ramus of a thoracic spinal nerve and its accompanying vessels, as these structures will clearly demarcate the separation of these two ligaments from one another [5].

6.18.2 Biomechanics

The major function of the accessory ligament is to strengthen the costovertebral joint [5].

6.19 Sacroiliac Joint

6.19.1 Anatomy

The sacroiliac joint is an extremely strong joint in the pelvis between the sacrum and the ilium of the pelvis joined by strong ligaments such as anterior, interosseous, and posterior sacroiliac ligaments [1]. The sacroiliac joints link and support the axial skeleton, i.e., the vertebral column, with the inferior appendicular skeleton, i.e., the skeleton of the lower limb [1]. These weight-bearing joints, located on the left and the right side of the body, consist of anterior synovial joints and posterior syndesmotic joints [1]. The anterior synovial joint is formed between the sacrum's ear-shaped auricular surfaces, which are irregular but have congruent elevations and depressions that interlock, and the ilium and is covered with articular cartilage [1]. The sacroiliac joints differ from most synovial joints in that very limited mobility is allowed, which is a consequence of their role in transmitting the weight of most of the body to the hipbones [1]. Meanwhile, the posterior syndesmosis joint is formed between the tuberosities of the same bones [1]. The sacroiliac joints are covered by two different kinds of cartilage: hyaline cartilage covering the sacral surface and fibrocartilage covering the ilial surface [33].

The surfaces of the sacroiliac joints start out flat or planar in early life; however, as we begin walking, the sacroiliac joint surfaces begin to form distinct angular orientations while losing their planar or flat landscape [34]. These joints will also develop an elevated ridge along the ilial surface and a depression along the sacral surface, which, along with the very strong ligaments, increase the sacroiliac joints' stability and make dislocations very rare [34].

6.19.2 Biomechanics

The sacroiliac joints' function is mainly that of shock absorption for the spine as well as weight transfer from the trunk and upper limbs to the lower limbs. However, the amount of this shock absorption depends on the amount of available motion at the sacroiliac joint [35]. Motion at the sacroiliac joint is limited by the interlocking of the articulating bones and the sacroiliac ligaments to slight gliding and rotary movements [1]. During weight-bearing exercises, tremendous force is transmitted through the lumbar vertebrae bodies to the superior end of the sacrum, which is pushed inferiorly and anteriorly because the weight transfer occurs anterior to the axis of the sacroiliac joint [1]. Despite the rotation of the superior sacrum, the sacrum's movement is counterbalanced by strong ligaments that anchor the inferior end of the sacrum to the ischium thus preventing any superior and posterior rotation of the inferior sacrum [1]. By preventing too much upward movement of the inferior sacrum relative to the hip bones, resilience is provided to the sacroiliac region when the vertebral columns sustain sudden increases in force or weight [1].

In addition to shock absorption, the sacroiliac joint also facilitates torque conversion, enabling transverse rotations in the lower limbs to be transmitted up the spine. This provides a "self-locking" mechanism that helps with stability during the push-off phase of walking as the joint will lock on one side as weight is transferred from one leg to the other through the sacrum to the other hip bone [35]. Motion of the sacroiliac joint is limited to minute amounts of rotation and translation about the three major axes with normal ranges for rotation equal to approximately 2° in males and 2–4° in females (allowing for increased mobility during parturition) [36]. Movements of the sacroiliac joint were identified using motion palpation, passive motion, and provocation tests, as analyzed in 25 patients with sacroiliac disorders [37]. Sturesson et al. determined that the mean maximal mobility between end points in flexion and extension on each sacroiliac joint was 2.5° ± 0.5° (1.6–3.9°), and a mean translation of 0.7 mm (0.1–1.6 mm) along the axes of rotation [37].

There are five major motions of the sacroiliac joint. Two of these movements are the anterior and posterior tilt of both hipbones on the sacrum, in which both the left and right coxal bones move together as a unit in the anterior or posterior direction, respectively [35]. Another movement is an anterior tilt of one hipbone while the opposite hipbone tilts posteriorly on the sacrum; this movement is seen during gait [35]. During sacral flexion, the motion of the sacrum will occur simultaneously with the motion of the ilium, while sacral extension involves opposite movements of the sacrum and the ilium [35].

6.20 Anterior Sacroiliac Ligament

6.20.1 Anatomy

The anterior sacroiliac ligament is the anterior part of the fibrous capsule of the synovial part of the joint [1]. This ligament is considered to be just an antero-inferior capsular thickening covering the anterior aspect of the joint [5, 6, 24]. While the ligament is mostly thin in nature, it is particularly well developed near the arcuate line and posterior inferior iliac spine, where it will connect the third sacral segment to the lateral side of the preauricular sulcus [5]. The ligament consists of long and transversely oriented fibers that extend from the ala and the anterior surface of the sacrum to the anterior surface of the ilium [6]. These ligamentous fibers are attached to these bony landmarks for considerable distances beyond the margins of the joint [6].

6.20.2 Biomechanics

While the anterior sacroiliac ligament binds the ilium to the sacrum, it can prevent diastasis of the sacroiliac joint due to its anterior location [6]. However during pregnancy, relaxation of the sacroiliac ligaments due to the effects of the hormone relaxin causes the interlocking mechanism of the sacroiliac joint to become less rigid thus allowing greater rotation of the pelvis during parturition; in addition, this relaxation will also help contribute to the lordotic posture assumed during pregnancy with the change in the center of gravity during childbirth [1], but this relaxation of the ligaments of the sacroiliac joint is not just limited to the pelvis because of the increased possibility of other joint dislocations late during pregnancy [1].

6.21 Interosseous Sacroiliac Ligament

6.21.1 Anatomy

While the interosseous sacroiliac ligament is not officially recognized as a true ligament, it may be the most important ligament of the sacroiliac joint [5, 6]. This is the largest syndesmotic joint, a fibrous articulation in which bony surfaces are bound together by an interosseous ligament, a slender fibrous cord, or an aponeurotic membrane that allows for slight movement between the attachments, in the body and lies deep in the narrow recess between the sacrum and ilium posterior to the cavity of the joint [5, 6]. This "ligament," which consists of a dense and thick collection of short collagen fibers, is the major bond between the ligamentous surfaces of the sacrum and ilium, filling the irregular space posterosuperior to the sacroiliac joint [5, 6]. While the posterior sacroiliac ligament covers this ligament superficially, its deeper part has superior and inferior bands that pass from depressions posterior to the sacral auricular surface to depressions on the iliac tuberosity [5]. The superior band of the interosseous sacroiliac ligament will connect the superior articular process and the lateral crest of the first two sacral segments to the neighboring ilium [5, 6]. This superior band is thusly termed the "short posterior sacroiliac ligament" as it acts in concert with the interosseous connection between the ilium and the sacrum to prevent posterior diastasis of the joint [5, 6]. To fully appreciate the actual thickness of this ligament, one must look at transverse sections of the sacrum and ilium where this ligament is most clearly evident grossly [6].

6.21.2 Biomechanics

The primary function of the interosseous sacroiliac ligament is to firmly bind the ilium to the sacrum to form a secure bony interlocking mechanism that inhibits excessive movement between the sacrum and the ilium [6]. Thus, this interosseous sacroiliac ligament tightly binds the primary structures involved in transferring the weight of the upper body from the axial skeleton (vertebral column and sacrum) to the two ilia of the appendicular skeleton [1].

6.22 Posterior Sacroiliac Ligament

6.22.1 Anatomy

The posterior sacroiliac ligament is the chief ligament involved in the union of the sacrum and the ilium [5]. While overlying the interosseous ligament, the posterior sacroiliac ligament has numerous fasciculi that run in multiple directions [5, 6]. It will connect the intermediate and the lateral sacral crests to the posterior superior iliac spine and the posterior end of the internal lip of the iliac crest [5, 6]. As a posterior external continuation of the same mass of fibrous tissue, fibers of the posterior sacroiliac ligament and the interosseous ligament run obliquely superolaterally from the sacrum [1].

The posterior sacroiliac ligament consists of an upper part, or a short posterior sacroiliac ligament, and a lower part, or a long posterior sacroiliac ligament (LPSL) [5]. The upper part consists of nearly horizontal fibers that pass from the first and second transverse tubercles on the back of the sacrum to the tuberosity of the ilium [5]. Meanwhile, the lower part's fibers are oblique in direction and run from the transverse tubercle between the third and fourth sacral segments on the back of the sacrum to the posterior superior spine of the ilium and the posterior end of the internal lip of the iliac crest [5, 6, 38]. The lower part or long posterior sacroiliac ligament is continuous laterally with part of the sacrotuberous ligament and medially with the thoracolumbar fascia's posterior lamina [5].

In 2009, McGrath et al. conducted histological experiments on the long posterior sacroiliac ligament, which showed that this part of the sacroiliac ligament is divided into three morphologically distinct regions [38]. Two of these regions were attached to osseous structures: the posterior superior iliac spine superiorly and the third sacral transverse tubercle inferiorly [38]. Between the proximal and distal regions of osseous attachment, the middle portion of the long posterior sacroiliac ligament, i.e., the third region of the long posterior sacroiliac ligament, was observed to be a confluence of three layers: the erectors spinae aponeurosis, the "deep fasical layer," and the gluteal aponeurosis [38]. The lateral branches of the posterior sacral rami (medial clunial nerves) were found to be within a layer of adipose and loose connective tissue that lies deep to the "deep fascial layer" with the middle posterior sacroiliac ligament providing a pathway for these rami between the posterior sacral region and the gluteal region [38]. With the discovery of these morphological findings, a possible pathoanatomical basis for localized pain in the posterior sacroiliac region due to an entrapment neuropathy of the lateral branches of the middle clunial nerves was discovered [38].

Running among the posterior sacroiliac ligaments are the posterior rami of the sacral spinal nerves, which innervate the ligament, and vessels with the lateral branches of the first three sacral posterior rami sharing an intimate relationship with the long posterior sacroiliac ligament and the sacrotuberous ligament [5, 38, 39]. The lateral division of the S1 nerve will pass deep into the long posterior sacroiliac ligament and run between this ligament and the sacroiliac joint [39]. Meanwhile, the lateral branches of S2 and S3 unite and pass through a tunnel created by the sacrotuberous ligament and an outer sheath of thoracolumbar fascia [39].

6.22.2 Biomechanics

The major function of the posterior sacroiliac ligament is to unite the sacrum and the ilium [1]. Due to the fibers of the interosseous and posterior sacroiliac ligaments being obliquely oriented superolaterally from the sacrum, the axial weight pushing down on the sacrum will actually pull the ilium medially so that the ligaments compress the sacrum between them [1]. This will lock the irregular but congruent surfaces of the sacroiliac joints together along with some help from the iliolumbar ligaments [1]. In fact, it is the long posterior sacroiliac ligament that prevents backward rocking (counter-nutation) of the sacrum with respect to the ilium [6].

6.23 Sacrotuberous Ligament

6.23.1 Anatomy

The sacrotuberous ligament attaches the sacrum, ilium, and the coccyx to the ischial tuberosity [24]. The posterior part of this ligament will originate cranially at the sacrum and insert caudally at the ischial tuberosity while the anterior part of this ligament will originate caudally at the sacrum and insert cranially at the ischial tuberosity; as a result, the sacrotuberous ligament is considered to be composed of two triangles that connect at their tips [40]. The sacrotuberous ligament is formed from the inferior portions of the posterior sacroiliac ligaments as well as fibers extending from the posterior margin of the ilium (between the posterior superior and posterior inferior iliac spines) and the base of the coccyx [1]. The sacrotuberous ligament arises from the transverse tubercles of the lower sacral segments, from the lateral margin of the sacrum where it will blend with the sacrospinous ligament, and broadly from the posterior superior iliac spine (PSIS) where it will blend with the long posterior sacroiliac ligament [5, 6]. From this very broad origin, the ligament's oblique fibers will descend laterally to form a thick, narrow band which will widen again as it traverses laterally to attach to the medial margin of the ischial ramus/tuberosity [5, 6]. As this ligament passes the posterior ilium and the lateral sacrum and coccyx on its way to its attachment on the ischial tuberosity, the sciatic notch of the hipbone is transformed into a large sciatic foramen [1]. Where the ligament attaches to the ischial tuberosity is called the "falciform process," whose concave edge blends with the fascial sheath of the internal vessels and pudendal nerve [5].

In 2009, Hammer et al. determined that the sacrotuberous ligament in men had a mean length of 64 mm and 70 mm in women [40].

There are various muscle fibers that are continuous with the sacrotuberous ligament. Superficial fibers of this ligament are continuous with the tendon of the biceps femoris, while fibers of the posterior surface of this ligament are attached to the lowest fibers of the gluteus maximus [5, 6, 41]. It was also found that a thin fascia covering the posterior aspect of the piriformis muscle was continuous with the sacrotuberous ligament [41]. The attachment of these muscles (gluteus maximus, biceps femoris long head) to the sacrotuberous ligaments can dynamically influence the movement and stability of sacroiliac joints [42].

The coccygeal branches of the inferior gluteal artery, the perforating cutaneous nerve, and filaments of the coccygeal plexus all perforate the sacrotuberous ligament [5]. In addition to sharing an intimate relationship with the long posterior sacroiliac ligament, the lateral branches of the first three sacral posterior rami are involved with the sacrotuberous ligament [39]. As mentioned earlier in the paper, the lateral division of S1 passes deep into long posterior sacroiliac ligament, coursing between it and the sacroiliac joint; however pressure on or swelling of the LPSL is not only capable of compressing the S1 nerve but also the S2 and S3 since these nerves also pass in close proximity to this ligament [39]. Such pressure could even compromise the microvasculature that accompanies these nerves, thus potentially creating ischemic zones, which could represent the origin of local tenderness when this LPSL ligament is palpated during physical examination [39]. The lateral branches of the S2 and S3 will unite and pass through a tunnel created by the sacrotuberous ligament internally and an outer sheath of thoracolumbar fascia externally; compression of this tunnel by congestion or edema could also potentially result in low back or buttock pain [39].

6.23.2 Biomechanics

Due to the orientation of the sacrotuberous ligament fibers, upward tilting of the lower end of the sacrum, i.e., nutation, is prevented due to its anchoring to the ischium along with the sacrospinous ligament [6, 42]. The sacrotuberous ligament rotates from its origin at the sacrum towards its insertion at the ischial tuberosity as cited by multiple authors such as Fick in 1904, Waldeyer and Fangha¨nel in 2003 and Kapandji and Koebke in 2006 [40]. An interesting fact about the sacrospinous and sacrotuberous ligaments is that both are remnants of tail muscles seen in primates [40]. Since the ligaments unroll like a contorted rope under tension, the sacrotuberous ligament will raise the ischium in relation to the sacrum while the sacrospinous will lower the ischium in relation to the sacrum; since these ligaments do not rotate in the same direction, it is assumed that the ligaments exert oppositional effects on the pelvis [40]. Even though these two ligaments have opposite effects, they are still considered to be a couple as both are very closely correlated with regard to the volumes and cross-sectional areas of both ligaments [40].

The sacrotuberous ligament can be tensed using the infamous straight leg raise test, which causes shortening of the muscles [41]. The straight leg raise test alters the position of the sacrum because the sacrotuberous ligament bridges the sacroiliac joint [41]. Lavignolle et al. demonstrated that the straight leg raise test causes distinct movements in the sacroiliac joint when the patient lies supine and the hip is flexed [41]. As a result, pain elicited by the straight leg raise test could be caused by a multitude of factors including a sacroiliac joint strain [41].

6.24 Sacrospinous Ligament

6.24.1 Anatomy

The sacrospinous ligament is a thin, triangular ligament that extends from broadly from the lateral margins of the sacrum and coccyx below the sacroiliac joint to ischial spine and, together with the sacrotuberous ligament, divides the greater sciatic notch into the greater sciatic foramen and the lesser sciatic notch into the lesser sciatic foramen [1, 5, 6, 24]. This ligament will attach to the coccyx anterior to the sacrotuberous ligament with which it will blend [5]. The lateral portion of the upper border of the sacrospinous ligament will form the lower border of the greater sciatic foramen. In comparison, the lateral portion of the lower border of this ligament will form the upper border of the lesser sciatic foramen [5]. While the posterior half of the sacrospinous ligament is covered by the sacrotuberous ligament, the anterior half of the sacrospinous ligament is muscular and constitutes the coccygeus muscle; in fact, many anatomists regard the sacrospinous ligament as the degenerate part of the coccygeus muscle [5].

A 2009 study by Hammer et al. found that the sacrospinous ligament, interspersed with coccygeus skeletal muscle fibers, in men had a mean length of 38 mm, whereas in women, the mean length was found to be 46 mm [40]. They described the sacrospinous ligament as a triangle with a medial base that attaches to the sacrum and coccyx and a lateral apex that attaches to the ischial spine [40].

6.24.2 Biomechanics

The sacrospinous ligament has fibers oriented to prevent upward tilting of the lower end of the sacrum; in order to accomplish this task, the sacrospinous ligament anchors to the ischium with the help of the sacrotuberous ligament [6]. As a result of this tilted orientation, these two ligaments oppose upward movement of the lower part of the sacrum under downward thrust at the sacrum's upper end [5]. Since these two ligaments do not rotate in the same direction, a suggestion has been made that these two ligaments have oppositional effects on the pelvis [40]. If these ligaments unroll like a "contorted rope under tension," then it can be considered that the sacrotuberous ligament will raise the ischium in relation to the sacrum while the sacrospinous ligament will lower the ischium in relation to the sacrum thus preventing any posterior rotation of the ilium with respect to the sacrum [40]. Even though these ligaments perform different functions, the two must be considered as a pair since they are closely correlated in terms of their volumes and cross-sectional areas [40].

6.25 Anterior Sacrococcygeal Ligament

6.25.1 Anatomy

The anterior sacrococcygeal ligament consists of irregular fibers that descend onto the pelvic surfaces of both the sacrum and coccyx [5]. It is the sacrococcygeal joint equivalent of the anterior longitudinal ligament as it attaches anterior to the sacrum and the coccyx [5].

6.25.2 Biomechanics

This ligament acts in concert with the posterior sacrococcygeal ligament to reinforce this joint [1].

6.26 Superficial Posterior Sacrococcygeal Ligament

6.26.1 Anatomy

The superficial posterior sacrococcygeal ligament is a flat ligament that passes from the margin of the sacral hiatus to the posterior coccygeal surface, thus forming the roof of the lower sacral canal [5]. This ligament is the sacral equivalent of the ligamentum flavum [5].

6.26.2 Biomechanics

This ligament acts in concert with the posterior sacrococcygeal ligament to reinforce this joint while also covering the lower portion of the sacral canal [1, 5].

6.27 Deep Dorsal Sacrococcygeal Ligament

6.27.1 Anatomy

The deep posterior sacrococcygeal ligament is the short part of the posterior sacrococcygeal ligament that passes from the back of the fifth sacral vertebral body to the dorsum of the coccyx [5]. This ligament is actually a continuation of the posterior longitudinal ligament [5].

6.27.2 Biomechanics

This ligament will connect the sacrum to the coccyx as well as acting in concert with the posterior sacrococcygeal ligament to reinforce this joint [1, 5].

6.28 Lateral Sacrococcygeal Ligament

6.28.1 Anatomy

There are two lateral sacrococcygeal ligaments, one on each side of the sacrum, that connect the first coccygeal transverse process to the inferolateral sacral angle [5]. These lateral sacrococcygeal ligaments will complete a foramen through which the fifth sacral spinal nerve will pass [5].

6.28.2 Biomechanics

Together with the anterior, posterior, and intercornual sacrococcygeal ligaments, the lateral sacrococcygeal ligaments help to stabilize the sacrococcygeal symphysis [43].

6.29 Intercornual Sacrococcygeal Ligaments

6.29.1 Anatomy

The intercornual ligaments will connect the sacral and coccygeal cornua on each side [5]. The cornua of the coccyx are superiorly projecting processes that arise from the upper part of coccyx [5]. The coccygeal cornua will articulate with the sacral cornua to form synovial joints [5]. There is also a fasciculus that will connect the sacral cornua to the coccygeal transverse processes [5].

6.29.2 Biomechanics

Together with the anterior, posterior, and lateral sacrococcygeal ligaments, the intercornual sacrococcygeal ligaments help to stabilize the sacrococcygeal symphysis [43].

References

1. Moore KL, Dalley AF, Agur AMR. Clinically oriented anatomy. 6th ed. Baltimore: Lippincott Williams & Wilkins; 2010.
2. Jaumard NV, Welch WC, Winkelstein BA. Spinal facet joint biomechanics and mechanotransduction in normal, injury and degenerative conditions. J Biomech Eng. 2011;133(7):071010.
3. Onan OA, Heggeness MH, Hipp JA. A motion analysis of the cervical facet joint. Spine. 1998;23(4):430–9.
4. Serhan HA, Varnavas G, Dooris AP, Patwardhan A, Tzsermiadonis M. Biomechanics of the posterior lumbar articulating elements. Neurosurg Focus. 2007;22(1):E1.
5. Bannister LH, Berry MM, Collins P, Dyson M, Dussek JE, Ferguson MWJ, editors. Gray's anatomy. 38th ed. New York: Churchill Livingston; 1996.
6. Bogduk N. Clinical anatomy of the lumbar spine and sacrum. 3rd ed. New York: Churchill Livingston; 1997.
7. Dickman CA, Rosenthal DJ, Perin NI. Thoracoscopic spine surgery. New York: Thieme Medical Publishers; 1999.
8. Lang J. Clinical anatomy of the cervical spine. New York: Thieme Medical Publishers; 1993.
9. Pintar FA, Yoganandan N, Myers T, Elhagediab A, Sances A Jr. Biomechanical properties of human lumbar spine ligaments. J Biomech. 1992;25(11):1351–6.
10. Neumann P, Keller TS, Ekstrom L, Perry L, Hansson TH, Spengler DM. Mechanical properties of the human lumbar anterior longitudinal ligament. J Biomech. 1992;25(10):1185–94.
11. Zander T, Rohlmann A, Bergmann G. Influence of ligament stiffness on the mechanical behavior of a functional spinal unit. J Biomech. 2004;37(7):1107–11.
12. Neumann P, Keller T, Ekstrom L, Hult E, Hansson T. Structural properties of the anterior longitudinal ligament. Spine. 1993;18(5):637–45.
13. Panjabi MM, Goel VK, Takata K. Physiologic strains in the lumbar spinal ligaments. Spine. 1982;7(3):192–203.
14. Chazal J, Tanguy A, Bourges M, Gaurel G, Escande G, Guillot M, Vanneuville G. Biomechanical properties of spinal ligaments and a histological study of the supraspinal ligament in traction. J Biomech. 1985;18(3):167–76.
15. Yong-Hing K, Reilly J, Kirkaldy-Willis WH. The ligamentum flavum. Spine. 1976;1(4):226–34.
16. Yahia LH, Garzon S, Strykowski H, Rivard CH. Ultrastructure of the human interspinous ligament and ligamentum flavum: a preliminary study. Spine. 1990;15(4):262–8.
17. Panjabi MM, Greenstein G, Duranceau J, Nolte LP. Three-dimensional quantitative morphology of lumbar spinal ligaments. J Spinal Disord. 1991;4(l):54–62.
18. Nachemson AL, Evans JH. Some mechanical properties of the third human lumbar interlaminar ligament (ligamentum flavum). J Biomech. 1968;1(3):211–20.
19. Heylings DJA. Supraspinous and interspinous ligaments of the human lumbar spine. J Anat. 1978;125(1):127–31.
20. Parke WW. The spine, vol. 1. Philadelphia/London/Toronto: W. B. Saunders Co; 1975.
21. Gudavalli MR, Triano JJ. An analytical model of lumbar motion segment in flexion. J Manip Physiol Ther. 1999;22:201–8.
22. Hindle RJ, Pearcy MJ, Cross A. Mechanical function of the human lumbar interspinous and supraspinous ligaments. J Biomed Eng. 1990;12:340–4.
23. Spalteholz W. Hand atlas of human anatomy, vol. 1. 7th ed. Philadelphia/London: JB Lippincott Co; 1943.
24. Agur AMR, Dalley AF. Grant's atlas of anatomy. 11th ed. Baltimore: Lippincott Williams and Wilkins; 2005.
25. Rissanen PM. The surgical anatomy and pathology of the supraspinous and interspinous ligaments of the lumbar spine, with special reference to ligament ruptures. Acta Orthop Scand. 1976;Suppl. 46:1–100.
26. Jiang H, Raso JV, Moreau MJ, Russell G, Hill DL, Bagnall KM. Quantitative morphology of the lateral ligaments of the spine: assessment of their importance in maintaining lateral stability. Spine. 1994;19(23):2676–82.
27. Hanson P, Magnusson SP, Sorensen H, Simonsen EB. Differences in the iliolumbar ligament and the transverse process of the L5 vertebra in young white and black people. Acta Anat. 1998;163(4):218–23.

28. Pool-Goudzwaard AL, Kleinrensink GJ, Snijders CJ, Entius C, Stoeckart R. The sacroiliac part of the iliolumbar ligament. J Anat. 2001;199:457–63.
29. Luk KDK, Ho HC, Leong JCY. The iliolumbar ligament: a study of its anatomy, development, and clinical significance. J Bone Joint Surg. 1986;68:197–200.
30. Sims JA, Moorman SJ. The role of the iliolumbar ligament in low back pain. Med Hypotheses. 1996;46:511–5.
31. Yamamoto I, Panjabi MM, Oxland TR, Crisco JJ. The role of the iliolumbar ligament in the lumbosacral junction. Spine. 1990;15:1138–41.
32. Pool-Goudzwaard AL, Hoek van Dijke G, Mulder P, Spoor C, Snijders CJ, Stoeckart R. The iliolumber ligament: its influence on stability of the sacroiliac joint. Clin Biomech. 2003;18(2):99–105.
33. Wilder DG, Pope MH, Frymoyer JW. The functional topography of the sacroiliac joint. Spine. 1980;5(6):575–9.
34. Alderink GJ. The sacroiliac joint: review of anatomy, mechanics, and function. J Orthop Sports Phys Ther. 1991;13(2):71–84.
35. DonTigny RL. Function and pathomechanics of the sacroiliac joint: a review. Phys Ther. 1985;65(1):35–44.
36. Goode A, Hegedus E, Sizer P Jr, Brismee JM, Linberg A, Cook CE. Three-dimensional movements of the sacroiliac joint: a systematic review of the literature and assessment of clinical utility. J Man Manip Ther. 2008;16(1):25–38.
37. Sturesson B, Selvik G, Uden A. Movements of the sacroiliac joints: a roentgen stereophotogrammetric analysis. Spine. 1989;14:162–5.
38. McGrath C, Nicholson H, Hurst (2009). The long posterior sacroiliac ligament: a histological study of morphological relations in the posterior sacroiliac region. Joint Bone Spine 76(1): 57–62.
39. Willard FH, Carreiro JE, Manko W. The long posterior interosseous ligament and the sacrococcygeal plexus. In: Proceedings of the third interdisciplinary world congress on low back and pelvic pain; 1998. p. 207–9.
40. Hammer N, Steinke H, Slowik V, Josten C, Stadler J, Bohme J, Spanel-Borowski K. The sacrotuberous and the sacrospinous ligament – a virtual reconstruction. Ann Anat. 2009;191(4):417–25.
41. Vleeming A, Stoeckart R, Snijders CJ. The sacrotuberous ligament: a conceptual approach to its dynamic role in stabilizing the sacroiliac joint. Clin Biomech. 1989;4(4):201–3.
42. Vleeming A, Van Wingerden JP, Snijders CJ, Stoeckart R, Stijnen T. Load application to the sacrotuberous ligament; influences on sacroiliac joint mechanics. Clin Biomech. 1989;4(4):204–9.
43. Morris CE. Low Back syndromes: integrated clinical management. New York: McGraw-Hill; 2005.

7 Neuroimaging of the Ligaments of the Craniocervical Junction

Ali Çağlar Turgut, Cenk Eraslan, and R. Shane Tubbs

7.1 Introduction

The craniocervical junction (CCJ) is a unique component of the osseous and ligamentous craniospinal axis with distinctive developmental characteristics and specific biomechanical requirements. The anatomy of the ligamentous structures in the CCJ region is complex. There are numerous ligaments, but only three of them are considered the main stabilizers: the tectorial membrane (TM), the transverse ligament, and the paired alar ligaments (ALs) [9]. Special and careful radiological evaluation is required in the event of trauma in this environment. Comprehensive knowledge by neuroradiologists and spine surgeons is a prerequisite for correct interpretation of the spinal ligaments of the CCJ region.

A review of the literature concluded that the following pathological conditions involving the spinal ligaments are extremely common today and have the potential to lead to a variety of serious consequences: traumatic lesions, inflammatory rheumatological arthropathies involving the CCJ region such as rheumatoid arthritis (RA) and spondyloarthritis (SpA), neoplastic lesions or infections of the spine or paraspinal region, and noninflammatory degenerative conditions of the spinal ligaments (calcifications/ossifications of the spinal ligaments and facet joint arthritis). These conditions can be diagnosed by neuroimaging methods such as plain radiography,

A. Ç. Turgut (✉)
Department of Radiology, Ege University Faculty of Medicine, Bornova, İzmir, Türkiye

Department of Histology and Embryology, Aydın Adnan Menderes University Institute of Health Sciences, Efeler, Aydın, Türkiye

International Joint Laboratory of Nervous System Malformations of Henan Province, Zhengzhou, Henan, China
e-mail: alicaglar304.at@gmail.com

C. Eraslan
Department of Radiology, Ege University Faculty of Medicine, Bornova, İzmir, Türkiye

International Joint Laboratory of Nervous System Malformations of Henan Province, Zhengzhou, Henan, China

R. S. Tubbs
Director of Surgical Anatomy, Program Director of Anatomical Research, Clinical Neuroscience Research Center, Tulane University School of Medicine, New Orleans, LA, USA

Departments of Neurosurgery, Neurology, Surgery, and Structural and Cellular Biology, Tulane University School of Medicine, Center for Clinical Neurosciences, New Orleans, LA, USA

Department of Neurosurgery and Ochsner Neuroscience Institute, Ochsner Health System, New Orleans, LA, USA

Department of Anatomical Sciences, St. George's University, School of Medicine, Grenada, West Indies

University of Queensland, Brisbane, Australia

M. Turgut et al. (eds.), *Ligaments of the Vertebral Column*,
https://doi.org/10.1007/978-3-032-09070-6_7

computed tomography (CT) or magnetic resonance imaging (MRI). Neuroradiological studies in these cases should be carefully evaluated by neuroradiologists to ensure correct diagnosis and treatment.

This chapter will focus on the fascinating yet complex anatomical features of the spinal ligaments, and will also touch upon different lesions involving the ligaments of the CCJ region. It is important for all physicians to be knowledgeable on this topic, including neuroradiologists, spine surgeons, neurosurgeons, orthopedic surgeons, neuroanatomists, rehabilitation physicians, and physiotherapists. They must recognize all clinical situations involving the spinal ligaments and decide the management of patients.

7.2 Ligaments of the Craniocervical Junction

7.2.1 Normal Anatomical Features of the Craniocervical

The CCJ, also known as the "cervicocranium," has three bony structures—the occipital bone (C0) surrounding the foramen magnum (FM), the atlas (C1), and the axis (C2) vertebrae; it has three joints (C0/C1, C1/C2, and C2/C3) between the skull and C3; and it has ligaments—the AL, the cruciate ligament, the apical ligament, the accessory atlanto-axial ligament (AAAL), the TM, the anterior atlanto-occipital membrane (AAOM), the posterior atlanto-occipital membrane (PAOM), the anterior atlanto-axial membrane (AAAM), the posterior atlanto-axial membrane (PAAM), and capsular joint ligaments, the atlantooccipital capsule (AOC) and the atlantoaxial capsule (AAC) [27]. Three of these ligaments (TM, transverse ligament and duplicate ALs) have a primary role in stabilizing the CCJ region [27]. The ligament complex that stabilizes craniocervical movements is divided into intrinsic and extrinsic ligaments.

(A) Intrinsic Ligaments

The intrinsic ligaments comprise three layers: odontoid ligaments, cruciate ligament, and TM (Fig. 7.1) [127, 164].

(a) Odontoid Ligaments

The odontoid ligaments are the apical ligament and ALs. The apical ligament extends from the apex of the odontoid process (OP) to the anterior edge of the FM (Figs. 7.2, 7.3 and 7.4) [164]. The ALs attach the apex of the OP of C2 to the ipsilateral edge of the occipital condyles and the lateral mass of C1 (Figs. 7.3, 7.5, 7.6 and 7.7) [9, 147, 152]. The ALs contribute to CCJ stability by limiting axial rotation of the head in the occipitoatlantoaxial complex [9]. Unfortunately, the complex anatomical features of these ligaments often lead to difficulties in their radiological examination [14, 132]. Radiologically, they exhibit low MRI signal intensity (hypointensity), but can also display a hyperintense signal in normal individuals due to changes in fiber compression due to fat and connective tissue between the fibers [74, 118]. It is reported that tightening the AL by application of axial tension to this anatomical structure with opposite flexion of the neck facilitates visibility [69].

(b) Cruciate Ligament

The cruciate ligament, also known as the cruciform ligament of C1, is a tight band-like sling that holds C2 against the anterior arch of C1 [29, 44, 62] (Figs. 7.1, 7.2, 7.8, 7.9 and 7.10). Flexion forces can cause a tear in the stiff, inelastic cruciate ligament, resulting in an "all or nothing" phenomenon, which can lead to C2 subluxation anterior to C1 [29]. On MRI, the normal cruciate ligament occurs as a uniform dark band on standard spin-echo pulse sequences, but increased signal intensity or an irregular contour suggests presence of structural damage; neuroradiological grading system: no lesions, mild, moderate or severe lesions (grades ranging from "0" to "3") [27, 30, 31, 62, 74, 76].

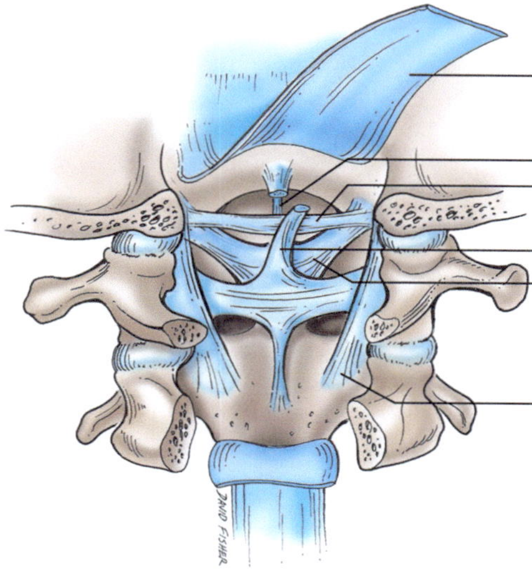

Fig. 7.1 Schematic illustration of the craniocervical junction (CCJ) ligaments from a posterior view. The tectorial membrane (TM) has been cut and reflected: Cruciate ligament (two transverse, one cranial and one caudal band), odontoid ligaments [alar ligament (AL) and apical ligament]. Importantly, the transverse ligament (band) of the cruciate ligament, called the "transverse ligament," is the thickest and strongest ligament in the CCJ; the cranio-caudal bands of the cruciate ligament and apical ligament are very thin and weak [77, 127, 159, 164]. Also shown are the accessory atlanto-axial ligaments (AAALs) and transverse occipital ligament (TOL)

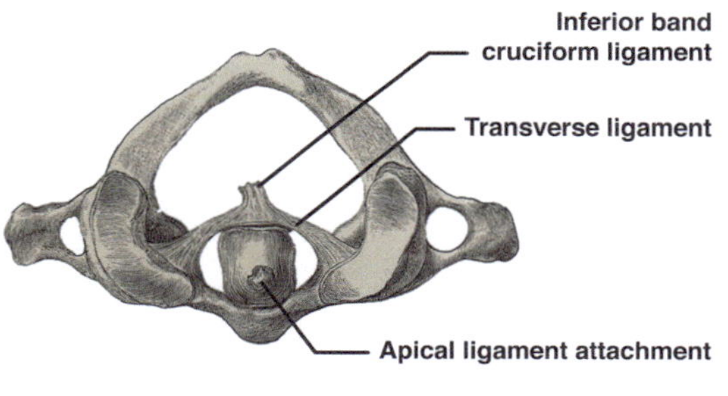

Fig. 7.2 Drawing of a superior view of the atlas (C1) and odontoid process (OP) with the transverse ligament and attachment site of the apical ligament shown. (After Morris)

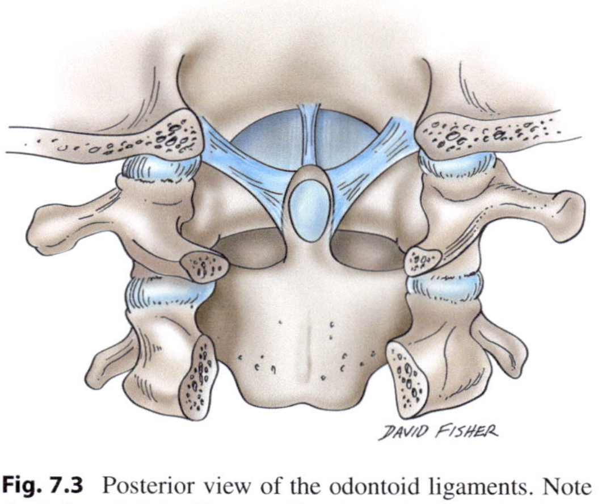

Fig. 7.3 Posterior view of the odontoid ligaments. Note the left and right ALs traveling laterally from the OP to attach onto the medial aspect of the occipital condyles. The apical ligament is seen arising from the apex of the OP and ascending to attach onto the basion of the foramen magnum (FM)

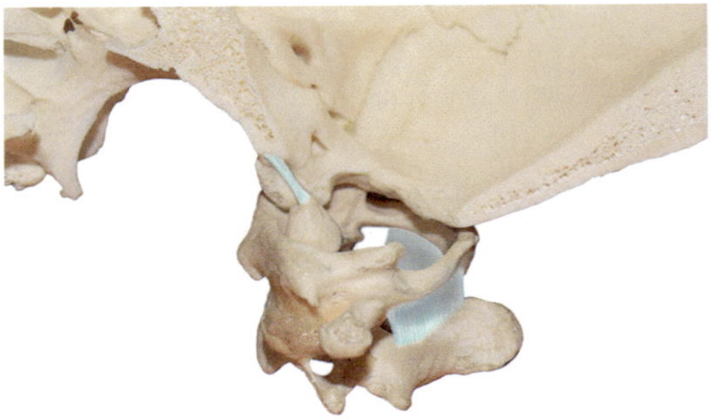

Fig. 7.4 Dry skull and C1-C2 specimen with overlaid apical ligament (blue) traveling from the odontoid apex to the basion. Also note the overlaid posterior atlantoaxial membrane (PAAM) (blue), uniting C1 and C2 vertebrae

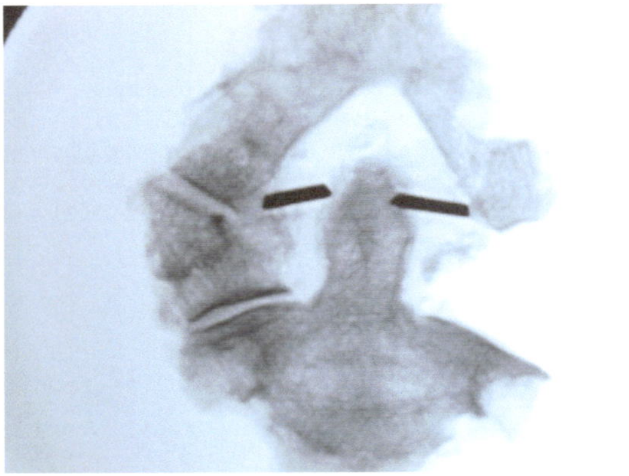

Fig. 7.5 Anteroposterior (AP) radiograph of the occipital bone, C1 and C2 vertebrae. Metal wires have been placed on the ALs to show their exact position on imaging

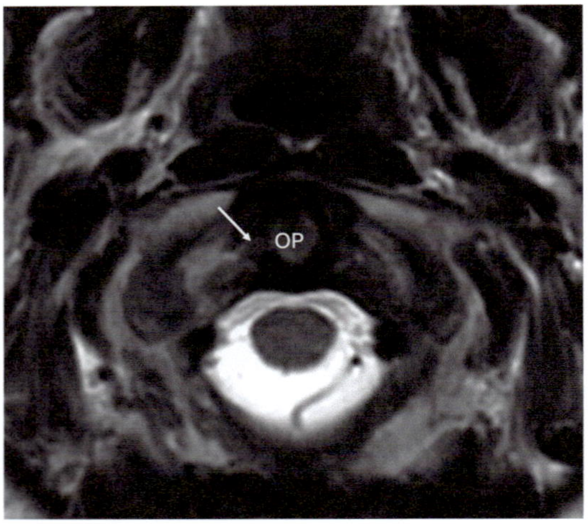

Fig. 7.6 Axial T2-weighted magnetic resonance imaging (MRI) through the CCJ. Note the apex of the OP and right-sided AL (arrow)

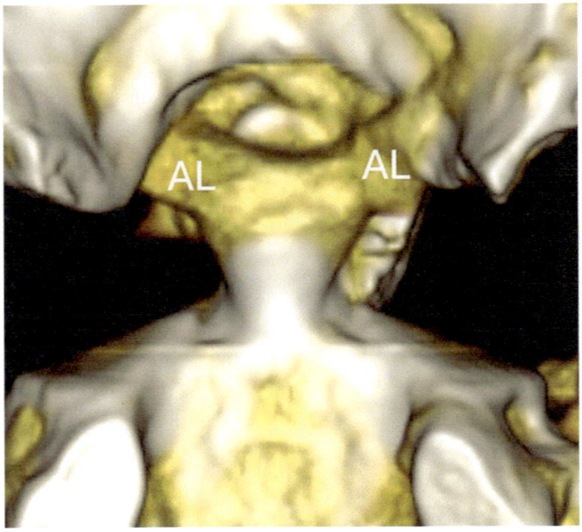

Fig. 7.7 Three-dimensional (3-D) reconstructed computed tomography (CT) of the alar ligament (AL)

(c) Tectorial Membrane

The TM, a cranial extension of the posterior longitudinal ligament (PLL), lies behind the cruciate ligament, extending from the posterior surface of C2 to the anterior edge of the FM, its cranial portion attaching to the dura mater (Figs. 7.1 and 7.10a) [108, 127, 159, 164].

(B) Extrinsic Ligaments

The extrinsic ligaments, the AAOM, PAOM, AAAM, and PAAM, are the anterior and posterior group of membranes with a marginal role in stabilizing the CCJ (Figs. 7.5 and 7.10a) [57]. Among these ligaments, the cranial continuation of the anterior longitudinal ligament (ALL) includes the AAOM and the AAAM; the lateral extensions covering the atlanto-occipital and atlanto-axial joints, the PAOM, and the PAAM, are considered cranial continuations of the ligamentum flavum (LF).

(a) Anterior Atlanto-Occipital Membrane

The AAOM attaches from the anterior arch of C1 to the anterior margin of the FM [164].

(b) Anterior Atlanto-Axial Membrane

The AAAM attaches from the anterior body of C2 to the anterior arch of C1 [164].

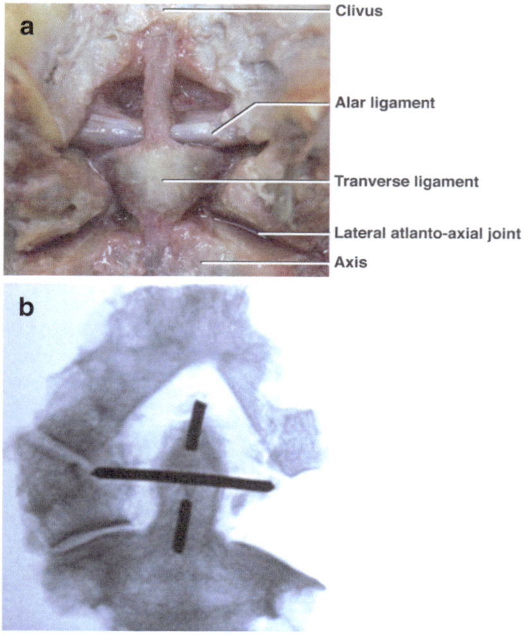

Fig. 7.8 A. Posterior cadaveric view noting the main part of the cruciform ligament, i.e., the transverse ligament. Note its superior and inferior crus. B. AP radiograph of the craniocervical bones with metal wires laid exactly onto the course of the cruciate ligament and its parts

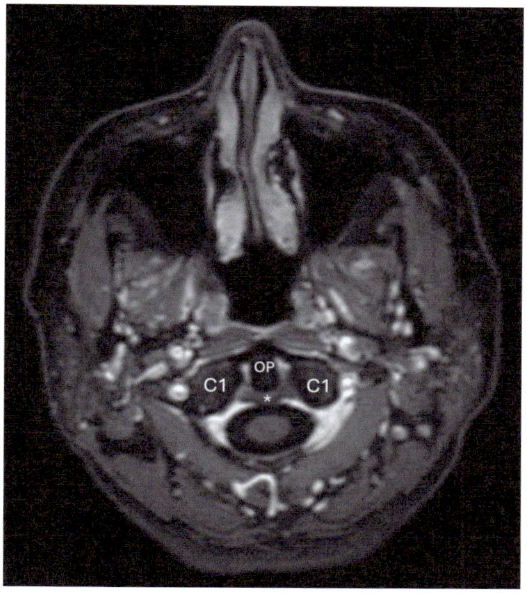

Fig. 7.9 Axial T1-weighted MRI of the CCJ noting the transverse ligament (*). Also note the odontoid process (OP) and lateral masses of C1

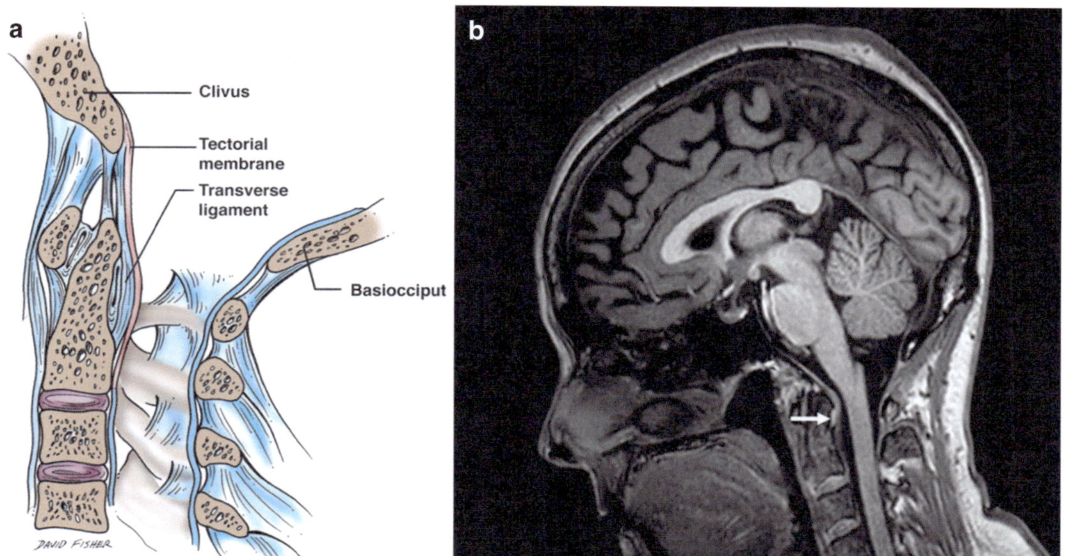

Fig. 7.10 (**a**) Schematic drawing of the ligaments of the CCJ in sagittal view and noting the position of the transverse atlantal ligament, called "transverse ligament". (**b**) Sagittal T1-weighted MRI noting the transverse ligament (arrow)

(c) Posterior Atlanto-Occipital Membrane

The PAOM extends from the posterior arch of C1 to the posterior margin of the FM [159, 164].

(d) Posterior Atlanto-Axial Membrane

The PAAM extends from the posterior margin of the body of C2 onto C1 [159, 164].

(e) Nuchal Ligament

The nuchal ligament (NL) is the cranial extension of the interspinous ligament (ISL) and supraspinous ligament (SSL) from C7 to the inion (Fig. 7.11) [127, 159, 164].

(f) Accessory Atlanto-Axial Ligament

A significant but often neglected ligament, the AAAL attaches medially to the dorsal surface of C2 and courses laterally and superiorly to attach behind the transverse ligament on the lateral mass of C1 [161, 175].

(g) Lateral Atlanto-Occipital Ligament

The lateral atlanto-occipital ligament (LAOL), which attaches to the anterolateral aspect of the transverse process of C1 and connects to the jugular process of the occipital bone, is lateral to the AAOM (Fig. 7.12) [126, 160, 162].

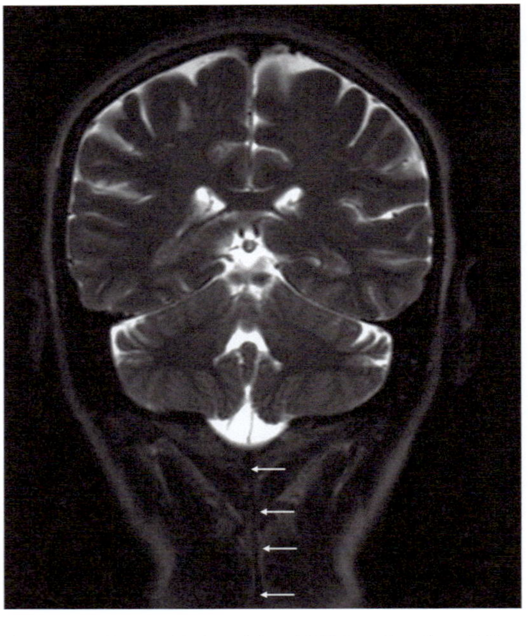

Fig. 7.11 Coronal T2-weighted MRI noting the midline nuchal ligament (NL) (arrows)

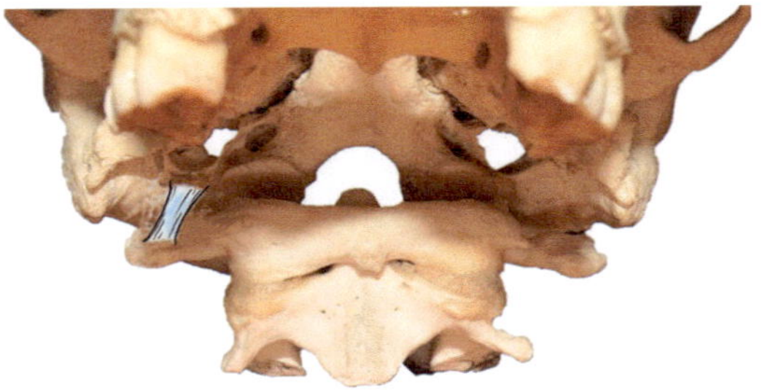

Fig. 7.12 Schematic drawing indicating the right-sided lateral atlanto-occipital ligament (LAOL). Note the attachment inferiorly to the anterior aspect of the transverse process of C1 and onto the occiput anterior to the jugular foramen

(h) Barkow's Ligament

Barkow's ligament is a horizontal band that attaches to the anteromedial side of the occipital condyles, anterior to the attachment site of the ALs [122, 156]. It is smaller than the transverse ligament, but it has a similar morphology and is close to the transverse ligament [122]. It has been reported that Barkow's ligament resists extension of the C0-C1 joint, synergistic with the AAOM [122].

(i) Transverse Occipital Ligament

The transverse occipital ligament (TOL) (Fig. 7.1), which connects to the inner part of the occipital condyles, lies superior to the AL and horizontally along the FM [81, 158].

(j) Capsular Joint Ligaments

The capsular joint ligaments, the AOC and the AAC (Fig. 7.13), contain synovial fluid in the C0-C2 articular joints (Fig. 7.3). They have a mechanical role in limiting rotatory movement of the CCJ.

Anatomically, the bony elements (C0, C1, and C2) of the CCJ region are supported by the integrity of the ligamentous and muscular elements [47]. Biomechanically, the primary stabilizers for the C0/C1 level are the AAOM and the PAOM, the TM, the paired ALs and the apical ligament from C2, and the joint capsular ligaments (AOC and AAC). The primary stabilizer for the C1/C2 level is the transverse ligament, with additional bands of the paired ALs coming from C2 [103]. Biomechanically, types of CCJ instability involv-

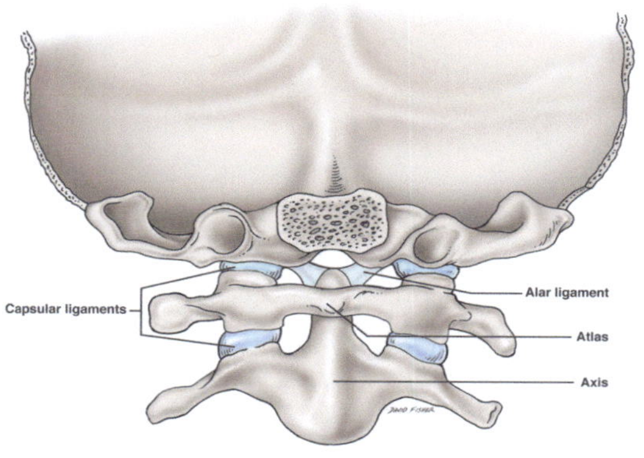

Fig. 7.13 Schematic anterior view of the capsular joint ligaments, atlanto-occipital capsule (AOC) and atlanto-axial capsule (AAC). Also, note the positioning of the ALs

ing the C0-C1, C1-C2, or C0-C1-C2 levels and related to the spinal ligaments are as follows: functional posture disorder with disorder of the proprioceptive system; ligamentous or capsule hypermobility or hyperlaxity under physiological load forces, characterized by increased range of motion due to excessive looseness in the ligamentous capsular structures, as in Ehlers-Danlos syndrome and Marfan syndrome; and true structural instability with structural injuries in the ligamentous capsular system such as traumatic rupture, elongation, or insufficiency [7, 85, 101, 170]. Other true structural etiologies of instability of the CCJ include congenital anomalies such as Chiari malformation, traumatic injuries, infections such as tuberculosis, bone defects on the joint surfaces such as Paget's disease, and inflammatory arthropathies involving the spine such as RA and SpAs, including "ankylosing spondylitis" (AS), "psoriatic arthritis" (PsA), "reactive arthritis" (ReA), "enteropathic arthritis," "juvenile (idiopathic) SpA," and "undifferentiated SpA."

Clinically, it is important to know that most of the flexion/extension movement of the neck takes place at the C0-C1-C2 levels, while the most of rotation movement occurs at C1-C2 level [47, 52]. If there is spinal instability, hyperlaxity of the ligaments results with neurological symptoms such as headaches, neck pain, double vision, vertigo, speech difficulties, difficulty in swallowing, sleep apnea, numbness in arms or legs, and unsteady walking and weakness in arms, hands or legs during head and neck movements due to compression of the brainstem, spinal cord, nerve roots, or the vertebral artery (VA) [46, 115]. In instability of the CCJ region, decompression and surgical stabilization is necessary to protect neural and vascular structures from compression.

7.2.2 Normal Imaging Properties of Ligaments of the Craniocervical Junction

The normal imaging features of the spinal ligaments in the CCJ are discussed in detail below, before the pathological aspects are considered in subsequent sections.

(a) Plain Radiography

In addition to plain radiographs in anteroposterior (AP), lateral, and oblique positions for visualizing the bony anatomy, open-mouth plain radiographs can reveal any asymmetry in the lateral masses of C1–2 (Fig. 7.14) [25].

(b) Computed Tomography

CT is the first best of choice imaging modality for evaluating the spinal ligaments of the CCJ (Figs. 7.15 and 7.16) [61, 62, 104]. Ideally, an axial source dataset with a thin section of 2 mm or less is advocated, from which suitable resolution multiplanar reformats can be obtained [68]. Coronal and sagittal reformats are required in addition to axial slices, and the use of angular/oblique reformats is also advocated in multidetector CT technology [62, 104]. However, CT is inadequate for evaluating the CCJ, and MRI is inadequate for evaluating the CCJ; an additional study to evaluate the spinal ligaments is mandatory, as described below.

(c) Computed Tomography Angiography

Computed tomography angiography (CTA) can be required for further evaluation of vascular structures in the CCJ. CTA should be included in imaging of the CCJ region because the internal carotid arteries (ICAs) and VAs are contiguous in

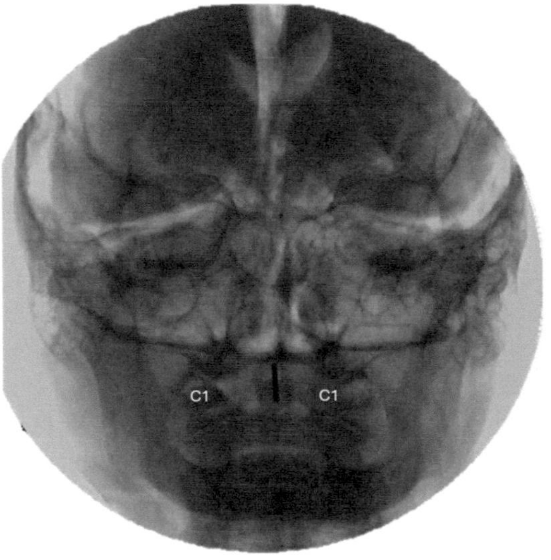

Fig. 7.14 AP radiograph of the skull and upper cervical spine. The lateral masses of C1 and the OP (vertical metal wire) are noted

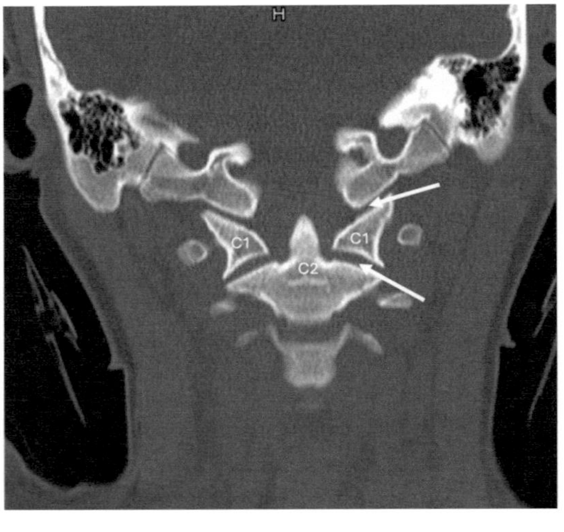

Fig. 7.15 Coronal CT of the CCJ. Note the normal alignment of the C1–2 joints. The lateral C0–1 joint (upper arrow) and C1–2 joint (lower arrow) are shown

this region [104]. A high suspicion of traumatic vascular dissection should be kept in mind by neuroradiologists [104].

(d) Magnetic Resonance Imaging

Nowadays, MRI is the best choice for imaging the spinal ligaments of the CCJ region and other

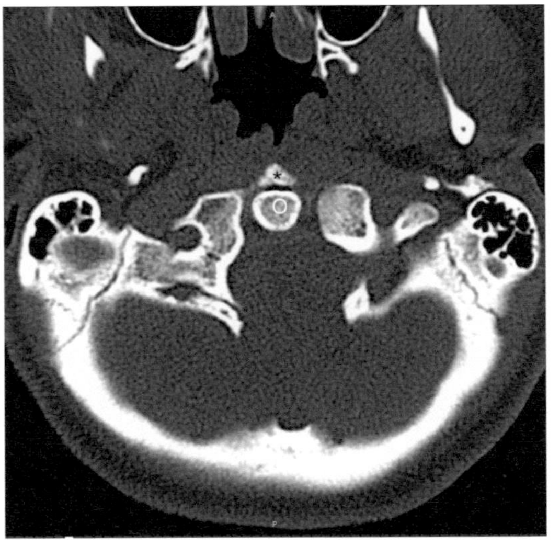

Fig. 7.16 Axial CT noting the normal positioning of the OP (O) at the CCJ and anterior arch of C1 (*)

surrounding soft tissues [17, 95, 113]. The inclusion of a T2-weighted sequence provides post-procedural evaluation of peri-ligamentous soft tissue and the ligamentous structures [104]. Normal spinal ligaments of the CCJ are hypointense on T1- and T2-weighted MRI (Fig. 7.17).

From a technical perspective, in addition to the field strength, coil design, gradient strength, and software features of the MRI system, appropriate sequence parameters for MRI are also very significant in imaging the spinal ligaments of the CCJ region [9, 61, 62]. Furthermore, it is significant to remember that cerebrospinal fluid (CSF) pulsatility artifacts may prevent evaluation of the spinal cord on T2-weighted MRI, and that fast spin-echo inversion-recovery (FSE-IR) sequences can be useful in such cases [9]. Radiologically, it has been reported that among the ligaments in the CCJ region, the normal TM and transverse ligament can be assessed on MRI, although the ALs are difficult to evaluate [9]. In similar, evaluation of the AAOM is also difficult because of fatty tissue surrounding the membrane, but it is easy to evaluate the PAOM in sagittal MRI sections because of the elastic fibers within the membrane [50, 75, 76].

Radiologically, it is generally impossible to demonstrate instability by plain radiography, but CCJ instability can be diagnosed using measure-

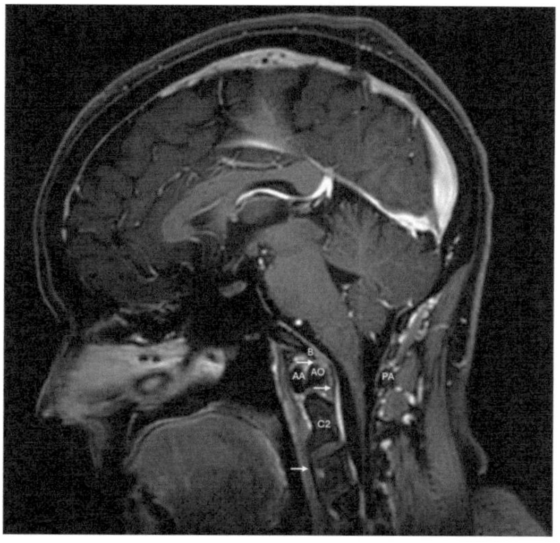

Fig. 7.17 T1-weighted and enhanced sagittal MRI of the head and upper cervical spine. Bony landmarks include the basion (B), anterior (AA) and posterior (PA) arches of C1, axis (C2), and apex of the OP (AO). The upper arrow indicates the space where the apical ligament would be located, the middle arrow points to the TM and the lower arrow shows the anterior longitudinal ligament (ALL)

ments of bone reference points on CT in about half of all cases, and MRI is the best of choice for identifying traumatic soft tissue injuries, including injuries to the spinal ligaments [61, 62, 90, 112]. Rojas et al. reported that the transverse ligament was involved in 36% of patients with AS [129]. Interestingly, it has also been reported that about 50% of RA patients with C1/C2 subluxation are asymptomatic, but surgical intervention is inevitable in such patients [99].

7.3 Imaging Properties of Various Lesions of the Ligaments of the Craniocervical Junction

Various pathological conditions involving the spinal ligaments of the CCJ, including traumatic lesions, inflammatory arthropathies (RA and SpAs), neoplastic lesions, various infections and noninflammatory degenerative conditions of the spinal ligaments (calcifications/ossifications of the spinal ligaments and facet joint arthritis) will be discussed in detail in the following sections.

7.3.1 Traumatic Lesions of the Ligaments of the Craniocervical Junction

In general, plain radiography and CT using a 0.75 mm thin-section axial source data set with coronal and sagittal reformations are the initial imaging modalities of choice for patients with trauma involving the CCJ adjacent to the VAs and CTA and should be used to assess possible vascular injuries [104]. Indications for MRI in such patients are as follows: (1) Patients with neurological symptoms or persistent neck and/or back pain, suspected ligament or spinal cord injury, negative plain radiographs and CT; (2) Patients who cannot be evaluated clinically for more than 48 h owing to changes in level of consciousness; (3) Findings on plain radiographs or CT indicating ligamentous injury, such as facet dislocation, widening of the intervertebral disc (IVD) space or interspinous space, bone fractures adjacent to the spinal ligaments, and prevertebral swelling; (4) Patients with spinal fractures or unstable injuries on plain radiographs or CT; and (5) MRI before closed reduction or open surgical intervention is helpful for diagnosing possible IVD herniation or extradural/subdural hematoma [43, 164].

7.3.1.1 Traumatic Lesions of the Ligaments in the Craniocervical Junction

Traumatic lesions of the cervical spine account for the vast majority of spinal injuries, approximately one third of which involve the CCJ [6, 13, 28, 96, 145, 164]. "Static" imaging techniques such as radiography in erect position and standard MRI in upright supine position can provide diagnoses of subluxations or anatomical abnormalities. However, it is difficult to diagnose patients with instability of the CCJ when the signs are of mild instability, or there are indirect signs of instability, or positional symptoms from images taken in a neutral position of the head-on-neck [127]. In such cases, "dynamic" imaging of the CCJ in flexion and extension and neck rotation is necessary for correct diagnosis. Otherwise, the MRI of patients with instability of the CCJ can be erroneously judged normal. It is essential to note that there may be potential medico-legal consequences if such injuries are not promptly detected.

Traumatic lesions of the CCJ region should be investigated using the following radiological measurements for diagnosis of potential instability: the basion-axial interval (BAI), the basion-dens interval (BDI of Wholey et al.), the clivo-axial angle (CXA), the anterior or posterior atlantodental interval (ADI), and the Grabb-Oakes line (GOL), as described below in detail (Figs. 7.18 and 7.19). In many cases, it is also important to perform a three-dimensional (3-D) bone CT scan of the CCJ region. Regardless of the imaging method, the following radiological criteria should be considered for evaluating CCJ instability:

(i) The BAI, called the "horizontal" Harris measurement, the distance between the basion and the posterior axial line drawn along the posterior aspect of the body of C2 and extended cranially, with normal values ≤ 12 mm [48, 49, 51, 61] (Fig. 7.18a). An increased BAI indicates anterior subluxation of C0-C1 [48, 49, 51].

(ii) The BDI, called the "vertical" Harris measurement, the distance from the posteroinferior basion to the superior line of the dens of the C2 in the midsagittal plane, with values ≤ 12 mm on radiographs and <8.5 mm on CT in normal individuals [48, 49, 61]. In children, however, it has normal values of <10 mm. An increased BDI indicates dissociation (distraction) of C0-C1, dislocation or subluxation [131].

(iii) For radiological evaluation of the C1-C2 relationship, the "anterior" ADI (predental space) has normal values of <3 mm in men and < 2.5 mm in women (up to 5 mm in children), while the "posterior" ADI has normal values of >18 mm [53, 61, 131] (Fig. 7.18a). An increased or decreased anterior or posterior ADI, respectively, indicates deficiency of the transverse ligament [131].

(iv) The CXA, also known as the "basion-axial angle" or the "clivo-canal angle" or the "craniovertebral angle" (of Wackenheim) or the "clivus canal angle" or the "clivus vertebral angle or the "the "clivus-cervical angle" or the "clivus-axial angle", is the angle between the bony part of the skull base (Wackenheim line) and the posterior part of the dens of the C2 (posterior axial or spinal line), with normal values in the range of 139–172° (Fig. 7.18b) [51]. A low CXA (< 135°) with kyphosis indicates the risk of CCJ instability and compression of the anterior brainstem, medulla oblongata, and upper spinal cord [51].

(v) The GOL, also known as the "Grabb-Mapstone-Oakes measurement", is a line drawn from the basion to the posteroinferior side of the body of C2, with normal values of < 9 mm [51] (Fig. 7.19). An increased length indicates a high risk of ventral compression of the brainstem and/or upper spinal cord [51].

(vi) Other radiological criteria can be used for determining CCJ instability:

(a) The "Powers ratio," the ratio of the distance from the tip of the basion (B) to the posterior arch of C1, also known as the spinolaminar line (C), to the distance between the midpoint of the posterior aspect of the anterior arch of C1 or anterior side of the dens of C2 (A) and the tip of the opisthion (O), with normal values of BC/AO <1. A higher ratio indicates anterior atlanto-occipital (C0-C1) dissociation (distraction) and C1-C2 instability (Fig. 7.18c) [119, 131].

(b) Crossing of the "McRae line" (the FM line joining the basion and opisthion) by the apex of the dens of C2, crossing of the "McGregor line" (line drawn from the posterosuperior margin of the hard palate to the lowest point of the midline occipital curve) by the apex of the OP of C2 > 4 mm, or crossing of the "Chamberlain line" (line drawn from the posterior end of the hard palate to the posterior margin of the FM, called the opisthion) >6 mm, indicates "basilar invagination," also known as "basilar impression or basilar/cranial settling" (Fig. 7.20) [91].

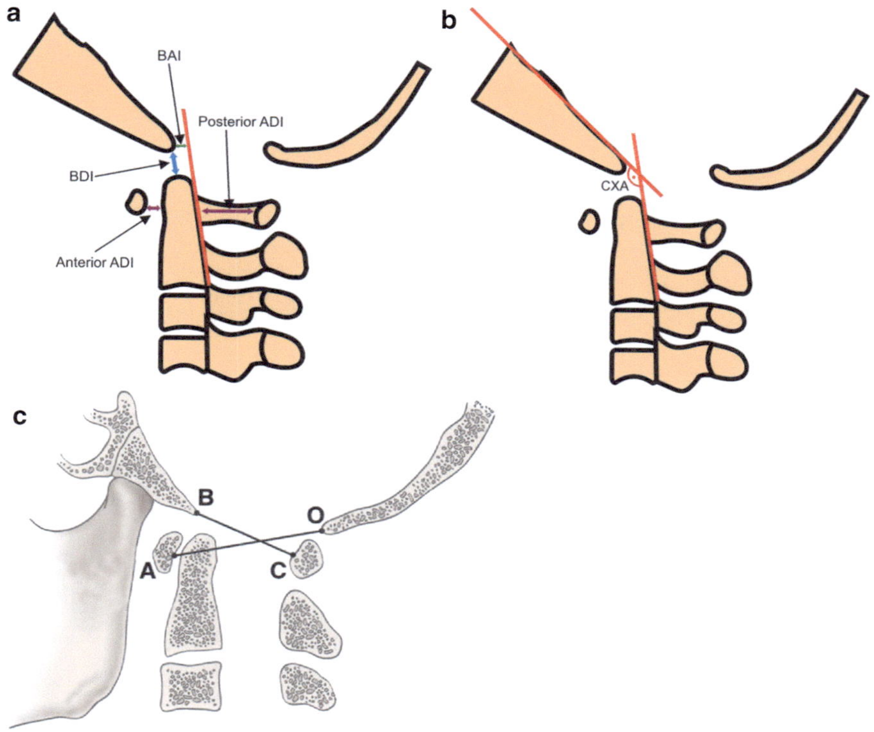

Fig. 7.18 Schematic illustrations of sagittal alignment of the CCJ demonstrating: (**a**) BAI (the distance between the basion and the posterior axial line drawn along the posterior aspect of the body of C2 and extended cranially), BDI (the distance from the most inferior portion of the basion to the closest point of the superior aspect of the dens of the C2), anterior ADI (the distance between the posterior aspect of the anterior arch of the C1 and the anterior cortex of the dens of the C2 in the midsagittal plane) and posterior ADI (the distance between the dens of the C2 and the posterior arch of C1 reflecting the width of the spinal cord on C1-C2 level); (**b**) CXA (a measure of the angle between the clivus, a bony part of the base of the skull and the spine); and (**c**) the Powers ratio calculated by dividing the distance between the tip of the basion (B) to the spinolaminar line, also known as posterior arch of C1, (C) by the distance from the tip of the opisthion (O) to the midpoint of the posterior aspect of the anterior arch of C1 (A) [48, 49, 51, 53, 61, 131]

(c) The interval from the posterior aspect of the dens of C2 to the posterior aspect of the C1 arch >13 mm; a shorter interval indicates “spinal stenosis” [59].
(d) Atlanto-occipital (C0-C1) interval < 1 mm, measured by drawing a line perpendicular to the articular surfaces of the occipital condyle (C0) and the lateral mass of C1; a longer interval suggests “distraction” [131].
(e) Axial rotation of C0-C1 and C1-C2 should be <8° and <45°, respectively, to each side; greater ranges of rotation indicate “instability” [12].
(f) Occipital condyle (C0)-C1 interval, normal value <2.5 mm; a longer interval indicates “instability” [61, 148].

“Spine instability” occurs when spinal ligaments lose their ability to maintain normal alignment under a physiological load. Atlanto-occipital (C0-C1) dissociation (distraction) injuries include dislocations (usually fatal) and subluxations (rarely fatal) [47, 62]. In children and adolescents, a traumatic injury to the capsular joint ligaments (AAC, AOC) due to forced rotation and forward flexion causes an increased range of motion of C1-C2 axial rotation, resulting in rotatory C1-C2 dislocation [25, 129]. In general, TM injury is accompanied by injuries of paired ALs,

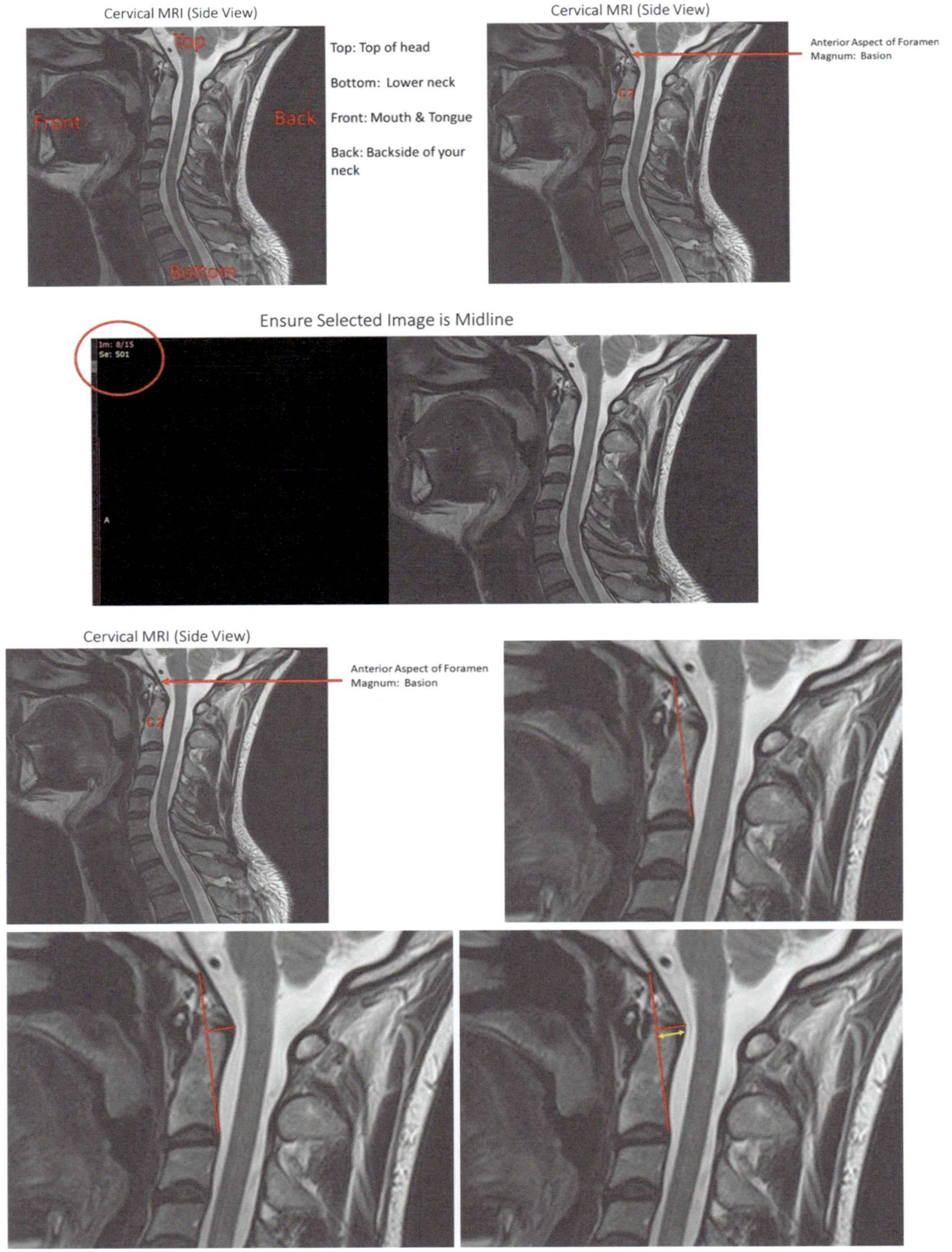

Fig. 7.19 The Grabb-Oakes line for measuring the correct placement of the OP on sagittal imaging. A vertical line is drawn from the basion to the posteroinferior border of the C2 vertebra. The perpendicular distance between the two arrows should not exceed 9 mm

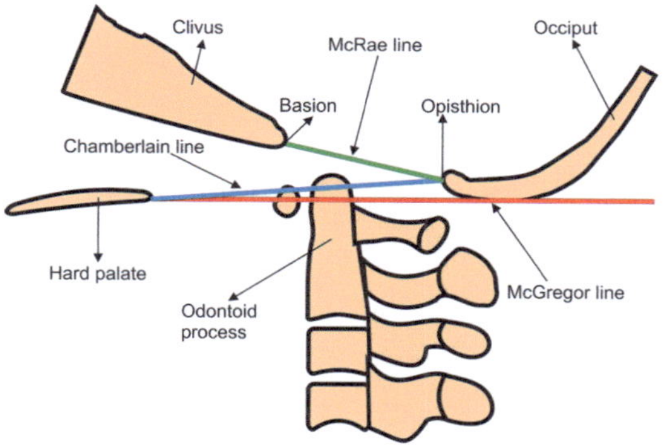

Fig. 7.20 Schematic illustration of sagittal alignment of the CCJ demonstrating the McRae line, McGregor line, and Chamberlain line used for diagnosing basilar invagination, also known as basilar impression or basilar cranial settling [91]

transverse ligament, and apical ligament associated with instability of the cervical spine [27, 39]. It is difficult to visualize these structures radiologically [142]. In contrast, traumatic injuries to the AAAL or apical ligament can be isolated; they have no role in the treatment of cervical spine trauma because they have no stability effects [157, 161].

Radiologically, in cases with traumatic injury to the CCJ region, fracture-dislocations of the C0, C1, and C2 can be diagnosed with plain radiography. In particular, "open-mouth" plain radiographs can reveal asymmetry of the lateral masses of C1-C2 [27]. Thin-section axial, coronal, and sagittal reformatted CT is the initial imaging modality of choice for acute traumatic injury to the CCJ [62, 104]. Osseous fracture apparent on CT and C1-C2 rotation of more than 47° in the axial plane are pathognomonic for rotatory C1-C2 dislocation [27, 34]. However, CT is not sufficient for complete radiological evaluation of the CCJ; MRI is suggested for evaluating the spinal ligaments. CTA can be indicated for traumatic injuries of the CCJ because the ICAs and VAs are close to the CCJ. A high index of suspicion is necessary for diagnosing traumatic vascular dissection injury in such cases [104]. As a general rule, MRI is valuable for the diagnosis, treatment, and outcome of certain types of ligamentous injuries at the CCJ [16, 62, 63, 68, 143]. In cases of C1-C2 dislocation with traumatic injury to the capsular joint ligaments, MRI can reveal injuries of the capsular joint ligaments and soft tissues [25, 55, 62, 129]. Technically, incorporating an isovolumetric T2-weighted sequence provides post-procedural evaluation for radiological assessment of the integrity of spinal ligaments and traumatic changes in the peri-ligamentous structures [104].

An ideal MRI standard for spinal ligament injury must include sagittal T1- and T2-weighted, gradient-echo (GRE), short TI inversion recovery, also known as short tau inversion recovery (STIR), axial GRE or T2-weighted, and optional coronal T1-weighted or GRE images. GRE and T2-weighted sequences are the most suitable sequences for evaluating ligaments, and STIR is the most sensitive to soft tissue injury in the CCJ [9]. Spinal ligaments are generally visualized on GRE and T2-weighted sequences, but T1-weighted images give the best anatomical detail for detecting any associated spinal fractures [9, 43]. The heterogeneity effect generated by GRE imaging techniques at high field strengths gives greater sensitivity in detecting blood products within the spinal cord, but it also diminishes signal intensity within the bone, making fractures more challenging to detect. At low field strength the GRE heterogeneity effect is weaker, so blood products are less easily detected but fracture detection is slightly improved [9]. On the other hand, T2-weighted and FSE-IR MRI sequences are the most sensitive for bone marrow edema (related to fracture or contusion), spinal cord injury, and soft tissue edema [9].

While acute injuries to the spinal ligaments are easily diagnosed by increased T2/STIR signals due to edema or hemorrhage, the ligaments of normal individuals appear hypointense on T1- and T2-weighted MRI; this hypointensity typically decreases over time, usually after 72 h. Therefore, in radiological evaluation of spinal ligaments using MRI, the ideal time interval between injury and MRI must be "less than 72 hours" [143, 144]. Within this interval, T2 signal hyperintensity due to edema or leakage of blood into injured extradural tissues gives a first-class contrast agent effect, improving the visualization of ligaments with low signal intensity on all MRI sequences [9]. After this period, absorption of edema or bleeding makes MRI less sensitive for disclosing various injuries [9].

Traumatic injuries to the transverse ligament produce an "all-or-nothing phenomenon" visualized by heterogeneous signal intensity or distortion of fibers on T2/GRE axial images [127, 144, 164]. The paired ALs are visualized in the coronal plane, and a symmetrical signal indicates unilateral ligament injury [144]. Blood or edema next to the AL tear improves visualization of the traumatic injury. On the other hand, evidence of injury to the ALs is the contralateral displacement of the OP resulting from hypermobility in the C1–2 joint, which leads to reduced blood flow in the contralateral VA [9]. TM injury caused by frontal hyperflexion with anterior translation in motor vehicle accidents, stripping of ligaments from underlying bone due to fluid, or discontinuity associated with avulsion fractures of the vertebral cartilage end plate (CEP), present as linear T2/STIR hyperintensity [33, 75, 76, 144, 160, 162, 164].

7.3.2 Involvement of Ligaments in the Craniocervical Junction by Inflammatory Rheumatological Arthropathies

Inflammatory rheumatological arthropathies involving the CCJ region, such as RA and SpAs (AS, PsA, ReA, enteropathic arthritis, juvenile SpA, and undifferentiated SpA), are described in detail below.

7.3.2.1 Rheumatoid Arthritis

Seropositive RA, an autoimmune arthritis, involves the synovia of the joints and the spine, particularly involving the cervical region, and particularly in women [167]. RA is the most common type of inflammatory arthropathy, and the C1-C2 joint is one of the most frequently involved anatomical regions. This condition can cause myelopathy with severe neurological deficits including loss of consciousness, radiculopathy, lower cranial nerve palsies, and occipital pain in patients with subluxation in the cervical spine, resulting from mechanical compression of the brainstem, spinal cord, spinal nerves or vessels [19, 73, 100, 109, 124, 167].

In RA patients, there is inflammation of the bone marrow (osteitis), discitis, (pseudo)spondylolisthesis, and synovitis, causing "pannus formation." There is also C1-C2 subluxation due to ligamental laxity and tears, with subsequent life-threatening spinal cord myelopathy or brainstem compression [73, 166]. Involvement of the vertebral bodies can result in enthesitis, collapse of the vertebrae, or an extension of the inflammatory process from the apophyseal joints [67, 83]. Involvement of the CCJ region and C1-C2 subluxation is particularly well described in RA patients, in contrast to involvement of other parts of the spine [67, 83, 137]. Hypermobility of the CCJ can also result in a pannus formation (Fig. 7.21).

Classical radiological findings for RA using plain radiography, CT, and MRI include demineralization of the bone, osseous erosion/destruction, bone marrow edema, cyst, subluxation, pannus formation, spondylolysis, ankylosis, ligament injury, and compression of neural structures (spinal cord, brainstem, or spinal nerves) [73]. Among these findings, pannus formation, osseous erosion/destruction, subluxation (anterior, posterior, lateral or vertical), and ligament injury

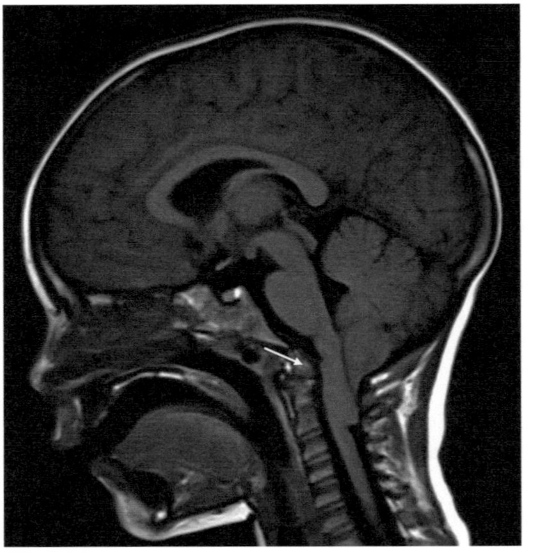

Fig. 7.21 Sagittal MRI noting a pannus formation (arrow) in a child with Chiari I malformation

at C1-C2 are seen in the vast majority of RA patients. In contrast, subaxial subluxation is encountered in only a few [73, 100]. In particular, CT or MRI is used for pannus formation, while MRI is the best option for visualizing bone marrow edema [73, 174].

7.3.2.2 Spondyloarthritis

SpA, called "spondylarthropathy" or "seronegative disease" (negative rheumatoid factor), is a group of chronic inflammatory diseases involving the joints and ligaments of the spine attaching to the vertebrae [167]. The following lesions are observed in the pathogenesis of SpA: Anterior/lateral ossification of the annulus fibrosus and various spinal ligaments (PLL, ALL, LF, NL, ISL, and SSL), called "syndesmophyte or parasyndesmophyte," and ankylosis and immobility of the spine, called "ankylosis or "vertebral squaring" [73, 123]. The typical lesions in SpAs include involvement of the annulus fibrosus of IVD tissue in the spine, called "enthesitis," bone marrow edema of the anterior vertebral edges, called "corner inflammatory lesions," vertebral erosions, called "Romanus lesions," triangular sclerosis, called "shiny corner," and chronic osteitis and remodeling of the anterior side of the vertebral body, called "vertebral squaring," in more advanced disease [3, 73]. Radiologically, MRI clearly shows bone marrow edema, fatty degeneration of vertebral corners, new syndesmophytes, spinal fractures, and spinal cord injury [73, 82, 155].

Clinical, laboratory, and imaging findings in SpAs are not specific for any of these diseases, although some imaging patterns suggest possible differential diagnoses [45, 167]. As a rule, they are called "axial SpA" when the spine and/or sacroiliac joints are involved, and "peripheral SpA" when other joints and tendons are involved [45, 167]. They are subclassified as AS, PsA, ReA, "enteropathic arthritis," and other kinds of SpA, such as "juvenile SpA" and "undifferentiated SpA" [73, 133]. They are characterized by human leukocyte antigen (HLA)-B27 antigen positivity. Involvement of the cervical spine is not common in patients with SpA, in advanced stage AS or in early stage PsA, in contrast to patients with RA [15, 73].

Ankylosing Spondylitis

In AS, called "Bechterew disease," a type of inflammatory spinal arthritis, several vertebrae are fused [3, 18, 26, 155, 167]. AS is a seronegative SpA characterized by chronic, progressive, and systemic inflammation of the axial skeleton, including the ligaments and joints of the spinal column and sacroiliac joints. Other organs (eye, lung, kidney, and heart) and joints (shoulder, knee, and hip) are also involved, but the sacroiliac joints are involved primarily [3, 36, 167]. Inflammation of the spine, called "spondylitis," results in fusion of vertebrae, called "ankylosis," kyphosis of the spine, and restriction of movements of the spinal column in advanced stages of this disabling disease owing to deposition of calcification/ossification in the spinal ligaments around the IVDs [3, 36, 155, 167]. Clinically, the symptoms of AS such as progressive pain in the lower back and buttock, stiffness, and loss of mobility (reduced flexibility of the spine) are related to synovitis and inflammation of the sacroiliac joint, called "sacroiliitis," forward curving of the thoracic spine, called "kyphotic deformity," and difficulty breathing during the late stage of the disease [3, 36, 155, 167]. The laboratory test used for diagnosing inflammation anywhere in the body is the erythrocyte sedimentation rate [167]. In patients with AS, which usually affects Caucasian men in their third decades rather than women, the rheumatoid factor is negative in blood tests [3, 18, 167]. Genetically, a positive blood test for HLA-B27 is diagnostic for AS if the patient presents with clinical findings of the condition [18, 167].

Radiologically, symmetrically deformed vertebral bodies with an abnormal square shape, called "bamboo spine appearance," are apparent in plain radiographs of the spine. They result from calcium deposition in the spinal ligaments and IVDs, spinal fusion, and spinal fractures in the advanced stages. Early findings include patchy osteoporosis, poorly defined joint margins, widening of the sacroiliac joint space, and erosions of the sacroiliac joint [36, 167]. It has been reported that about half of patients with AS, in particular those in advanced age and with long duration of the disease, have radiological findings

[36]. About 1 in 5 have an anterior C1-C2 dislocation [83, 155]. About half of AS patients exhibit syndesmophytes, and about 1/4 of AS patients have ankylosis of the facet joints [88]. The PLL is ossified (called OPLL), causing myelopathy, in 10–20% [123].

Treatment of AS is usually conservative. It includes non-steroidal anti-inflammatory drugs (NSAIDs), sulfasalazine, corticosteroids, or immunosuppressive agents, as well as physical therapy, exercise, and surgical intervention, for the appropriate management of both inflammation and pain. Physical therapy for spinal mobility and an exercise program can help alleviate pain in AS patients [167]. Surgical interventions such as spinal osteotomy or artificial hip replacement can be necessary if the patient has a kyphotic deformity or if the hip joints are injured by arthritis, respectively [167]. In summary, a detailed clinical history and physical examination, radiography, and laboratory tests are necessary for diagnosing AS.

Psoriatic Arthritis

PsA, an autoimmune disorder, is associated with psoriasis that develops before arthritis; it can involve the spinal column [167]. In patients with PsA, involvement of the cervical spine can be "ankylosing," characterized by ankylosis, syndesmophytis, and ligamental calcification; or "rheumatoid-like," an erosive type with C1-C2 subluxation [58]. Although the C1-C2 level is involved in the vast majority of PsA patients, a thick and irregular asymmetric syndesmophyte, called "parasyndesmophyte," is found in the thoraco-lumbar spine [150].

Reactive Arthritis

ReA, also known as "Reiter syndrome," is characterized by inflammation of the joints and spinal ligaments following an infection of the bowel or genitals [167].

Enteropathic Arthritis

Enteropathic arthritis involving the CCJ region is associated with inflammatory bowel disease (IBD) and is referred to as "IBD-related arthritis" [167].

Other Kinds of Spondyloarthritis

Other kinds of arthritis or SpA are "juvenile (idiopathic) SpA" and "undifferentiated SpA" [73, 133, 167]. Juvenile SpA, the most common inflammatory arthritis of autoimmune and autoinflammatory origin in children, is characterized primarily by peripheral joint arthritis, though the cervical spine can also be involved [38]. In juvenile SpA cases, the following findings are observed: ankylosis of apophyseal joints at the C2-C3 level, vertebral hypoplasia, dens erosions, anterior C1-C2 subluxation, subaxial subluxation, and ossification of the spinal ligaments [80]. RA involving the CCJ region may cause development of instability and myelopathy, whereas SpA patients produce typical radiological findings, such as syndesmophytes and bone ankylosis [73].

Imaging is diagnostic for inflammatory arthropathies, although their clinical findings are nonspecific [8, 64, 73, 149]. Plain radiography, lateral (flexion, extension, and neutral views) and AP projections, is useful for evaluating various vertebral lesions and cervical spine alignment and subluxations, especially at the C1-C2 level, despite the superimposition of anatomical structures in the CCJ [64, 73]. Specifically, AP projection plain radiography with an open mouth is useful for evaluating this complex region. The "Fischgold-Metzger's line" is used to assess vertical subluxation at the C1-C2 level, although CT and/or MRI have been used more recently [73]. CT of the cervical spine with 3-D reconstruction for visualization of anomalies, fractures, and subluxations demonstrates the complex anatomy of the CCJ region, including the C0-C1 joint, C1-C2 joint, IVDs, uncovertebral (Luschka) joints, and apophyseal joints [73]. CT is more effective than plain radiography for assessing soft tissue involvement, but less effective than MRI for visualizing the involvement of brainstem, spinal cord, and nerve roots [73]. MRI clearly shows various osseous lesions and CEPs of the vertebrae, but it is useful for visualizing neural structures such as the brainstem, spinal cord, and nerve roots. Sagittal post-contrast T1-weighted and fluid-sensitive MRI sequences with fat saturation are useful for evaluating active inflammatory lesions and bone marrow edema, respectively [149]. Recently, it has been reported that functional MRI studies in flexion, extension, and neutral positions can be used for further evaluation of patients with inflammatory rheumatological arthropathies [10].

Overall, the inflammatory rheumatological arthropathies, including RA and SpAs, have common imaging features, including subluxations (horizontal anterior or posterior, lateral, or vertical) and spinal canal stenosis involving the C1-C2 level [73]. In anterior C1-C2 subluxation, the "anterior ADI" exceeds 3 mm in adults; it exceeds 5 mm in children owing to skeletal immaturity [53, 61, 73, 131]. In posterior C1-C2 subluxation, the "posterior ADI" is less than 14 mm [53, 61, 73, 131]. In lateral C1-C2 subluxation, a displacement or asymmetry of C2 in relation to C1 is ≥2 mm [73]. In patients with C1-C2 subluxation, neurological deficits develop as a result of spinal cord compression. In vertical C1-C2 subluxation, called "basilar invagination" or "basilar impression or basilar/cranial settling", vertical migration of the dens into the FM is caused by ligamentous destruction or erosion at the C0-C1-C2 level. Measurement results in plain radiography, CT or MRI are positive using "Ranawat's method" (line between central part of C2 pedicle and intersection of horizontal line drawn along C2; length < 15 mm in males, <13 mm in females), "Redlunde Johnell's line" (line between McGregor's line and midpoint of caudal edge of C2 body; length < 34 mm in males, <29 mm in females), or "Clark's method" (division of the dens of the C2 into three equal stations on sagittal projection from superior to inferior; anterior arch of C1 is adjacent to II or III station) [11, 73, 83, 88, 128]. In normal individuals, values of the "cervicomedullary angle," the angle between lines drawn parallel to the anterior border of the upper cervical spinal cord and the medulla oblongata, are in the range 135°-175° (Fig. 7.22) [27, 102].

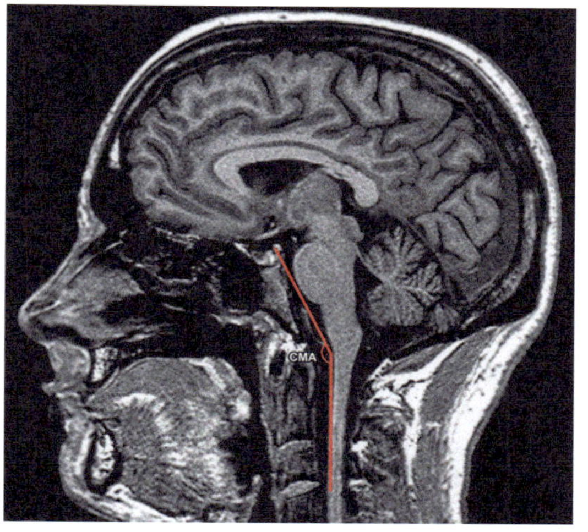

Fig. 7.22 Sagittal MRI of the CCJ demonstrating the cervicomedullary angle (CMA) between the line parallel to the ventral side of the medulla oblongata and the line parallel to the ventral side of the upper cervical spinal cord [19, 73]

7.3.3 Noninflammatory Degenerative Conditions of the Spinal Ligaments

7.3.3.1 Osteoarthritis of the Spine

Osteoarthritis, also known as "facet joint arthritis/syndrome" or "facet disease," is a noninflammatory or degenerative arthritis, the most common form of spinal arthritis, and it frequently affects the lower back [78, 167]. Pain related to inflammation develops in these osteoarthritis patients due to involvement of the facet joints between the vertebrae, IVDs, and the spinal ligaments [78, 167]. If these changes occur in the upper cervical region of the spine, including the C1-C2 joint of CCJ region, this condition is called "CCJ spondylosis" [167]. For neuroradiologists to ensure a correct diagnosis and proper management of patients with facet joint disease, it is essential to recognize its characteristic imaging findings.

7.3.3.2 Calcifications/Ossifications of Spinal Ligaments of the Craniocervical Junction

Noninflammatory degenerative conditions with calcifications/ossifications of the spinal ligaments, including the AL, PLL, SSL, ISL, and NL, and diffuse idiopathic skeletal hyperostosis (DISH), can result in ankylosis of the spine [35, 71, 98, 125, 167].

Calcification/Ossification of the Alar Ligament

Sometimes, the paired AL is calcified/ossified, which can simulate a type I fracture of the odontoid process of C2 or a type III fracture of the occipital condyle (C0). Rarely, this causes a difficult imaging choice in severe trauma patients who are unconscious and/or intubated, with increased risk for injuries involving the CCJ region. Calcification typically appears as well-defined calcification or ossification in the region of the AL on CT [147].

Diffuse Idiopathic Skeletal Hyperostosis

DISH, also known as "Forestier's disease," is characterized by anterior and lateral osteophytes of the vertebral body in male adults. It results from increased activity of osteoblasts in the spinal ligaments [20, 37, 79]. In patients with DISH, spinal stenosis and C1-C2 subluxation in the CCJ region develop as a result of reduced flexibility of the spinal column due to calcification/ossification of the spinal ligaments [20]. When such patients show progressive severe clinical symptomatology, surgical intervention to remove the osteophytes is indicated [94, 105].

Calcification/Ossification of the Posterior Longitudinal Ligament

Heterotopic calcification or ossification of the PLL, called "OPLL," a distinct condition attributable to genetic and environmental factors, leads to compression of the spinal cord [65, 72, 100, 107, 111, 117, 174]. In plain radiography, radiological classification of OPLL is as follows: "continuous type" (ligamentous calcification in two or more vertebrae), "segmental type" (calcification/ossification located behind one or more vertebrae), "mixed type" (composed of both continuous and segmented types), and "restricted type" (characterized by arch-shaped ossification/ossification behind the IVD) [114, 139].

On CT, there are two types of calcified/ossified lesions of the PLL, referred to as OPLL, which can be classified as bridge or non-bridge (sagittal classification) and central or lateral (axial classification), depending on their anatomical location [66, 139]. On the other hand, calcified/ossified lesions of the PLL, called "OPLL", are classified as square, mushroom, or hill type on MRI (axial classification) [114, 139]. The value of MRI is limited because the calcified/ossified PLL, called OPLL, is similar to CSF and the vertebral cortex on T1-weighted sequences, although proton density imaging can be useful for diagnosis owing to the contrast between the PLL, CSF, and calcification/ossification of vertebral bodies [114, 172].

Calcifications/Ossifications of Other Ligaments

Apart from calcification/ossification of the AL and PLL, the other ligaments (the SSL, ISL and NL) in the CCJ region can be calcified/ossified [117, 173]. In some patients, various combinations of calcification or ossification of these ligaments in the upper cervical spine, or even other spinal ligaments (the ALL and LF) in the thoracic or lumbar spine, have been reported [93, 140, 173]. In this context, it is also useful to remember various cystic lesions (such as synovial, cyst, ganglion cyst, juxta-facet cyst, or hemorrhagic/granulomatous cyst) as well as hematomas of other spinal ligaments, in addition to calcifications/ossifications of spinal ligaments in the CCJ region [1, 2, 4, 21, 22, 32, 41, 42, 60, 70, 84, 87, 89, 92, 106, 116, 121, 130, 136, 138, 141, 146, 151, 153, 154, 163, 165, 171]. Surgical decompression can be indicated for patients with myelopathy caused by calcified/ossified spinal ligaments [72, 117].

7.3.4 Involvement of Spinal Ligaments Secondary to Infections of the Spine or Paraspinal Region

All of the spinal ligaments can be affected secondary to various infections of the CCJ region or surrounding soft tissue. Spondylodiscitis involving the spinal ligaments in the CCJ region is a rare infectious disorder that is typically encountered in immunocompromised elderly patients [24, 56, 86, 167]. In these infections caused by bacteria or fungi, different parts of the spine, including the spinal ligaments, are also involved via the following three routes: hematogenous spread from a remote area, direct external contamination from trauma or surgery, or external spread from an adjacent tissue [5]. In patients with infections in the CCJ region or paraspinal region, clinical symptoms and laboratory tests are nonspecific; however, tissue sampling for microbiological tests is necessary for a definitive diagnosis and appropriate antibiotic treatment [56, 120, 167]. However, radiological evaluation of patients with spinal infections using plain radiographs of the spine and MRI following the administration of contrast material is helpful for accurate diagnosis [56, 167]. On MRI, hypointense vertebral bodies on T1-weighted images, hyperintense vertebral bodies on T2-weighted or STIR images, and increased contrast enhancement in the IVD and vertebral body are typical findings. Surgical intervention is indicated for patients if conservative treatment has failed and there is spinal instability, abscesses in the spinal canal or paravertebral region, and progressive neurological deficits caused by compression of spinal cord or nerve root [135].

7.3.5 Involvement of Spinal Ligaments Secondary to Neoplastic Lesions of the Spine or Paraspinal Region

All of the ligaments in the CCJ region can be affected secondary to various neoplasms of the spinal column, spinal cord, or surrounding soft tissue [17, 95, 113]. The vast majority of these tumors are caused by metastatic dissemination of a malignant tumor from another part of the body [17, 114, 169]. Therefore, knowledge of the anatomy of the CCJ region and paraspinal region, as well as understanding of the imaging characteristics of these neoplasms, is of great importance for accurate diagnosis and adequate management. Fortunately, only 0.5% of all spinal metastases affect the CCJ region; however, their management is complex, requiring various radiological studies and different surgical approaches [23, 110, 113, 134, 168]. In patients with metastatic disease, breast carcinoma is the most common primary site, but other primary lesions such as thyroid, lung, renal, and prostate carcinoma are possible [97, 110, 168, 169]. Clinical evaluation of a patient with neck pain can reveal early-stage metastatic disease with a stable CCJ, and MRI is the gold standard imaging modality for detecting any pathological process, with nuclear bone scan for distinguishing benign from malignant ones [113, 168, 169]. In patients with involvement of neoplastic lesions in the spinal ligaments in the CCJ region, neoplastic C1-C2 instability and progressive neurological deficits are indications for surgery [113, 169]. In such complex cases, a multidisciplinary approach involving neuroradiologists, spinal surgeons, neurosurgeons, orthopedic surgeons, and medical and radiation oncologists is necessary.

7.4 Conclusion

The ligaments of the human spine are highly complex and important anatomical structures that provide spinal stability, especially in the CCJ, which is an interesting and complex region of the spine. In recent years, advancements in anatomical knowledge of the spinal ligaments have led to significant improvements in neuroradiology and spine surgery. Current imaging techniques of spinal ligamentous structures include plain radiography, CT, and MRI, where there is a significant bone injury or suspicion of injury to the spinal ligaments with any traumatic signal change [104]. In particular, MRI using a special imaging protocol provides excellent visualization of the spinal ligaments and adjacent soft tissue elements in the CCJ region [40, 75–77].

Importantly, the optimal time interval between injury and MRI should be less than 72 h, using special radiological criteria for diagnosing potential traumatic instability of CCJ [9, 143]. Neuroradiological tools such as CT and MRI are useful for diagnosing other lesions, including the inflammatory rheumatological arthropathies involving the spine (RA and SpAs), noninflammatory degenerative conditions (calcifications/ossifications of the spinal ligaments, including the AL and the PLL, and DISH, and facet joint arthritis), and neoplastic lesions or infections of the spine or paraspinal region involving spinal ligaments of the CCJ region. These are causes of various neurological deficits secondary to compression of the spinal cord and/or nerve roots due to degenerative spinal canal stenosis and/or neoplastic or infectious instability [54]. Further long-term, multicenter, prospective, and randomized controlled trials are needed to provide more definitive guidance for clinical practice on this topic.

References

1. Abdullah AF, Chambers RW, Daut DP. Lumbar nerve root compression by synovial cysts of the ligamentum flavum. Report of four cases. J Neurosurg. 1984;60:617–20.
2. Akhaddar A. Posterior longitudinal ligament cysts. In: Akhaddar A, editor. Atlas f Sciatica; 2024. p. 857–9.
3. Aufdermaur M. Pathogenesis of square bodies in ankylosing spondylitis. Ann Rheum Dis. 1989;48:628–31.
4. Baba H, Furusawa N, Maezawa Y, Uchida K, Kokubo Y, Imura S, Noriki S. Ganglion cyst of the posterior longitudinal ligament causing lumbar radiculopathy: case report. Spinal Cord. 1997;35(9):632–5.
5. Babic M, Simpfendorfer C. Infections of the spine. Infect Dis Clin N Am. 2017;31:279–97.
6. Barrey C, Afathi M, Broussolle T, Dauleac C, Bancel P. Craniovertebral junction instability and mechanisms of injury. In: Tessitore E, Dehdashti A, Schonauer C, Thomé C, editors. Surgery of the cranio-vertebral junction. Cham: Springer; 2020.
7. Belhassen S, Mat Q, Ferret C, Clavel R, Renaud B, Cabaraux P. Post-traumatic craniocervical disorders from a postural control perspective: a narrative review. Brain Neurorehabil. 2023;16:e15.
8. Bell GR, Stearns KL. Flexion-extension MRI of the upper rheumatoid cervical spine. Orthopedics. 1991;14:969–73.
9. Benedetti PF, Fahr LM, Kuhns LR, Hayman LA. MR imaging findings in spinal ligamentous injury. AJR Am J Roentgenol. 2000;175:661–5.
10. Benny BV, Nagpal AS, Singh P, Smuck M. Vascular causes of radiculopathy: a literature review. Spine J. 2011;11(1):73–85.
11. Blau RH, Kaufman RL. Erosive and subluxing cervical spine disease in patients with psoriatic arthritis. J Rheumatol. 1987;14:111–7.
12. Bogduk N, Mercer S. Biomechanics of the cervical spine I: Normal kinematics. Clin Biomech (Bristol, Avon). 2000;15(9):633–48.
13. Bogner E. Imaging of cervical spine injuries in athletes. Sports Health. 2009;1:384–91.
14. Borchgrevink G, Smevik O, Haave I, Haraldseth O, Nordby A, Lereim I. MRI of cerebrum and cervical column within two days after whiplash neck sprain injury. Injury. 1997;28(5–6):331–5.
15. Braun J, Bollow M, Remlinger G, Eggens U, Rudwaleit M, Distler A, Sieper J. Prevalence of spondylarthropathies in HLA-B27 positive and negative blood donors. Arthritis Rheum. 1998;41(1):58–67.
16. Brightman RP, Miller CA, Rea GL, Chakeres DW, Hunt WE. Magnetic resonance imaging of trauma to the thoracic and lumbar spine: the importance of the posterior longitudinal ligament. Spine. 1992;17:541–50.
17. Brihaye J, Ectors P, Lemort Van Houtte P. The management of spinal epidural metastases. Adv Tech Stand Neurosurg. 1988;16:121–76.
18. Brown MA, Laval SH, Brophy S, Calin A. Recurrence risk modelling of the genetic susceptibility to ankylosing spondylitis. Ann Rheum Dis. 2000;59(11):883–6.
19. Bundschuh C, Modic MT, Kearney F, Morris R, Deal C. Rheumatoid arthritis of the cervical spine: surface-coil MR imaging. AJR Am J Roentgenol. 1988;151(1):181–7.
20. Cammisa M, Serio D, Guglielmi G. Diffuse idiopatic skeletal hyperostosis. Eur J Radiol. 1997;27:7–11.
21. Chiba K, Toyama Y, Matsumoto M, Maruiwa H, Watanabe M, Nishizawa T. Intraspinal cyst communicating with the intervertebral disc in the lumbar spine: discal cyst. Spine (Phila Pa 1976). 2001;26:2112–8.
22. Cho SM, Rhee WT, Lee SY, Lee SB. Ganglion cyst of the posterior longitudinal ligament causing lumbar radiculopathy. J Korean Neurosurg Soc. 2010;47:298–301.
23. Constans JP, de Divitiis E, Donzelli R, Spaziante R, Meder JF, Haye C. Spinal metastases with neurological manifestations. Review of 600 cases. J Neurosurg. 1983;59:111–8.
24. Creze M, Ghaouche J, Missenard G, Lazure T, Cluzel G, Devilder M, Briand S, Soubeyrand M, Lew DP, Waldvogel FA. Osteomyelitis Lancet. 2004;364:369–79.
25. Crisco JJ III, Oda T, Panjabi MM, Bueff HU, Dvorak J, Grob D. Transactions of the C1-C2 joint

capsular ligaments in the cadaveric spine. Spine. 1991;16(10S):474–9.
26. Dean LE, Jones GT, MacDonald AG, Downham C, Sturrock RD, Macfarlane GJ. Global prevalence of ankylosing spondylitis. Rheumatology (Oxford). 2014;53(4):650–7.
27. Debernardi A, D'Aliberti G, Talamonti G, Villa F, Piparo M, Collice M. The craniovertebral junction area and the role of the ligaments and membranes. Neurosurgery. 2011;68:291–301.
28. Denis F. The three-column spine and its significance in the classification of acute thoracolumbar spinal injuries. Spine. 1983;8:817–31.
29. Dickman CA, Crawford NR. Surgery of the Craniovertebral junction. New York: Thieme; 1998.
30. Dickman CA, Greene CA, Sonntag VKH. Injuries involving the transverse atlantal ligament: classifications and treatment guidelines based upon experience with 39 injuries. Neurosurgery. 1996;38:44–50.
31. Dickman CA, Mamourian A, Sonntag VKH, Drayer BP. Magnetic resonance imaging of the transverse atlantal ligament for the evaluation of atlanto-axial instability. J Neurosurg. 1991;75:221–7.
32. DiMario S, Marmor E, Albrecht S, Mohr G. Ligamentum flavum cysts causing incapacitating lumbar spinal stenosis. Can J Neurol Sci. 2005;32:237–42.
33. Dundamadappa S, Cauley K. MR imaging of acute cervical spinal ligamentous and soft tissue trauma. Emerg Radiol. 2012;19:277–86.
34. Dvorak J, Panjabi M, Gerber M, Wichmann W. CT functional diagnostics of the rotatory instability of upper cervical spine. 1. An experimental study on cadavers. Spine (Phila Pa 1976). 1987;12:197–205.
35. Ehara S, Shimamura T, Nakamura R, Yamazaki K. Paravertebral ligamentous ossification: DISH. OPLL and OLF Eur J Radiol. 1998;27(3):196–205.
36. El Maghraoui A, Bensabbah R, Bahiri R, Bezza A, Guedira N, Hajjaj-Hassouni N. Cervical spine involvement in ankylosing spondylitis. Clin Rheumatol. 2003;22(2):94–8.
37. el Miedany YM, Wassif G, el Baddini M. Diffuse idiopathic skeletal hyperostosis (DISH): is it of vascular aetiology? Clin Exp Rheumatol. 2000;18:193–200.
38. Elhai M, Wipff J, Bazeli R, Freire V, Feydy A, Drapé JL, Quartier P, Kahan A, Job-Deslandre C. Radiological cervical spine involvement in young adults with polyarticular juvenile idiopathic arthritis. Rheumatology (Oxford). 2013;52(2):267–75.
39. Farley FA, Gebarski SS, Garton HL. Tectorial membrane injuries in children. J Spinal Disord Tech. 2005;18:136–8.
40. Farooki S, Seeger LL. Magnetic resonance imaging in the evaluation of ligament injuries. Skeletal Radiol. 1999;28:61–74.
41. Finkelstein SD, Sayegh R, Watson P, Knuckey N, Juxta-facet cysts. Report of two cases and review of the clinicopathologic features. Spine (Phila Pa 1976). 1993;18:779–82.
42. Gazzeri R, Galarza M, Gorgoglione L, Bisceglia M, D'Angelo V. Cervical cyst of the ligamentum flavum and C7-T1 subluxation: case report. Eur Spine J. 2005;14:807–9.
43. Goradia D, Linnau KF, Cohen WA, Mirza S, Hallam DK, Blackmore CC. Correlation of MR imaging findings with intraoperative findings after cervical spine trauma. Am J Neuroradiol. 2007;28:209–15.
44. Greene KA, Dickman CA, Marciano FF, Drabier J, Drayer BP, Sonntag VK. Transverse atlantal ligament disruption associated with odontoid fractures. Spine (Phila Pa 1976). 1994;19:2307–14.
45. Grigoryan M, Roemer FW, Mohr A, Genant HK. Imaging in spondyloarthropathies. Curr Rheumatol Rep. 2004;6(2):102–9.
46. Gupta V, Khandelwal N, Mathuria SN, Singh P, Pathak A, Suri S. Dynamic magnetic resonance imaging evaluation of craniovertebral junction abnormalities. J Comput Assist Tomogr. 2007;31:354–9.
47. Harris JH Jr. The cervicocranium: its radiographic assessment. Radiology. 2001;218:337–51.
48. Harris JH Jr, Carson G, Wagner L. Radiologic diagnosis of traumatic occipitovertebral dissociation: 1. Normal occipitovertebral relationships on lateral radiographs of supine subjects. Am J Roentgenol. 1994;162:881–6.
49. Harris JH Jr, Carson GC, Wagner LK, Kerr N. Radiologic diagnosis of traumatic occipitovertebral dissociation: 2. Comparison of three methods of detecting occipitovertebral relationships on lateral radiographs of supine subjects. AJR Am J Roentgenol. 1994;162(4):887–92.
50. Harris MB, Duval MJ, Davis JA, Bernini PM. Anatomical and roentgenographic features of atlanto-occipital instability. J Spinal Disord. 1993;6:5–10.
51. Henderson F Sr, Rosenbaum R, Narayanan M, Mackall J, Koby M. Optimizing alignment parameters during craniocervical stabilization and fusion: a technical note. Cureus. 2020;12:e7160.
52. Henderson FC, Wilson WA, Mott S, Mark A, Schmidt K, Berry JK, Vaccaro A, Benzel E. Deformative stress associated with an abnormal clivo-axial angle: a finite element analysis. Surg Neurol Int. 2010;1:30.
53. Hinck VC, Hopkins CE. Measurement of the atlanto-dental interval in the adult. Am J Roentgenol Radium Therapy, Nucl Med. 1960;84:945–51.
54. Hirabayashi S. Ossification of the ligamentum flavum. Spine Surg Relat Res. 2017;1:158–63.
55. Hodak JA, Mamourian A, Dean BL. Surgery of the craniovertebral junction. New York: Thieme; 1998.
56. Hong SH, Choi JY, Lee JW, Kim NR, Choi JA, Kang HS. MR imaging assessment of the spine: infection or an imitation? Radiographics. 2009;29(2):599–612.
57. Jea A, Tatsui C, Farhat H, Vanni S, Levi AD. Vertically unstable type III odontoid fractures: case report. Neurosurgery. 2006;58:797–8.

58. Jenkinson T, Armas J, Evison G, Cohen M, Lovell C, McHugh NJ. The cervical spine in psoriatic arthritis: a clinical and radiological study. Br J Rheumatol. 1994;33(3):255–9.
59. Joaquim AF, Baum G, Tan LA, Riew KD. C1 stenosis-an easily missed cause for cervical myelopathy. Neurospine. 2019;16(3):456–61.
60. Kao CC, Uihlein A, Bickel WH, Soule EH. Lumbar intraspinal extradural ganglion cyst. J Neurosurg. 1968;29:168–72.
61. Kassem MW, Tubbs RS. Injuries to the craniocervical ligaments: radiological diagnosis. In: Tubbs RS, Iwanaga J, Loukas M, Oskouian RJ, editors. Clinical anatomy of the ligaments of the Craniocervical junction. Newcastle upon Tyne: Cambridge Scholars Publishing; 2019. p. 89–110.
62. Kassem MW, Tubbs RS. The cruciform ligament. In: Tubbs RS, Iwanaga J, Loukas M, Oskouian RJ, editors. Clinical anatomy of the ligaments of the craniocervical junction. Newcastle upon Tyne: Cambridge Scholars Publishing; 2019. p. 155–85.
63. Katzberg RW, Benedetti PF, Drake CM, Ivanovic M, Levine RA, Beatty CS, Nemzek WR, McFall RA, Ontell FK, Bishop DM, Poirier VC, Chong BW. Acute cervical spine injuries: prospective MR imaging assessment at a level 1 trauma center. Radiology. 1999;213(1):203–12.
64. Kauppi M, Neva MH. Sensitivity of lateral view cervical spine radiographs taken in the neutral position in atlantoaxial subluxation in rheumatic diseases. Clin Rheumatol. 1998;17:511–4.
65. Kawaguchi H, Kurokawa T, Machida H, Hoshino Y, Hirabayashi S, Ohnishi I, Katoh M, Mamada T. Roentgenological manifestation of ossification of the posterior longitudinal ligament in the cervical spine causing severe spinal canal stenosis—a group comparison with and without marked spinal cord dysfunction (in Japanese). J Jpn Orthop Assoc. 1991;65:173–80.
66. Kawaguchi Y, Matsumoto M, Iwasaki M, Izumi T, Okawa A, Matsunaga S, Chiba K, Tsuji T, Yamazaki M, Fujimori T, Yoshii T, Toyama Y. New classification system for ossification of the posterior longitudinal ligament using CT images. J Orthop Sci. 2014;19(4):530–6.
67. Kawaguchi Y, Matsuno H, Kanamori M, Ishihara H, Ohmori K, Kimura T. Radiologic findings of the lumbar spine in patients with rheumatoid arthritis, and a review of pathologic mechanisms. J Spinal Disord Tech. 2003;16:38–43.
68. Keiper ZRA, Bilaneui LT. MRI assessment of the supportive soft tissues of the cervical spine in acute trauma in children. Neuroradiology. 1998;40:359–63.
69. Kim H-J, Jun B-Y, Kim W, Cho YK, Lim MK, Suh CH. MR imaging of the alar ligament: morphology changes during axial rotation of the head in asymptomatic young adults. Skeletal Radiol. 2002;31:637–42.
70. Kobayashi S, Miyazaki T, Yayama T, Baba H. Microsurgical excision of hematoma of the lumbar ligamentum flavum. Joint Bone Spine. 2010;77(4):351–4.
71. Koga H, Sakou T, Taketomi E, Hayashi K, Numasawa T, Harata S, Yone K, Matsunaga S, Otterud B, Inoue I, Leppert M. Genetic mapping of ossification of the posterior longitudinal ligament of the spine. Am J Hum Genet. 1998;62(6):1460–7.
72. Kotani Y, Takahata M, Abumi K, Ito M, Sudo H, Minami A. Cervical myelopathy resulting from combined ossification of the ligamentum flavum and posterior longitudinal ligament: report of two cases and literature review. Spine J. 2013;13(1):e1–6.
73. Kotecki M, Sotniczuk M, Gietka P, Gasik R, Sudoł-Szopińska I. Imaging of cervical spine involvement in inflammatory arthropathies: a review. Pol J Radiol. 2021;86:e620–9.
74. Krakanes J, Kaale BR, Moen G, Nordli H, Gilhus NE, Rorvik J. MRI assessment of the alar ligaments in the late stage of whiplash injury: a study of structural abnormalities and observer agreement. Neuroradiology. 2002;44:617–24.
75. Krakanes J, Kaale BR, Moen G, Nordhi H, Gilhus NE, Rorvik J. MRI of the tectorial and posterior atlanto-occipital membranes in the late stage of whiplash injury. Neuroradiology. 2003;45:585–91.
76. Krakenes J, Kaale BR, Nordli H, Moen G, Rorvik J, Gilhus NE. MR analysis of the transverse ligament in the late stage of whiplash injury. Acta Radiol. 2003;44:637–44.
77. Krakenes J, Kaale B, Rorvik J, Gilhus N. MRI assessment of normal ligamentous structures in the craniovertebral junction. Neuroradiology. 2001;43:1089–97.
78. Kwee RM, Kwee TC. Imaging of facet joint diseases. Clin Imaging. 2021;80:167–79.
79. Ladenheim SE, Marlowe FI. Dysphagia secondary to cervical osteophytes. Am J Otolaryngol. 1999;20:184–9.
80. Laiho K, Kauppi M. The cervical spine in patients with psoriatic arthritis. Ann Rheum Dis. 2002;61:650–2.
81. Lang J. Craniocervical region, osteology, and articulations. Neuro-Orthopedics. 1986;1:67–92.
82. Lazennec JY, d'Astorg H, Rousseau MA. Cervical spine surgery in ankylosing spondylitis: review and current concept. Orthop Traumatol Surg Res OTSR. 2015;101:507–13.
83. Lee JS, Lee S, Bang SY, Choi KS, Joo KB, Kim YB, Sung IL, Kim TH. Prevalence and risk factors of anterior atlantoaxial subluxation in ankylosing spondylitis. J Rheumatol. 2012;39(12):2321–6.
84. Liu HP, Chen CL, Chen NF, Liao CY, Ou CY. Ligamentum flavum hematoma due to stretching exercise. Am J Emerg Med. 2016;34(10):2058.e3–6.

85. Lohkamp L-N, Marathe N, Fehlings MG. Craniocervical instability in Ehlers-Danlos syndrome-a systematic review of diagnostic and surgical treatment criteria. Glob Spine J. 2022;12:1862–71.
86. Loibl M, Stoyanov L, Doenitz C, Brawanski A, Wiggermann P, Krutsch W, Nerlich M, Oszwald M, Neumann C, Salzberger B, Hanses F. Outcome-related co-factors in 105 cases of vertebral osteomyelitis in a tertiary care hospital. Infection. 2014;42(3):503–10.
87. Lyons MK, Atkinson JL, Wharen RE, Deen HG, Zimmernan RS, Lemens SM. Surgical evaluation and management of lumbar synovial cysts: the Mayo Clinic experience. J Neurosurg. 2000;93:53–7.
88. Maas F, Spoorenberg A, Brouwer E, van der Veer E, Bootsma H, Bos R, Wink FR, Arends S. Radiographic damage and progression of the cervical spine in ankylosing spondylitis patients treated with TNF-α inhibitors: facet joints vs. vertebral bodies. Semin Arthritis Rheum. 2017;46(5):562–8.
89. Mahallati H, Wallace K, Hunter M, Bilbao J, Clark A. MR imaging of a hemorrhagic and granulomatous cyst of the ligamentum flavum with pathologic correlation. AJNR. 1999;20:1166–8.
90. Mantripragada S, Kannivelu A, Peh WC. Magnetic resonance imaging of cervical ligamentous anatomy and traumatic ligamentous injuries. J Med Imaging Radiat Oncol. 2020;64:368–76.
91. Marathe NA, Dahapute AA, Desai JR, Dhole KP, Bhaladhare S, Shah S. X-ray and computed tomography scan-based morphometric analysis of skull baselines in Indian population. Asian J Neurosurg. 2019;14(4):1116–21.
92. Marshman LA, Benjamin JC, David KM, King A, Chawda SJ. “Disc cysts” and “posterior longitudinal ligament ganglion cysts”: synonymous entities? Report of three cases and literature review. Neurosurgery. 2005;57:E818.
93. Maruta K, Ichimura K, Matsui H, Yamagami T, Sano A, Tsuji H. Calcification inhibitors in human ligamentum flavum. J Orthop Res. 1993;11(1):92–103.
94. Meeks LW, Renshaw TS. Vertebral osteophytes and dysphagia. Ann Otol Rhinol Laryngol. 1970;79:1091–7.
95. Meyrignac O, Carlier RY, Court C, Bouthors C. Understanding a mass in the paraspinal region: an anatomical approach. Insights Imaging. 2023;14(1):128.
96. Mirvis SE, NessAiver M. The radiology of acute cervical spine trauma. Baltimore: William and Wilkins; 1996.
97. Nakamura M, Toyama Y, Suzuki N, Fujimura Y. Metastases to the upper cervical spine. J Spinal Disord. 1996;9:195–201.
98. Nascimento FA, Gatto LA, Lages RO, Neto HM, Demartini Z, Koppe GL. Diffuse idiopathic skeletal hyperostosis: a review. Surg Neurol Int. 2014;5(Suppl 3):S122–5.
99. Neva MH, Häkkinen A, Mäkinen H, Hannonen P, Kauppi M, Sokka T. High prevalence of asymptomatic cervical spine subluxation in patients with rheumatoid arthritis waiting for orthopaedic surgery. Ann Rheum Dis. 2006;65:884–8.
100. Nguyen HV, Ludwig SC, Silber J, Gelb DE, Anderson PA, Frank L, Vaccaro AR. Rheumatoid arthritis of the cervical spine. Spine J. 2004;4(3):329–34.
101. Nishikawa M, Bolognese PA, Yamagata T, Naito K, Sakamato H, Hara M, Ohata K, Goto T. Surgical management of Chiari malformation type I and instability of the craniocervical junction based on its pathogenesis and classification. Neurol Med Chir. 2022;62:400–15.
102. Nizamani WM. Ligamentum flavum cyst: an uncommon but recognizable and surgically correctable category of juxtafacet cyst. Radiol Case Rep. 2017;13:302–4.
103. Offiah CE. Craniocervical junction and cervical spine anatomy. Neuroimaging Clin. 2022;32:875–88.
104. Offiah CE, Day E. The craniocervical junction: embryology, anatomy, biomechanics and imaging in blunt trauma. Insights Imaging. 2017;8:29–47.
105. Oga M, Mashima T, Iwakuma T, Sugioka Y. Dysphagia complications in ankylosing spinal hyperostosis and ossification of the posterior longitudinal ligament. Roentgenographic findings of the developmental process of cervical osteophytes causing dysphagia. Spine (Phila Pa 1976). 1993;18:391–4.
106. Ogawa Y, Kumano K, Hirabayashi S, Aota Y. A ganglion cyst in the lumbar spinal canal: a case report. Spine (Phila Pa 1976). 1992;17:1429–31.
107. Ohtsuka K, Terayama K, Yanagihara M, Wada K, Kasuga K, Machida T, Matsushima S. A radiological population study on the ossification of the posterior longitudinal ligament in the spine. Arch Orthop Trauma Surg (1978). 1987;106(2):89–93.
108. Ojuma N, Tubbs RS. The tectorial membrane. In: Tubbs RS, Iwanaga J, Loukas M, Oskouian RJ, editors. Clinical anatomy of the ligaments of the Craniocervical junction. Newcastle upon Tyne: Cambridge Scholars Publishing; 2019. p. 120–31.
109. Oláh C, Kardos Z, Kostyál L, Hodosi K, Tamási L, Bereczki D, Szekanecz Z. Assessment of cervical spine involvement in rheumatoid arthritis patients in the era of biologics: a real-life, cross-sectional MRI study. Rheumatol Int. 2020;40(6):915–21.
110. Ortiz Gómez JA. The incidence of vertebral body metastases. Int Orthop. 1995;19:309–11.
111. Osborn AG, editor. Diagnostic neuroradiology. St Louis: Mosby Yearbook, Inc; 1994. p. 836–75.
112. Osmotherly PG, Rivett DA, Rowe LJ. The anterior shear and distraction tests for craniocervical instability. An evaluation using magnetic resonance imaging. Man Ther. 2012;17:416–21.
113. O’Sullivan MD, Lyons F, Morris S, Synnott K, Munigangaiah S, Devitt A. Metastasis affecting craniocervical junction: current concepts and an update on surgical management. Global Spine J. 2018;8(8):866–71.
114. Otake S, Matsuo M, Nishizawa S, Sano A, Kuroda Y. Ossification of the posterior longitudinal ligament: MR evaluation. AJNR Am J Neuroradiol. 1992;13(4):1059–67.

115. Oxland TR. Fundamental biomechanics of the spine–what we have learned in the past 25 years and future directions. J Biomech. 2016;49:817–32.
116. Ozdemir B, Kanat A, Batcik OE, Gucer H, Yolas C. Ligamentum flavum hematomas: why does it mostly occur in old Asian males? Interesting point of reported cases: review and case report. J Craniovertebr Junct Spine. 2016;7(1):7–12.
117. Park JY, Chin DK, Kim KS, Cho YE. Thoracic ligament ossification in patients with cervical ossification of the posterior longitudinal ligaments: tandem ossification in the cervical and thoracic spine. Spine (Phila Pa 1976). 2008;33(13):E407–10.
118. Pfirmann CWA, Binkert CA, Zanetti M, Boos N, Hodler J. MR morphology of alar ligaments and occipito-atlanto-axial joints: study in 50 asymptomatic subjects. Radiology. 2001;18:133–7.
119. Powers B, Miller MD, Kramer RS, Martinez S, Gehweiler JA Jr. Traumatic anterior atlanto-occipital dislocation. Neurosurgery. 1979;4(1):12–7.
120. Prodi E, Grassi R, Iacobellis F, Cianfoni A. Imaging in spondylodiskitis. Magn Reson Imaging Clin N Am. 2016;24(3):581–600.
121. Radatz M, Jakubowski J, Cooper J, Powell T. Synovial cysts of the lumbar spine: a review. Br J Neurosurg. 1997;11:520–4.
122. Rai R, Tubbs RS. Barkow's ligament. In: Tubbs RS, Iwanaga J, Loukas M, Oskouian RJ, editors. Clinical anatomy of the ligaments of the craniocervical junction. Newcastle upon Tyne: Cambridge Scholars Publishing; 2019. p. 213–9.
123. Ramos-Remus C, Gomez-Vargas A, Guzman-Guzman JL, Jimenez-Gil F, Gamez-Nava JI, Gonzalez-Lopez L, Farrera-Gamboa H, Maksymowych WP, Suarez-Almazor ME. Frequency of atlantoaxial subluxation and neurologic involvement in patients with ankylosing spondylitis. J Rheumatol. 1995;22(11):2120–5.
124. Reijnierse M, Dijkmans BA, Hansen B, Pope TL, Kroon HM, Holscher HC, Breedveld FC, Bloem JL. Neurologic dysfunction in patients with rheumatoid arthritis of the cervical spine. Predictive value of clinical, radiographic and MR imaging parameters. Eur Radiol. 2001;11(3):467–73.
125. Resnick D, Niwayama G. Radiographic and pathologic features of spinal involvement in diffuse idiopathic skeletal hyperostosis (DISH). Radiology. 1976;119(3):559–68.
126. Rhoton AL Jr. The posterior cranial fossa: microsurgical anatomy and surgical approaches. Neurosurgery. 2000;47(Suppl):S5–S298.
127. Riascos R, Bonfante E, Cotes C, Guirguis M, Hakimelahi R, West C. Imaging of atlanto-occipital and atlantoaxial traumatic injuries: what the radiologist needs to know. Radiographics. 2015;35:2121–34.
128. Riew KD, Hilibrand AS, Palumbo MA, Sethi N, Bohlman HH. Diagnosing basilar invagination in the rheumatoid patient. The reliability of radiographic criteria. J Bone Joint Surg Am. 2001;83(2):194–200.
129. Robertson PA, Swan HA. Traumatic bilateral rotatory facet dislocation of the atlas on the axis. Spine (Phila Pa 1976). 1992;(17):1252–4.
130. Roh SW, Rhim SC, Lee HK, Kang SK. Spinal ganglion cyst of lumbar posterior longitudinal ligament. J Korean Neurosurg Soc. 2000;29:543–9.
131. Rojas CA, Bertozzi JC, Martinez CR, Whitlow J. Reassessment of the craniocervical junction: normal values on CT. Am J Neuroradiol. 2007;28:1819–23.
132. Ronnen HR, de Korte PJ, Brink PR, van der Bijl HJ, Tonino AJ, Franke CL. Acute whiplash injury: is there a role for MR imaging? — a prospective study of 100 patients. Radiology. 1996;201:93–6.
133. Rudwaleit M, van der Heijde D, Landewé R, Listing J, Akkoc N, Brandt J, Braun J, Chou CT, Collantes-Estevez E, Dougados M, Huang F, Gu J, Khan MA, Kirazli Y, Maksymowych WP, Mielants H, Sørensen IJ, Ozgocmen S, Roussou E, Valle-Oñate R, Weber U, Wei J, Sieper J. The development of assessment of SpondyloArthritis international society classification criteria for axial spondyloarthritis (part II): validation and final selection. Ann Rheum Dis. 2009;68(6):777–83.
134. Sabo RA, Tracy PT, Weinger JM. A series of 60 juxtafacet cysts: clinical presentation, the role of spinal instability, and treatment. J Neurosurg. 1996;85:560–5.
135. Saeed K, Esposito S, Ascione T. Hot topics on vertebral osteomyelitis from the International Society of Antimicrobial Chemotherapy. Int J Antimicrob Agents. 2019;54:125–33.
136. Sahri IE, Tlemcani ZC, Abide Z, Obame FLO, Ramdani H, Mohammed M, Dokponou YCH, Elmi SM, Imbunhe N, Akroud SE, Cherif EA, Miloudi G. Ligamentum flavum hematoma in the lumbar spine mimicking spinal tumor: a case report and review of the literature. Radiol Case Rep. 2023;18(9):3060–4.
137. Sakai T, Sairyo K, Hamada D, Katoh S, Takata Y, Shinomiya F, Yasui N. Radiological features of lumbar spinal lesions in patients with rheumatoid arthritis with special reference to the changes around intervertebral discs. Spine J. 2008;8:605–11.
138. Salmon B, Martin D, Lenelle J, Stevenaert A. Juxtafacet cyst of the lumbar spine. Clinical, radiological and therapeutic aspects in 28 cases. Acta Neurochir. 2001;143:129–34.
139. Sartip KA, Dong T, Ndukwe M, East JE, Graves JA, Davis B, Midyett FA, Duerinckx A. Ossification of the posterior longitudinal ligament: imaging findings in the era of cross-sectional imaging. J Comput Assist Tomogr. 2015;39(6):835–41.
140. Sato T, Kokubun S, Ishii Y. Choice of operative method for ossification of ligamentum flavum based on CT findings (in Japanese). Rinshoseikeigeka. 1996;31:541–5.

141. Schräder PK, Grob D, Rahn BA, Cordey J, Dvorak J. Histology of the ligamentum flavum in patients with degenerative lumbar spinal stenosis. Eur Spine J. 1999;8(4):323–8.
142. Schweitzer ME, Hodler J, Cervilla V, Resnick D. Craniovertebral junction: normal anatomy with MR correlation. Am J Roentgenol. 1992;158:1087–90.
143. Selden NR, Quint DJ, Patel N, d'Arcy HS, Papadopoulos SM. Emergency magnetic resonance imaging of cervical spinal cord injuries: clinical correlation and prognosis. Neurosurgery. 1999;44:785–92.
144. Shen P, Nidecker A. Magnetic resonance imaging of the craniovertebral junction ligaments: normal anatomy and traumatic injury. J Neurol Surg Part B Skull Base. 2016;77:388–95.
145. Sherk HH. Lesions of the atlas and axis. Clin Orthop Relat Res. 1975;109:33–41.
146. Shiono T, Yoshikawa K, Aota Y, Euguchi M, Teshima Y, Tanaka J, et al. Two cases of the ganglion cysts in the lumbar spinal canal. Radiat Med. 1994;12:125–8.
147. Sim KB, Park JK. A nodular calcification of the alar ligament simulating a fracture in the craniovertebral junction. AJNR Am J Neuroradiol. 2006;27(9):1962–3.
148. Smith P, Linscott LL, Vadivelu S, Zhang B, Leach JL. Normal development and measurements of the occipital condyle-C1 interval in children and young adults. AJNR Am J Neuroradiol. 2016;37(5):952–7.
149. Sudoł-Szopińska I, Jurik AG, Eshed I, Lennart J, Grainger A, Østergaard M, Klauser A, Cotten A, Wick MC, Maas M, Miese F, Egund N, Boutry N, Rupreht M, Reijnierse M, Oei EH, Meier R, O'Connor P, Feydy A, Mascarenhas V, Plagou A, Simoni P, Platzgummer H, Rennie WJ, Mester A, Teh J, Robinson P, Guglielmi G, Åström G, Schueller-Weiderkamm C. Recommendations of the ESSR arthritis subcommittee for the use of magnetic resonance imaging in musculoskeletal rheumatic diseases. Semin Musculoskelet Radiol. 2015;19(4):396–411.
150. Sudoł-Szopińska I, Matuszewska G, Kwiatkowska B, Pracoń G. Diagnostic imaging of psoriatic arthritis. Part I: etiopathogenesis, classifications and radiographic features. J Ultrason. 2016;16(64):65–77.
151. Taha H, Bareksei Y, Albanna W, Schirmer M. Ligamentum flavum cyst in the lumbar spine: a case report and review of the literature. J Orthop Traumatol. 2010;11:117–22.
152. Takahashi M, Satomi K, Hasegawa A, Hasegawa M, Taki N, Ichimura S. Ligamentum flavum hematoma in the lumbar spine. J Orthop Sci. 2012;17(3):308–12.
153. Takahashi H, Wada A, Yokoyama Y, Fukushi S, Sakurai T, Shibuya K, Suguro T. Ligamentum flavum haematoma: a report of two cases. J Orthop Surg (Hong Kong). 2009;17(2):212–5.
154. Takeno K, Tamura T, Sakai T, Sairyo K, Takao S, Kagawa S, Katoh S, Yasui N. Hematoma in the cervical ligamentum flavum. Report of a case and review of the literature. Skeletal Radiol. 2010;39(3):289–93.
155. Tan S, Wang R, Ward MM. Syndesmophyte growth in ankylosing spondylitis. Curr Opin Rheumatol. 2015;27:326–32.
156. Tubbs RS, Dixon J, Loukas M, Shoja MM, Cohen-Gadol AA. Ligament of Barkow of the craniocervical junction: its anatomy and potential clinical and functional significance. J Neurosurg Spine. 2010;12:619–22.
157. Tubbs SR, Grabb P, Spooner A, Wilson W, Oakes J. The apical ligament: anatomy and functional significance. J Neurosurg. 2000;92(2 Suppl):197–200.
158. Tubbs RS, Griessenauer CJ, McDaniel JG, Burns AM, Kumbla A, Cohen-Gadol AA. The transverse occipital ligament: anatomy and potential functional significance. Neurosurgery. 2010;66(3 Suppl Operative):1–3.
159. Tubbs RS, Hallock JD, Radcliff V, Naftel RP, Mortazavi M, Shoja MM, Loukas M, Cohen-Gadol AA. Ligaments of the craniocervical junction. J Neurosurg Spine. 2011;14(6):697–709.
160. Tubbs RS, Kelly DR, Humphrey ER, Chua GD, Shoja MM, Salter EG, Acakpo-Satchivi L, Wellons JC 3rd, Blount JP, Oakes WJ. The tectorial membrane: anatomical, biomechanical, and histological analysis. Clin Anat. 2007;20(4):382–6.
161. Tubbs RS, Salter GE, Oakes WJ. The accessory atlantoaxial ligament. Neurosurgery. 2004;55:400–4.
162. Tubbs RS, Stetler W, Shoja MM, Loukas M, Hansasuta A, Liechty P. The lateral atlantooccipital ligament. Surg Radiol Anat. 2007;29:219–23.
163. Vasani SS, Demetriades AK, Joshi SM, Yeh J, Ellamushi H. Traumatic intraspinal extradural ganglion cyst in a teenager: case report and review of the literature. Clin Neurol Neurosurg. 2007;109:88–91.
164. Vassiou K, Eftichia K, Marinos K, Kotrogianni F, Fanariotis M, Fezoulidis I, Arvanitis D. Magnetic resonance imaging of the ligaments of the craniocervical region at 3Tesla magnetic resonance unit: quantitative and qualitative assessment. J Biomed Sci Eng. 2012;5:901–9.
165. Vernet O, Frankhauser H, Schnyder P, Déruaz JP. Cyst of the ligamentum flavum: report of six cases. Neurosurgery. 1991;29:277–83.
166. Wasserman BR, Moskovich R, Razi AE. Rheumatoid arthritis of the cervical spine–clinical considerations. Bull NYU Hosp Jt Dis. 2011;69:136–48.
167. Wolf M, Weber MA. Inflammatory and infectious disorders of the spine. In: Barkhof F, Jager R, Thurnher M, Rovira Cañellas A, editors. Clinical Neuroradiology. Cham: Springer; 2019. https://doi.org/10.1007/978-3-319-61423-6_80-1.
168. Wong DA, Fornasier VL, MacNab I. Spinal metastases: the obvious, the occult, and the impostors. Spine (Phila Pa 1976). 1990;15:1–4.
169. Xu R, Sciubba DM, Gokaslan ZL, Bydon A. Metastasis to the occipitocervical junction: a case report and review of the literature. Surg Neurol Int. 2010;1:16.

170. Yalçinkaya F, Parlak Sağol Ş, Azizova A, Bilgin E, Karli Oğuz K, Kalyoncu U. Craniocervical junction involvement in inflammatory arthritis: a single-center radiologic study. Turk J Med Sci. 2023;53:1713–21.
171. Yamamoto A, Nishiura I, Handa H, Kondo A. Ganglion cyst in the ligamentum flavum of the cervical spine causing myelopathy: report of two cases. Surg Neurol. 2001;56(6):390–5.
172. Yamashita Y, Takahashi M, Matsuno Y, Sakamoto Y, Yoshizumi K, Oguni T, Kojima R. Spinal cord compression due to ossification of ligaments: MR imaging. Radiology. 1990;175(3):843–8.
173. Yoshii T, Hirai T, Iwanami A, Nagoshi N, Takeuchi K, Mori K, Yamada T, Seki S, Tsuji T, Fujiyoshi K, Furukawa M, Nishimura S, Wada K, Koda M, Furuya T, Matsuyama Y, Hasegawa T, Takeshita K, Kimura A, Abematsu M, Haro H, Ohba T, Watanabe M, Katoh H, Watanabe K, Ozawa H, Kanno H, Imagama S, Ando K, Fujibayashi S, Matsumoto M, Nakamura M, Yamazaki M, Okawa A, Kawaguchi Y. Co-existence of ossification of the nuchal ligament is associated with severity of ossification in the whole spine in patients with cervical ossification of the posterior longitudinal ligament -a multi-center CT study. J Orthop Sci. 2019;24(1):35–41.
174. Younes M, Belghali S, Kriâa S, Zrour S, Bejia I, Touzi M, Golli M, Gannouni A, Bergaoui N. Compared imaging of the rheumatoid cervical spine: prevalence study and associated factors. Joint Bone Spine. 2009;76(4):361–8.
175. Yuksel M, Heiserman JE, Sonntag VK. Magnetic resonance imaging of the craniocervical junction at 3-T: observation of the accessory atlantoaxial ligaments. Neurosurgery. 2006;59:888–93.

Neuroimaging of the Ligaments of the Subaxial Cervical, Thoracic, and Lumbosacral Spine

8

Ali Çağlar Turgut, Cenk Eraslan, and Fuyou Guo

8.1 Introduction

The subaxial C3-C7 segments, thoracic spine, and lumbar spine are unique components of the osseous and ligamentous vertebral column, characterized by unusual embryological origins and specific biomechanical requirements. The essential ligaments of the spine are the anterior longitudinal ligament (ALL), the posterior longitudinal ligament (PLL), and the posterior ligamentous complex (PLC). Therefore, it requires a special and careful radiological evaluation in the trauma environment. Therefore, a comprehensive understanding of neuroradiologists and spine surgeons is a prerequisite for accurately interpreting all spinal ligaments in clinical practice.

A review of the literature concluded that the following pathological conditions involving the spinal ligaments, including traumatic lesions, noninflammatory degenerative conditions (calcification/ossifications of the spinal ligaments and facet joint arthritis), neoplastic or infections lesions of the spine or paraspinal region and as well as the inflammatory rheumatological arthropathies involving the spine like rheumatoid arthritis (RA) and spondyloarthritis (SpA), including ankylosing spondylitis (AS) and psoriatic arthritis (PsA), are among the clinical conditions that are extremely common today and have the potential to lead to a variety of serious consequences. These conditions can be diagnosed with neuroimaging studies such as X-rays, computed tomography (CT), or magnetic resonance imaging (MRI). Therefore, it is clear that neuroradiological studies of these cases should be carefully evaluated by neuroradiologists for correct diagnosis and appropriate treatment.

This chapter will pay attention to the intriguing yet complicated anatomical features of the spinal ligaments in the subaxial C3-C7 segments, as well as the thoracic and lumbosacral spine, and will also cover different lesions involving

A. Ç. Turgut (✉)
Department of Radiology, Ege University Faculty of Medicine, Bornova, İzmir, Türkiye

Department of Histology and Embryology, Aydın Adnan Menderes University Institute of Health Sciences, Efeler, Aydın, Türkiye

International Joint Laboratory of Nervous System Malformations of Henan Province, Zhengzhou, Henan, China
e-mail: alicaglar304.at@gmail.com

C. Eraslan
Department of Radiology, Ege University Faculty of Medicine, Bornova, İzmir, Türkiye

International Joint Laboratory of Nervous System Malformations of Henan Province, Zhengzhou, Henan, China

F. Guo
International Joint Laboratory of Nervous System Malformations of Henan Province, Zhengzhou, Henan, China

Department of Neurosurgery, The First Affiliated Hospital of Zhengzhou University, Zhengzhou, Henan, China

M. Turgut et al. (eds.), *Ligaments of the Vertebral Column*,
https://doi.org/10.1007/978-3-032-09070-6_8

these ligamentous structures. Of course, every physician needs to be knowledgeable on this subject, including neuroradiologists, spine surgeons, neurosurgeons, orthopedic surgeons, neuroanatomists, rehabilitation physicians, and physiotherapists, who must recognize and appreciate the management of patients in all clinical situations involving the spinal ligaments.

8.2 Ligaments of the Subaxial C3-C7 Segments, Thoracic, and Lumbosacral Spine

8.2.1 Normal Anatomical Features of the Spinal Ligaments

A detailed knowledge of the ligamentous anatomy in the subaxial C3-C7 segments, thoracic, and lumbosacral spine is a prerequisite for accurate interpretation of spinal ligaments.

(a) *Nuchal Ligament*

The nuchal ligament has been described as the cranial extension of the interspinous ligament (ISL) and supraspinous ligament (SSL), from the C7 to the inion [136, 170, 176].

(b) *Anterior Longitudinal Ligament*

The ALL extending from the anterior margins of the vertebral bodies to the sacrum is responsible for spinal stability [34, 176].

(c) *Posterior Longitudinal Ligament*

The PLL extending from the posterior margins of the vertebral bodies to the sacrum is responsible for spinal stability [34, 176].

(d) *Posterior Ligamentous Complex*

The PLC consists of the following ligaments: (a) the ligamentum flavum (LF), called yellow ligament or interlaminar ligament, as a caudal continuation of the posterior atlanto-axial membrane; (b) the ISL; (c) the SSL; (d) the "facet joint capsules" which annex the back portion of the vertebra, mainly in the thoracic and lumbar areas; and (e) the "intertransverse ligament" attaching adjacent vertebral transverse processes for restriction of lateral flexion of the spine [26, 176]. The PLC has a mechanical role in the movements of the subaxial C3-C7 segments, thoracic, and lumbosacral spine.

Among these ligamentous structures, the LF bridges the adjacent lamina, while the ISL and SSL bridge the spinous processes [14, 34]. The LF, consisting of about 80% elastic fibers and 20% collagen but weak vascularization, is a long ligament structure from C2 to the lumbosacral region, extending down the lamina of the corresponding anatomical segment and extending laterally to merge with the facet capsule [11]. From a biomechanical point of view, the LF, the thinnest in the cervical vertebrae and largest in the lumbar area, is important for maintaining the body's upright position [11]. Pathologically, various sequential pathological changes of the LF, such as hypertrophy, calcification, ossification, and cyst formation, may develop, ensuing in compression of the spinal cord [87]. Hypertrophy of the LF can occur in conjunction with chronic degenerative processes. It may lead to spinal stenosis, a narrowing of the size of the spinal canal where the nerve roots exit laterally, called "foramina" [59]. Stenosis caused by hypertrophy of the LF is usually affliated with bulging of the intervertebral discs (IVDs) and facet hypertrophy, and when stenosis from these processes is serious sufficient to induce compression of neural structures, encroachment may result in "radiculopathy" or "myelopathy," as a result of the involvement of neural structures.

8.2.2 Normal Imaging Findings of the Spinal Ligaments

Normal imaging features of the ligaments of the subaxial C3-C7 segments, thoracic, and lumbosacral spine will be discussed in detail below before considering the pathological aspects in the following sections.

(a) ***X-rays***

X-rays in anterior-posterior (AP), lateral, and oblique positions are used for visualization of the bone anatomy adjacent to the ligaments in the subaxial C3-C7 segments, thoracic, and lumbosacral spine.

(b) *Computed Tomography*

CT is the primary imaging modality for evaluating spinal ligaments in the subaxial C3-C7 segments, thoracic spine, and lumbar spine due to its high sensitivity and availability [111, 176]. Appropriate resolution multiplanar reformats can be obtained using an axial source data set with thin sections of 2 mm or less [111]. In addition to axial slices, coronal and sagittal reformats can be obtained using multidetector CT technology, and the application of angular or oblique reformats may be necessary, as did in the evaluation of spinal ligaments of the CCJ region including the transverse atlantal ligament, the cruciform ligament, the tectorial membrane, the alar ligament, the apical ligament, the transverse occipital ligament, and Barkow's ligament [30, 31, 40, 46, 49-56, 58, 60, 62, 64, 65, 84, 88, 94, 108, 110, 111, 116, 130, 139, 155, 157, 167, 168, 171].

(c) *Computed Tomography Angiography*

In some cases, CT angiography may be necessary due to the proximity of the thoracic and abdominal aorta and its roots to the thoracic and lumbar spine [111].

(d) *Magnetic Resonance Imaging*

In addition to CT, MRI is required to evaluate the subaxial C3-C7 segments and ligaments in the thoracic and lumbar spine. Nowadays, MRI is the best choice for imaging the spinal ligaments [15, 17, 32, 41, 48, 66, 71, 72, 78, 93, 120, 126, 150, 172, 173, 188]. Radiologically, subaxial C3-C7 segments and normal spinal ligaments of the thoracic and lumbar spine are hypointense on T1- and T2-weighted MRIs. Furthermore, there is no doubt that for an individualized approach, the use of pertinent sequence parameters of MRI is significant consistent with the coil design and strength of field and gradient, in addition to software capabilities of the MRI system [10, 41, 78, 93, 126, 150, 188]. Additionally, selecting various parameters, such as field of view, slice thickness, matrix, and signal averages, can compensate for effects on signal-to-noise ratio (SNR), spatial resolution, and imaging times, thereby improving MRI scan quality [10]. Additionally, it should be kept in mind that cerebrospinal fluid (CSF) pulsatility artifacts may prevent evaluation of the spinal cord in T2-weighted and fast spin-echo inversion-recovery (FSE-IR) sequences [10].

8.3 Imaging Properties of Various Lesions of the Ligaments of the Subaxial C3-C7 Segments, Thoracic, and Lumbosacral Spine

Various pathological conditions affecting the ligaments of the subaxial C3-C7 segments, as well as the thoracic and lumbosacral spine, including traumatic lesions, calcifications and ossifications, cysts, neoplastic lesions, infections, and inflammatory arthropathies, will be discussed in detail in the following sections.

8.3.1 Traumatic Lesions of the Ligaments of the Subaxial C3-C7 Segments, Thoracic, and Lumbosacral Spine

In general, X-rays and CT using a 0.75 mm thin-section axial source data set with coronal and sagittal reformations are the initial imaging modalities of choice in patients with trauma involving the C3-C7 segments, thoracic, and lumbosacral spine [111]. Indications for MRI in such patients are as follows: (1) Patients with neurological symptoms or persistent neck and/or back pain, suspected ligament or spinal cord injury, negative X-rays and CT; (2) Patients who cannot be evaluated clinically for more than 48 h due to change in level of consciousness; (3) Findings on X-rays or CT indicating ligamentous injury, such as facet dislocation, widening of the IVD space or interspinous space, bone fractures adjacent to the spinal ligaments, and prevertebral swelling; (4) Patients with spinal bone fractures or unstable injuries on X-rays or CT; and (5) MRI before closed fastal reduction or open surgical intervention is helpful in the diagnosis of possible IVD herniation or extradural/subdural hematoma [45, 176].

Anatomically, the stability of the spinal column is covered by solid composition of ligamentous and osseous structures. In clinical practice, instability of the spine, referred to as "spinal instability," develops when the spinal ligaments and vertebral structures lose their capability to provide adjustment between osseous spinal segments underneath normal anatomical loads [7, 8, 10, 13, 35, 123, 127, 137, 153]. Flexion, extension, axial loading, and rotational injuries cause instability of the spine [10, 14, 136, 140, 170]. Denis's "three-column" concept applies to the decision of an unstable spine in injuries involving the C3-C7 segments, thoracic, and lumbosacral spine (Fig. 8.1) [29, 176]. The "anterior column" is composed of the anterior vertebral body, ALL, and anterior anulus fibrosus. The "middle column" includes the posterior vertebral body, PLL, and posterior anulus fibrosus. The "posterior column" consists of the posterior elements of the spine, the LF, ISLs, SSLs, and facet joint capsules. Hyperextension may cause injury to the anterior column with/without the middle column ("compression fracture"), while hyperflexion can cause injury to the middle and posterior column ("compression fracture") [10]. Disruption of all three columns due to axial and rotational forces results in "burst fractures," bilateral interface dislocations, and teardrop fractures [10]. As a rule, injury to any two adjacent columns, including the middle column, will result in instability that requires stabilization as a management measure, because such cases may lead to further injury.

Radiological point of view, an unstable spine is considered when there is (1) involvement of two adjacent columns, including the "middle column"; (2) >2 mm offset; (3) Widening of the facet joint and interspinous space; (4) Distortion of the posterior vertebral body border; and (5) >50% loss of vertebral body height or > 20° kyphotic deformity [176].

At present, MRI is the selected imaging method for detecting ligamentous injuries in the spine, particularly in patients with neurological deficits and normal CT scans [10, 34, 45, 136, 140, 176]. However, MRI needs to be evaluated in conjunction with other imaging methods, such as X-rays and CT [45, 176]. Technically, selecting appropriate array parameters, field of view, slice thickness, matrix, and signal averages to balance effects on SNR, spatial resolution, and

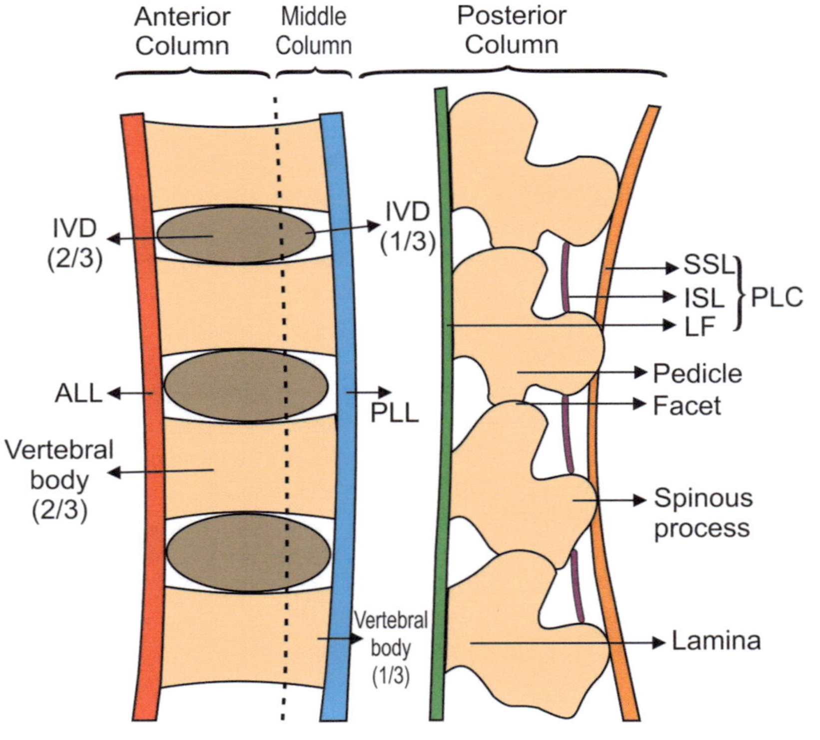

Fig. 8.1 Schematic illustration of sagittal alignment of the spine demonstrating the Denis' three-column concept of spinal stability for the C3–7 segments, thoracic, and lumbar spine [176]. Abbreviations: *ALL* anterior longitudinal ligament, *ISL* interspinous ligament, *IVD* intervertebral disc, *LF* ligamentum flavum, *PLC* posterior ligamentous complex, *PLL* posterior longitudinal ligament, *SSL* supraspinous ligament

imaging times based on coil design, strengths of field and gradient, in addition to software capabilities. The MRI system is also important [10]. In such cases, a typical MRI standard for spinal ligament injury should include the following sequences in the sagittal plane: T1-weighted, fast spin-echo T2-weighted, gradient-echo (GRE), and FSE-IR images [10]. In the axial plane, the standard should cover GRE or T2-weighted images for optimal visualization of the spinal ligaments; T1-weighted images, on the other hand, provide the best anatomical detail, exactly show alignment, and are helpful for detection of the fracture [10].

Importantly, MRI must be performed "within 72 hours of injury" for acute traumatic soft tissue edema to be identified as an increased-intensity signal on T2-weighted MRI sequences. However, MRI performed following 72 h may give false negative results for acute injuries because acute edema may diminish "after 72 hours" [10, 81, 103]. Within 72 h after spinal trauma, the presence of T2 signal hyperintensity, mimicking the effect of a contrast agent, is caused by edema or leakage of hemorrhage into traumatized extradural tissues, similar to the effect of a contrast agent. Additionally, ligaments appear at low signal intensity on all MRI sequences [10]. However, the presence of spinal ligaments showing the intermediate signal called "gray ligament" may result from the low fiber density of the ligament or anatomical ligament variation [28].

MRI has been reported to have high sensitivity in detecting PLL (93%) and interspinous injuries (100%), but is less sensitive in ALL (71%) and LF (67%) injuries [45]. ALL injury presents with separation of ligaments from underlying bone due to PLL, linear T2/short TI inversion recovery (STIR) hyperintensity, fluid, or discontinuity [176]. These are associated with avulsion fractures of the vertebral cartilage end plate (CEP) [34, 152]. Similarly, LF injuries manifest as T2/STIR edema, discontinuity, or flexure on sagittal MRIs. In contrast, ISL and SSL injuries are best appreciated on midsagittal STIR images as hyperintense areas between and at the ends of the spinous processes. These ligament injuries are associated with fractures of posterior spinal structures [34, 151]. Although fractures of the spinous processes and widening of the interspinous space are useful indicators, there is a potential for overestimating the extent of destructive ligamentous damage, which can lead to unnecessary surgical intervention [45, 176].

Spinal surgery is based on those with "spinal instability," incurable pain, or neurological involvement like motor weakness or loss of spincter control of bladder or bowel. The mode of surgical intervention, including laminectomy, discectomy, spinal fusion, corpectomy, and foraminotomy, is primarily based upon the underlying pathology and each of these different surgical techniques can be carried out in various ways.

8.3.2 Non-inflammatory Degenerative Conditions of the Spinal Ligaments

8.3.2.1 Osteoarthritis of the Spine

Osteoarthritis, also known as "facet joint arthritis" or "facet joint syndrome" or "facet disease," is a noninflammatory or degenerative arthritis, the most frequent kind of spinal arthritis, and it frequently involves the lower back, including the lumbar region of the spine [181]. As a result of the involvement of the facet joints between the vertebrae, IVDs, and the spinal ligaments, pain related to inflammation develops in these patients with osteoarthritis of the spine [181]. According to the localization of the involvement in the subaxial C3–7 segments, thoracic, and lumbosacral spinal column, these changes are called "cervical spondylosis," "thoracic spondylosis," or "lumbosacral spondylosis" [181].

8.3.2.2 Calcifications/Ossifications of the Spinal Ligaments

Noninflammatory degenerative conditions with calcifications/ossifications of the spinal ligaments such as calcification/ossification of the PLL (CPLL/OPLL), calcification/ossification of the LF (CLF/OLF), calcifications/ossifications of the other ligaments (ALL, NL, ISL and SSL), and diffuse idiopathic skeletal hyperostosis

(DISH) may cause ankylosis of the spine [36, 74, 106, 133, 155, 181].

Calcification/Ossification of the Posterior Longitudinal Ligament

Heterotopic CPLL/OPLL, a distinct entity related with both genetic and environmental elements, compresses the spinal cord, leading to myelopathy [117, 125]. Its etiology is unclear, but the prevalence of CPLL/OPLL, dependent on lateral X-rays of the spine, varies between 0.1% and 1.7% in Europe and the United States, 0.4% and 3% in Asia, and 1.9% and 4.3% in Japan [86, 99, 156]. Li et al. stated that the CPLL/OPLL is a common cause of thoracic myelopathy in the Japanese people [86]. There will undoubtedly be a higher prevalence of the CPLL/OPLL based on CT [43, 104, 117, 158]. The original classification was based on lateral X-rays of the spine in 1981; however, the new classification is based on CT scans in 2014. Nowadays, radiologists can identify incidental CPLL/OPLL in asymptomatic patients [69, 147].

In X-rays or CT, the CPLL/OPLL has been classified into the following four types depending on length: continuous, segmental, mixed, and limited (Figs. 8.2 and 8.3) [122, 147]: (a) "continuous type," ligamentous calcification/ossification in two or more vertebrae; (b) "segmental type," calcification/ossification located behind one or more vertebrae; (c) "mixed type" consisting of both continuous and segmented types; and (d) the "restricted type," characterized by an arch-shaped ossification behind the IVD. The most common type is segmental CPLL/OPLL, and the most frequent type in the thoracic spine is continuous CPLL/OPLL [43, 104, 115, 147].

A more detailed evaluation of the CPLL/OPLL on X-ray is possible with the help of CT. The continuity of the CPLL/OPLL over multiple vertebral segments is much better defined on CT [147]. The central and lateral location of the CPLL/OPLL in the spinal canal can be evaluated by cross-sectional imaging of CT [147]. Today, CT is the best of choice for detecting CPLL/OPLL and for preoperative planning. In clinical practice, the type of CPLL/OPLL, its thickness, the length of the affected segments, and related diseases, such as common DISH. On CT, "double density or double

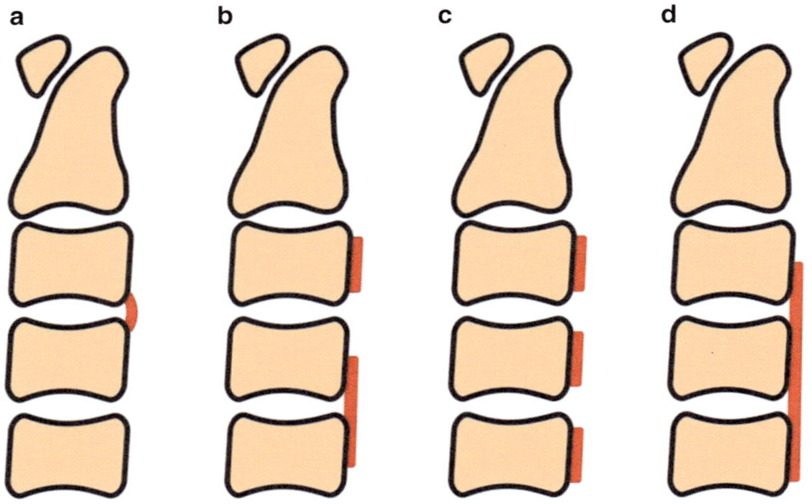

Fig. 8.2 Schematic illustration of sagittal alignment of the spine demonstrating the calcification/ossification of PLL (CPLL/OPLL) classification based on X-ray or computed tomography (CT). (**a**) "Circumscribed type" is characterized by a bow-shaped CPLL/OPLL behind an IVD. (**b**) "Mixed type" is characterized by the presence of continuous and segmental types of CPLL/OPLL. (**c**) "Segmental type" is characterized by the CPLL/OPLL located behind one or more vertebrae. (**d**) "Continuous type" is characterized by the presence of CPLL/OPLL spans across 2 or more vertebral bodies [147]

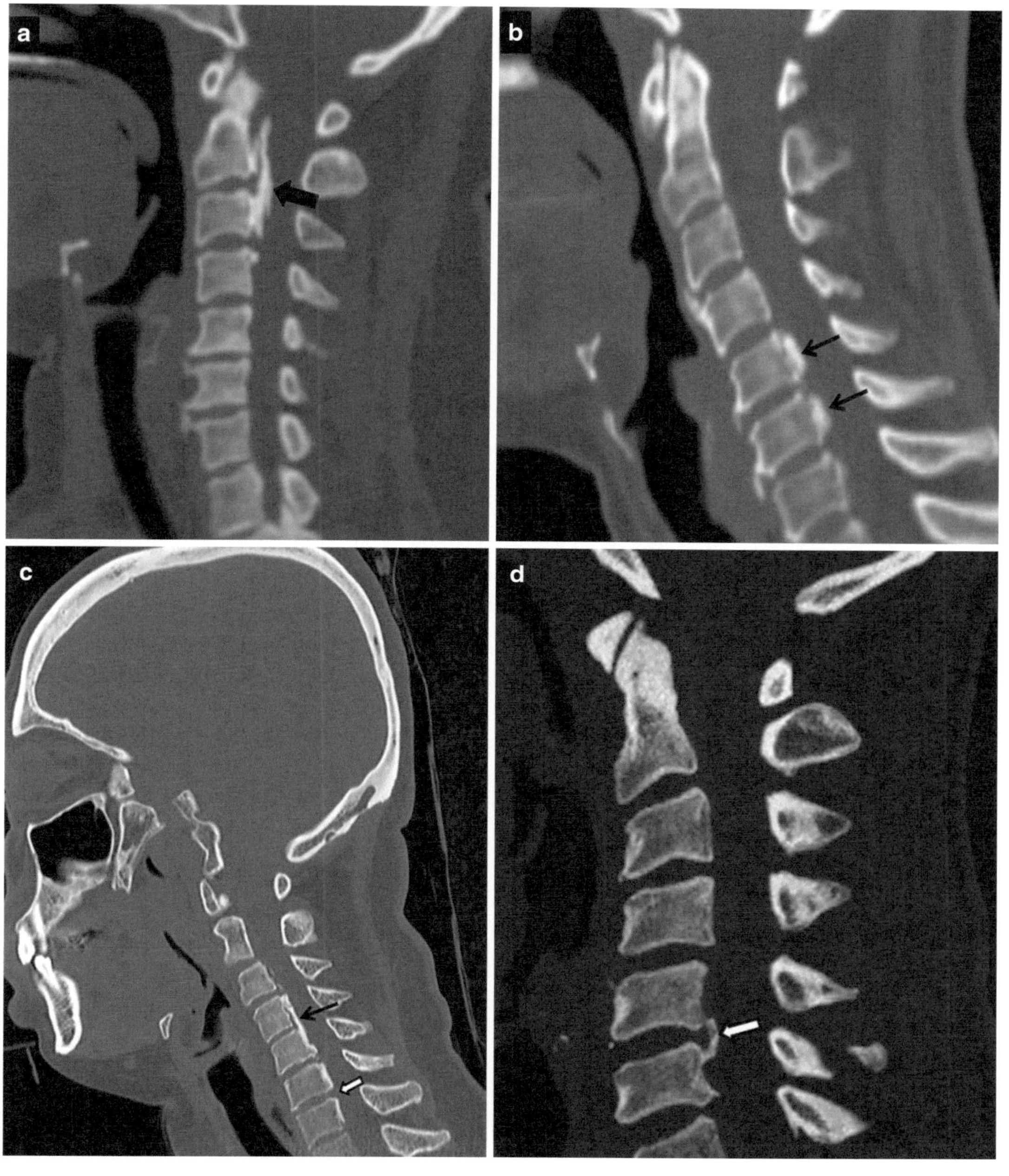

Fig. 8.3 (**a**) The CPLL/OPLL, when extended to two or more vertebral bodies, is classified as "continuous type" (black thick arrow). (**b**) The CPLL/OPLL is located posterior to one or more vertebrae and is classified as "segmental type" (black thin arrows). (**c**) It is classified as "mixed type" when "continuous type" (black thin arrow) and "segmental type" (thick white arrow) CPLL/OPLL is present. (**d**) The "circumscribed type" is defined as an arch-shaped calcification/ossification behind an IVD [147]

layer sign" on bone window axial CT as two separate calcified/ossified rings separated by a non-calcified/non-ossified mass representing a hypertrophic PLL and dural penetration or tight adhesion of calcification/ossification is seen. It has been reported that the presence of CPLL/OPLL causes a higher rate of dural tears (ranging from 52.6% to 83.3%) during anterior decompression [39, 55, 102, 147]. A normal PLL is often seen on CT because of its thin appearance and central location; the cut-off point for distinguishing between normal and the CPLL/OPLL is 2 mm [45].

The new classification system based on CT is as follows [69, 147]: (a) "Classification A" (ossified lesion, 2 types: bridge and non-bridge) depends on the adjacent posterior edge of calcification/ossification (Fig. 8.4). It is important to distinguish between excess vertebral level and bridging and non-bridging CPLL/OPLL because vertebral body segmental motion is lost in cases where bridge-type CPLL/OPLL leads to instability [69, 147]; (b) "Classification B"; and (c) "Axial classification" (there are 2 types, central or lateral, depending on the location of the CPLL/OPLL) (Fig. 8.5).

On axial CT or MRI as a complement to CT, the CPLL/OPLL is identified as square, mushroom, or hill type based on tangential lines drawn at the edges of the calcification/ossification (Figs. 8.6 and 8.7) [122, 147]. Recent studies

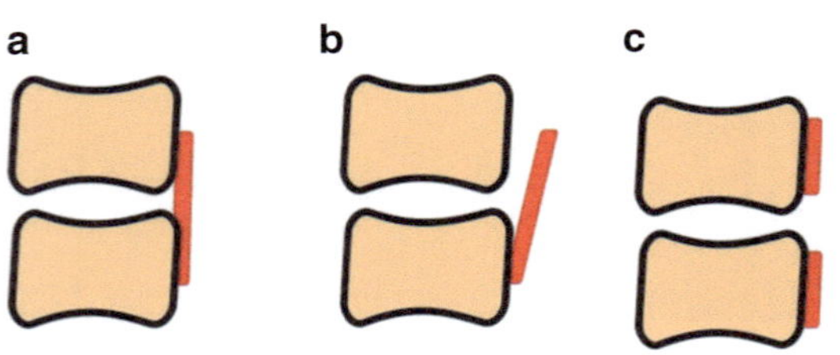

Fig. 8.4 Schematic illustration of sagittal alignment of the spine demonstrating the CPLL/OPLL classification based on sagittal CT. (**a**) "Bridge type" is characterized by the CPLL/OPLL abutting the posterior aspect of two or more vertebral bodies. (**b**) and (**c**) "Non-bridged type" is characterized by the presence of the CPLL/OPLL adjacent to the posterior aspect of only one vertebral level [147]

have revealed that the sensitivity of MRI is limited to 44% on sagittal T2-weighted images and 32% on sagittal T1-weighted images because the signal intensity of the CPLL/OPLL on T1-weighted sequences is similar to that of CSF and the vertebral cortex on T1-weighted sequences. On T2-weighted images [122, 185], "proton density imaging" is superior to T1- and T2-weighted images owing to the superior contrast between PLL, CSF, and calcification/ossification of vertebral bodies [122]. It is possible to evaluate the cord signal using MRI in the assessment of CPLL/OPLL and hyperintense T2 spinal cord signal abnormalities, which can occur with various neurological deficits and may be secondary to edema or myelomalacia [77].

Based on data obtained from axial MRI at the maximum neural compression level, Matsuyama et al. classified spinal cord shape as "boomerang," "teardrop," or "triangle" as a prognostic factor for clinical recovery [98]. Specifically, the teardrop type had focal indentation in the spinal cord, whereas the triangle type had flattening and findings consistent with spinal cord compression [98]. They found that the triangular shape was the worst for healing and the teardrop shape was the best; patients with spinal cord expansion on postoperative MRI in axial section following decompression demonstrated the most significant neurological recovery [98]. It is essential to note that the radiologically classified systems above must be combined with other imaging findings, like the degree of spinal stenosis and clinical observations. In such cases, axial MRI may also be used for estimation of degree of the spinal canal stenosis through the CPLL/OPLL, an important determinant of myelopathy [147]. From a surgical perspective, CPLL/OPLL, when involving three or more segments, has complication rates associated with posterior decompression and anterior approach due to technical difficulties [147]. Surgical intervention is necessary for the treatment of patients with anterior extradural compressive lesions caused by CPLL/OPLL [86].

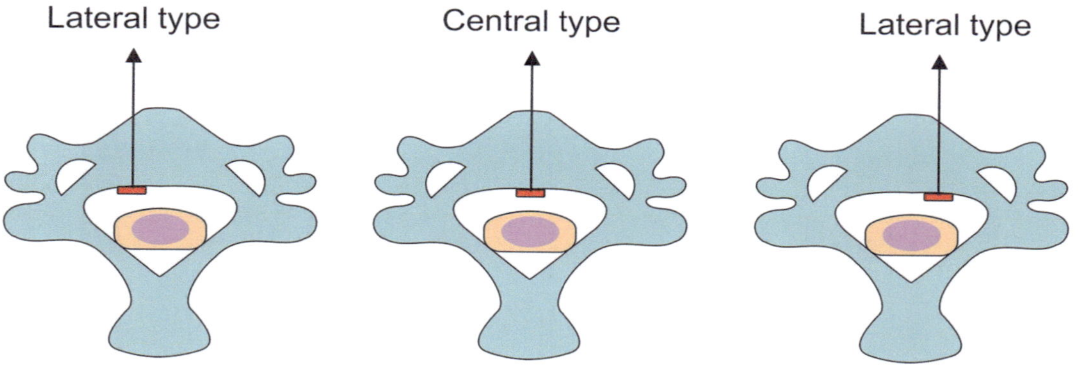

Fig. 8.5 Schematic illustration of axial alignment of the spine demonstrating the CPLL/OPLL classification based on axial CT. "Central type" is characterized by the CPLL/OPLL abuts the posterior aspect of the vertebral body. "Lateral type" is characterized by the presence of the CPLL/OPLL, which is adjacent to the lateral aspect of the vertebral body [147]

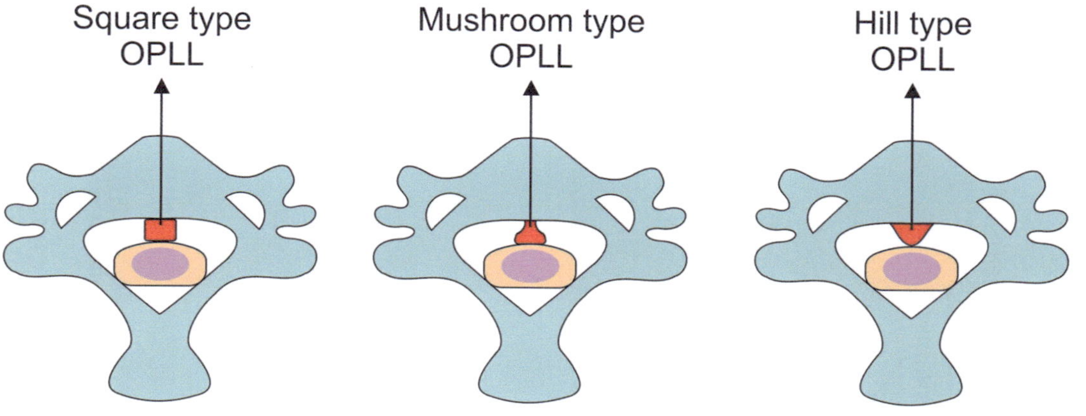

Fig. 8.6 Schematic illustration of axial alignment of the spine demonstrating the CPLL/OPLL classification based on axial CT or magnetic resonance imaging (MRI). "Square type" is characterized by the presence of lines parallel or tangential to the CPLL/OPLL margins. "Mushroom type" is characterized by the presence of lines drawn parallel to the CPLL/OPLL margins crossing anterior to the CPLL/OPLL lesion. "Hill type" is characterized by the presence of the lines drawn parallel to the CPLL/OPLL margins, crossing posterior to the CPLL/OPLL lesion [147]. Abbreviations: OPLL, ossification of the PLL

Calcification/Ossification of the Ligamentum Flavum

Calcification/ossification of the LF (CLF/OLF) in the lumbar spine causes a variety of neurological symptoms due to compression of the spinal cord, conus medullaris, cauda equina, and/or spinal nerves [57, 86, 162]. Pathophysiologically, focal or diffuse CLF/OLF may develop as a result of aging and inflammation, leading to loss of elasticity and thickening of the LF, as well as tophaceous deposition of calcium pyrophosphate crystals and inhibition of fibroblastic-like cell production [96, 149, 161]. This process may be related to previous degeneration of the LF due to any traumatic event that predisposes to calcium deposition [33]. This may be followed by the process of chondroid metaplasia and eventually ssification of the LF [161]

Clinically, the diagnosis of CLF/OLF is based on neurological findings, and it is important to know that the level at which the CLF/OLF is most prominent is responsible for the compression of the spinal cord and nerves in patients with the CLF/OLF at multiple levels using imaging

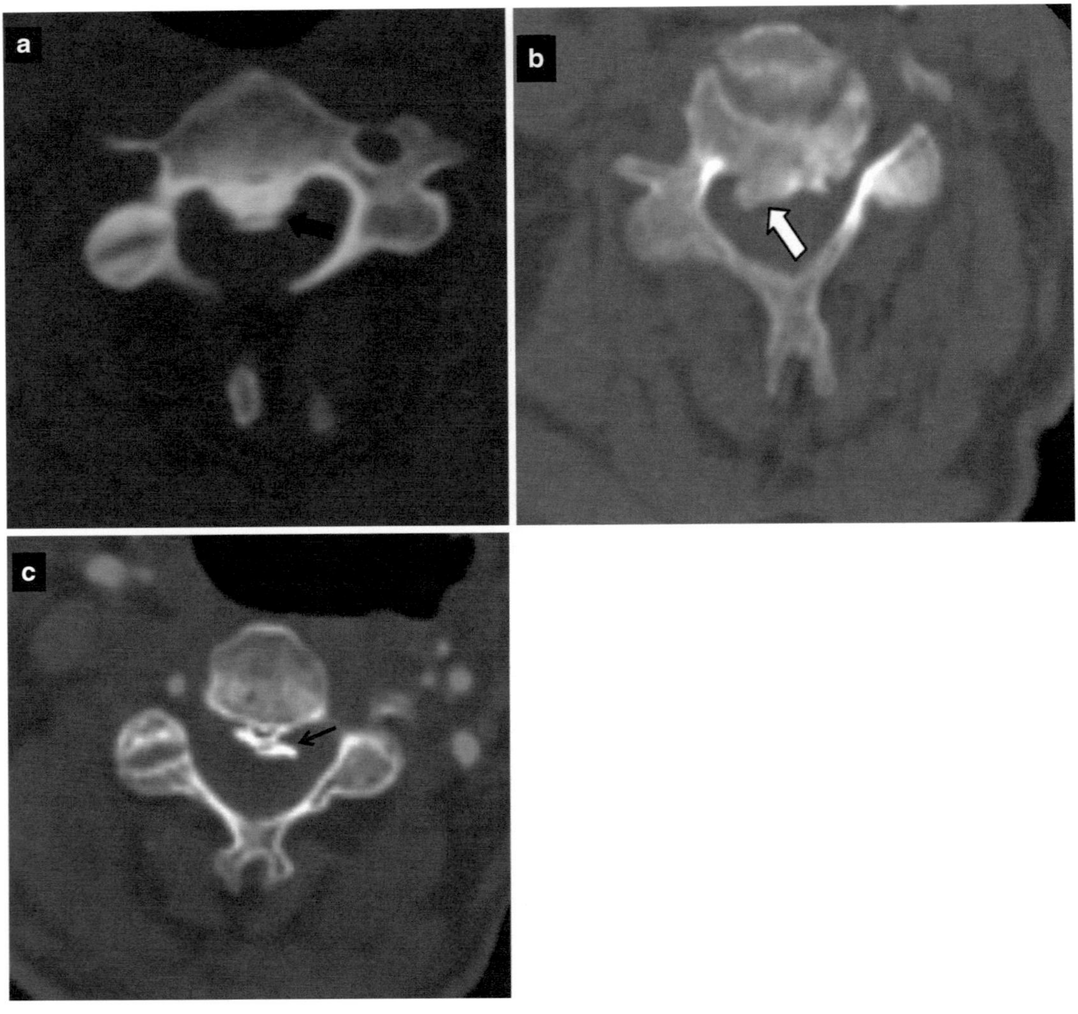

Fig. 8.7 Non-contrast axial CT images demonstrate (**a**) "Hill type CPLL/OPLL," lines drawn parallel to the calcification/ossification of the PLL edges pass dorsal to the CPLL/OPLL lesion. (**b**) "Square type CPLL/OPLL," lines are parallel or tangential to the calcification/ossification of the PLL edges. (**c**) "Mushroom type CPLL/OPLL," lines drawn parallel to the calcification/ossification of the PLL edges pass ventral to the CPLL/OPLL lesion [109]

techniques like X-rays, CT, and MRI [57, 68, 125, 162]. Early surgical treatment is recommended in cases where there are serious neurological deficits, such as motor and/or sensory loss and bladder-intestinal disorder, especially in cases where the CLF/OLF is combined at the same level and causes severe compression on the spinal cord [57, 162].

Radiologically, assessment of the CLF/OLF at the middle and lower thoracic levels is possible with lateral plain radiographs, but is difficult at the upper thoracic level due to overlapping of shoulder shadows [57]. However, sagittal CT images are very useful because evaluation of the CLF/OLF is possible at all levels of the spine without any difficulty [148] (Fig. 8.8). The CLF/OLF is now based on CT images performed at the mid-level of the facet joint, although the CLF/OLF was previously based on lateral X-rays at the thoracic level [148]. In 1996, Sato et al. divided the configuration of CLF/OLF into five types; bilateral calcifications/ossifications

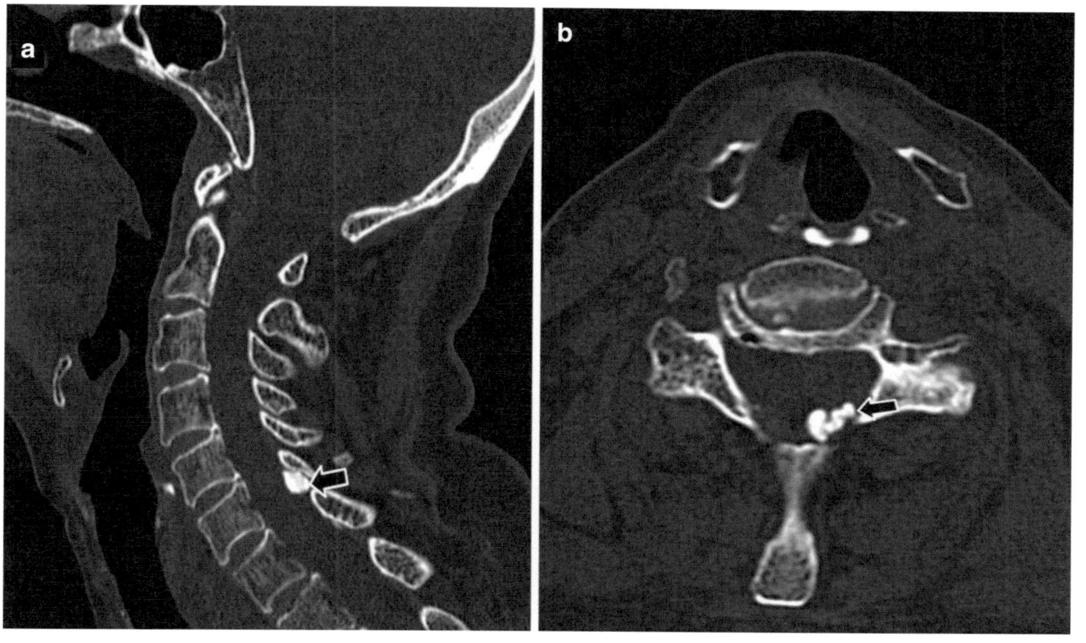

Fig. 8.8 (**a**) Sagittal unenhanced CT image shows calcification/ossification of the LF, called CLF/OLF (black thick arrow) just beneath the C6 spinous process. (**b**) Axial CT image demonstrates focal left-sided CLF/OLF in the same patient

do not fuse in the center of the lamina in lateral, extended, and enlarged types, whereas bilateral calcifications/ossifications fuse in the center in fused and tuberous types. The calcification/ossification of the dura mater spreads to more than one level [148]. From a radiological perspective, MRI is the best modality for imaging soft tissues, including the spinal cord; however, there is no clear correlation between the degree of spinal cord compression and the severity of neurological findings [68, 162]. Many different surgical procedures have been used for the treatment of patients with posterior extradural compressive lesions caused by CLF/OLF, although the possibility of postoperative paraplegia remains a significant risk in the postoperative period in patients with involvement of the thoracic spine [86],

Calcifications/Ossifications of Other Spinal Ligaments

In addition to the CPLL/OPLL and CLF/OLF, calcifications/ossifications of the other ligaments (the ALL, SSL, ISL, and NL) sometimes are seen in the same patients as combination or alone, especially in the cervical and thoracic spine as a cause of myelopathy [114, 125, 186]. The anatomical levels of calcifications/ossifications in the spine may be different, and calcified/ossified ligaments in the cervical spine may coexist with those localized in the thoracic or lumbar regions [86, 114]. Furthermore, it has been reported that the most frequently reported combination is the CPLL/OPLL and calcification/ossification of the ALL (CALL/OALL) or CLF/OLF [75, 86, 114, 125]. However, combinations of calcification/ossification of other spinal ligaments, such as CLF/OLF, calcification/ossification of the SSL (CSSL/OSSL), calcification/ossification of the ISL (CISL/OISL), and calcification/ossification of the nuchal ligament (CNL/ONL) have been reported in the literature [86, 114, 155, 186]. Various dynamic factors of the spinal column, such as increased mechanical stress at the junction regions, have been proposed as causative factors in the pathogenesis of calcification and ossification of the spinal ligaments [75]. Decompressive surgery (laminectomy and laminoplasty) is useful in patients with anterior/posterior extradural compressive lesions caused by calcified/ossified spinal ligaments [75, 125].

Diffuse Idiopathic Skeletal Hyperostosis

DISH, also known as Forestier's disease, is characterized by the formation of osteophytes on the anterior and lateral sides of the vertebral body in male adults with systemic diseases, such as diabetes mellitus (DM), obesity, hypervitaminosis A, and hyperuricemia [21, 82, 134]. In 2006, Atzeni et al. found high insulin and growth hormone levels in patients with DISH [3]. Pathophysiologically, calcification and ossification develop as a result of increased activity of osteoblastic cells in the spinal ligaments related to stimulation of alkaline phosphatase activity and type II collagen production by insulin-like growth factor 1 [38, 178]. Clinically, neck pain and restriction of neck motions are rarely encountered symptoms and signs in these patients with DISH. However, dysphagia is the most frequent symptom caused by compression, inflammation of the esophagus by anterior osteophytes in the spinal column, particularly at the C4-5 level. DISH is characterized by calcification/ossification of the spinal ligaments in the cervical spine, in addition to those in other parts of the skeletal system [21]. Neurological findings develop in patients with DISH as a result of spinal stenosis caused by the calcification or ossification of spinal ligaments, such as the PLL and ALL) in the cervical spine, and C1-C2 subluxation in the CCJ, which is attributed to the reduced flexibility of the spinal column [21]. Radiological point of view, presence of flowing new bone formation on at least four contiguous vertebral bodies despite absence of degenerative IVD disease and inflammatory changes in facet or sacroiliac joints and preservation of IVD height suggest the diagnosis of DISH [21] (Fig. 8.9). In patients with DISH with progressive severe clinical symptomatology, surgical intervention for removal of the osteophytes is performed. However, a conservative approach, including NSAIDs and corticosteroids, is sufficient in the vast majority of these patients [100, 112].

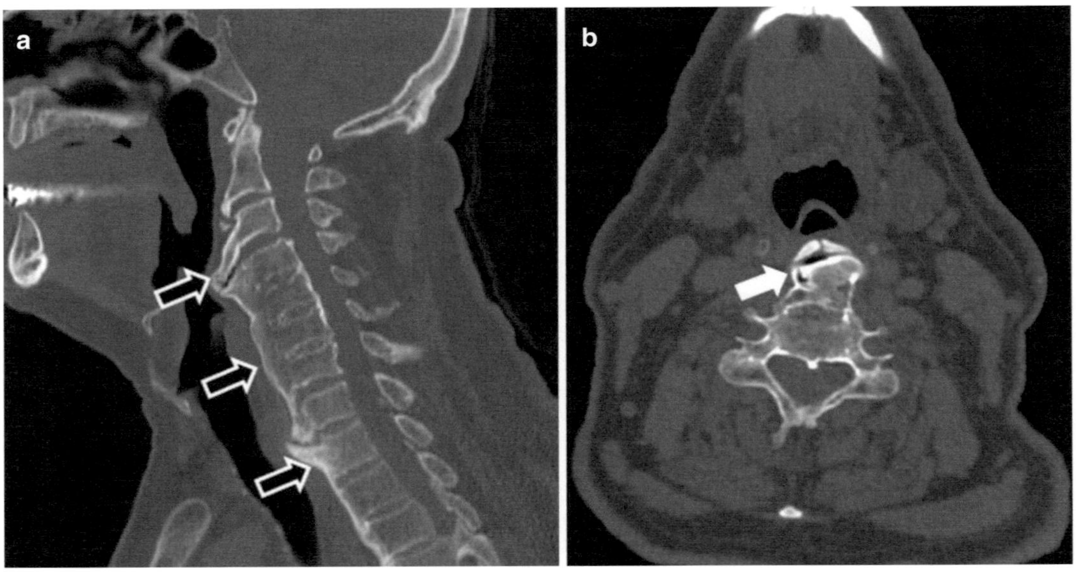

Fig. 8.9 (**a**) Sagittal non-enhanced contrast CT demonstrating calcifications of the ALL (thick black arrows) adjacent to vertebral bodies compatible with diffuse idiopathic skeletal hyperostosis, called "Forestier disease". (**b**) Axial image showing osteophytic bone formation (thick white arrow) anterior to C5 vertebral body, compressing neighbouring structures

8.3.3 Cysts of the Spinal Ligaments

8.3.3.1 Cyst of the Posterior Longitudinal Ligament

A PLL cyst is a small, benign collection of fluid that develops within the layers of the spinal PLL. Extradural cysts within the spinal canal in the lumbosacral region are generally classified as follows, according to their location, origin and pathological characteristics: (1) "synovial cyst," called juxtafacet cyst; (2) PLL cyst, which is called "ganglion cyst" even though it is not related to the posterior nerve root ganglia; or (3) LF cyst [1, 2, 23, 42, 63, 177].

Typically, any cystic lesion located in the periarticular region and not in continuity with the facet joint synovium but not its epithelial lining and PLL is classified as a "PLL cyst," a rare entity [23, 95, 129]. On the contrary, the cystic lesion located on the inner and posterolateral side of the spinal canal, lined with epithelial tissue and continuing with facet joints, is classified as a "synovial cyst" [129, 142]. Unlike the synovial cyst, the PLL cyst does not arise from synovial joints or tendon sheaths covered with synovium [23]. The exact pathogenesis of PLL cysts is unclear. Still, there are different etiologies, including multitraumatic events, spondylolisthesis, facet arthropathy, soft tissue degeneration, and accumulation of viscous material due to hyaluronidase production [5, 175]. It has been suggested that the adverse effect of degenerated IVD on PLL may be responsible for the development of PLL cysts containing serous or mucinous material, blood, or gas [22, 138, 175]. Clinically, most cases of PLL cysts are reported in athletic males in the third to fourth decades of life with a history of recurrent traumatic spinal cord injuries [113, 138, 142]. These lesions usually cause the following symptoms: radiculopathy, neurological claudication, myelopathy, neurological deficit, and even cauda equina syndrome [90]. Therefore, PLL cyst should be considered in the differential diagnosis of intraspinal lesions causing radiculopathy/neurogenic claudication.

On CT scans, these lesions appear as round masses in the anterior epidural space, have a low density compared to the adjacent IVD, and do not show enhancement following contrast administration [113]. Radiologically, MRI is the best choice for visualizing the PLL cyst as hypointense on T1 and hyperintense on T2-weighted MRIs [5, 23, 77, 119, 142, 154] (Fig. 8.10). Additionally, there is a peripheral enhancement of the cyst after gadolinium injection on MRI [5, 154]. Typically, all these lesions are hypointense on T1-weighted MRIs, hyperintense on T2-weighted MRIs, and often exhibit rim contrast enhancement after intravenous gadolinium administration [77, 113].

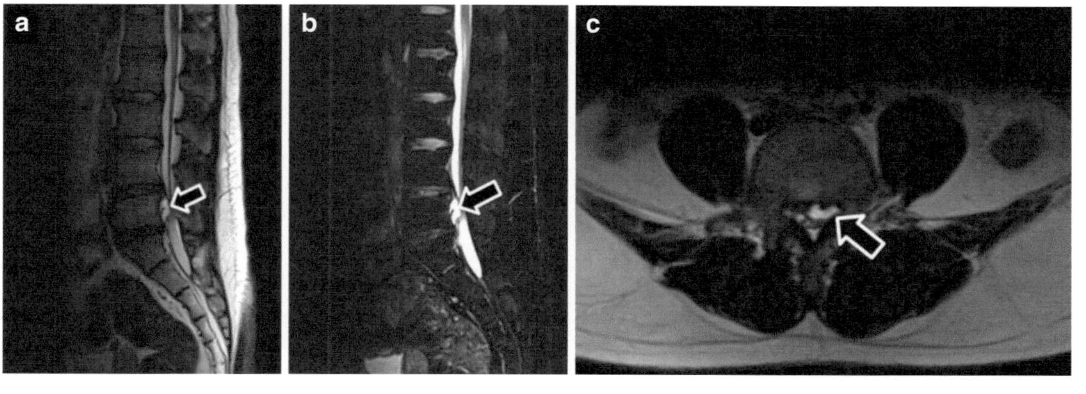

Fig. 8.10 (**a**) Sagittal T2-weighted MRI demonstrates a hyperintense lesion (thick black arrow) at the L5 vertebral level, located on the left side of the PLL. (**b**) Sagittal fat-suppressed image further delineates the lesion (thick black arrow) with a hyperintense signal, confirming its cystic nature and ruling out fat-containing components. (**c**) Axial T2-weighted MRI shows the lesion (thick black arrow) at the left side of the PLL of the spinal canal

Treatment of PLL cyst includes conservative treatment (bed rest, oral analgesics, and physical therapy) and/or surgical cyst excision in patients with persistent radicular pain and/or neurological deficits [90, 129, 142, 146].

8.3.3.2 Cyst of the Ligamentum Flavum

A cyst or pseudocyst of the LF, a rare cystic lesion, is an unusual cause of neurological signs and symptoms in older individuals, as a result of compression of the nerve root or spinal cord [161, 177]. They are enclosed in the inner surface of the LF without any epithelial lining or continuity with the facet joint synovium [1]. Pathophysiologically, the LF cyst is secondary to tissue degeneration and hypermobility in the transition zones between the mobile and fixed parts of the spinal column [44]. These cysts may contain hematomas as a result of ruptured vessels in degenerated LF and may develop secondary to tensile forces resulting from acute or chronic trauma [92]. They are frequently located as a category of juxtafacet cysts in the lower lumbar region and subaxial C3-C7 segments. Still, they rarely can also be localized in the remaining parts of the spine [1, 42, 63, 109, 161, 177]. In the numerous cases of the LF cyst, they are localized at L4-L5, a segment known to be very mobile in the lumbar spine, often associated with degenerative spondylolisthesis [161]. There are no pathognomonic clinical symptoms and/or signs for an LF cyst, and cysts within the spinal canal can lead to neurological symptoms (radiculopathy or myelopathy), including motor or sensory disorders and abnormal reflexes as a result of displacement of neural structures and spinal stenosis [161].

Radiologically, these lesions are diagnosed as intraspinal extradural masses on myelography and CT myelography [184]. MRI is the most effective method for diagnosing LF cysts accurately. It is a variable signal on T1-weighted images and a high-intensity signal on T2-weighted MRIs [44, 92] (Fig. 8.11). It is essential to note that LF cyst, as well as IVD herniation and facet joint diseases, can also cause radiculopathy or myelopathy [109]. Complete removal of the LF cyst results in resolution of the radiculopathy [176].

8.3.4 Ligamentum Flavum Hematoma

Anatomically, LF hematoma mainly affects the lumbar and thoracic spine, and the underlying pathogenetic mechanism of this entity remains unclear [124]. However, without any history of

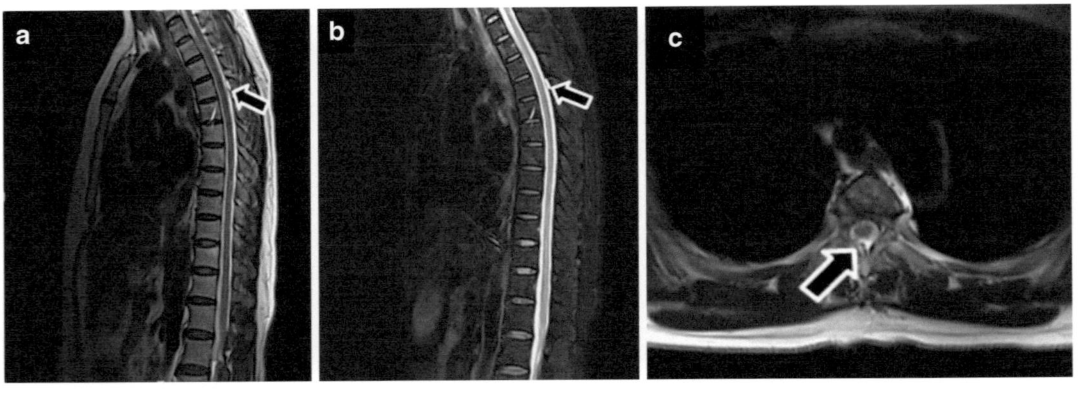

Fig. 8.11 (**a**) Sagittal T2-weighted MRI demonstrates a hyperintense lesion (white arrow) at the T4 vertebral level, located posterior to the right side of the LF. (**b**) Sagittal fat-suppressed image further delineates the lesion (white arrow) with hyperintense signal, confirming its cystic nature and ruling out fat-containing components. (**c**) Axial T2-weighted MRI shows the lesion (white arrow) at the right posterior aspect of the spinal canal, with no significant spinal cord compression observed

traumatic events, a partial tear in a degenerate or hypertrophic LF with vascular proliferation following a minor trauma, such as flexion of the back during a lumbar puncture, has been hypothesized to cause bleeding, fibrinolytic, and hemolytic changes in the LF. It causes symptoms of neural compression due to an increase in volume in the LF mass [11, 73, 163, 164].

Clinically, LF hematoma occurs with similar common symptomatology as an IVD herniation or other space-occupying spinal lesions, but is an extremely rare cause of low back pain, radiculopathy, weakness, urinary incontinence, and constipation as a result of spinal nerve compression [11]. Therefore, the preoperative diagnosis of LF hematoma remains challenging in most cases due to its rarity and clinical similarity to other conditions; a high index of suspicion for LF hematoma is crucial for clinicians [73, 144].

Radiologically, a postmyelographic CT scan is a preferred choice for diagnosing epidural mass lesions associated with LF [11]. MRI is the best option for the correct diagnosis of LF hematoma, as it shows blood-consistent signaling characteristics that can develop over time due to the degradation of oxy-hemoglobin to hemosiderin, resulting in a heterogeneous density of the mass adjacent to the lesion with LF [87, 144]. Therefore, due to the dynamic nature of the hematoma density, it may be challenging to image the LF hematoma using MRI [124]. Although rare, an increase in contrast has also been observed occasionally in LF hematoma. However, when present, it typically manifests as mild to moderate contrast around the lesion [163–165]. Early diagnosis and complete surgical removal of LF hematoma provides a positive result with instant resolution of clinical symptoms in patients [11, 144].

8.3.5 Involvement of Ligaments Secondary to Neoplastic Spinal and/or Paraspinal Lesions

All of the spinal ligaments can be affected secondary to various neoplasms of the spine, spinal cord, or surrounding soft tissue in the complex paraspinal region, including the retroperitoneum, pleura, or extradural compartment [18, 101, 121]. Most spinal tumors are caused by metastatic cancer spreading to the spine from another part of the body, and all neoplasms of the vertebral column and paraspinal region may involve spinal ligaments [18, 121]. Therefore, knowledge of the anatomy of the spinal and paraspinal regions, as well as an understanding of the imaging characteristics of spinal neoplasms, whether benign or malignant, is of great importance for accurate diagnosis and adequate patient management.

Nowadays, it is well known that spinal metastasis is the third most frequent anatomical site of metastasis in the skeletal system of the body, with most cases involving the thoracic spine, accounting for only 10–20% of cases in the cervical spine [18, 24, 118, 182]. It has been found that breast carcinoma is usually the most common primary site. Still, other common primary lesion sites such as thyroid, lung, breast, renal, and prostate carcinoma are possible [105]. MRI is the gold standard imaging modality for detection of any pathological process, with a nuclear bone scan used to distinguish between benign and malignant ones [101, 121]. In such patients, the presence of neoplastic instability and progressive neurological deficits is a relative indication for spinal surgery [121]. In most cases, radiologists present a challenging diagnostic and treatment problem that requires a multidisciplinary approach with neuroradiologists, spinal surgeons, neurosurgeons, orthopedic surgeons, and medical and radiation oncologists.

8.3.6 Involvement of the Ligaments Secondary to Infections of the Spine and/or Paraspinal Region

All of the spinal ligaments can be affected as a result of various infections of the spine or surrounding soft tissue. Spondylodiscitis is an infectious disorder of the spine encountered in immunocompromised elderly patients [25, 59, 89, 181]. In these infections caused by bacterial or fungal microorganisms, different parts of the spine are affected, including the ligaments of the spine [6]. In spinal infections, bacteria can arrive the spine and infect the spine in the following three ways: (1) hematogenous spread from a remote area, (2) direct external contamination from trauma or surgery, and (3) external spread from an adjacent tissue [6]. Given the vascular system of the spine, the same vascular pedicle forks feed the CEPs of two adjacent vertebrae; therefore, in most cases, the infection involves two adjacent vertebral bodies [6]. The CEPs of the spine are the first to be infected, and then the infection spreads to the adjacent IVD or vertebral body, causing discitis and spondylitis, respectively.

Imaging plays a pivotal role in diagnosis, particularly in patients with nonspecific clinical symptoms. Laboratory tests and tissue sampling for microbiological analysis may be useful for definitive diagnosis and appropriate antibiotic treatment [59, 89, 128, 181]. The imaging evaluation of patients with spinal infection should include X-rays of the spine and an MRI with the application of contrast media. MRI is the best choice for correct diagnosis [59, 181]. Typical MRI findings for spondylodiscitis include hypointense vertebral bodies on T1-weighted images and IVD with CEP loss, hyperintense vertebral bodies with CEP loss on T2-weighted images or STIR images, and increased contrast in IVD and vertebral body (Fig. 8.12). Approximately 50% of patients with spinal infections will undergo some type of surgery with the following indications: failure of conservative treatment, septic condition, infectious spinal instability, spinal canal abscesses, >2.5 cm paravertebral abscess, and progressive neurological deficits caused by compression of spinal cord or nerve root [143]. In most cases, radiologists present a challenging diagnostic and treatment problem that requires a multidisciplinary approach with neuroradiologists, spinal surgeons, neurosurgeons, orthopedic surgeons, and infectious disease specialists.

8.3.7 Involvement of the Spinal Ligaments in Inflammatory Rheumatological Arthropathies

The inflammatory rheumatological arthropathies involving the subaxial C3-C7 segments, thoracic, and lumbar spine, such as RA and SpAs, including AS, and PsA, are briefly given below:

8.3.7.1 Rheumatoid Arthritis

RA, an inflammatory arthropathy, may affect the joints of the whole body, including various elements of the spinal column, such as ligamentous structures and capsular joints localized in the subaxial C3-C7 segments, thoracic, and lumbar spine, apart from the C1-C2 joint [181]. Involvement of the cervical spine is frequent in patients with RA, although involvement of the thoracic and lumbar regions of the spine is rare [70, 145]. Histopathologically, it is characterized by synovitis, discitis, and osteitis, leading to ligamentous laxity and (pseudo)spondylolisthesis, resulting in collapse of the vertebrae and compressive myelopathic changes involving the spinal cord and spinal nerves [70, 76, 179]. From a clinical perspective, back pain and various neurological findings related to myelopathy and radiculopathy develop [20, 76, 132, 181]. Radiological findings such as X-rays, CT, and MRI reveal a variety of osseous findings, including destruction, bone marrow edema, spondylolysis, subluxation, and ankylosis, as well as ligament damage, in addition to compression of the spinal cord and/or spinal nerve [20, 70, 76] (Fig. 8.13). In particular, MRI is the best choice for evaluation of patients with RA involving the subaxial C3-C7 segments, thoracic, and lumbar spine [20, 70, 76, 107,187].

8.3.7.2 Spondyloarthritis

Axial SpA, a seronegative arthropathy group, involves the joints and the spinal ligaments, resulting with fusion of the capsular joints, also known as "syndesmophyte," and calcification/

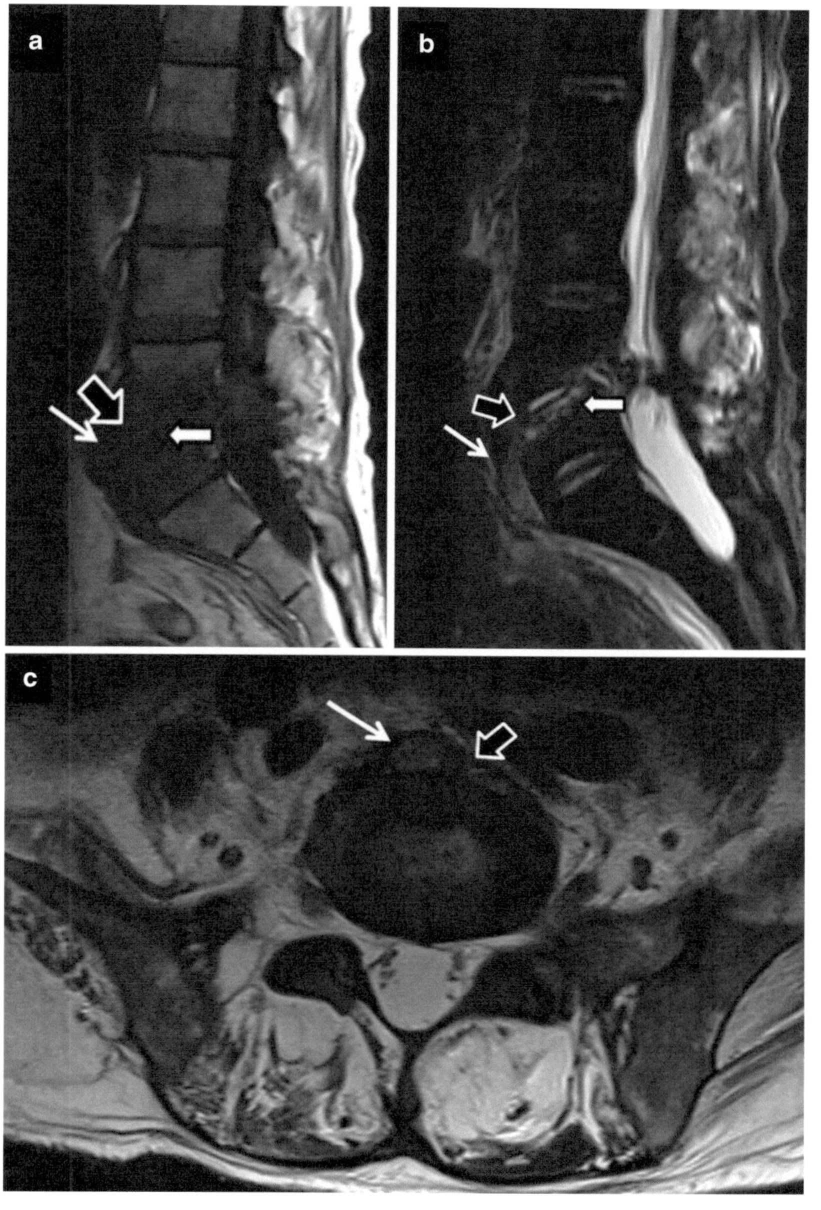

Fig. 8.12 (**a**, **b**) Sagittal T1- and T2-weighted STIR MRIs demonstrate L4 and L5 vertebral bodies as T1 hypointense T2 hyperintense signal changes and L4–5 IVD T2 hyperintensity compatible with acute spondylodiscitis (white thick arrows). (**a**, **b**, **c**) Sagittal T1- and T2-weighted STIR, axial T2-weighted images show that there is a prevertebral collection located in close proximity to L4 and L5 vertebral bodies (white arrow), and ALL (black thick arrow) can not be discriminated easily at those levels

ossification of anulus fibrosus and various spinal ligaments (PLL, ALL, LF, NL, ISL, and SSL), causing ankylosis of the spine [37, 76, 131, 181]. Unfortunately, clinical findings of SpAs are nonspecific, but their laboratory (human leukocyte antigen (HLA)-B27 antigen positivity) and radiological findings may be useful in the differential diagnosis of this group [47, 141, 181]. Unlike RA, involvement of the cervical spine is uncommon in patients with SpAs [16, 76]. Radiological point of view, bone marrow edema, and osseous erosion of the anterior sides of vertebrae, and involvement of

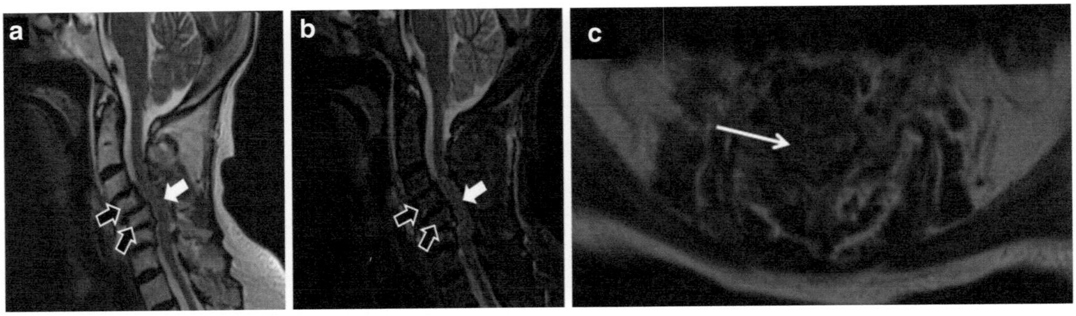

Fig. 8.13 Sagittal T2 (**a**) and T2 STIR (**b**) MRIs showing spinal canal narrowing secondary to grade 1 spondylolisthesis (thick black arrow) at the levels of C3-C5 and myelopathic signal changes (thick white arrow). C5 vertebral body height decreased moderately as a result of a chronic compression fracture. Axial T2 MRI (**c**) showing obliteration of the right subarachnoid space and spinal stenosis (thin white arrow) at the C5–6 level in a patient with rheumatoid arthritis

the anulus fibrosus of IVD, also known as "corner inflammatory lesions," "Romanus lesions," and "enthesitis," respectively, are characteristic findings of these patients in early stage SpA disease [4, 76]. On the other hand, the presence of triangular sclerosis, chronic osteitis, and remodelling of the anterior aspect of the vertebrae, also known as "shiny corner" and "vertebral squaring," respectively, are typical findings in these patients with more advanced SpA disease [4, 76].

Ankylosing Spondylitis

AS, called "Bechterew disease," a *seronegative* inflammatory spondylitis, is a chronic, progressive systemic inflammation of the axial skeleton, including the spinal ligaments, and fusion of the spine, in addition to arthritis of major joints (sacroiliac, hip, shoulder, and knee) and many vital organs in the human body, including the heart, lung, kidney, and heart [4, 19, 181, 183]. Histopathologically, it is characterized by deposition of calcification/ossification in the spinal ligaments around the IVDs of the spine, resulting in bony growths within the spinal ligaments and ankylosing of the vertebrae with restriction of movements of the spinal column, known as "syndesmophyte," in the advanced stage of the AS [37, 85, 166, 181]. It is well-known that the rheumatoid factor is negative in patients with AS [27, 181]. Clinical symptoms of AS include low back and buttock pain, stiffness, sacroiliitis, iritis, and kyphotic deformity [37, 181]. On X-rays of the spine, "bamboo spine appearance" of symmetrically deformed vertebral bodies, a diagnostic imaging finding, is related with calcium deposition in the spinal ligaments and IVDs, resulting with spinal fusion, and spinal fractures in advanced stage [181] (Fig. 8.14). Radiologically, approximately 1/4 of patients with AS have ankylosis of the facet joints and only 1/5 of patients with AS have the CPLL/OPLL as a cause of myelopathy [37, 91, 132, 166]. Conservative treatment, including corticosteroids or non-steroidal anti-inflammatory drugs, immunosuppressive agents, and physical therapy, is necessary before surgery for correction of kyphotic deformity and decompression of the neural structures in patients with AS [37, 181].

Psoriatic Arthritis

PsA, an autoimmune arthritis, involves the thoraco-lumbar spine of patients with psoriasis, resulting in ligamental calcification, syndesmophytes, parasyndesmophytes, ankylosis, and sacroiliitis [12, 61, 83, 159, 160, 181] (Fig. 8.15).

Overall, the inflammatory rheumatological arthropathies, including RA and SpAs, share common imaging features, including subluxations (horizontal anterior or posterior, lateral, or

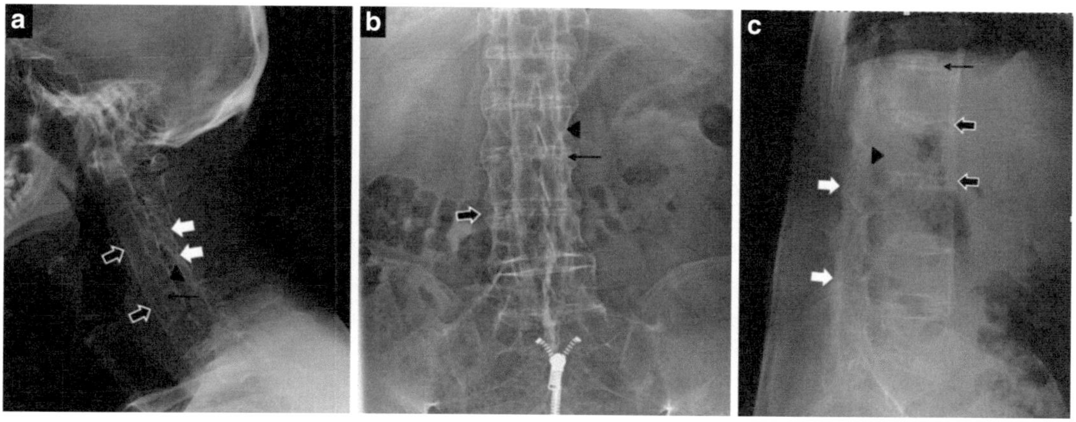

Fig. 8.14 In a patient with ankylosing spondylosis, respectively sagittal cervical (**a**), coronal (**b**) and sagittal lomber (**c**) X-ray images showing narrowing of IVD spaces (thin black arrows) and facet joint spaces (thick white arrows), squaring of vertebral bodies (black arrowhead), bridging desmophytes and fusion of vertebral bodies ("bamboo spine appearence") (thick black arrow)

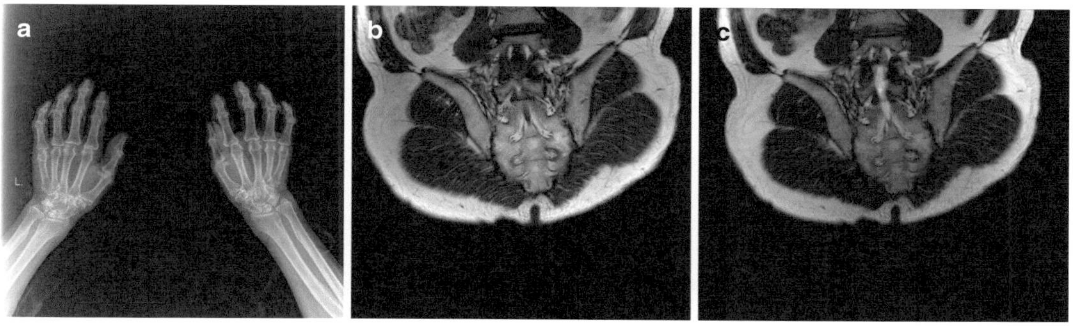

Fig. 8.15 (**a**) An X-ray of a patient with psoriatic arthritis shows abnormal bone structure of both hands, narrowing of interphalangeal and metacarpophalangeal joint spaces, bilateral first metacarpophalangeal joint deformation, and soft tissue swelling of interphalangeal joints (white arrow). (**b**) The fat-suppressed image further delineates the lesion (white arrow) with hyperintense signal, suggesting the presence of inflammation and ruling out fat-containing components. (**c**) T2-weighted MRI shows roughness of the articular surface at the lesion (white arrow), suggesting sacroiliitis

vertical) and spinal canal stenosis involving the ligaments of the subaxial C3-C7 segments, as well as the thoracic and lumbar spine [12]. Radiological point of view, X-ray study, lateral (flexion, extension, and neutral views) and AP projections, is necessary for evaluation of spinal alignment and paravertebral soft tissue including the spinal ligaments as well as diagnosis of various vertebral lesions related with inflammatory rheumatological arthropathies involving the ligaments of the subaxial C3-C7 segements, thoracic and lumbar spine [67, 76]. For example, the cut-off values for prevertebral thickness on X-rays are 7 mm and 21 mm at the C2-C3 and C6-C7 levels, respectively [97]. In lateral projection, the measurement of AP diameter of the canal in the cervical spine is below 10 mm ("absolute stenosis") and between 10 and 13 mm ("relative stenosis") [76, 174]. Similarly, CT of the spine with 3-D reconstruction is more effective than X-rays in assessing IVDs, uncovertebral (Luschka) joints, apophyseal joints, fractures/dislocations, various spinal anomalies, and involvement of the soft tissue [76]. The criterion for subluxation of subaxial C3-C7 segments caused by damage to the IVD, uncovertebral, and facet joints is a greater than 2.0–3.5 mm displacement of adjacent vertebrae [180]. MRI is useful for visualization of neural structures, the spinal ligaments, and CEPs of the vertebrae as well as various osseous lesions of the spinal column. Specifically, it has been reported that sagittal post-contrast T1-weighted and fluid-sensitive MRI sequences with fat saturation provide perfect visualization of active inflammatory lesions and bone marrow edema [159]. Moreover, functional MRI study in flexion, extension, and neutral positions is useful for further evaluation of patients with inflammatory rheumatological arthropathies involving the spinal ligaments [9].

8.4 Conclusion

The ligaments of the human spine are highly complex and important anatomical structures that provide spinal stability. In recent years, anatomical knowledge of ligaments of the subaxial C3-C7 segments, thoracic, and lumbosacral spine has led to dramatic advances in neuroradiology and spine surgery. Current imaging techniques for spinal ligamentous structures include X-rays, CT scans, and MRI, which are used when there is a significant bone injury or suspicion of injury to the spinal ligaments with any traumatic signal change [111]. In particular, MRI using a special imaging protocol provides excellent visualization of the spinal ligaments and adjacent soft tissue elements in the subaxial C3-C7 segments and the CCJ region [15, 17, 32, 41, 48, 66, 71, 72, 78-81, 93, 120, 126, 150, 172, 173, 188]. Importantly, the optimal time interval between injury and MRI should possibly be less than 72 h using special radiological criteria for diagnosis of potential traumatic instability [10, 151]. On the other hand, other lesions, including noninflammatory degenerative conditions of the spinal ligaments (calcification/ossifications of the spinal ligaments and facet joint arthritis), neoplastic lesions or infections or inflammatory rheumatological arthropathies of the spine or paraspinal region, involving certain ligaments of the cervical spine and lower thoracic or lumbar spine have nonspecific findings and clinical evaluation of these patients does not provide adequate information about these diseases, but they may cause spinal instability and severe neurological findings secondary to compression of the spinal cord and/or nerve roots [57]. Therefore, imaging of such patients using CT and MRI is very useful for adequate management of these pathologies. Large, multicenter, prospective, randomized controlled trials will be needed in the future to draw strong guidance on this topic. There is no doubt that microneurosurgical anatomical studies related to spinal ligaments, just as there are microsurgical anatomy of the posterior cranial fossa, are also necessary to develop new surgical approaches to improve the care of patients with affected spinal ligaments [30, 108, 135].

References

1. Abdullah AF, Chambers RW, Daut DP. Lumbar nerve root compression by synovial cysts of the ligamentum flavum. Report of four cases. J Neurosurg. 1984;60:617–20.
2. Akhaddar A. Posterior longitudinal ligament cysts. In: Akhaddar A, editor. Atlas f Sciatica; 2024. p. 857–9.
3. Atzeni F, Sarzi-Puttini P, Bevilacqua M. Calcium deposition and associated chronic diseases (atherosclerosis, diffuse idiopathic skeletal hyperostosis, and others). Rheum Dis Clin N Am. 2006;32:413–26.
4. Aufdermaur M. Pathogenesis of square bodies in ankylosing spondylitis. Ann Rheum Dis. 1989;48:628–31.
5. Baba H, Furusawa N, Maezawa Y, Uchida K, Kokubo Y, Imura S, Noriki S. Ganglion cyst of the posterior longitudinal ligament causing lumbar radiculopathy: case report. Spinal Cord. 1997;35(9):632–5.
6. Babic M, Simpfendorfer C. Infections of the spine. Infect Dis Clin N Am. 2017;31:279–97.
7. Barrey C, Afathi M, Broussolle T, Dauleac C, Bancel P. Craniovertebral junction instability and mechanisms of injury. In: Tessitore E, Dehdashti A, Schonauer C, Thomé C, editors. Surgery of the cranio-vertebral junction. Cham: Springer; 2020.

8. Belhassen S, Mat Q, Ferret C, Clavel R, Renaud B, Cabaraux P. Post-traumatic craniocervical disorders from a postural control perspective: a narrative review. Brain Neurorehabil. 2023;16:e15.
9. Bell GR, Stearns KL. Flexion-extension MRI of the upper rheumatoid cervical spine. Orthopedics. 1991;14:969–73.
10. Benedetti PF, Fahr LM, Kuhns LR, Hayman LA. MR imaging findings in spinal ligamentous injury. AJR Am J Roentgenol. 2000;175:661–5.
11. Benny BV, Nagpal AS, Singh P, Smuck M. Vascular causes of radiculopathy: a literature review. Spine J. 2011;11(1):73–85.
12. Blau RH, Kaufman RL. Erosive and subluxing cervical spine disease in patients with psoriatic arthritis. J Rheumatol. 1987;14:111–7.
13. Bogduk N, Mercer S. Biomechanics of the cervical spine. I: normal kinematics. Clin Biomech (Bristol, Avon). 2000;15(9):633–48.
14. Bogner E. Imaging of cervical spine injuries in athletes. Sports Health. 2009;1:384–91.
15. Borchgrevink G, Smevik O, Haave I, Haraldseth O, Nordby A, Lereim I. MRI of cerebrum and cervical column within two days after whiplash neck sprain injury. Injury. 1997;28(5–6):331–5.
16. Braun J, Bollow M, Remlinger G, Eggens U, Rudwaleit M, Distler A, Sieper J. Prevalence of spondylarthropathies in HLA-B27 positive and negative blood donors. Arthritis Rheum. 1998;41(1):58–67.
17. Brightman RP, Miller CA, Rea GL, Chakeres DW, Hunt WE. Magnetic resonance imaging of trauma to the thoracic and lumbar spine: the importance of the posterior longitudinal ligament. Spine. 1992;17:541–50.
18. Brihaye J, Ectors P, Lemort Van Houtte P. The management of spinal epidural metastases. Adv Tech Stand Neurosurg. 1988;16:121–76.
19. Brown MA, Laval SH, Brophy S, Calin A. Recurrence risk modelling of the genetic susceptibility to ankylosing spondylitis. Ann Rheum Dis. 2000;59(11):883–6.
20. Bundschuh C, Modic MT, Kearney F, Morris R, Deal C. Rheumatoid arthritis of the cervical spine: surface-coil MR imaging. AJR Am J Roentgenol. 1988;151(1):181–7.
21. Cammisa M, Serio D, Guglielmi G. Diffuse idiopatic skeletal hyperostosis. Eur J Radiol. 1997;27:7–11.
22. Chiba K, Toyama Y, Matsumoto M, Maruiwa H, Watanabe M, Nishizawa T. Intraspinal cyst communicating with the intervertebral disc in the lumbar spine: discal cyst. Spine (Phila Pa 1976). 2001;26:2112–8.
23. Cho SM, Rhee WT, Lee SY, Lee SB. Ganglion cyst of the posterior longitudinal ligament causing lumbar radiculopathy. J Korean Neurosurg Soc. 2010;47:298–301.
24. Constans JP, de Divitiis E, Donzelli R, Spaziante R, Meder JF, Haye C. Spinal metastases with neurological manifestations. Review of 600 cases. J Neurosurg. 1983;59:111–8.
25. Creze M, Ghaouche J, Missenard G, Lazure T, Cluzel G, Devilder M, Briand S, Soubeyrand M, Lew DP, Waldvogel FA. Osteomyelitis Lancet. 2004;364:369–79.
26. Crisco JJ III, Oda T, Panjabi MM, Bueff HU, Dvorak J, Grob D. Transactions of the C1-C2 joint capsular ligaments in the cadaveric spine. Spine. 1991;16(10S):474–9.
27. Dean LE, Jones GT, MacDonald AG, Downham C, Sturrock RD, Macfarlane GJ. Global prevalence of ankylosing spondylitis. Rheumatology (Oxford). 2014;53(4):650–7.
28. Debernardi A, D'Aliberti G, Talamonti G, Villa F, Piparo M, Collice M. The craniovertebral junction area and the role of the ligaments and membranes. Neurosurgery. 2011;68:291–301.
29. Denis F. The three-column spine and its significance in the classification of acute thoracolumbar spinal injuries. Spine. 1983;8:817–31.
30. Dickman CA, Crawford NR. Surgery of the craniovertebral junction. New York: Thieme; 1998.
31. Dickman CA, Greene CA, Sonntag VKH. Injuries involving the transverse atlantal ligament: classifications and treatment guidelines based upon experience with 39 injuries. Neurosurgery. 1996;38:44–50.
32. Dickman CA, Mamourian A, Sonntag VKH, Drayer BP. Magnetic resonance imaging of the transverse atlantal ligament for the evaluation of atlanto-axial instability. J Neurosurg. 1991;75:221–7.
33. DiMario S, Marmor E, Albrecht S, Mohr G. Ligamentum flavum cysts causing incapacitating lumbar spinal stenosis. Can J Neurol Sci. 2005;32:237–42.
34. Dundamadappa S, Cauley K. MR imaging of acute cervical spinal ligamentous and soft tissue trauma. Emerg Radiol. 2012;19:277–86.
35. Dvorak J, Panjabi M, Gerber M, Wichmann W. CT functional diagnostics of the rotatory instability of upper cervical spine. 1. An experimental study on cadavers. Spine (Phila Pa 1976). 1987;12:197–205.
36. Ehara S, Shimamura T, Nakamura R, Yamazaki K. Paravertebral ligamentous ossification: DISH. OPLL and OLF Eur J Radiol. 1998;27(3):196–205.
37. El Maghraoui A, Bensabbah R, Bahiri R, Bezza A, Guedira N, Hajjaj-Hassouni N. Cervical spine involvement in ankylosing spondylitis. Clin Rheumatol. 2003;22(2):94–8.
38. el Miedany YM, Wassif G, el Baddini M. Diffuse idiopathic skeletal hyperostosis (DISH): is it of vascular aetiology? Clin Exp Rheumatol. 2000;18:193–200.
39. Epstein NE. Identification of ossification of the posterior longitudinal ligament extending through the dura on preoperative computed tomographic examinations of the cervical spine. Spine (Phila Pa 1976). 2001;26:182–6.
40. Farley FA, Gebarski SS, Garton HL. Tectorial membrane injuries in children. J Spinal Disord Tech. 2005;18:136–8.

41. Farooki S, Seeger LL. Magnetic resonance imaging in the evaluation of ligament injuries. Skeletal Radiol. 1999;28:61–74.
42. Finkelstein SD, Sayegh R, Watson P, Knuckey N, Juxta-facet cysts. Report of two cases and review of the clinicopathologic features. Spine (Phila Pa 1976). 1993;18:779–82.
43. Fujimori T, Le H, Hu SS, Chin C, Pekmezci M, Schairer W, Tay BK, Hamasaki T, Yoshikawa H, Iwasaki M. Ossification of the posterior longitudinal ligament of the cervical spine in 3161 patients: a CT-based study. Spine (Phila Pa 1976). 2015;40(7):E394–403.
44. Gazzeri R, Galarza M, Gorgoglione L, Bisceglia M, D'Angelo V. Cervical cyst of the ligamentum flavum and C7-T1 subluxation: case report. Eur Spine J. 2005;14:807–9.
45. Goradia D, Linnau KF, Cohen WA, Mirza S, Hallam DK, Blackmore CC. Correlation of MR imaging findings with intraoperative findings after cervical spine trauma. Am J Neuroradiol. 2007;28:209–15.
46. Greene KA, Dickman CA, Marciano FF, Drabier J, Drayer BP, Sonntag VK. Transverse atlantal ligament disruption associated with odontoid fractures. Spine (Phila Pa 1976). 1994;19:2307–14.
47. Grigoryan M, Roemer FW, Mohr A, Genant HK. Imaging in spondyloarthropathies. Curr Rheumatol Rep. 2004;6(2):102–9.
48. Gupta V, Khandelwal N, Mathuria SN, Singh P, Pathak A, Suri S. Dynamic magnetic resonance imaging evaluation of craniovertebral junction abnormalities. J Comput Assist Tomogr. 2007;31:354–9.
49. Harris JH Jr. The cervicocranium: its radiographic assessment. Radiology. 2001;218:337–51.
50. Harris JH Jr, Carson G, Wagner L. Radiologic diagnosis of traumatic occipitovertebral dissociation: 1. Normal occipitovertebral relationships on lateral radiographs of supine subjects. Am J Roentgenol. 1994;162:881–6.
51. Harris JH Jr, Carson GC, Wagner LK, Kerr N. Radiologic diagnosis of traumatic occipitovertebral dissociation: 2. Comparison of three methods of detecting occipitovertebral relationships on lateral radiographs of supine subjects. AJR Am J Roentgenol. 1994;162(4):887–92.
52. Harris MB, Duval MJ, Davis JA, Bernini PM. Anatomical and roentgenographic features of atlanto-occipital instability. J Spinal Disord. 1993;6:5–10.
53. Henderson F Sr, Rosenbaum R, Narayanan M, Mackall J, Koby M. Optimizing alignment parameters during craniocervical stabilization and fusion: a technical note. Cureus. 2020;12:e7160.
54. Henderson FC, Wilson WA, Mott S, Mark A, Schmidt K, Berry JK, Vaccaro A, Benzel E. Deformative stress associated with an abnormal clivo-axial angle: a finite element analysis. Surg Neurol Int. 2010;1:30.
55. Hida K, Iwasaki Y, Koyanagi I, Abe H. Bone window computed tomography for detection of dural defect associated with cervical ossified posterior longitudinal ligament. Neurol Med Chir (Tokyo). 1997;37(2):173–5.
56. Hinck VC, Hopkins CE. Measurement of the atlanto-dental interval in the adult. Am J Roentgenol Radium Therapy, Nucl Med. 1960;84:945–51.
57. Hirabayashi S. Ossification of the ligamentum flavum. Spine Surg Relat Res. 2017;1:158–63.
58. Hodak JA, Mamourian A, Dean BL. Surgery of the Craniovertebral junction. New York: Thieme; 1998.
59. Hong SH, Choi JY, Lee JW, Kim NR, Choi JA, Kang HS. MR imaging assessment of the spine: infection or an imitation? Radiographics. 2009;29(2):599–612.
60. Jea A, Tatsui C, Farhat H, Vanni S, Levi AD. Vertically unstable type III Odontoid fractures: case report. Neurosurgery. 2006;58:797–8.
61. Jenkinson T, Armas J, Evison G, Cohen M, Lovell C, McHugh NJ. The cervical spine in psoriatic arthritis: a clinical and radiological study. Br J Rheumatol. 1994;33(3):255–9.
62. Joaquim AF, Baum G, Tan LA, Riew KD. C1 stenosis-An easily missed cause for cervical myelopathy. Neurospine. 2019;16(3):456–61.
63. Kao CC, Uihlein A, Bickel WH, Soule EH. Lumbar intraspinal extradural ganglion cyst. J Neurosurg. 1968;29:168–72.
64. Kassem MW, Tubbs RS. Injuries to the craniocervical ligaments: radiological diagnosis. In: Tubbs RS, Iwanaga J, Loukas M, Oskouian RJ, editors. Clinical anatomy of the ligaments of the craniocervical junction. Newcastle upon Tyne: Cambridge Scholars Publishing; 2019. p. 89–110.
65. Kassem MW, Tubbs RS. The cruciform ligament. In: Tubbs RS, Iwanaga J, Loukas M, Oskouian RJ, editors. Clinical anatomy of the ligaments of the craniocervical junction. Newcastle upon Tyne: Cambridge Scholars Publishing; 2019. p. 155–85.
66. Katzberg RW, Benedetti PF, Drake CM, Ivanovic M, Levine RA, Beatty CS, Nemzek WR, McFall RA, Ontell FK, Bishop DM, Poirier VC, Chong BW. Acute cervical spine injuries: prospective MR imaging assessment at a level 1 trauma center. Radiology. 1999;213(1):203–12.
67. Kauppi M, Neva MH. Sensitivity of lateral view cervical spine radiographs taken in the neutral position in atlantoaxial subluxation in rheumatic diseases. Clin Rheumatol. 1998;17:511–4.
68. Kawaguchi H, Kurokawa T, Machida H, Hoshino Y, Hirabayashi S, Ohnishi I, Katoh M, Mamada T. Roentgenological manifestation of ossification of the posterior longitudinal ligament in the cervical spine causing severe spinal canal stenosis—a group comparison with and without marked spinal cord dysfunction (in Japanese). J Jpn Orthop Assoc. 1991;65:173–80.
69. Kawaguchi Y, Matsumoto M, Iwasaki M, Izumi T, Okawa A, Matsunaga S, Chiba K, Tsuji T, Yamazaki M, Fujimori T, Yoshii T, Toyama Y. New classification system for ossification of the posterior longitudinal ligament using CT images. J Orthop Sci. 2014;19(4):530–6.

70. Kawaguchi Y, Matsuno H, Kanamori M, Ishihara H, Ohmori K, Kimura T. Radiologic findings of the lumbar spine in patients with rheumatoid arthritis, and a review of pathologic mechanisms. J Spinal Disord Tech. 2003;16:38–43.
71. Keiper ZRA, Bilaneui LT. MRI assessment of the supportive soft tissues of the cervical spine in acute trauma in children. Neuroradiology. 1998;40:359–63.
72. Kim H-J, Jun B-Y, Kim W, Cho YK, Lim MK, Suh CH. MR imaging of the alar ligament: morphology changes during axial rotation of the head in asymptomatic young adults. Skeletal Radiol. 2002;31:637–42.
73. Kobayashi S, Miyazaki T, Yayama T, Baba H. Microsurgical excision of hematoma of the lumbar ligamentum flavum. Joint Bone Spine. 2010;77(4):351–4.
74. Koga H, Sakou T, Taketomi E, Hayashi K, Numasawa T, Harata S, Yone K, Matsunaga S, Otterud B, Inoue I, Leppert M. Genetic mapping of ossification of the posterior longitudinal ligament of the spine. Am J Hum Genet. 1998;62(6):1460–7.
75. Kotani Y, Takahata M, Abumi K, Ito M, Sudo H, Minami A. Cervical myelopathy resulting from combined ossification of the ligamentum flavum and posterior longitudinal ligament: report of two cases and literature review. Spine J. 2013;13(1):e1–6.
76. Kotecki M, Sotniczuk M, Gietka P, Gasik R, Sudoł-Szopińska I. Imaging of cervical spine involvement in inflammatory arthropathies: a review. Pol J Radiol. 2021;86:e620–9.
77. Koyanagi I, Iwasaki Y, Hida K, Imamura H, Abe H. Magnetic resonance imaging findings in ossification of the posterior longitudinal ligament of the cervical spine. J Neurosurg. 1998;88(2):247–54.
78. Krakanes J, Kaale BR, Moen G, Nordli H, Gilhus NE, Rorvik J. MRI assessment of the alar ligaments in the late stage of whiplash injury: a study of structural abnormalities and observer agreement. Neuroradiology. 2002;44:617–24.
79. Krakanes J, Kaale BR, Moen G, Nordhi H, Gilhus NE, Rorvik J. MRI of the tectorial and posterior atlanto-occipital membranes in the late stage of whiplash injury. Neuroradiology. 2003;45:585–91.
80. Krakenes J, Kaale BR, Nordli H, Moen G, Rorvik J, Gilhus NE. MR analysis of the transverse ligament in the late stage of whiplash injury. Acta Radiol. 2003;44:637–44.
81. Krakenes J, Kaale B, Rorvik J, Gilhus N. MRI assessment of normal ligamentous structures in the craniovertebral junction. Neuroradiology. 2001;43:1089–97.
82. Ladenheim SE, Marlowe FI. Dysphagia secondary to cervical osteophytes. Am J Otolaryngol. 1999;20:184–9.
83. Laiho K, Kauppi M. The cervical spine in patients with psoriatic arthritis. Ann Rheum Dis. 2002;61:650–2.
84. Lang J. Craniocervical region, osteology, and articulations. Neuro-Orthopedics. 1986;1:67–92.
85. Lazennec JY, d'Astorg H, Rousseau MA. Cervical spine surgery in ankylosing spondylitis: review and current concept. Orthop Traumatol Surg Res OTSR. 2015;101:507–13.
86. Li M, Meng H, Du J, Tao H, Luo Z, Wang Z. Management of thoracic myelopathy caused by ossification of the posterior longitudinal ligament combined with ossification of the ligamentum flavum-a retrospective study. Spine J. 2012;12(12):1093–102.
87. Liu HP, Chen CL, Chen NF, Liao CY, Ou CY. Ligamentum flavum hematoma due to stretching exercise. Am J Emerg Med. 2016;34(10):2058.e3–6.
88. Lohkamp L-N, Marathe N, Fehlings MG. Craniocervical instability in Ehlers-Danlos syndrome-a systematic review of diagnostic and surgical treatment criteria. Glob Spine J. 2022;12:1862–71.
89. Loibl M, Stoyanov L, Doenitz C, Brawanski A, Wiggermann P, Krutsch W, Nerlich M, Oszwald M, Neumann C, Salzberger B, Hanses F. Outcome-related co-factors in 105 cases of vertebral osteomyelitis in a tertiary care hospital. Infection. 2014;42(3):503–10.
90. Lyons MK, Atkinson JL, Wharen RE, Deen HG, Zimmernan RS, Lemens SM. Surgical evaluation and management of lumbar synovial cysts: the Mayo Clinic experience. J Neurosurg. 2000;93:53–7.
91. Maas F, Spoorenberg A, Brouwer E, van der Veer E, Bootsma H, Bos R, Wink FR, Arends S. Radiographic damage and progression of the cervical spine in ankylosing spondylitis patients treated with TNF-α inhibitors: facet joints vs. vertebral bodies. Semin Arthritis Rheum. 2017;46(5):562–8.
92. Mahallati H, Wallace K, Hunter M, Bilbao J, Clark A. MR imaging of a hemorrhagic and granulomatous cyst of the ligamentum flavum with pathologic correlation. AJNR. 1999;20:1166–8.
93. Mantripragada S, Kannivelu A, Peh WC. Magnetic resonance imaging of cervical ligamentous anatomy and traumatic ligamentous injuries. J Med Imaging Radiat Oncol. 2020;64:368–76.
94. Marathe NA, Dahapute AA, Desai JR, Dhole KP, Bhaladhare S, Shah S. X-ray and computed tomography scan-based morphometric analysis of skull baselines in Indian population. Asian J Neurosurg. 2019;14(4):1116–21.
95. Marshman LA, Benjamin JC, David KM, King A, Chawda SJ. "Disc cysts" and "posterior longitudinal ligament ganglion cysts": synonymous entities? Report of three cases and literature review. Neurosurgery. 2005;57:E818.
96. Maruta K, Ichimura K, Matsui H, Yamagami T, Sano A, Tsuji H. Calcification inhibitors in human ligamentum flavum. J Orthop Res. 1993;11(1):92–103.
97. Matar LD, Doyle AJ. Prevertebral soft-tissue measurements in cervical spine injury. Australas Radiol. 1997;41:229–37.

98. Matsuyama Y, Kawakami N, Yanase M, Yoshihara H, Ishiguro N, Kameyama T, Hashizume Y. Cervical myelopathy due to OPLL: clinical evaluation by MRI and intraoperative spinal sonography. J Spinal Disord Tech. 2004;17(5):401–4.
99. Matsunaga S, Sakou T, Taketomi E, Komiya S. Clinical course of patients with ossification of the posterior longitudinal ligament: a minimum 10-year cohort study. J Neurosurg. 2004;100(3 Suppl Spine):245–8.
100. Meeks LW, Renshaw TS. Vertebral osteophytes and dysphagia. Ann Otol Rhinol Laryngol. 1970;79:1091–7.
101. Meyrignac O, Carlier RY, Court C, Bouthors C. Understanding a mass in the paraspinal region: an anatomical approach. Insights Imaging. 2023;14(1):128.
102. Min JH, Jang JS, Lee SH. Significance of the double-layer and single-layer signs in the ossification of the posterior longitudinal ligament of the cervical spine. J Neurosurg Spine. 2007;6:309–12.
103. Mirvis SE, NessAiver M. The radiology of acute cervical spine trauma. Baltimore: William and Wilkins; 1996.
104. Mori K, Imai S, Kasahara T, Nishizawa K, Mimura T, Matsusue Y. Prevalence, distribution, and morphology of thoracic ossification of the posterior longitudinal ligament in Japanese: results of CT-based cross-sectional study. Spine (Phila Pa 1976). 2014;39(5):394–9.
105. Nakamura M, Toyama Y, Suzuki N, Fujimura Y. Metastases to the upper cervical spine. J Spinal Disord. 1996;9:195–201.
106. Nascimento FA, Gatto LA, Lages RO, Neto HM, Demartini Z, Koppe GL. Diffuse idiopathic skeletal hyperostosis: a review. Surg Neurol Int. 2014;5(Suppl 3):S122–5.
107. Neva MH, Häkkinen A, Mäkinen H, Hannonen P, Kauppi M, Sokka T. High prevalence of asymptomatic cervical spine subluxation in patients with rheumatoid arthritis waiting for orthopaedic surgery. Ann Rheum Dis. 2006;65:884–8.
108. Nishikawa M, Bolognese PA, Yamagata T, Naito K, Sakamato H, Hara M, Ohata K, Goto T. Surgical management of Chiari malformation type I and instability of the craniocervical junction based on its pathogenesis and classification. Neurol Med Chir. 2022;62:400–15.
109. Nizamani WM. Ligamentum flavum cyst: an uncommon but recognizable and surgically correctable category of juxtafacet cyst. Radiol Case Rep. 2017;13:302–4.
110. Offiah CE. Craniocervical junction and cervical spine anatomy. Neuroimaging Clin. 2022;32:875–88.
111. Offiah CE, Day E. The craniocervical junction: embryology, anatomy, biomechanics and imaging in blunt trauma. Insights Imaging. 2017;8:29–47.
112. Oga M, Mashima T, Iwakuma T, Sugioka Y. Dysphagia complications in ankylosing spinal hyperostosis and ossification of the posterior longitudinal ligament. Roentgenographic findings of the developmental process of cervical osteophytes causing dysphagia. Spine (Phila Pa 1976). 1993;18:391–4.
113. Ogawa Y, Kumano K, Hirabayashi S, Aota Y. A ganglion cyst in the lumbar spinal canal: a case report. Spine (Phila Pa 1976). 1992;17:1429–31.
114. Ohara Y. Ossification of the ligaments in the cervical spine, including ossification of the anterior longitudinal ligament, ossification of the posterior longitudinal ligament, and ossification of the ligamentum flavum. Neurosurg Clin N Am. 2018;29(1):63–8.
115. Ohtsuka K, Terayama K, Yanagihara M, Wada K, Kasuga K, Machida T, Matsushima S. A radiological population study on the ossification of the posterior longitudinal ligament in the spine. Arch Orthop Trauma Surg (1978). 1987;106(2):89–93.
116. Ojuma N, Tubbs RS. The tectorial membrane. In: Tubbs RS, Iwanaga J, Loukas M, Oskouian RJ, editors. Clinical anatomy of the ligaments of the Craniocervical junction. Newcastle upon Tyne: Cambridge Scholars Publishing; 2019. p. 120–31.
117. Okumura T, Ohhira M, Kumei S, Nozu T. A higher frequency of lumbar ossification of the posterior longitudinal ligament in elderly in an outpatient clinic in Japan. Int J Gen Med. 2013;6:729–32.
118. Ortiz Gómez JA. The incidence of vertebral body metastases. Int Orthop. 1995;19:309–11.
119. Osborn AG, editor. Diagnostic neuroradiology. St Louis: Mosby Yearbook, Inc; 1994. p. 836–75.
120. Osmotherly PG, Rivett DA, Rowe LJ. The anterior shear and distraction tests for craniocervical instability. An evaluation using magnetic resonance imaging. Man Ther. 2012;17:416–21.
121. O'Sullivan MD, Lyons F, Morris S, Synnott K, Munigangaiah S, Devitt A. Metastasis affecting craniocervical junction: current concepts and an update on surgical management. Global Spine J. 2018;8(8):866–71.
122. Otake S, Matsuo M, Nishizawa S, Sano A, Kuroda Y. Ossification of the posterior longitudinal ligament: MR evaluation. AJNR Am J Neuroradiol. 1992;13(4):1059–67.
123. Oxland TR. Fundamental biomechanics of the spine–what we have learned in the past 25 years and future directions. J Biomech. 2016;49:817–32.
124. Ozdemir B, Kanat A, Batcik OE, Gucer H, Yolas C. Ligamentum flavum hematomas: why does it mostly occur in old Asian males? Interesting point of reported cases: review and case report. J Craniovertebr Junct Spine. 2016;7(1):7–12.
125. Park JY, Chin DK, Kim KS, Cho YE. Thoracic ligament ossification in patients with cervical ossification of the posterior longitudinal ligaments: tandem ossification in the cervical and thoracic spine. Spine (Phila Pa 1976). 2008;33(13):E407–10.
126. Pfirmann CWA, Binkert CA, Zanetti M, Boos N, Hodler J. MR morphology of alar ligaments and occipito-atlanto-axial joints: study in 50 asymptomatic subjects. Radiology. 2001;18:133–7.

127. Powers B, Miller MD, Kramer RS, Martinez S, Gehweiler JA Jr. Traumatic anterior atlanto-occipital dislocation. Neurosurgery. 1979;4(1):12–7.
128. Prodi E, Grassi R, Iacobellis F, Cianfoni A. Imaging in spondylodiskitis. Magn Reson Imaging Clin N Am. 2016;24(3):581–600.
129. Radatz M, Jakubowski J, Cooper J, Powell T. Synovial cysts of the lumbar spine: a review. Br J Neurosurg. 1997;11:520–4.
130. Rai R, Tubbs RS. Barkow's ligament. In: Tubbs RS, Iwanaga J, Loukas M, Oskouian RJ, editors. Clinical anatomy of the ligaments of the Craniocervical junction. Newcastle upon Tyne: Cambridge Scholars Publishing; 2019. p. 213–9.
131. Ramos-Remus C, Gomez-Vargas A, Guzman-Guzman JL, Jimenez-Gil F, Gamez-Nava JI, Gonzalez-Lopez L, Farrera-Gamboa H, Maksymowych WP, Suarez-Almazor ME. Frequency of atlantoaxial subluxation and neurologic involvement in patients with ankylosing spondylitis. J Rheumatol. 1995;22(11):2120–5.
132. Reijnierse M, Dijkmans BA, Hansen B, Pope TL, Kroon HM, Holscher HC, Breedveld FC, Bloem JL. Neurologic dysfunction in patients with rheumatoid arthritis of the cervical spine. Predictive value of clinical, radiographic and MR imaging parameters. Eur Radiol. 2001;11(3):467–73.
133. Resnick D, Niwayama G. Radiographic and pathologic features of spinal involvement in diffuse idiopathic skeletal hyperostosis (DISH). Radiology. 1976;119(3):559–68.
134. Resnick D, Shaul SR, Robins JM. Diffuse idiopathic skeletal hyperostosis (DISH): Forestier's disease with extraspinal manifestations. Radiology. 1975;115:513–24.
135. Rhoton AL Jr. The posterior cranial fossa: microsurgical anatomy and surgical approaches. Neurosurgery. 2000;47(Suppl):S5–S298.
136. Riascos R, Bonfante E, Cotes C, Guirguis M, Hakimelahi R, West C. Imaging of atlanto-occipital and atlantoaxial traumatic injuries: what the radiologist needs to know. Radiographics. 2015;35:2121–34.
137. Robertson PA, Swan HA. Traumatic bilateral rotatory facet dislocation of the atlas on the axis. Spine Phila Pa 1976. 1992;17:1252–4.
138. Roh SW, Rhim SC, Lee HK, Kang SK. Spinal ganglion cyst of lumbar posterior longitudinal ligament. J Korean Neurosurg Soc. 2000;29:543–9.
139. Rojas CA, Bertozzi JC, Martinez CR, Whitlow J. Reassessment of the craniocervical junction: normal values on CT. Am J Neuroradiol. 2007;28:1819–23.
140. Ronnen HR, de Korte PJ, Brink PR, van der Bijl HJ, Tonino AJ, Franke CL. Acute whiplash injury: is there a role for MR imaging? – A prospective study of 100 patients. Radiology. 1996;201:93–6.
141. Rudwaleit M, van der Heijde D, Landewé R, Listing J, Akkoc N, Brandt J, Braun J, Chou CT, Collantes-Estevez E, Dougados M, Huang F, Gu J, Khan MA, Kirazli Y, Maksymowych WP, Mielants H, Sørensen IJ, Ozgocmen S, Roussou E, Valle-Oñate R, Weber U, Wei J, Sieper J. The development of assessment of SpondyloArthritis international society classification criteria for axial spondyloarthritis (part II): validation and final selection. Ann Rheum Dis. 2009;68(6):777–83.
142. Sabo RA, Tracy PT, Weinger JM. A series of 60 juxtafacet cysts: clinical presentation, the role of spinal instability, and treatment. J Neurosurg. 1996;85:560–5.
143. Saeed K, Esposito S, Ascione T. Hot topics on vertebral osteomyelitis from the International Society of Antimicrobial Chemotherapy. Int J Antimicrob Agents. 2019;54:125–33.
144. Sahri IE, Tlemcani ZC, Abide Z, Obame FLO, Ramdani H, Mohammed M, Dokponou YCH, Elmi SM, Imbunhe N, Akroud SE, Cherif EA, Miloudi G. Ligamentum flavum hematoma in the lumbar spine mimicking spinal tumor: a case report and review of the literature. Radiol Case Rep. 2023;18(9):3060–4.
145. Sakai T, Sairyo K, Hamada D, Katoh S, Takata Y, Shinomiya F, Yasui N. Radiological features of lumbar spinal lesions in patients with rheumatoid arthritis with special reference to the changes around intervertebral discs. Spine J. 2008;8:605–11.
146. Salmon B, Martin D, Lenelle J, Stevenaert A. Juxtafacet cyst of the lumbar spine. Clinical, radiological and therapeutic aspects in 28 cases. Acta Neurochir. 2001;143:129–34.
147. Sartip KA, Dong T, Ndukwe M, East JE, Graves JA, Davis B, Midyett FA, Duerinckx A. Ossification of the posterior longitudinal ligament: imaging findings in the era of cross-sectional imaging. J Comput Assist Tomogr. 2015;39(6):835–41.
148. Sato T, Kokubun S, Ishii Y. Choice of operative method for ossification of ligamentum flavum based on CT findings (in Japanese). Rinshoseikeigeka. 1996;31:541–5.
149. Schräder PK, Grob D, Rahn BA, Cordey J, Dvorak J. Histology of the ligamentum flavum in patients with degenerative lumbar spinal stenosis. Eur Spine J. 1999;8(4):323–8.
150. Schweitzer ME, Hodler J, Cervilla V, Resnick D. Craniovertebral junction: normal anatomy with MR correlation. Am J Roentgenol. 1992;158:1087–90.
151. Selden NR, Quint DJ, Patel N, d'Arcy HS, Papadopoulos SM. Emergency magnetic resonance imaging of cervical spinal cord injuries: clinical correlation and prognosis. Neurosurgery. 1999;44:785–92.
152. Shen P, Nidecker A. Magnetic resonance imaging of the craniovertebral junction ligaments: normal anatomy and traumatic injury. J Neurol Surg Part B Skull Base. 2016;77:388–95.
153. Sherk HH. Lesions of the atlas and axis. Clin Orthop Relat Res. 1975;109:33–41.

154. Shiono T, Yoshikawa K, Aota Y, Euguchi M, Teshima Y, Tanaka J, et al. Two cases of the ganglion cysts in the lumbar spinal canal. Radiat Med. 1994;12:125–8.
155. Sim KB, Park JK. A nodular calcification of the alar ligament simulating a fracture in the craniovertebral junction. AJNR Am J Neuroradiol. 2006;27(9):1962–3.
156. Smith ZA, Buchanan CC, Raphael D, et al. Ossification of the posterior longitudinal ligament: pathogenesis, management, and current surgical approaches. A review. Neurosurg Focus. 2011;30:E10.
157. Smith P, Linscott LL, Vadivelu S, Zhang B, Leach JL. Normal development and measurements of the occipital condyle-C1 interval in children and young adults. AJNR Am J Neuroradiol. 2016;37(5):952–7.
158. Sohn S, Chung CK, Yun TJ, Sohn CH. Epidemiological survey of ossification of the posterior longitudinal ligament in an adult Korean population: three-dimensional computed tomographic observation of 3,240 cases. Calcif Tissue Int. 2014;94(6):613–20.
159. Sudoł-Szopińska I, Jurik AG, Eshed I, Lennart J, Grainger A, Østergaard M, Klauser A, Cotten A, Wick MC, Maas M, Miese F, Egund N, Boutry N, Rupreht M, Reijnierse M, Oei EH, Meier R, O'Connor P, Feydy A, Mascarenhas V, Plagou A, Simoni P, Platzgummer H, Rennie WJ, Mester A, Teh J, Robinson P, Guglielmi G, Åström G, Schueller-Weiderkamm C. Recommendations of the ESSR arthritis Subcommittee for the use of magnetic resonance imaging in musculoskeletal rheumatic diseases. Semin Musculoskelet Radiol. 2015;19(4):396–411.
160. Sudoł-Szopińska I, Matuszewska G, Kwiatkowska B, Pracoń G. Diagnostic imaging of psoriatic arthritis. Part I: etiopathogenesis, classifications and radiographic features. J Ultrason. 2016;16(64):65–77.
161. Taha H, Bareksei Y, Albanna W, Schirmer M. Ligamentum flavum cyst in the lumbar spine: a case report and review of the literature. J Orthop Traumatol. 2010;11:117–22.
162. Takahashi T, Hanakita J, Minami M. Pathophysiology of calcification and ossification of the ligamentum flavum in the cervical spine. Neurosurg Clin N Am. 2018;29(1):47–54.
163. Takahashi M, Satomi K, Hasegawa A, Hasegawa M, Taki N, Ichimura S. Ligamentum flavum hematoma in the lumbar spine. J Orthop Sci. 2012;17(3):308–12.
164. Takahashi H, Wada A, Yokoyama Y, Fukushi S, Sakurai T, Shibuya K, Suguro T. Ligamentum flavum haematoma: a report of two cases. J Orthop Surg (Hong Kong). 2009;17(2):212–5.
165. Takeno K, Tamura T, Sakai T, Sairyo K, Takao S, Kagawa S, Katoh S, Yasui N. Hematoma in the cervical ligamentum flavum. Report of a case and review of the literature. Skeletal Radiol. 2010;39(3):289–93.
166. Tan S, Wang R, Ward MM. Syndesmophyte growth in ankylosing spondylitis. Curr Opin Rheumatol. 2015;27:326–32.
167. Tubbs RS, Dixon J, Loukas M, Shoja MM, Cohen-Gadol AA. Ligament of Barkow of the craniocervical junction: its anatomy and potential clinical and functional significance. J Neurosurg Spine. 2010;12:619–22.
168. Tubbs SR, Grabb P, Spooner A, Wilson W, Oakes J. The apical ligament: anatomy and functional significance. J Neurosurg. 2000;92(2 Suppl):197–200.
169. Tubbs RS, Griessenauer CJ, McDaniel JG, Burns AM, Kumbla A, Cohen-Gadol AA. The transverse occipital ligament: anatomy and potential functional significance. Neurosurgery. 2010;66(3 Suppl Operative):1–3.
170. Tubbs RS, Hallock JD, Radcliff V, Naftel RP, Mortazavi M, Shoja MM, Loukas M, Cohen-Gadol AA. Ligaments of the craniocervical junction. J Neurosurg Spine. 2011;14(6):697–709.
171. Tubbs RS, Kelly DR, Humphrey ER, Chua GD, Shoja MM, Salter EG, Acakpo-Satchivi L, Wellons JC 3rd, Blount JP, Oakes WJ. The tectorial membrane: anatomical, biomechanical, and histological analysis. Clin Anat. 2007;20(4):382–6.
172. Tubbs RS, Salter GE, Oakes WJ. The accessory atlantoaxial ligament. Neurosurgery. 2004;55:400–4.
173. Tubbs RS, Stetler W, Shoja MM, Loukas M, Hansasuta A, Liechty P. The lateral atlantooccipital ligament. Surg Radiol Anat. 2007;29:219–23.
174. Ulbrich EJ, Schraner C, Boesch C, Hodler J, Busato A, Anderson SE, Eigenheer S, Zimmermann H, Sturzenegger M. Normative MR cervical spinal canal dimensions. Radiology. 2014;271(1):172–82.
175. Vasani SS, Demetriades AK, Joshi SM, Yeh J, Ellamushi H. Traumatic intraspinal extradural ganglion cyst in a teenager: case report and review of the literature. Clin Neurol Neurosurg. 2007;109:88–91.
176. Vassiou K, Eftichia K, Marinos K, Kotrogianni F, Fanariotis M, Fezoulidis I, Arvanitis D. Magnetic resonance imaging of the ligaments of the craniocervical region at 3Tesla magnetic resonance unit: quantitative and qualitative assessment. J Biomed Sci Eng. 2012;5:901–9.
177. Vernet O, Frankhauser H, Schnyder P, Déruaz JP. Cyst of the ligamentum flavum: report of six cases. Neurosurgery. 1991;29:277–83.
178. Vetter U, Zapf J, Heit W, Helbing G, Heinze E, Froesch ER, Teller WM. Human fetal and adult chondrocytes. Effect of insulinlike growth factors I and II, insulin, and growth hormone on clonal growth. J Clin Invest. 1986;77(6):1903–8.
179. Wasserman BR, Moskovich R, Razi AE. Rheumatoid arthritis of the cervical spine-clinical considerations. Bull NYU Hosp Jt Dis. 2011;69:136–48.
180. White AA 3rd, Johnson RM, Panjabi MM, Southwick WO. Biomechanical analysis of clinical stability in the cervical spine. Clin Orthop Relat Res. 1975;109:85–96.

181. Wolf M, Weber MA. Inflammatory and infectious disorders of the spine. In: Barkhof F, Jager R, Thurnher M, Rovira Cañellas A, editors. Clinical neuroradiology. Cham: Springer; 2019. https://doi.org/10.1007/978-3-319-61423-6_80-1.
182. Wong DA, Fornasier VL, MacNab I. Spinal metastases: the obvious, the occult, and the impostors. Spine. 1990;Phila Pa 1976(15):1–4.
183. Yalçinkaya F, Parlak Sağol Ş, Azizova A, Bilgin E, Karli Oğuz K, Kalyoncu U. Craniocervical junction involvement in inflammatory arthritis: a single-center radiologic study. Turk J Med Sci. 2023;53:1713–21.
184. Yamamoto A, Nishiura I, Handa H, Kondo A. Ganglion cyst in the ligamentum flavum of the cervical spine causing myelopathy: report of two cases. Surg Neurol. 2001;56(6):390–5.
185. Yamashita Y, Takahashi M, Matsuno Y, Sakamoto Y, Yoshizumi K, Oguni T, Kojima R. Spinal cord compression due to ossification of ligaments: MR imaging. Radiology. 1990;175(3):843–8.
186. Yoshii T, Hirai T, Iwanami A, Nagoshi N, Takeuchi K, Mori K, Yamada T, Seki S, Tsuji T, Fujiyoshi K, Furukawa M, Nishimura S, Wada K, Koda M, Furuya T, Matsuyama Y, Hasegawa T, Takeshita K, Kimura A, Abematsu M, Haro H, Ohba T, Watanabe M, Katoh H, Watanabe K, Ozawa H, Kanno H, Imagama S, Ando K, Fujibayashi S, Matsumoto M, Nakamura M, Yamazaki M, Okawa A, Kawaguchi Y. Co-existence of ossification of the nuchal ligament is associated with severity of ossification in the whole spine in patients with cervical ossification of the posterior longitudinal ligament -a multi-center CT study. J Orthop Sci. 2019;24(1):35–41.
187. Younes M, Belghali S, Kriâa S, Zrour S, Bejia I, Touzi M, Golli M, Gannouni A, Bergaoui N. Compared imaging of the rheumatoid cervical spine: prevalence study and associated factors. Joint Bone Spine. 2009;76(4):361–8.
188. Yuksel M, Heiserman JE, Sonntag VK. Magnetic resonance imaging of the craniocervical junction at 3-T: observation of the accessory atlantoaxial ligaments. Neurosurgery. 2006;59:888–93.

Part II

The Ligaments of the Vertebral Bodies

9 The Anterior Longitudinal Ligament

Keishiro Kikuchi and Joe Iwanaga

9.1 Introduction

The anterior longitudinal ligament (ALL) is a robust band of collagenous fibers that extends along the anterior surface of the vertebral column [1–4]. It is composed of densely packed collagen fibers oriented longitudinally and interwoven at acute angles, with a small number of elastic fibers interspersed throughout [2, 4, 5]. Despite its anatomical significance, histological studies on the ALL are limited and have yielded inconsistent interpretations among anatomists and spine surgeons. This chapter reviews available anatomical, histological, and biomechanical data to clarify the current understanding of the ALL.

9.2 General Morphology

The ALL originates from the basilar part of the occipital bone, attaching to the anterior tubercle of the atlas (C1), continuing along the anterior surfaces of the vertebral bodies, and terminating at the anterior aspect of the sacrum [1]. It may merge with the prevertebral layer of the deep cervical fascia [6]. The ALL is narrower and thicker over vertebral bodies than over intervertebral (IV) discs [1, 3]. In the thoracic region, it is generally thicker and narrower than in the cervical and lumbar regions, gradually widening as it descends caudally [1]. Structurally, the ALL is composed of two to three fiber layers: superficial,

K. Kikuchi
Department of Orthopaedic Surgery, Kurume University School of Medicine, Kurume, Fukuoka, Japan

Division of Gross and Clinical Anatomy, Department of Anatomy, Kurume University School of Medicine, Kurume, Fukuoka, Japan

J. Iwanaga (✉)
Division of Gross and Clinical Anatomy, Department of Anatomy, Kurume University School of Medicine, Kurume, Fukuoka, Japan

Department of Neurosurgery, Clinical Neuroscience Research Center, Tulane Center for Clinical Neurosciences, Tulane University School of Medicine, New Orleans, LA, USA

Department of Neurology, Clinical Neuroscience Research Center, Tulane University School of Medicine, New Orleans, LA, USA

Department of Structural & Cellular Biology, Tulane University School of Medicine, New Orleans, LA, USA

Department of Neurosurgery and Ochsner Neuroscience Institute, Ochsner Health System, New Orleans, LA, USA

Dental and Oral Medical Center, Kurume University School of Medicine, Kurume, Fukuoka, Japan
e-mail: jiwanaga@tulane.edu

M. Turgut et al. (eds.), *Ligaments of the Vertebral Column*,
https://doi.org/10.1007/978-3-032-09070-6_9

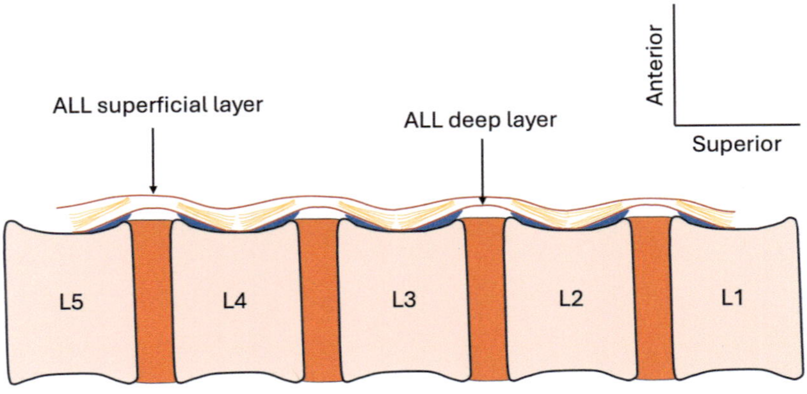

Fig. 9.1 Schematic drawing of the lumbar anterior longitudinal ligament (ALL)

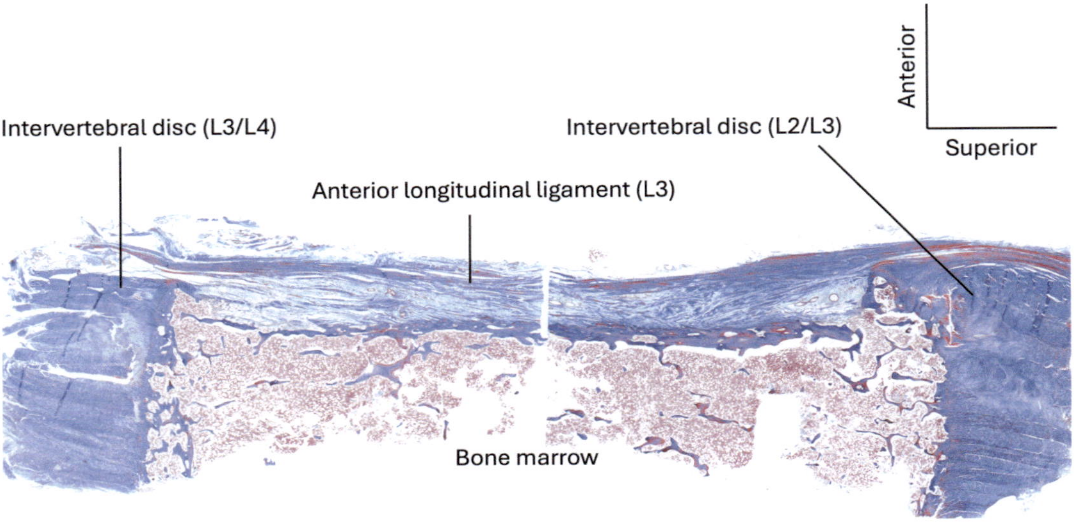

Fig. 9.2 Sagittal histological section of the ALL on L3. Masson trichrome staining

intermediate, and deep [1, 2, 4]. Superficial fibers span three to five vertebrae, intermediate fibers span two to three, and deep fibers connect adjacent vertebrae [1, 4]. Histological descriptions of the ALL vary across sources. Some texts describe three layers: superficial fibers spanning three to four vertebrae, intermediate fibers bridging two to three vertebrae, and deep fibers connecting adjacent vertebral bodies [6] (Figs. 9.1, 9.2 and 9.3).

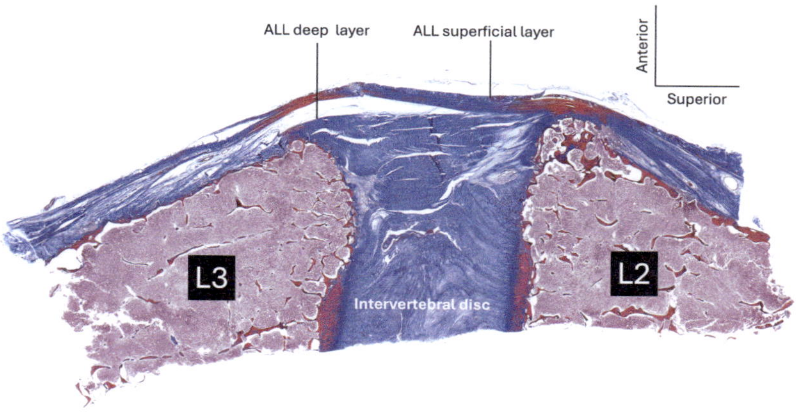

Fig. 9.3 Sagittal histological section of the ALL between L2 and L3. Note that there are at least two layers of ALL anterior to the intervertebral disc. Masson's trichrome staining

9.3 Relationship to Adjacent Structures

The longitudinal fibers of the ALL attach firmly to discs and the anterior margins of vertebral bodies [1–3], while forming looser connections to the mid-body surfaces, filling the concavities and flattening the anterior contour of the vertebral column [2]. Some authors described the ALL as attaching to the anterior contour of the vertebral column and the disc [7]. The deep fibers integrate with the periosteum, while the superficial fibers bridge across these concave surfaces [2]. The ALL also blends with the outer surface of the anulus fibrosus, which has led to differing views regarding the classification of these fibers. Some regard them as part of the anulus or a "disc capsule," but Bogduk [2] clarified that these should not be considered part of the anulus fibrosus due to distinct embryologic origins. While the ALL attaches to cortical bone, a defining feature of ligaments, the anulus attaches to the vertebral end plate and ring apophysis, not cortical bone [2]. The longus colli arises from the cervical and upper three thoracic bodies lateral to the ALL (Figs. 9.4 and 9.5). In contrast, in the lumbar region, some believe the ALL is partially formed by the caudal extension of the crura of the diaphragm [2] (Fig. 9.6). This has led to the suggestion that the lumbar ALL may, in part, represent a continuation of tendinous rather than purely ligamentous tissue [2].

Embryologically, the ALL develops in association with cortical bone, while the anulus fibrosus connects to the vertebral endplate. Fibers of the adult anulus that do attach to bone are incorporated secondarily into the ring apophysis—further supporting the distinction between the ALL and the anulus fibrosus [2].

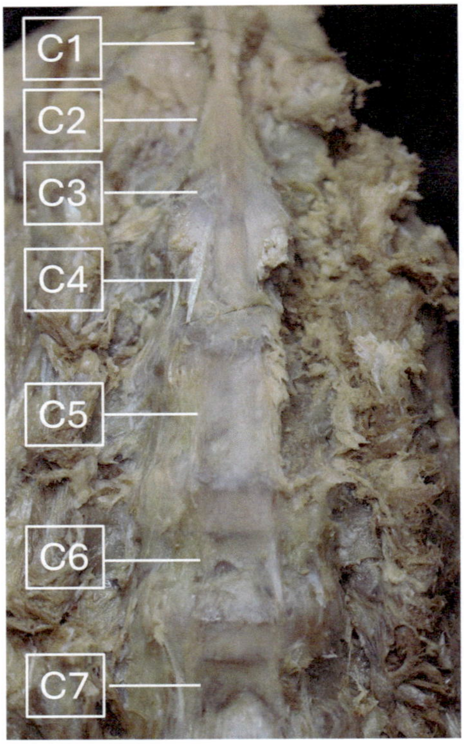

Fig. 9.4 Anterior view of the cervical ALLs after removal of majority of the prevertebral muscles

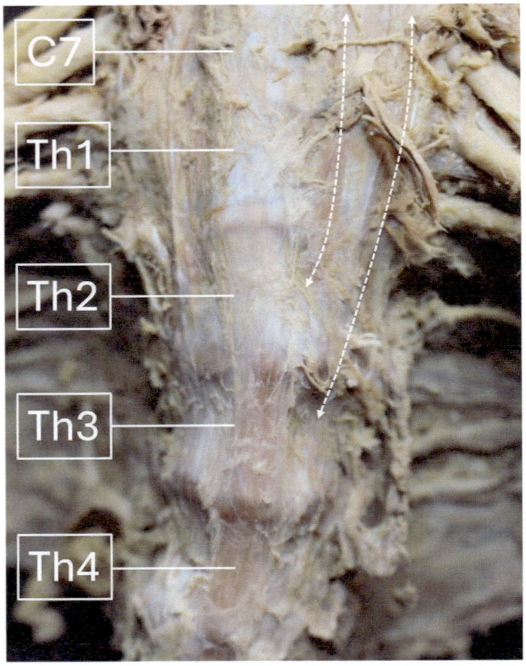

Fig. 9.5 Anterior view of the seventh cervical and upper thoracic ALLs. Note that the fourth thoracic ALL is not related to the longus colli (dotted lines)

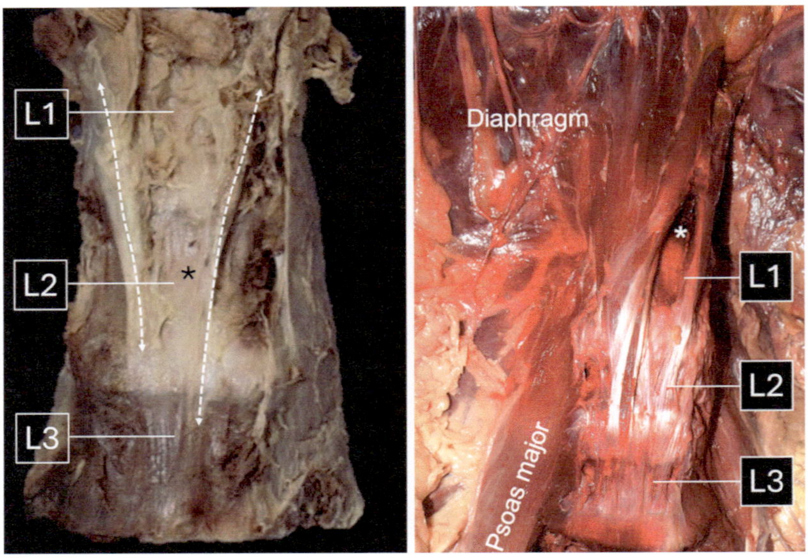

Fig. 9.6 Anterior view of the lumbar ALLs (*) with only crura (dotted lines) preserved in the left image, and with other muscles intact in the right image

9.4 Morphometrics

Limited data are available on the morphometrics of the ALL. In a cadaveric study of 25 lumbar spine specimens, the average width of the ALL was 37.1 mm with a mean cross-sectional area of 32.4 mm^2, ranging from 10.6 to 52.5 mm^2 [8]. Tkaczuk [9] reported that the mean width of the ALL at the level of L2, L3, and L5 was 2.3 mm, 2.5 mm, and 2 mm, respectively, and the mean thickness of the of the ALL at the level of L2, L3, and L5 was 0.9 mm, 2.1 mm, and 1.9 mm, respectively.

9.5 Function and Biomechanics

The ALL contributes to spinal stability by limiting hyperextension of the vertebral column [2, 10]. While Neumann et al. [5] proposed its involvement in extension, lateral bending, and axial rotation, Zander et al. [11] concluded that the ALL is engaged only during extension. It is the strongest and largest spinal ligament, uniquely limiting extension, whereas other ligaments constrain flexion [5, 10, 11]. Neumann et al. [5] found the stiffness of the ALL to be significantly higher than that of posterior ligaments like the ligamenta flava. They also observed a slight decline in tensile strength in specimens aged 21–43. Their 1993 study reported a mean failure load of 802 N for bone-ALL-bone complexes—markedly higher than the 330–473 N reported in earlier studies [12]. The discrepancy was attributed to the use of younger, more active cadaveric donors in Neumann's study. They further suggested that bone mineral content is a better predictor of ligament strength than age alone. In another study, Pintar et al. [8] reported a mean stiffness of 33.0 ± 15.7 N/mm. The ALL and supraspinous ligament (SSL) demonstrated the highest energy-to-failure values: 0.82–8.68 J for the ALL and 3.18–11.64 J for the SSL. Panjabi et al. [13] linked these values to the functional need for these ligaments to endure greater mechanical loads. Failure stress values for the ALL and posterior longitudinal ligament (PLL) were similar, ranging from 8.2–16.1 MPa and 7.2–28.4 MPa, respectively [8]. These findings were consistent with earlier values reported by Chazal et al. [14].

9.6 Clinical Relevance and Pathology

The ALL is vulnerable to injury during whiplash, where hyperextension forces stretch the ligament beyond its limits [10]. Another notable condition is diffuse idiopathic skeletal hyperostosis (DISH), also known as Forestier disease, which involves ossification of the ALL, most often in the cervical spine [4, 15–17] (Fig. 9.7). This rare pathology may co-occur with ossification of other spinal ligaments. In advanced cases, the ossified ALL may compress the esophagus, leading to dysphagia, and contribute to radiculomyelopathy by narrowing the cervical spinal canal [18]. Mizuno

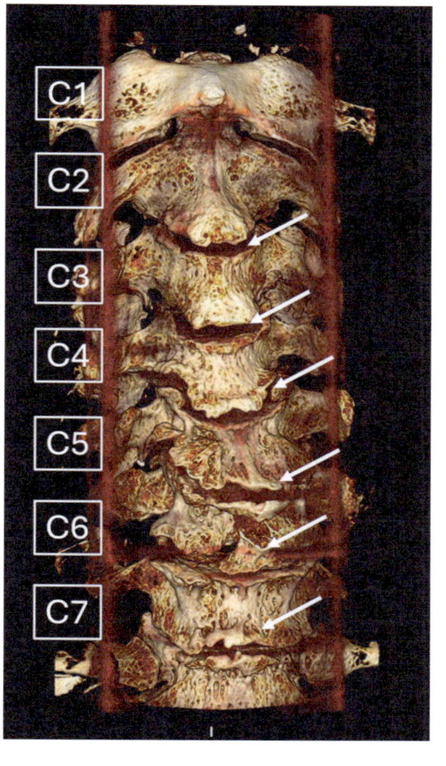

Fig. 9.7 Anterior view of the cervical vertebrae with diffuse idiopathic skeletal hyperostosis (DISH, arrows) in the 3D reconstructed computed tomography image

et al. [18] also noted that DISH-related ossification of the cervical ALL is most often found at C4–C5.

As the ALL is the only major spinal ligament that limits extension, it must be considered to be incised or preserved during the anterior cervical discectomy and fusion (ACDF) or anterior lumbar interbody fusion (ALIF). Katzman et al. [19] evaluated the relationship between DISH and kyphosis in 2767 patients, concluding that DISH may slow the long-term progression of kyphosis. In contrast, other studies argue that DISH does not represent ossification of the ALL, but rather the formation of new bone [20].

9.7 Conclusions

The ALL is a key structural element of the vertebral column, extending from the occiput to the sacrum and uniquely functioning to limit spinal extension. Its distinct morphology, layered fiber arrangement, and firm attachments to cortical bone distinguish it from adjacent structures such as the anulus fibrosus. Biomechanically, it exhibits high stiffness and tensile strength, particularly in younger individuals. Clinically, the ALL is relevant in trauma, degenerative conditions such as DISH, and anterior spinal surgeries where its preservation or resection may influence postoperative stability. A thorough understanding of its anatomy, biomechanics, and pathology is essential for spine clinicians and surgeons.

References

1. Bannister LH, Berry MM, Collins P, Dyson M, Dussek JE, Ferguson MWJ, editors. Gray's anatomy. 38th ed. New York: Churchill Livingston; 1996.
2. Bogduk N. Clinical anatomy of the lumbar spine and sacrum. 3rd ed. New York: Churchill Livingston; 1997.
3. Dickman CA, Rosenthal DJ, Perin NI. Thoracoscopic spine surgery. New York: Thieme Medical Publishers; 1999.
4. Lang J. Clinical anatomy of the cervical spine. New York: Thieme Medical Publishers; 1993.
5. Neumann P, Keller T, Ekstrom L, Hult E, Hansson T. Structural properties of the anterior longitudinal ligament. Spine. 1993;18(5):637–45.
6. Standring S. Gray's anatomy 42nd edition the anatomical basis of clinical practice. London: Elsevier; 2020.
7. Kapandji I. The physiology of the joints, vol. 3. Edinburgh: Churchill Livingstone; 1984.
8. Pintar FA, Yoganandan N, Myers T, Elhagediab A, Sances A Jr. Biomechanical properties of human lumbar spine ligaments. J Biomech. 1992;25(11):1351–6.
9. Tkaczuk H. Tensile properties of human lumbar longitudinal ligaments. Acta Orthop Scand. 1968;39(sup115):1–69.
10. Moore KL, Dalley AF, Agur AMR. Clinically oriented anatomy. 6th ed. Baltimore: Lippincott Williams & Wilkins; 2010.
11. Zander T, Rohlmann A, Bergmann G. Influence of ligament stiffness on the mechanical behavior of a functional spinal unit. J Biomech. 2004;37(7):1107–11.
12. Nachemson AL, Evans JH. Some mechanical properties of the third human lumbar interlaminar ligament (ligamentum flavum). J Biomech. 1968;1(3):211–20.
13. Panjabi MM, Goel VK, Takata K. Physiologic strains in the lumbar spinal ligaments. Spine. 1982;7(3):192–203.
14. Chazal J, Tanguy A, Bourges M, Gaurel G, Escande G, Guillot M, Vanneuville G. Biomechanical properties of spinal ligaments and a histological study of the supraspinal ligament in traction. J Biomech. 1985;18(3):167–176.
15. Hirasawa A, Wakao N, Kamiya M, Takeuchi M, Kawanami K, Murotani K, Matsuo T, Deie M. The prevalence of diffuse idiopathic skeletal hyperostosis in Japan – the first report of measurement by CT and review of the literature. J Orthop Sci. 2016 May;21(3):287–90. https://doi.org/10.1016/j.jos.2016.02.001.
16. Horváth F, Forgács S, Sillár P, Lengyel E. Verkalkungen ventraler Wirbelligamente im Alter (Forestiersche Krankheit) [Calcification of the ligament. ant. of the spina (disease of Forestier) (author's transl)]. Aktuelle Gerontol. 1979;9(9):405–10. German
17. Nascimento FA, Gatto LA, Lages RO, Neto HM, Demartini Z, Koppe GL. Diffuse idiopathic skeletal hyperostosis: a review. Surg Neurol Int. 2014;5(Suppl 3):S122–5. https://doi.org/10.4103/2152-7806.130675. PMID: 24843807; PMCID: PMC4023007
18. Mizuno J, Nakagawa H, Song J. Symptomatic ossification of the anterior longitudinal ligament with stenosis of the cervical spine: a report of seven cases. J Bone Joint Surg. 2005;87:1375–9.
19. Katzman WB, Parimi N, Mansoori Z, Nardo L, Kado DM, Cawthon PM, Marshall LM, Schousboe JT, Lane NE. Osteoporotic fractures in men study research group and the study of osteoporotic fractures. Cross-sectional and longitudinal associations of diffuse idiopathic skeletal hyperostosis and thoracic kyphosis in older men and women. Arthritis Care Res (Hoboken). 2017;69(8):1245–52. https://doi.org/10.1002/acr.23115.
20. Kuperus JS, Smit EJM, Pouran B, van Hamersvelt RW, van Stralen M, Seevinck PR, Buckens CF, Bleys RLAW, Weinans HH, Oner FC, de Jong PA, Verlaan JJ. Anterior longitudinal ligament in diffuse idiopathic skeletal hyperostosis: ossified or displaced? J Orthop Res. 2018 Sep;36(9):2491–6. https://doi.org/10.1002/jor.24020.

Posterior Longitudinal Ligament 10

Bin Yu and Fuyou Guo

10.1 Introduction

10.1.1 Overview of Posterior Longitudinal Ligament

The posterior longitudinal ligament (PLL) is a long and narrow structure, yet it is strong. It extends along the backs of the vertebral bodies from behind the body of the axis, continues with the tectorial membrane covering the vertebral body behind the axis, and reaches down to the sacrum. It consists mainly of elastin and fibrillin-1 [1, 2]. The shape and structure of the PLL exhibit distinct features in different areas of the spine. It is wider in the cervical and upper thoracic spine, particularly at the site of the intervertebral disc, but narrower in the lower thoracic and lumbar spine, specifically at the site of the vertebral body. It is closely connected to the annulus fibrosus of the intervertebral disc and the upper and lower edges of the vertebral body, but the connection with the vertebral body is relatively loose. Vertebral veins pass through it. The part if the PLL that is combined with the vertebral body is narrower, but the ligament expands and widens on both sides at the intervertebral disc. This limits excessive forward flexion of the spine and prevents the intervertebral disc from prolapsing backward.

B. Yu (✉) · F. Guo
Department of Neurosurgery, The First Affiliated Hospital of Zhengzhou University, Zhengzhou, Henan, China

International Joint Laboratory of Nervous System Malformation, Zhengzhou, China
e-mail: fccyub@zzu.edu.cn

10.1.2 Importance of Understanding Developmental Anatomy and Histology

In clinical practice, a deep comprehension of the anatomy and histology of the PLL is necessary so that the characteristics and development of PLL-related disease can be thoroughly understood. Surgeons performing spine operations must understand the anatomy and histology of these regions in depth to achieve more thorough decompression, better surgical results, and fewer complications such as disc herniation and spinal stenosis. For spinal trauma assessment, knowledge of the anatomy of the spinal ligaments enables medical professionals to precisely assess the stability of the spine and manage related injuries effectively.

Radiologists utilize their knowledge of the anatomy of the PLL to accurately interpret the results of imaging studies, such as CT scans and MRIs, thereby enabling the correct diagnosis of PLL-related diseases. Knowledge of PLL anatomy also allows pathologists to deepen their understanding of the histopathology of the ligament and abnormalities related to it, such as PLL ossification.

M. Turgut et al. (eds.), *Ligaments of the Vertebral Column*,
https://doi.org/10.1007/978-3-032-09070-6_10

10.2 Embryonic Origins of the Posterior Longitudinal Ligament

The PLL is composed of collagen and elastin fibers arranged in the head-to-tail direction [3]. It originates from the mesenchymal cells of the osteogenic ganglion, which have differentiated from the mesodermal somite. The initial ligament begins to appear during the late embryonic or early fetal stage. The PLL starts to develop during the tenth gestational week and then gradually matures [4].

10.3 Posterior Longitudinal Ligament Anatomy

10.3.1 Posterior Longitudinal Ligament Anatomy

The PLL is a long, narrow, tough ligament located behind the vertebral bodies. It is thick in the central section and broad at both ends, tapering to a thin point. It continues upward with the tectorial membrane covering the vertebral body behind the axis, and then migrates downward with the deep posterior sacrococcygeal ligament. It consists mainly of elastin and fibrillin-1 [1, 2]. The morphology and structure of the PLL differ in different segments of the spine. Overall, it narrows gradually from top to bottom. In the cervical and upper thoracic regions, it is uniformly broad (10–15 mm wide), but becomes almost saw-toothed in appearance as it reaches the lower thoracic and lumbar regions [5–7]. This is because it narrows as it passes over the vertebral bodies and expands over the intervertebral discs caudally, particularly in the lumbar 4-sacral 1 segment [8], where there is significant PLL narrowing (Fig. 10.1). The PLL is closely connected to the anulus fibrosus of the intervertebral disc and the upper and lower edges of the vertebral body. However, its junctions with the vertebral body are relatively loose because the basivertebral vein, nutrient artery, and the branches of

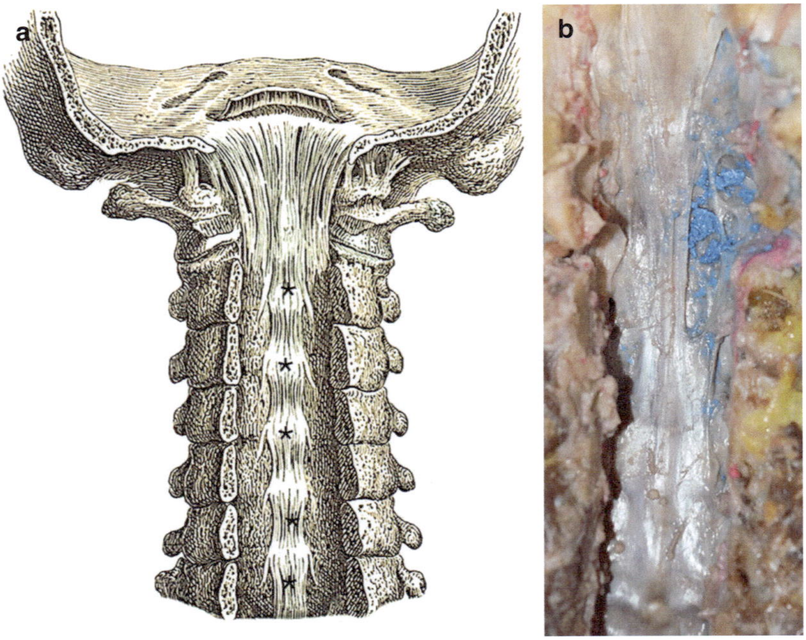

Fig. 10.1 Posterior longitudinal ligament (PLL) (*) in the cervical spine. Note its extension cranially as the tectorial membrane. (**a**) In this drawing, laminectomies have been performed, and the spinal dura and its contents have been removed. From Bock's Hand-Atlas der Anatomie des Menschen (Verlag der Rengerschen Buchhandlung, Berlin, 1860). (**b**) Cadaveric dissection noting the PLL in the cervical spine. Note the most cranial part, which represents the tectorial membrane. Also observe the internal vertebral venous plexus (blue latex) that travels between the layers of the PLL

sinuvertebral nerve (basivertebral nerves) pass through them. It then enters and exits the vertebral body through the basivertebral vein foramen; here, the part that combines with the vertebral body is narrow. However, at the intervertebral disc, it expands and widens on both sides.

The PLL can be divided into three layers under the microscope [9, 10]: superficial, middle, and deep. The superficial fibers span several intervertebral spaces and are divided into a central longitudinal traveling portion and expanded parts on each side. The expanded part runs obliquely outward and is connected to the upper border of the pedicle and the nerve root sheath. The middle layer is a longitudinal fiber that spans a single intervertebral disc. It begins below the basivertebral vein foramen of the upper vertebral body and terminates above the basivertebral vein foramen of the lower vertebral body and is loosely connected to the superficial PLL, which is easily separated. The deep fibers span a single intervertebral space, starting and ending at the posterior edge of the bony endplates of the upper and lower vertebral bodies immediately adjacent to the intervertebral disc, and adhere tightly to the anulus fibrosus of the intervertebral disc and the epiphyseal annulus of the vertebral body. It is also divided into a central longitudinal traveling portion and an expanded part on each side, which travels obliquely outward and downward, ending behind uncovertebral cervical vertebrae 3–7 and forming the perivertebral ligaments (Fig. 10.2).

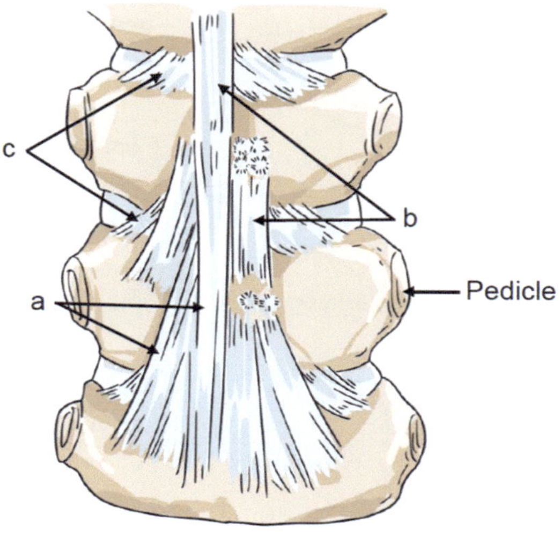

Fig. 10.2 A schematic sketch of the components of the PLL. (**a**) Superficial fibers and their lateral extensions, (**b**) intermediate fibers, (**c**) deep fibers and their thin alar extensions toward the uncinate process

10.3.2 Innervation of the Posterior Longitudinal Ligament

The PLL is innervated by the descending branch of the sinuvertebral nerve. After exiting the foramen, the spinal nerve sends out a small branch known as the sinuvertebral nerve, which returns to the vertebral canal. It is jointly emitted by the ventral branch of the spinal nerve and the gray ramus communicans, and along the PLL, it divides into ascending, descending, and transverse branches. The ascending branch emits the basivertebral nerve near each pedicle to innervate the vertebral body, the descending branch innervates the PLL and the intervertebral disc, and the transverse branch innervates the intervertebral disc [5] (Figs. 10.3 and 10.4).

10.3.3 Blood Supply to the Posterior Longitudinal Ligament

The blood supply to the PLL originates mainly from the segmental spinal artery that supplies the vertebral body. The segmental spinal artery divides into a posterior branch on the side of the vertebral body, which sends a spinal branch into the intervertebral foramen. The spinal branch is divided into the anterior branch of the spinal canal, the radicular artery, and the posterior branch of the spinal canal. This posterior branch is divided into ascending and descending terminal branches, which run obliquely upward and downward, respectively. They run deep to the PLL and distribute to the corresponding ligament area (Fig. 10.5) [11].

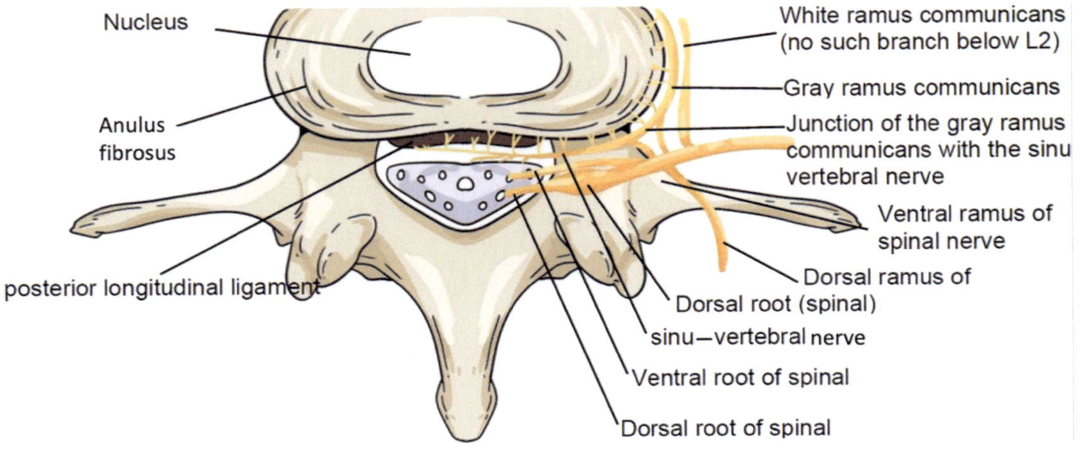

Fig. 10.3 A schematic diagram of the innervation of the PLL

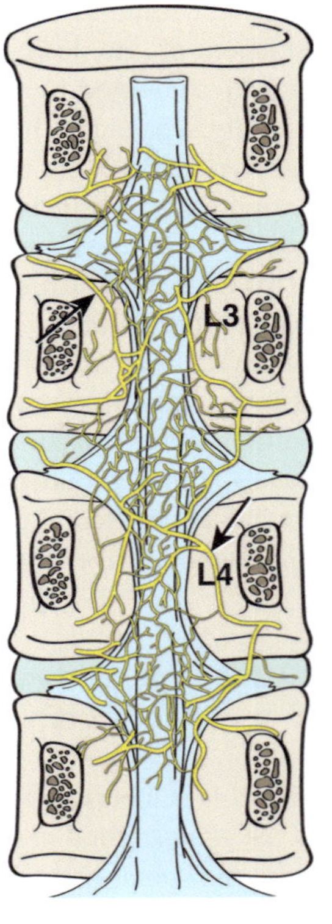

Fig. 10.4 Drawing of the PLL and the overlying nervous plexus contributed to by the sinuvertebral nerves (arrow). Note that the posterior elements of the vertebrae have been removed as well as the spinal dura and spinal cord. (After Bogduk)

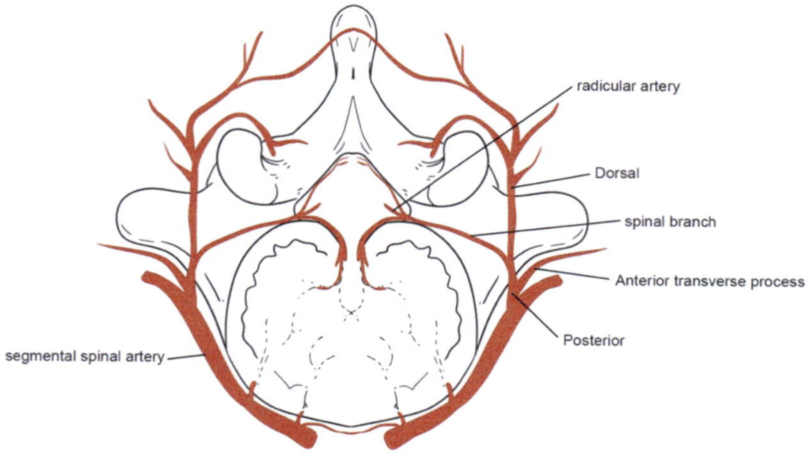

Fig. 10.5 A schematic diagram of the blood supply to the PLL

10.4 Clinical Significance of the Posterior Longitudinal Ligament

The PLL is important in humans, its main physiological functions being as follows. It is located behind each vertebral body, connecting the vertebral body and the intervertebral disc, and functions to limit excessive forward flexion of the spine and to maintain spinal stability. This is of great significance for maintaining the physiological curvature of the spine and limiting its range of motion [5]. Hence, the PLL is vital for maintaining the stability of the spine. It also functions to prevent intervertebral disc prolapse. It covers the backs of the vertebral bodies and is closely attached to the fibrous ring that helps to prevent intervertebral disc prolapse during activity. However, the central portion of the PLL is thicker and the expanded part on each side is wide and thin; there are more patients with disc herniation to the outer posterior (Fig. 10.6), particularly in the lumbar 4-sacral 1 segment. The PLL narrows rapidly, and lumbar 4-sacral 1 has become a high-risk segment for intervertebral disc herniation [8]. 3. The ligament also isolates the spinal cord and dura from the anterior vertebral body, reducing the stimulation of the spinal cord by the hard bone in front of it during activity or trauma [5].

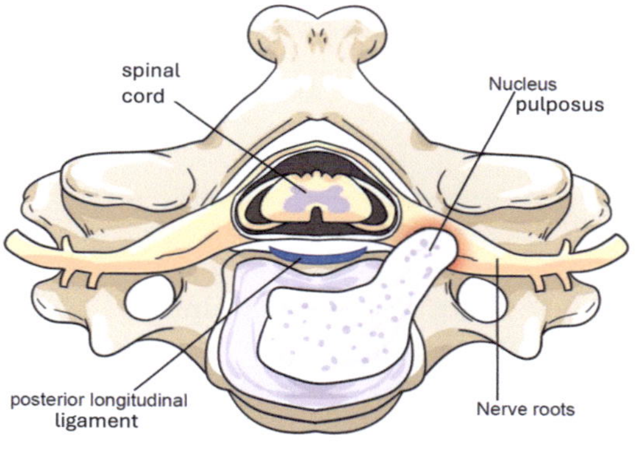

Fig. 10.6 A schematic diagram of intervertebral disc prolapse and the relationship to the PLL

The PLL can develop calcifications owing to increasing age or other factors, and these localized calcium deposits can cause the ligament to exhibit ossification features on imaging (Fig. 10.7). This change hardens it and can lead to various clinical symptoms, including spinal stenosis and nerve compression [12, 13].

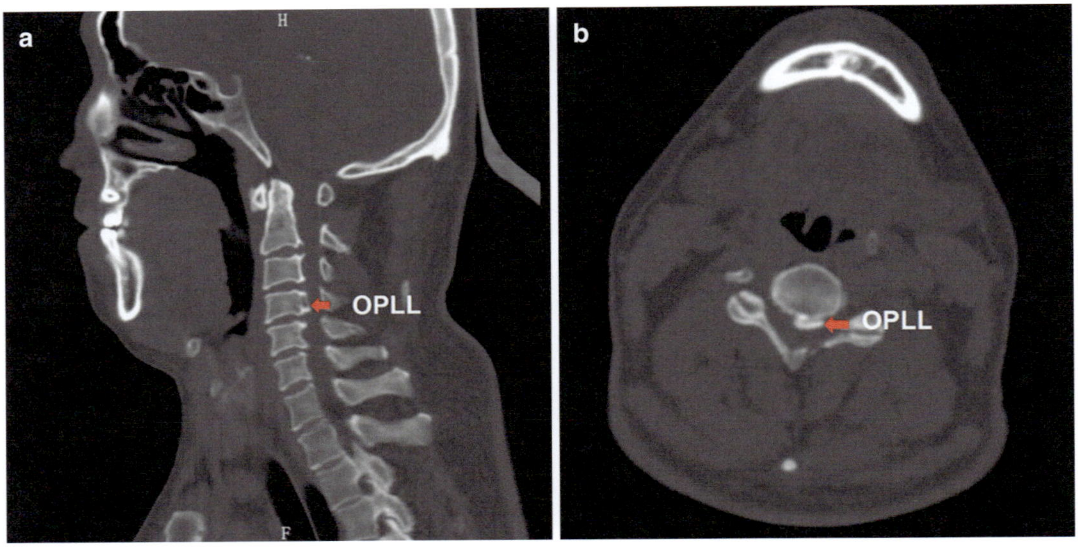

Fig. 10.7 Bone imaging by computed tomography showing ossification of the PLL

10.5 Conclusion

10.5.1 Summary of Key Points Regarding the Developmental Anatomy and Histology of the Posterior Longitudinal Ligament

1. Embryonic origin: During embryo development, the PLL originates in the mesoderm and begins to develop during the late embryonic or early fetal period.
2. PLL histology: The PLL can be divided into three layers: superficial, medium, and deep. All three of these layers consist mainly of elastin and fibrillin-1, but their attachment sites and travel directions are different.
3. Developmental changes over time: The PLL begins to develop during the late embryonic or early fetal period, approximately 10 weeks into gestation. Its elasticity gradually diminishes with age, making it more susceptible to mechanical stress injury.
4. Clinical significance: The PLL is one of the structures that maintain the stability of the spine, limiting its excessive forward flexion and preventing backward prolapse of the intervertebral disc. The degree of PLL injury is an important indicator for assessing spinal injury and determining the modality of surgery required. Age or other factors can lead to calcification of the PLL, ultimately causing spinal stenosis and nerve compression. The length, thickness, and shape of calcified areas are important for determining the surgical approach.

10.5.2 Importance of This Knowledge in Clinical Practice

Understanding the developmental anatomy and histology of the PLL is crucial for healthcare professionals in several specialties, particularly for spinal surgeons. Its degeneration is closely related to the occurrence and development of diseases, such as ligament ossification. In clinical management, recognizing the status of the PLL is vital for surgical selection and therapeutic efficacy.

References

1. Hayes AJ, et al. Colocalization in vivo and association in vitro of perlecan and elastin. Histochem Cell Biol. 2011;136(4):437–54.
2. Nakagawa H, et al. Elastin in the human posterior longitudinal ligament and spinal dura. A histologic and biochemical study. Spine. 1994;19(19):2164–9.
3. Butt AM, et al. A comprehensive review of the sub-axial ligaments of the vertebral column: part II histology and embryology. Childs Nerv Syst. 2015;31(7):1061–6.
4. Misawa H, et al. Embryological study of the spinal ligaments in human fetuses. J Spinal Disord. 1994;7(6):495–8.
5. Aryal V, et al. Anatomy, back, posterior longitudinal ligament. *StatPearls*. StatPearls Publishing; 2023.
6. Plaisant O, et al. The lumbar anterior epidural cavity: the posterior longitudinal ligament, the anterior ligaments of the dura mater and the anterior internal vertebral venous plexus. Acta Anat. 1996;155(4):274–81.
7. Butt AM, et al. A comprehensive review of the subaxial ligaments of the vertebral column: part I anatomy and function. Child Nerv Syst. 2015;31(7):1037–59.
8. Salaud C, et al. Morphometric study of the posterior longitudinal ligament at the lumbar spine. Surg Radiol Anat. 2018;40(5):563–9.
9. Loughenbury PR, et al. The posterior longitudinal ligament and peridural (epidural) membrane. Clin Anat. 2006;19(6):487–92.
10. Mercer S, Bogduk N. The ligaments and annulus fibrosus of human adult cervical intervertebral discs. Spine. 1999;24(7):619–26; discussion 627–8
11. Menck J, Lierse W. Zur arteriellen Gefässversorgung des thorakalen und lumbalen Bewegungssegmentes beim Neugeborenen [The arterial supply of the thoracic and lumbar spine in newborns]. Acta Anat. 1990;137(2):170–4.
12. Smith ZA, et al. Ossification of the posterior longitudinal ligament: pathogenesis, management, and current surgical approaches. A review. Neurosurg Focus. 2011;30(3):E10.
13. Saetia K, et al. Ossification of the posterior longitudinal ligament: a review. Neurosurg Focus. 2011;30(3):E1.

Part III

The Ligaments of the Vertebral Arches

The Ligamentum Flavum

11

Joe Iwanaga

11.1 Introduction

The ligamenta flava (singular: ligamentum flavum), which translates to "yellow ligaments" in Latin, are a series of strong, elastic ligaments that interconnect the laminae of adjacent vertebrae, forming alternating segments along the posterior wall of the vertebral canal [1, 3, 7, 22] (Fig. 11.1). Clinically, the lumbar segment of the ligamenta flava is of particular interest in the context of epidural analgesia, especially concerning the "loss of resistance" technique. These ligaments have been thoroughly investigated with regard to their anatomy, function, and associated pathologies. Nonetheless, the literature presents considerable variation and inconsistencies among authors. This chapter aims to synthesize and examine the previous findings and observations related to the ligamenta flava.

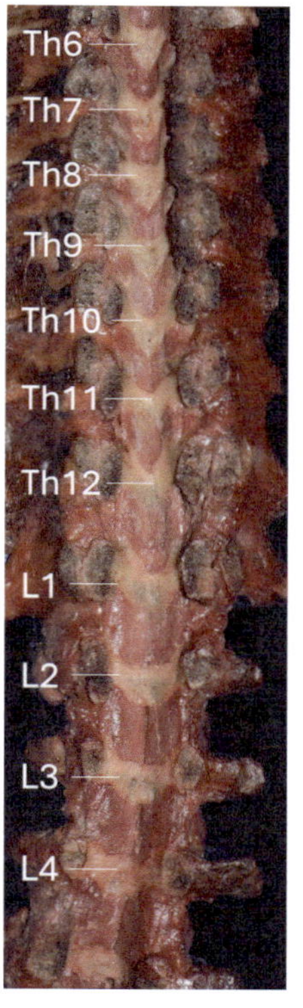

Fig. 11.1 Anterior view of the ligamenta flavum (LF) in the posterior wall of the vertebral canal (T6 to L4)

J. Iwanaga (✉)
Department of Neurosurgery, Clinical Neuroscience Research Center, Tulane University School of Medicine, New Orleans, LA, USA

Department of Neurology, Clinical Neuroscience Research Center, Tulane University School of Medicine, New Orleans, LA, USA

Department of Structural & Cellular Biology, Tulane University School of Medicine, New Orleans, LA, USA

Department of Neurosurgery and Ochsner Neuroscience Institute, Ochsner Health System, New Orleans, LA, USA

Dental and Oral Medical Center, Kurume University School of Medicine, Fukuoka, Japan

Division of Gross and Clinical Anatomy, Department of Anatomy, Kurume University School of Medicine, Fukuoka, Japan
e-mail: jiwanaga@tulane.edu

M. Turgut et al. (eds.), *Ligaments of the Vertebral Column*,
https://doi.org/10.1007/978-3-032-09070-6_11

11.2 General Morphology

The morphology of the ligamentum flavum has been described with significant variability across published studies, and no universal consensus has been established. Extending from the second cervical vertebra (C2) to the first sacral vertebra (S1), the ligamentum flavum contributes to spinal stability in combination with intervertebral discs, spinal musculature, fascial layers, and the vertebrae themselves [2, 6, 8, 10] (Fig. 11.2). Among spinal regions, the lumbar ligamentum flavum is the thickest and most robust, while the cervical ligamentum flavum is thinner and broader; the thoracic ligament displays intermediate thickness [29] (Fig. 11.3). Notably, the thickness of the ligamentum flavum is dynamic, and it changes with spinal flexion and extension, may vary between sides, and is affected by pathological processes [27].

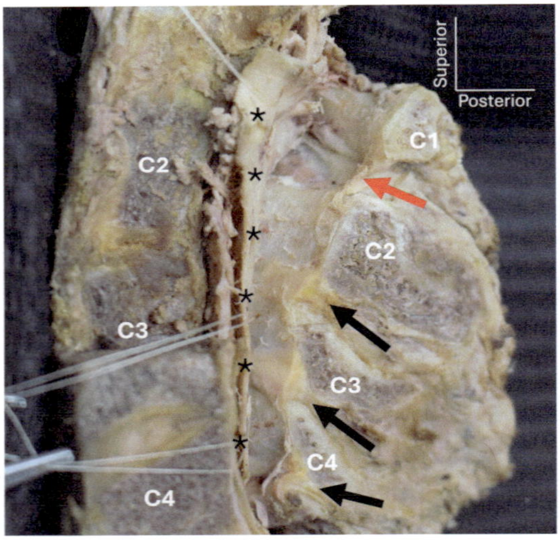

Fig. 11.2 Para midsagittal medial view (right side) of the cervical LF. Note that the dura (*) covered the posterior wall of the vertebral canal was turned anteriorly

At every vertebral level, ligamenta flava are found bilaterally and typically meet at the midline [3, 22]. However, a central gap between the right and left ligamenta flava has been documented [18–20].

11.3 Relationship to Adjacent Ligaments

The fibers of the ligamentum flavum extend perpendicularly, attaching superiorly to the anterior surface of the lamina and inferior pedicle of the vertebra above, and descending to insert on the posterior surface of the upper edge of the lamina below [1, 3, 7, 22, 32]. As the ligament courses downward, it divides into medial and lateral segments. The medial portion extends to the dorsal aspect of the adjacent lower lamina, whereas the lateral portion passes anterior to the zygapophysial joint [3]. Inferiorly, this lateral component reaches the midpoint between adjacent pedicles, where it contributes to the anterior capsule of the zygapophysial joint and attaches to the corresponding articular processes [1, 3, 13, 32]. The outermost fibers may extend along the superior articular process as far as the next lower pedicle [3, 13]. At the posterior midline, where the ligament merges toward the spinous processes, small venous channels traverse from the internal to the external vertebral venous plexuses through intervening gaps [1]. Iwanaga et al. [13] further noted that the lumbar ligamentum flavum is continuous with the interspinous ligament, with no distinct demarcation (Figs. 11.4, 11.5, and 11.6).

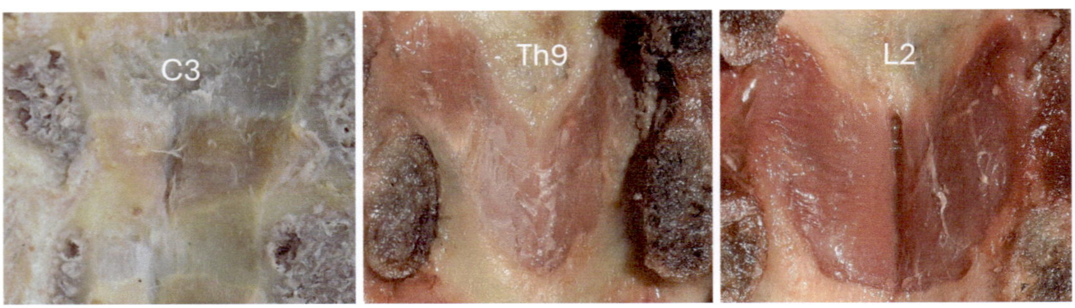

Fig. 11.3 LF in cervical (C3), thoracic (T9), and lumbar (L2) levels

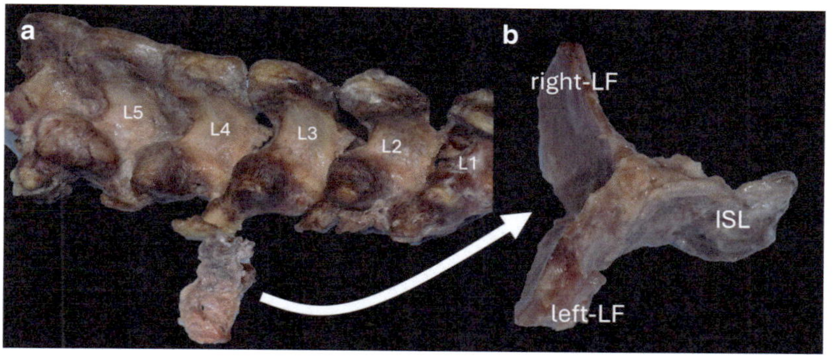

Fig. 11.4 Observation of the LF and interspinous ligament (ISL). (**a**) Harvesting the ligaments en bloc from the intervertebral space of the lumbar spine. (**b**) Superolateral view of the ligaments

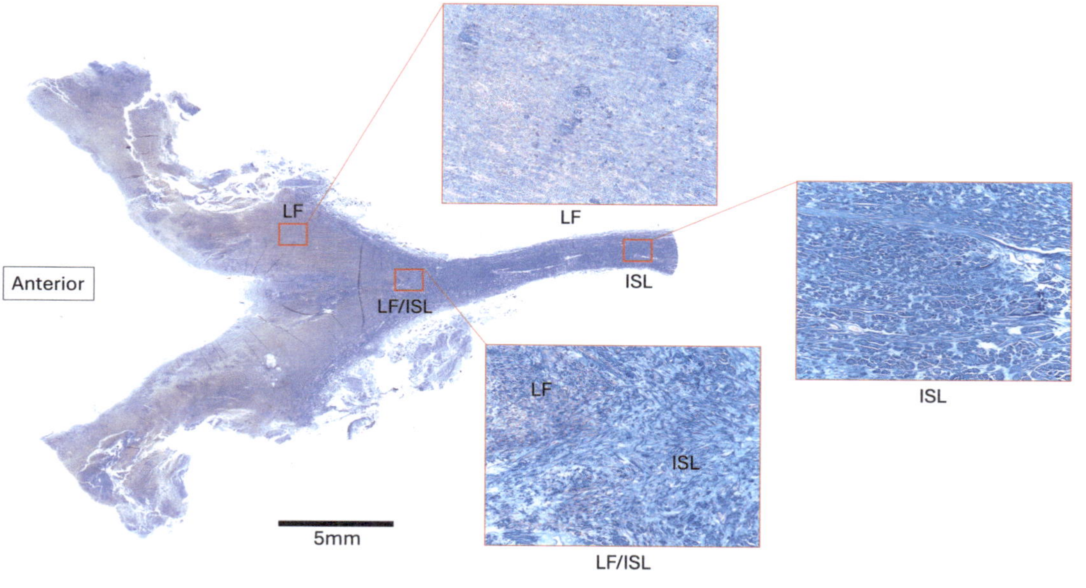

Fig. 11.5 Histological observations of the ISL and LF with Masson's trichrome staining. Rectangular images are shown at 100× magnification

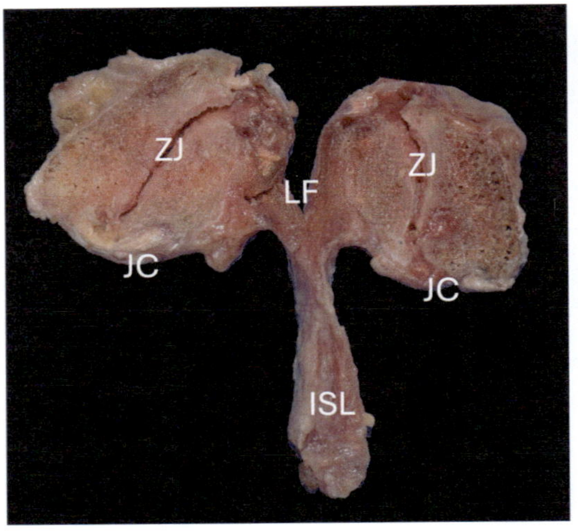

Fig. 11.6 Axial section of the lumbar LF, ISL, zygapophysial joint (ZJ), and joint capsule (JC)

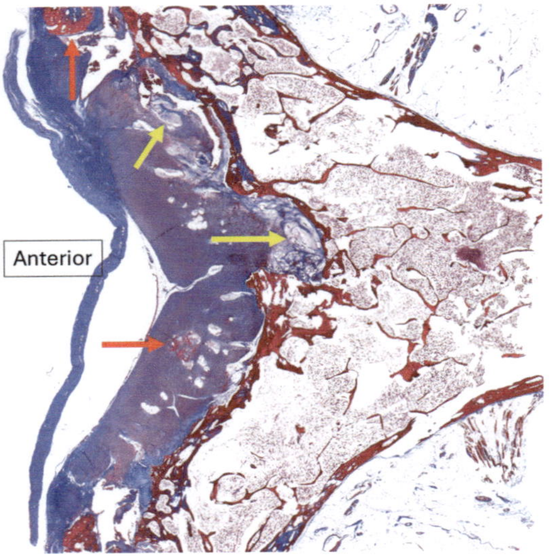

Fig. 11.7 Ossification (red arrows) and cartilaginous change (yellow arrows) in the axial histological section of the cervical LF (Masson's trichrome staining)

11.4 Histology

Macroscopically, the ligamentum flavum presents as a broad, pale yellow structure [1, 7, 22]. Histologically, it consists of approximately 80% elastin and 20% collagen, with the elastic fibers running longitudinally [3, 30, 31]. In 1976, Yong-Hing and colleagues examined 51 specimens using Gomori's aldehyde fuchsin stain and reported elastin and collagen compositions ranging from 50% to 80% and 20% to 50%, respectively. The anterior portion of the ligament is thinner, primarily due to its elastin-rich composition, whereas the posterior aspect is thicker due to a higher concentration of collagen [31]. Ultrastructural studies have identified two distinct types of elastic fibers: conventional elastic fibers found centrally, and elaunin fibers, which are defined by sparse elastin and embedded microtubules, located near the ligament's bony attachments [3, 30]. Additionally, fibroblasts are rare and predominantly spindle-shaped [30]. Among the spinal ligaments, the ligamentum flavum is unique due to its predominance of elastin [3]. Interestingly, elastin content does not appear to diminish with age. Yong-Hing et al. reported no correlation between elastin levels and age, symptom duration, or degenerative changes such as spondylosis. Moreover, they observed no evidence of hypertrophy, hyperplasia, or elastin degeneration in aging specimens [31]. Nevertheless, ossification and cartilaginous transformation of the ligamentum flavum become increasingly observed in histological slides with advanced age (Fig. 11.7).

11.5 Morphometrics

Pintar et al. [26] performed morphometric analysis on the lumbar ligamentum flavum using 22 cadaveric specimens, reporting a mean length of 15.2 mm and a mean cross-sectional area of 84.2 mm^2. The ligament shows progressive thickening from the cervical to the lumbar regions, with the latter being most developed [1, 22]. Yong-Hing et al. [31] measured average thicknesses of 2–3 mm at both the midline and lateral aspects [32]. Simonds et al. [28] described the presence of a midline interlaminar ligament within the gap separating the left and right ligamenta flava in the majority of lumbar samples [21, 28].

11.6 Function and Biomechanics

The ligamentum flavum plays a pivotal role in resisting separation of the laminae during spinal flexion, thereby contributing to vertebral stability and promoting return to an upright posture [1, 3, 7, 22]. Its elastic nature minimizes buckling during extension, thus safeguarding the spinal canal [3]. The lateral portion protects the zygapophysial joint capsule from entrapment during motion [3]. The ligament exerts an estimated disc pressure of 0.7 kg/cm^2, although the functional significance of this pressure is not fully understood [3]. Some investigators have proposed that the ligamentum flavum contributes to spinal extension, working in conjunction with the erector spinae muscles; however, this view has been questioned by Bogduk [3] and Zander et al. [32]. In terms of mechanical properties, Pintar et al. [26] noted that the ligamentum flavum has the greatest cross-sectional area among spinal ligaments, with the lowest failure stress (1.3–4.1 MPa). These findings align with the work of Panjabi et al. [25], Nachemson and Evans [23], and Chazal et al. [5]. Panjabi et al. also reported lengths ranging from 11.6 to 16.0 mm, consistent with the 13.0–18.0 mm range observed by Pintar et al. [26]. The mean stiffness of the ligament was determined to be 27.2 ± 9.2 N/mm [26].

11.7 Clinical Relevance and Pathology

Excision of the ligamentum flavum, even across multiple levels, has not been shown to cause significant disability, likely due to its proximity rather than critical functional role [3]. The ligament's lateral extensions provide elasticity to the anterior and medial capsules of the posterior facet joints, thereby complementing the elasticity of intervertebral discs [32]. During hyperextension, the ligamentum flavum may protrude into the spinal canal, potentially compressing the spinal cord, particularly in patients with spinal stenosis, ossification of the posterior longitudinal ligament, or ligamentum flavum ossification [15]. In spinal dissection, it was previously believed by spine surgeons that the ligamenta flava consisted of two distinct layers, i.e., superficial and deep [4, 24]. However, Iwanaga et al. [13] demonstrated that such a two-layered structure was a dissection bias [13, 14].

Ossification of the ligamentum flavum (OLF) represents a pathological condition characterized by ectopic bone formation within the ligament. Although OLF can occur at any spinal level, it is most frequently seen in the lower thoracic spine (T9–T12) [11, 12, 16, 17, 33]. According to Li et al. [17], more than 50% of associated dural ossification cases occurred between T9 and T12. A study by Fujimori [9] involving 1500 Japanese patients found that the incidence of thoracic OLF and lumbar OLF was 12% and 0.3%, respectively.

11.8 Conclusions

The ligamenta flava are key stabilizing structures of the spine, extending from C2 to S1 and contributing to vertebral alignment, spinal recoil, and protection of neural elements. Their unique elastin-rich composition distinguishes them from other spinal ligaments, particularly in the lumbar region, where they are thickest and most clinically relevant. Age-related changes, including hypertrophy and ossification, especially in the lower thoracic spine, can lead to spinal canal narrowing and neurological symptoms. A clear understanding of their anatomy, biomechanics, and pathology is essential for effective diagnosis and surgical management of related spinal conditions.

References

1. Bannister LH, Berry MM, Collins P, Dyson M, Dussek JE, Ferguson MWJ, editors. Gray's anatomy. 38th ed. New York: Churchill Livingston; 1996.
2. Blain M, Bedretdinova D, Bellin MF, Rocher L, Gagey O, Soubeyrand M, Creze M. Influence of thoracolumbar fascia stretching on lumbar back muscle stiffness: a supersonic shear wave elastography approach. Clin Anat. 2019;32:73–80.

3. Bogduk N. Clinical anatomy of the lumbar spine and sacrum. 3rd ed. New York: Churchill Livingston; 1997.
4. Chau AM, Pelzer NR, Hampton J, Smith A, Seex KA, Stewart F, Gragnaniello C. Lateral extent and ventral laminar attachments of the lumbar ligamentum flavum: cadaveric study. Spine J. 2014;14:2467–71.
5. Chazal J, Tanguy A, Bourges M, Gaurel G, Escande G, Guillot M, Vanneuville G. Biomechanical properties of spinal ligaments and a histological study of the supraspinal ligament in traction. J Biomech. 1985;18(3):167–76.
6. Creze M, Soubeyrand M, Yue JL, Gagey O, Maitre X, Bellin MF. Magnetic resonance elastography of the lumbar back muscles: a preliminary study. Clin Anat. 2018;31:514–20.
7. Dickman CA, Rosenthal DJ, Perin NI. Thoracoscopic spine surgery. New York: Thieme Medical Publishers; 1999.
8. Fan C, Fede C, Gaudreault N, Porzionato A, Macchi V, De Caro R, Stecco C. Anatomical and functional relationships between external abdominal oblique muscle and posterior layer of thoracolumbar fascia. Clin Anat. 2018;31:1092–8.
9. Fujimori T, Watabe T, Iwamoto Y, Hamada S, Iwasaki M, Oda T. Prevalence, concomitance, and distribution of ossification of the spinal ligaments: results of whole spine CT scans in 1500 Japanese patients. Spine (Phila Pa 1976). 2016;41(21):1668–76. https://doi.org/10.1097/BRS.0000000000001643.
10. Ghannam M, Jumah F, Mansour S, Samara A, Alkhdour S, Alzuabi MA, Aker L, Adeeb N, Massengale J, Oskouian RJ, Tubbs RS. Surgical anatomy, radiological features, and molecular biology of the lumbar intervertebral discs. Clin Anat. 2017;30:251–66.
11. Guo JJ, Luk KD, Karppinen J, Yang H, Cheung KM. Prevalence, distribution, and morphology of ossification of the ligamentum flavum: a population study of one thousand seven hundred thirty-six magnetic resonance imaging scans. Spine (Phila Pa 1976). 2010;35(1):51–6. https://doi.org/10.1097/BRS.0b013e3181b3f779.
12. Hur H, Lee JK, Lee JH, Kim JH, Kim SH. Thoracic myelopathy caused by ossification of the ligamentum flavum. J Korean Neurosurg Soc. 2009;46(3):189–94. https://doi.org/10.3340/jkns.2009.46.3.189.
13. Iwanaga J, Ishak B, Saga T, Singla A, Impastato D, Chapman JR, Oskouian RJ, David G, Porzionato A, Reina MA, Macchi V, de Caro R, Tubbs RS. The lumbar ligamentum flavum does not have two layers and is confluent with the interspinous ligament: anatomical study with application to surgical and interventional pain procedures. Clin Anat. 2020;33(1):34–40. https://doi.org/10.1002/ca.23437.
14. Iwanaga J, Kikuchi K, Hur MS, Kawai H, Tabira Y, Reina MA, LaPrade RF, Watanabe K. What do we know about ligaments? Clin Anat. 2025. https://doi.org/10.1002/ca.24289.
15. Lang J. Clinical anatomy of the cervical spine. New York: Thieme Medical Publishers; 1993.
16. Lang N, Yuan HS, Wang HL, Liao J, Li M, Guo FX, et al. Epidemiological survey of ossification of the ligamentum flavum in thoracic spine: CT imaging observation of 993 cases. Eur Spine J. 2013;22(4):857–62. https://doi.org/10.1007/s00586-012-2492-8.
17. Li B, Qiu G, Guo S, Li W, Li Y, Peng H, Wang C, Zhao Y. Dural ossification associated with ossification of ligamentum flavum in the thoracic spine: a retrospective analysis. BMJ Open. 2016;6(12):e013887. https://doi.org/10.1136/bmjopen-2016-013887. PMID: 27998902; PMCID: PMC5223670.
18. Lirk P, Kolbitsch C, Putz G, Colvin J, Colvin HP, Lorenz I, Keller C, Kirchmair L, Rieder J, Moriggl B. Cervical and high thoracic ligamentum flavum frequently fails to fuse in the midline. Anesthesiology. 2003;99:1387–90.
19. Lirk P, Moriggl B, Colvin J, Keller C, Kirchmair L, Rieder J, Kolbitsch C. The incidence of lumbar ligamentum flavum midline gaps. Anesth Analg. 2004;98:1178–80.
20. Lirk P, Colvin J, Steger B, Colvin HP, Keller C, Rieder J, Kolbitsch C, Moriggl B. Incidence of lower thoracic ligamentum flavum midline gaps. Br J Anaesth. 2005;94:852–5.
21. Millhuff A, Haddad H, Draper MS, Motzko M, Glueck E, Holland B, Wright B. The midline interlaminar ligament of the spine: an anatomical study. Clin Anat. 2023;36(4):618–23. https://doi.org/10.1002/ca.24003.
22. Moore KL, Dalley AF, Agur AMR. Clinically oriented anatomy. 6th ed. Baltimore: Lippincott Williams & Wilkins; 2010.
23. Nachemson AL, Evans JH. Some mechanical properties of the third human lumbar interlaminar ligament (ligamentum flavum). J Biomech. 1968;1(3):211–20.
24. Olszewski AD, Yaszemski MJ, White AA. The anatomy of the human lumbar ligamentum flavum. New observations and their surgical importance. Spine (Phila Pa 1976). 1996;21:2307–12.
25. Panjabi MM, Greenstein G, Duranceau J, Nolte LP. Three-dimensional quantitative morphology of lumbar spinal ligaments. J Spinal Disord. 1991;4(l):54–62.
26. Pintar FA, Yoganandan N, Myers T, Elhagediab A, Sances A Jr. Biomechanical properties of human lumbar spine ligaments. J Biomech. 1992;25(11):1351–6.
27. Reina MA, Lirk P, Puigdellívol-Sánchez A, Mavar M, Prats-Galino A. Human lumbar ligamentum flavum anatomy for epidural anesthesia: reviewing a 3D MR-based interactive model and postmortem samples. Anesth Analg. 2016;1:903–7.
28. Simonds E, Iwanaga J, Ishak B, Reina MA, Oskouian RJ, Tubbs RS. Discovery of a new ligament of the lumbar spine: the midline interlaminar ligament. Spine J. 2020;20(7):1134–7. https://doi.org/10.1016/j.spinee.2019.12.003.

29. Standring S. Gray's anatomy: the anatomical basis of clinical practice. London: Elsevier Health Sciences; 2015.
30. Yahia LH, Garzon S, Strykowski H, Rivard CH. Ultrastructure of the human interspinous ligament and ligamentum flavum: a preliminary study. Spine. 1990;15(4):262–8.
31. Yong-Hing K, Reilly J, Kirkaldy-Willis WH. The ligamentum flavum. Spine. 1976;1(4):226–34.
32. Zander T, Rohlmann A, Bergmann G. Influence of ligament stiffness on the mechanical behavior of a functional spinal unit. J Biomech. 2004;37(7):1107–11.
33. Zhang C, Chang Y, Shu L, Chen Z. Pathogenesis of thoracic ossification of the ligamentum flavum. Front Pharmacol. 2024;15:1496297. https://doi.org/10.3389/fphar.2024.1496297.

12 The Interspinous Ligament

Joe Iwanaga

12.1 Introduction

The interspinous ligaments are thin, short, membrane-covered structures that connect adjacent spinous processes. Their mechanical stiffness is attributed to interactions between collagen fibers [7]. The interspinous ligaments span from the root to the apex of each spinous process and connect posteriorly to the supraspinous ligament and anteriorly to the ligamenta flava [3, 8, 24]. Composed of collagen and elastic fibers, the interspinous ligaments typically exhibit parallel fiber orientation. With aging, these fibers may thicken and occasionally ossify, potentially leading to pain or instability [4, 25, 34]. The interspinous ligaments play a role in spinal stabilization [25], though their fan-like collagen arrangement, parallel to the spinous processes, suggests limited resistance to lumbar flexion [12]. Degeneration of these ligaments with age is a known contributor to spinal pain and mechanical instability [4].

J. Iwanaga (✉)
Department of Neurosurgery, Clinical Neuroscience Research Center, Tulane University School of Medicine, New Orleans, LA, USA

Department of Neurology, Clinical Neuroscience Research Center, Tulane University School of Medicine, New Orleans, LA, USA

Department of Structural & Cellular Biology, Tulane University School of Medicine, New Orleans, LA, USA

Department of Neurosurgery and Ochsner Neuroscience Institute, Ochsner Health System, New Orleans, LA, USA

Dental and Oral Medical Center, Kurume University School of Medicine, Fukuoka, Japan

Division of Gross and Clinical Anatomy, Department of Anatomy, Kurume University School of Medicine, Fukuoka, Japan
e-mail: jiwanaga@tulane.edu

12.2 General Morphology

Von Richter [39] was the first to describe the interspinous ligaments as broad, thin membranes composed of irregular, typically horizontal fibers. These membranes span the interspinous space from the base to the tip of the spinous process. As early as the nineteenth century, D'Alton and von Richter debated their function ([6]; [39]). Subsequently, various authors have proposed differing fiber orientations: Fick [9] described a diagonal anterosuperior–posteroinferior course; Kajava [17] described posterosuperior–anteroinferior orientation; Woerdeman [40] reported vertical fibers; and Tandler [37] described a dorsally open U-shaped configuration. D'Alton [6] further observed that these diagonal fibers separate radially during spinal flexion, exposing interfiber openings.

Fick [9] also noted that the interspinous ligaments resemble square plates with distinct margins and multiple laminae, each containing

M. Turgut et al. (eds.), *Ligaments of the Vertebral Column*,
https://doi.org/10.1007/978-3-032-09070-6_12

vascular and adipose elements. While fiber orientation has been variably described, many agree that it follows an anterosuperior to posteroinferior direction [31]. However, Iwanaga et al. [14] found that in the lumbar spine, ISL fibers run horizontally in a slightly curved anteroposterior course, suggesting fiber orientation may vary by vertebral level due to changes in spinous process angulation (Figs. 12.1 and 12.2).

Anatomical variation is also evident in gross morphology: lumbar interspinous ligaments are typically thicker, rhomboid or quadrilateral, and often appear as paired structures [36]. In *Gray's Anatomy*, the lumbar interspinous ligaments are shown with oblique anterior-to-posterior fibers running from the superior margin of the caudal spinous process to the cranial one [34, 36]. Netter's Atlas of Anatomy similarly depicts an oblique anterior-to-posterior orientation.

Scapinelli et al. [34] emphasized the inconsistency in ISL depictions and confirmed through dissection that lumbar interspinous ligaments generally follow an anterior-to-posterior, caudal-to-cranial direction, with the middle portion being the thickest. The posterior fibers run obliquely backward and upward. According to Rissanen [31], the lumbar interspinous ligaments can be divided into four parts based on their attachments and fiber trajectories. The ISL is described as membranous, connecting adjacent spinous processes [3, 5, 8, 24], being poorly developed in the cervical spine (Fig. 12.3), narrow in the thoracic region, and broad and thick in the lumbar spine [3, 8].

Fiber direction also varies: many describe a posterocaudal direction [3, 28, 35], while others observe a posterocranial course in the lumbar region, where anteriorly the ISL may appear paired with a central fat-filled cavity, which is

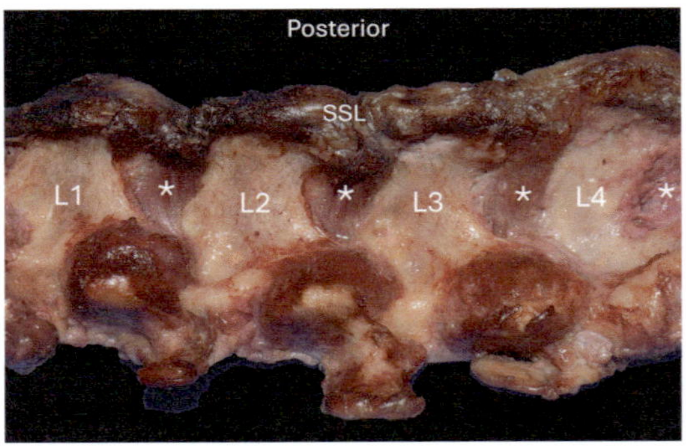

Fig. 12.1 Lateral view of the lumbar interspinous ligaments (ISLs) (*) and supraspinous ligaments (SSLs)

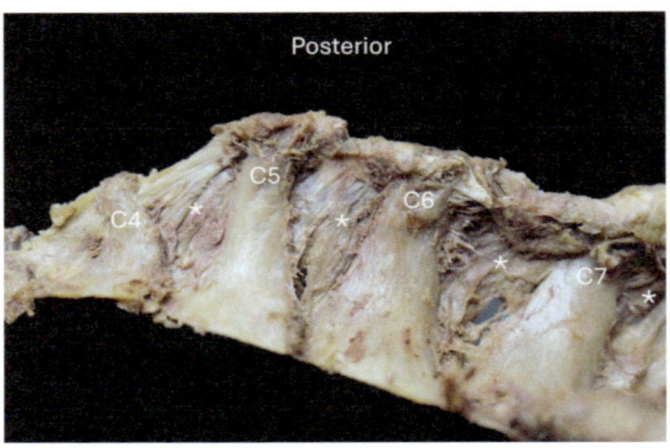

Fig. 12.2 Lateral view of the cervical ISLs (*)

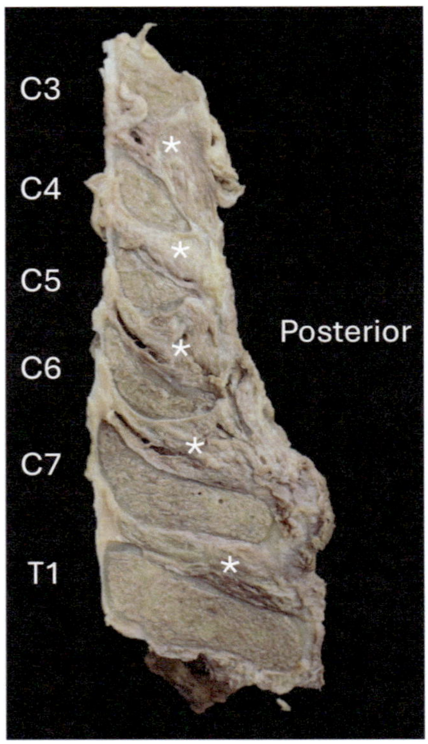

Fig. 12.3 Sagittal section of the cervical ISLs (*)

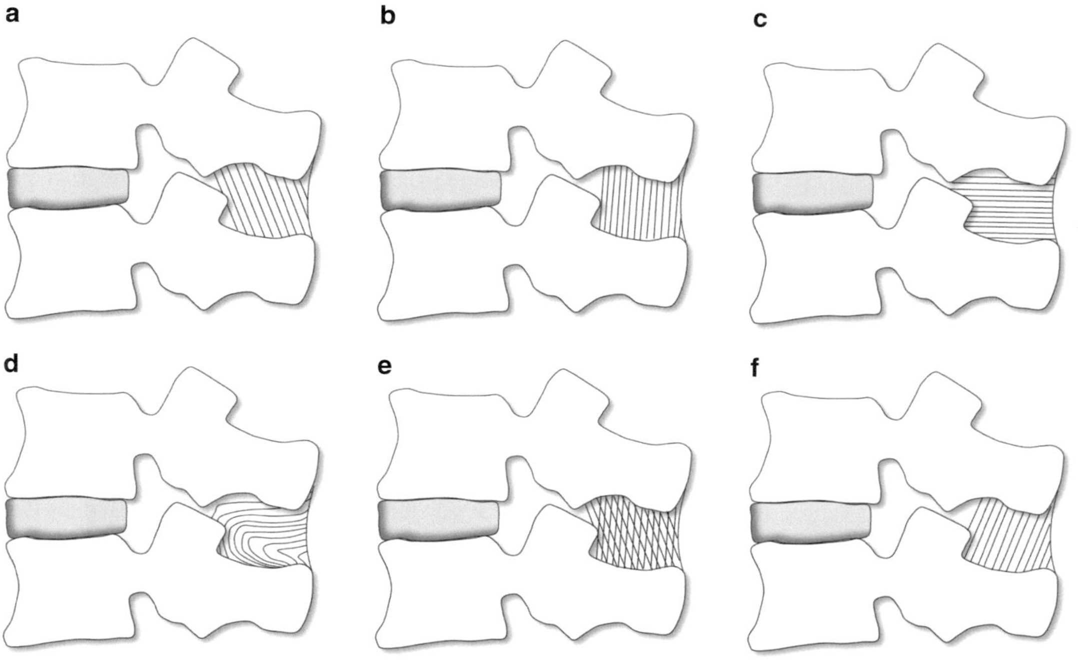

Fig. 12.4 Schematic drawings of the fiber directions of the ISL as described in various research articles. (After Scapinelli [34]). (**a**) anterosuperior to posteroinferior, (**b**) vertical, (**c**) horizontal, (**d**) C-shaped, (**e**) obliquely posterocaudal from the inferior margin of the overlying spinous process, and as obliquely posterocranial from the superior margin of the subjacent spinous process, and thus decussate at the center of the ligament, and (**f**) anteroinferior to posterosuperior

absent posteriorly [2, 5, 10, 32] (Fig. 12.4). The interspinous ligaments may ossify, particularly in the cervical and thoracic regions [25], and are richly vascularized and innervated, especially dorsally and laterally [34].

12.3 Morphometrics

Pintar et al. [29] reported a mean lumbar ISL length of 16 mm (SD 3.2 mm) and a mean cross-sectional area of 35.1 mm^2 (SD 15.0 mm). Iwanaga et al. [14] found that the mean anteroposterior length, anterior height, and posterior height of the ISL were 11.56 ± 2.32 mm, 12.01 ± 2.23 mm, and 21.42 ± 2.97 mm, respectively.

12.4 Relationship to Adjacent Ligaments

The ISL's anterior fibers are partly continuous with the ligamentum flavum, partly originating from the vertebral laminae, and partly from the caudal spinous process [34] (Fig. 12.5). Descriptions vary considerably, especially for the cervical interspinous ligaments, which are either considered part of the nuchal ligament or as distinct fascicles [3]. Iwanaga et al. [15] clearly showed that the lumber ISL is a continuation of the ligamentum flavum with no clear border. Histologically, the cervical ISL is less distinct than its lumbar counterpart (Fig. 12.6). Discrepancies also exist in descriptions of the lumbar supraspinous and interspinous ligaments [10].

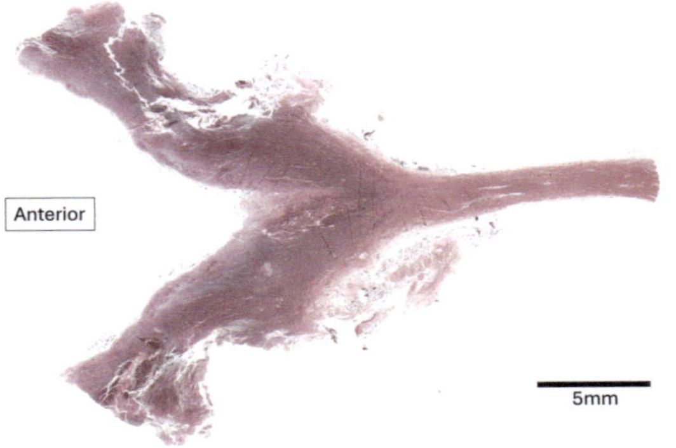

Fig. 12.5 Axial histological section of the lumbar ISL. Van-Gieson staining

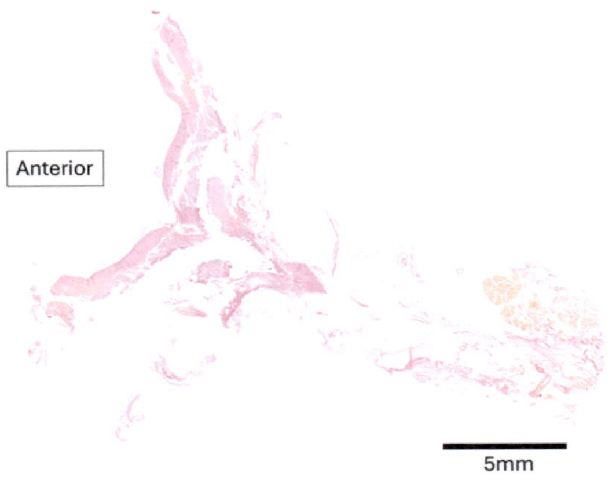

Fig. 12.6 Axial histological section of cervical ISL. The majority of the ISL is replaced with adipose tissue. Van-Gieson staining

12.5 Function and Biomechanics

The ISL fibers help limit lumbar flexion and may resist hyperextension [30]. Kallio noted ISL degeneration in nearly all cases of intervertebral disc prolapse [31]. Collagen fiber orientation contributes to stiffness and links the interspinous ligaments to thoracolumbar fascia [12]. Their fan-like collagen arrangement suggests limited resistance to spinal flexion [12]. The S-shaped fiber course provides reserve length [34].

Heylings [10] argued that fibers must run radially from the axis of motion—posterocranial in this case—to balance control and flexibility. Posterocaudal fibers would either limit motion too early or provide insufficient control during extension. The interspinous ligaments, in collaboration with the ligamenta flava and supraspinous ligaments, provide joint stabilization and energy storage [41]. Though weak flexion limiters, their near-perpendicular fiber alignment resists spinous process separation [5, 10]. Hindle et al. [11] found that the interspinous ligaments resist a minimal load during early flexion, but contribute significantly more toward the end, particularly when the supraspinous ligaments are absent. The interspinous ligaments are unloaded during lateral bending of the spine [42] and exhibit the lowest stiffness (11.5 ± 6.6 N/mm), compared to the joint capsule (33.9 ± 10.7 N/mm), and lowest stress (1.8–5.9 MPa) [29]. Tensile strength varies by level: 162 N (L1/2), 86 N (L2/3), and 79 N (L3/4) [14]. Strength declines with age [13]. Kotani et al. [22] studied the ISL tensile strength in sheep, but they also included the supraspinous ligament, which complicates their interpretations. Adams et al. [1] reported that the ISL and SSL contribute to up to 19% of lumbar flexion resistance.

12.6 Histology

The ISL comprises anterior, middle, and posterior portions, composed of type I collagen and rows of cells between bundles [5, 8, 27]. The anterior portion, an extension of the ligamentum flavum, contains elastic fibers and passes posterocranially to the anterior lower border of the superior spinous process [5, 8, 41]. The middle portion, purely collagenous, connects the anterior upper border of one spinous process to the posterior lower border of the one above. The posterior portion, also collagenous, attaches to the posterior upper border below and merges with the supraspinous ligament or erector spinae tendons [5, 10]. Only the anterior and middle portions are considered true ligaments due to their bony attachments. The ISL contains more cells than the ligamentum flavum, with fibroblasts between central collagen bundles and chondrocytes near bony attachments [41] (Fig. 12.7).

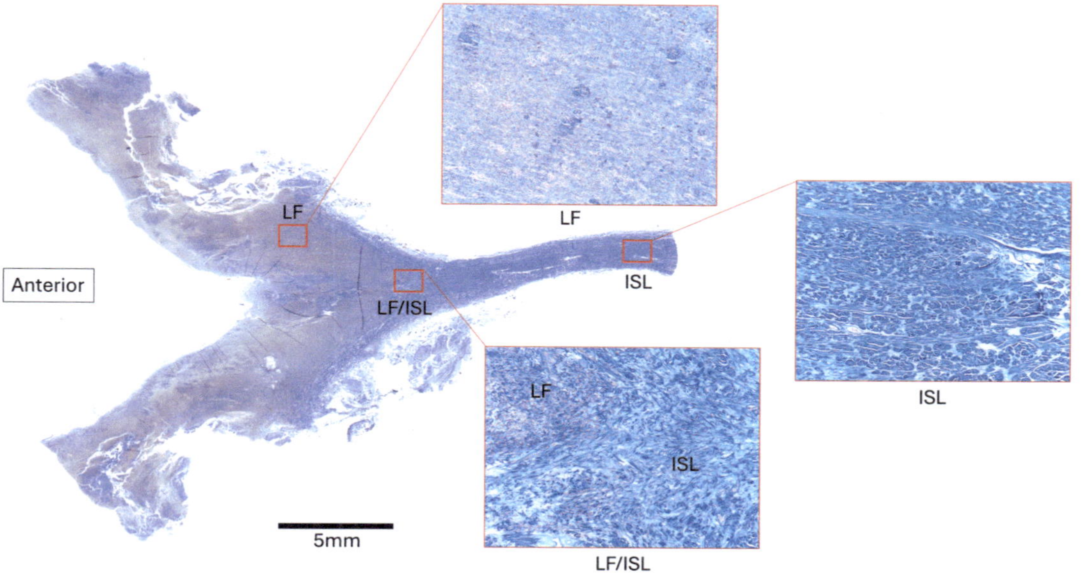

Fig. 12.7 Histological observations of the ISL and ligamentum flavum (LF). Rectangular images shown at 100× magnification

12.7 Clinical Relevance

ISL injuries have been implicated in the development of low back pain and disc herniation [18–21, 23, 33, 38, 43]. Knowledge of tensile strength by lumbar level may improve spinal fixation designs and inform injury risk assessment in trauma. Whiplash can sprain the ISL, often requiring weeks of recovery focused on reducing tears and swelling. ISL damage decreases spinal stability, with T5–L3 most commonly affected. Clinically, these injuries present as localized thickening and tenderness. Neumann et al. [26] suggested that an interspinous distance >7 mm in the lumbar region warrants imaging for potential ISL rupture. Jang and Park [16] found L3/L4 and L4/L5 had the widest interspinous spaces, which may relate to injury risk.

12.8 Conclusion

The interspinous ligaments play a key role in limiting spinal flexion and maintaining vertebral alignment, particularly in the lumbar spine. Despite their simple appearance, interspinous ligaments exhibit notable anatomical and histological complexity, with variations in fiber orientation and structure across spinal levels. Their biomechanical contribution becomes more significant in late flexion and in conjunction with adjacent ligaments. Clinically, ISL degeneration or injury may lead to pain and instability. A better understanding of their morphology and mechanical properties can support improved diagnosis, surgical planning, and treatment of spinal disorders.

References

1. Adams MA, Green TP, Dolan P. The strength in anterior bending of lumbar intervertebral discs. Spine. 1994;19:2197–203.
2. Agur AMR, Dalley AF. Grant's atlas of anatomy. 11th ed. Baltimore: Lippincott Williams and Wilkins; 2005.
3. Bannister LH, Berry MM, Collins P, Dyson M, Dussek JE, Ferguson MWJ, editors. Gray's anatomy. 38th ed. New York: Churchill Livingston; 1996.
4. Barros EM, Rodrigues CJ, Rodrigues NR, Oliveira RP, Barros TE, Rodrigues AJ Jr. Aging of the elastic

and collagen fibers in the human cervical interspinous ligaments. Spine J. 2002;2(1):57–62.
5. Bogduk N. Clinical anatomy of the lumbar spine and sacrum. 3rd ed. New York: Churchill Livingston; 1997.
6. D'Alton. Handbuch der Menschlichen. Leipzig, Germany; 1850.
7. Dickey JP, Bednar DA, Dumas GA. New insight into the mechanics of the lumbar interspinous ligament. Spine (Phila Pa 1976). 1996;21(23):2720–7.
8. Dickman CA, Rosenthal DJ, Perin NI. Thoracoscopic spine surgery. New York: Thieme Medical Publishers; 1999.
9. Fick R. Handbuch der Anatomie und Mechanik der Gelenke. In: Handbuch der Anatomie des Menschen. Jena: Fischer; 1904.
10. Heylings DJA. Supraspinous and interspinous ligaments of the human lumbar spine. J Anat. 1978;125(1):127–31.
11. Hindle RJ, Pearcy MJ, Cross A. Mechanical function of the human lumbar interspinous and supraspinous ligaments. J Biomed Eng. 1990;12:340–4.
12. Hukins DW, Kirby MC, Sikoryn TA, Aspden RM, Cox AJ. Comparison of structure, mechanical properties, and functions of lumbar spinal ligaments. Spine (Phila Pa 1976). 1990;15(8):787–95.
13. Iida T, Abumi K, Kotani Y, Kaneda K. Effects of aging and spinal degeneration on mechanical properties of lumbar supraspinous and interspinous ligaments. Spine J. 2002;2:95–100.
14. Iwanaga J, Simonds E, Yilmaz E, Schumacher M, Patel M, Tubbs RS. Anatomical and biomechanical study of the lumbar interspinous ligament. Asian J Neurosurg. 2019;14(4):1203–6. https://doi.org/10.4103/ajns.AJNS_87_19. PMID: 31903363; PMCID: PMC6896651.
15. Iwanaga J, Ishak B, Saga T, Singla A, Impastato D, Chapman JR, Oskouian RJ, David G, Porzionato A, Reina MA, Macchi V, de Caro R, Tubbs RS. The lumbar ligamentum flavum does not have two layers and is confluent with the interspinous ligament: anatomical study with application to surgical and interventional pain procedures. Clin Anat. 2020;33(1):34–40. https://doi.org/10.1002/ca.23437. Epub 2019 Aug 9. PMID: 31325341.
16. Jang D, Park S. A morphometric study of the lumbar interspinous space in 100 Stanford university medical center patients. J Korean Neurosurg Soc. 2014;55:261–6.
17. Kajava. Ihmisen anatomía Sderström. Porvoo, Finland; 1911.
18. Keorochana G, Taghavi CE, Tzeng ST, Morishita Y, Yoo JH, Lee KB, Liao JC, Wang JC. Magnetic resonance imaging grading of interspinous ligament degeneration of the lumbar spine and its relation to aging, spinal degeneration, and segmental motion. J Neurosurg Spine. 2010a;13:494–9.
19. Keorochana G, Taghavi CE, Tzeng ST, Lee KB, Liao JC, Yoo JH, Wang JC. MRI classification of interspinous ligament degeneration of the lumbar spine: intraobserver and interobserver reliability and the frequency of disagreement. Eur Spine J. 2010b;19:1740–5.
20. Kohler R. Contrast examination of the lumbar interspinous ligaments; preliminary report. Acta Radiol. 1959;1959(52):21–7.
21. Kong MH, Morishita Y, He W, Miyazaki M, Zhang H, Wu G, Hymanson HJ, Wang JC. Lumbar segmental mobility according to the grade of the disc, the facet joint, the muscle, and the ligament pathology by using kinetic magnetic resonance imaging. Spine (Phila Pa 1976). 2009;34:2537–44.
22. Kotani Y, Cunningham BW, Cappuccino A, Kaneda K, McAfee PC. The effects of spinal fixation and destabilization on the biomechanical and histologic properties of spinal ligaments: an in vivo study. Spine. 1998;23(6):672–82.
23. Maes R, Morrison WB, Parker L, Schweitzer ME, Carrino JA. Lumbar interspinous bursitis (Baastrup disease) in a symptomatic population: prevalence on magnetic resonance imaging. Spine (Phila Pa 1976). 2008;33:E211–5.
24. Moore KL, Dalley AF, Agur AMR. Clinically oriented anatomy. 6th ed. Baltimore: Lippincott Williams & Wilkins; 2010.
25. Mori K, Yoshii T, Hirai T, Iwanami A, Takeuchi K, Yamada T, et al. Prevalence and distribution of ossification of the supra/interspinous ligaments in symptomatic patients with cervical ossification of the posterior longitudinal ligament of the spine: a CT-based multicenter cross-sectional study. BMC Musculoskelet Disord. 2016;17(1):492. https://doi.org/10.1186/s12891-016-1350-y.
26. Neumann P, Wang Y, Kärrholm J, Malchau H, Nordwall A. Determination of inter-spinous process distance in the lumbar spine. Evaluation of reference population to facilitate detection of severe trauma. Eur Spine J. 1999;8:272–8.
27. Paniabi MM, Goel VK, Takata K. Phvsiologic strains in the lumbar spinal ligaments. Spine. 1982;7(3):192–203.
28. Parke WW. The spine, vol. 1. Philadelphia, London, Toronto: W. B. Saunders Co; 1975.
29. Pintar FA, Yoganandan N, Myers T, Elhagediab A, Sances A Jr. Biomechanical properties of human lumbar spine ligaments. J Biomech. 1992;25(11):1351–6.
30. Prestar FJ. Morphology and function of the interspinal ligaments and the supraspinal ligament of the lumbar portion of the spine. Morphol Med. 1982;2(1):53–8.
31. Rissanen PM. The surgical anatomy and pathology of the supraspinous and interspinous ligaments of the lumbar spine with special reference to ligament ruptures. Acta Orthop Scand. 1960;Suppl. 46:1–100.
32. Rissanen PM. The surgical anatomy and pathology of the supraspinous and interspinous ligaments of the lumbar spine, with special reference to ligament ruptures. Acta Orthop Scand. 1976;Suppl. 46:1–100.

33. Sartoris DJ, Resnick D, Tyson R, Haghighi P. Age-related alterations in the vertebral spinous processes and intervening soft tissues: radiologic-pathologic correlation. AJR Am J Roentgenol. 1985;145:1025–30.
34. Scapinelli R, Stecco C, Pozzuoli A, Porzionato A, Macchi V, De Caro R. The lumbar interspinous ligaments in humans: anatomical study and review of the literature. Cells Tissues Organs. 2006;183(1):1–11. https://doi.org/10.1159/000094901.
35. Spalteholz W. Hand atlas of human anatomy, vol. 1. 7th ed. Philadelphia, London: JB Lippincott Co; 1943.
36. Standring. Gray's anatomy: The anatomical basis of clinical practice. London: Elsevier; 2015.
37. Tandler. Lehrbuch der Systematischen Anatomie. Leipzig Germany Vogel. 1926.
38. Tsao H, Tucker KJ, Coppieters MW, Hodges PW. Experimentally induced low back pain from hypertonic saline injections into lumbar interspinous ligament and erector spinae muscle. Pain. 2010;150:167–72.
39. von Richter. Encyclopadie der menschlichen anatomie. Leipzig Germany; 1836.
40. Woerdeman MW. Standard-Atlas der Anatomie des Menschen, Bd I. Stuttgart: Medica Verlag; 1955.
41. Yahia LH, Garzon S, Strykowski H, Rivard CH. Ultrastructure of the human interspinous ligament and ligamentum flavum: a preliminary study. Spine. 1990;15(4):262–8.
42. Zander T, Rohlmann A, Bergmann G. Influence of ligament stiffness on the mechanical behavior of a functional spinal unit. J Biomech. 2004;37(7):1107–11.
43. Zhang C, Chang Y, Shu L, Chen Z. Pathogenesis of thoracic ossification of the ligamentum flavum. Front Pharmacol. 2024;15:1496297. https://doi.org/10.3389/fphar.2024.1496297.

13 The Supraspinous Ligament

George H. Bourdages and Walter A. Hall

13.1 Introduction

The numerous components of the spinal column include bones, ligaments, tendons, muscles, and neural tissue, which collectively provide stability and allow functional movement and ambulation in humans. The supraspinous ligament is a long posterior ligamentous support structure for the thoracolumbar spine, which is particularly involved during flexion and rotational movements. Various pathologies can have negative effects on the structure and subsequent function of the supraspinous ligament, resulting in clinically relevant alterations of patient mobility.

13.2 Embryology and Development of the Supraspinous Ligament

Spinal development and the genesis of the supraspinous ligament begin during gastrulation when the mesoderm differentiates from ectoderm and endoderm [1]. During the third week of development, somites begin to form from the mesodermal layer [2]. Every future spinal level has somites on each side of the neural tube. Somite formation begins rostrally and progresses caudally [3]. The somites then serve as deployment stations for subsequent mesodermal cells to generate the sclerotome, which forms the ligamentous tissues of the spine as they migrate ventromedially away from the somite [2, 4].

A sub-compartment of the sclerotome called the syndetome is responsible for vertebral tendon formation [5]. The supraspinous ligament is located posteriorly; accordingly, the syndetome is a dorsolateral component of the sclerotome located adjacent to the myotome. Placement at the border between the myotome and sclerotome allows the syndetome to develop into the musculoskeletal junctions of the spine [5].

Anatomical studies have revealed the progressive development of specific spinal ligaments corresponding to a range of gestational ages; anterior ligaments develop before posterior ones [6]. These findings suggest that the supraspinous ligament, being located posteriorly, will be detectable as an independent structure later in gestation (at around 12–15 weeks) than the anterior ligaments, which develop earlier, beginning at 8 weeks [6].

Hox genes encode features that facilitate specialized differentiation among the developing cervical, thoracic, and lumbar spinal segments, entailing differences in the supraspinous ligament among the various spinal levels after development is complete [7]. Many other signaling

G. H. Bourdages · W. A. Hall (✉)
Department of Neurosurgery, SUNY Upstate University Hospital, Syracuse, NY, USA
e-mail: hallw@upstate.edu

M. Turgut et al. (eds.), *Ligaments of the Vertebral Column*,
https://doi.org/10.1007/978-3-032-09070-6_13

pathways are thought to contribute to the distinctive specialization of each spinal level, including Sonic hedgehog, BMP, hairy, Wnt, retinoic acid, Pax, and fibroblast growth factors 4 and 8 [1–3, 8]. The Sonic hedgehog pathway promotes anterior movement while Wnt and BMP promote posterior alignment [8]. The signaling pathway specific to the supraspinous ligament remains unclear.

13.3 Supraspinous Ligament Anatomy

The supraspinous ligament (Fig. 13.1) connects the posterior aspects of the spinous processes extending from C7 to the lumbar spine; it can terminate between L3 and L5 with minimal variability [9–11]. In a series of 100 cases, the supraspinous ligament terminated 73% of the time at L4, 22% at L3, and 5% at L5 [12]. Although it was once thought to extend to the sacrum, multiple studies have demonstrated a much weaker, loose array of midline fibers connecting L5 to S1 after the supraspinous ligament has terminated superiorly [9, 11]. At C7, as its fibers extend rostrally, it becomes the nuchal ligament (Fig. 13.2), which inserts onto the inion. The supraspinous ligament is considered a vertebral arch ligament, in contrast to a vertebral body ligament. It is the most posteriorly located ligament of the spinal column [1].

The supraspinous ligament comprises three sections: a superficial posterior part, a middle component, and a deep anterior portion [9–11]. Various characteristics of it change as it traverses the thoracolumbar spine (Figs. 13.3 and 13.4). The superficial layer remains a longitudinal collagen-based tissue, ranging from <1 mm to approximately 6 mm in width. It is several millimeters thick, depending on the vertebral level, and traverses 3–4 spinous processes [10, 12]. In contrast, the middle layer consists of only thin fibers that connect the posterior thoracolumbar fascia across two to three spinous processes [11, 12]. Comprising numerous tendinous fibers from the longissimus muscle, the deep anterior layer is the strongest part; it connects

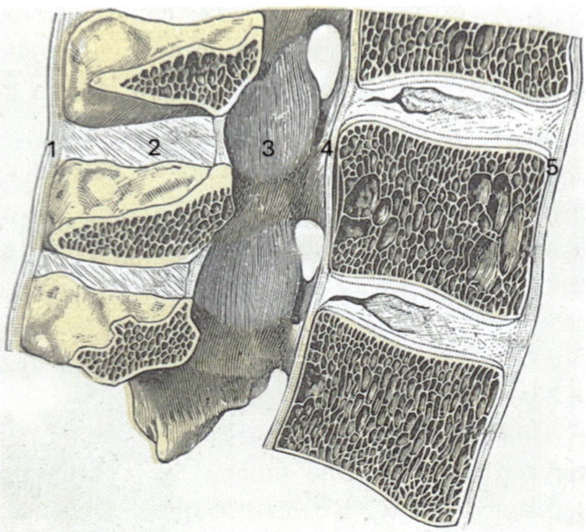

Fig. 13.1 Schematic drawing of the ligaments of the lumbar spine in sagittal section. Note the supraspinous ligament (SSL) (*1*), interspinous ligament (*2*), ligamentum flavum (*3*), posterior longitudinal ligament (*4*), and anterior longitudinal ligament (*5*). (After Testut)

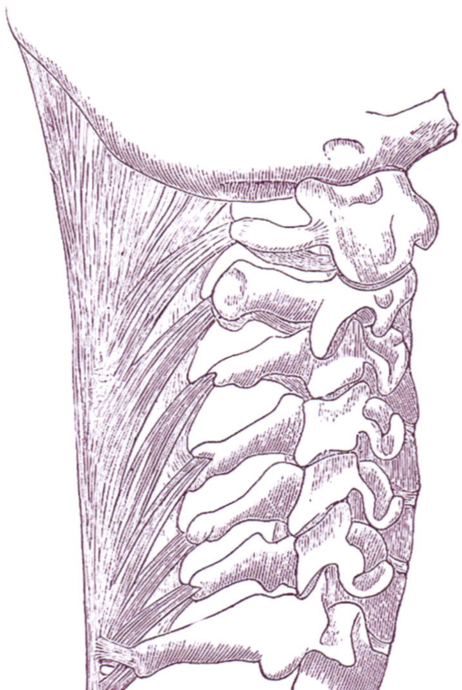

Fig. 13.2 Sagittal view of the nuchal ligament. (After Henle)

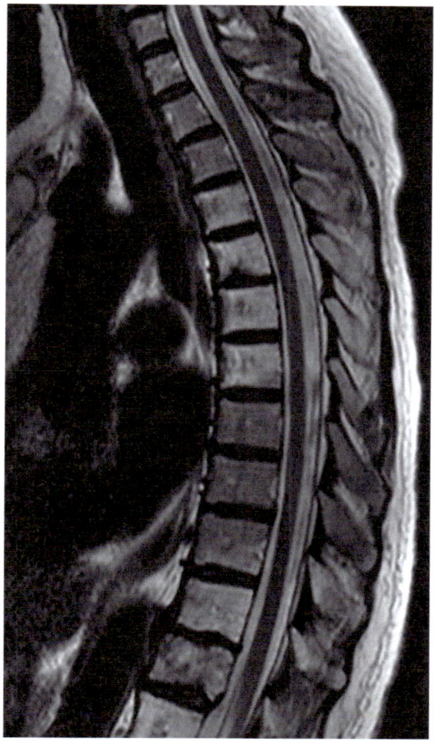

Fig. 13.3 On T2-weighted MR imaging, the SSLs are the dark hypointense band along the posterior aspect of the thoracolumbar spinous processes

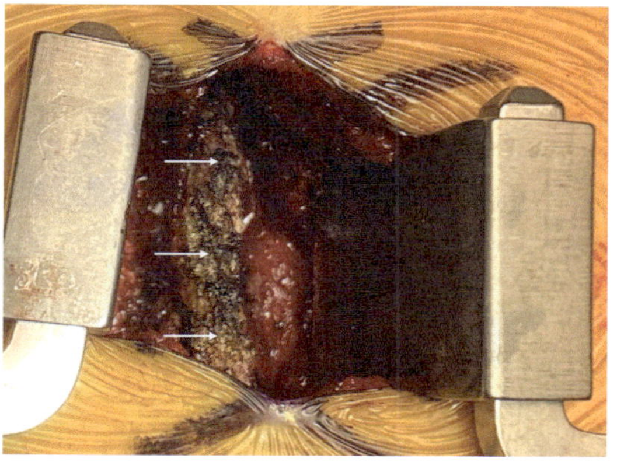

Fig. 13.4 An intraoperative view of a posterior lumbar exposure. The SSLs are indicated by the arrows

two spinous processes [12]. Because the longissimus muscle forms segments of the middle and deep layers, some authors remain skeptical as to whether the supraspinous ligament is a true ligament [10, 11].

In the upper thoracic spine from T1 to T5, the supraspinous ligament receives attachments from the trapezius, rhomboid major and splenius cervicis muscles along its deepest layer [13]. In the lower thoracic spine from T6 to T12, the thoracolumbar fascia attaches to the lateral aspect of the spinous process tip; it can be seen microscopically to form a fibrous layer around the longitudinal supraspinous ligament [13]. Heylings observed that the erector spinae musculature was inserted on the lateral aspect of the respective spinous process at levels where the supraspinous ligament was present. However, at L5 and S1, where the ligament had ended rostrally, he saw that tendons crossed the midline and attached to the contralateral posterior aspect of the spinous process [9]. More recent studies have produced similar results: the posterior thoracolumbar fascia, longissimus thoracis muscle, and multifidus muscle intersect in the lumbar spine to form parts of the supraspinous and interspinous ligaments [13]. Robertson et al. demonstrated in a study of 30 human cadavers that the anterior aspect of the supraspinous ligament was significantly firmer than the posterior aspect under higher stress before failure. Also, stiffness and stress tolerance were greater when the vector of force was applied longitudinally rather than transversely or perpendicularly [14].

13.4 Biomechanics

The primary biomechanical role of the supraspinous ligament is to limit hyperflexion, although it also provides stability during rotation [1, 9–13]. In combination with the ligamentum flavum and the interspinous ligament, it forms the posterior ligamentous complex (PLC). The PLC is responsible for 25–40% of stability, much of the contribution coming from the ligamentum flavum [15]. Approximately 6–6.6% of spinal flexion stiffness arises from a combination of the supraspinous and interspinous ligaments [16, 17]. However, other studies suggest that the supraspinous ligament typically handles the largest force-load during the later parts of flexion and contributes more than any other posterior ligament to resisting hyperflexion [10]. Animal studies also confirm that the supraspinous and interspinous ligaments provide the most resistance to flexion, with a 35.9% contribution in a porcine model [18]. Isolated removal of spinal ligaments and evaluation of the range of motion (ROM) and location of instantaneous axes of rotation (IAR) have shown that removal of the supraspinous ligament causes the greatest change in ROM and IAR with flexion movements [19]. This finding suggests that some studies have underreported the contribution of the supraspinous ligament, depending on the final amount of flexion force that was analyzed. No studies have clearly evaluated the full tensile properties of the isolated supraspinous ligament [15].

Flexion of the lower lumbar spine is significantly greater than flexion of the upper lumbar spine [9]. This correlates well with the anatomical termination of the supraspinous ligament at L3 or L4 in most people, suggesting that any additional lumbosacral flexion could be attributed to its absence. Cornaz et al. demonstrated that the initial tension and ultimate strength of the supraspinous ligament do not decrease during aging, in contrast to the ligamentum flavum, where aging correlates with a significant reduction in tension and strength, probably because the ligamentum flavum contains more elastin [20]. However, these authors determined that intervertebral disc degeneration correlated significantly with the reduced stiffness and ultimate strength of the supraspinous ligament [20].

13.5 Clinical Relevance and Importance

Numerous pathologies influence the structure and overall function of the supraspinous ligament. These include degenerative diseases, traumatic injury, ankylosing spondylitis, and ossification of the ligament.

The spine is subject to numerous stages of degeneration with repeated use over time, and the supraspinous ligament and posterior ligamentous complex can be involved. As intervertebral discs degenerate and dehydrate, load transmission and translation of the immediate axis of rotation increase the general stability of adjacent structures such as the PLC [21]. The increased load and force requirements can contribute to back pain in a patient. Surgical interventions can further affect the location of the instantaneous axis of rotation, resulting in increased load or stress on adjacent segments of the vertebral column [21]. During subsequent surgical interventions, it is prudent to maintain the PLC, when possible, to minimize additional stress on adjacent segments. Degeneration of the lower lumbar spine, particularly at the lumbosacral junction, can also result in pain. Increased mobility and ongoing micromotion of the lumbosacral spine, due to the absence of the supraspinous ligament at this level, is thought to contribute specifically to the high prevalence of low back pain [10].

Traumatic injuries can cause direct disruption, increased loading, and strain on the supraspinous ligament. One of the most important clinical questions in acute traumatic spinal injuries is whether the spine is stable or unstable at the affected level, and the PLC is often a crucial variable in determining this. Pizones et al. demonstrated that as the inciting traumatic force increases, a common stepwise sequence of ligamentous rupture is seen on post-injury magnetic resonance imaging (MRI) [22]. Further studies confirmed that the supraspinous ligament was the most important variable in determining incompetence of the PLC, because the high level of force required to injure it and its tendency for delayed rupture suggested that when it was injured, the rest of the PLC was also violated [23]. Although MRI remains the gold standard for preoperative diagnosis of ligamentous injury (Fig. 13.5), ultrasound has proven to be an alternative option for evaluating supraspinous ligament disruption, with 99% sensitivity and 75% specificity [24]. Ultrasound assessment is particularly useful when there are absolute contraindications to MRI, or for patients who cannot tolerate MRI, or in resource-limited regions without access to MRI.

Ossification of the supraspinous ligament and associated ankylosing spondylitis (AS) of the spine can also alter the biomechanical

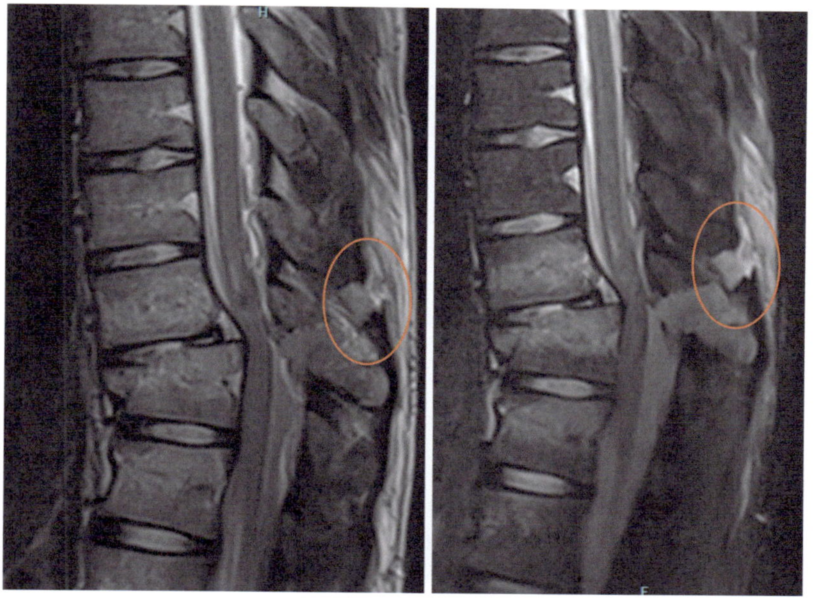

Fig. 13.5 A sagittal view of a T2 (left) and STIR (right) MRI for a patient who suffered a traumatic flexion distraction injury. The ovals show focal discontinuity of the SSL and complete disruption of the posterior ligamentous complex, indicating a highly unstable injury requiring surgical fixation

characteristics of the ligament. Ankylosing spondylitis is a chronic inflammatory autoimmune disease resulting in chronic pain, progressive stiffness, and fusion of the spinal joints [25]. Pathological calcium deposition in the supraspinous ligament and other spinal ligaments contributes to the stiffness and the decreased range of motion seen in AS (Fig. 13.6). Polymerase chain reaction analysis has shown that the expression of genes sampled from the supraspinous ligament differs between patients with AS and patients without AS, with corresponding changes in the protein composition of the ligament [26]. As the functional outcome of AS is generally poor and treatments are limited, identification of these differentially expressed genes and other associated proteins could generate novel treatment modalities for these patients. Ossification of the ligament from other sources is thought to be attributable to a fibroblast or chondrocyte response to a particular stimulus (autoimmune, traumatic, etc.), followed by the formation of a fibril network producing acidic mucopolysaccharides and capillary invasion, mesenchymal cell invasion, and transformation into osteoblasts,

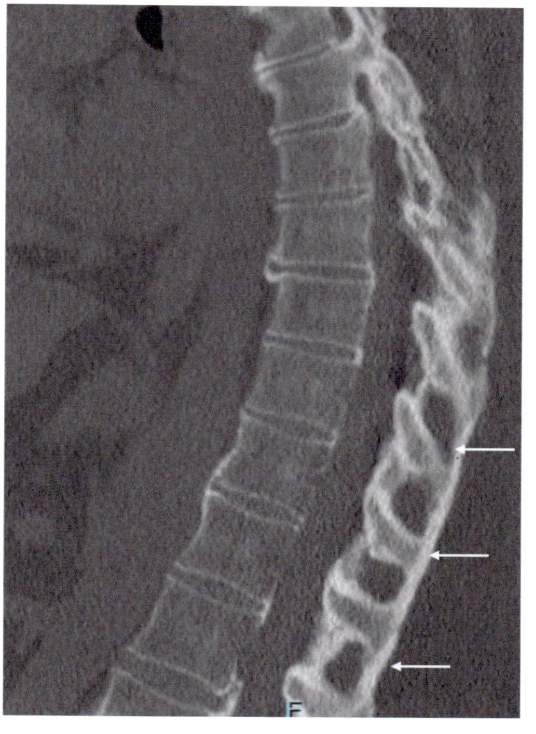

Fig. 13.6 An ossified SSLs (arrows) as seen on a sagittal view CT

ultimately causing osteogenesis [27]. There is a lack of studies on the ossification of the supraspinous ligament; however, clinical series suggest a greater predilection for calcification in the thoracic region than in the lumbar region [28]. Procedurally, ossification of the supraspinous ligament can pose a technical challenge for lumbar puncture or therapeutic epidural injections in patients with concomitant back pain, as it necessitates passing through the supraspinous ligament to access the thecal sac.

13.6 Conclusion

The supraspinous ligament extends from C7 to L4 in most humans and consists of three layers: superficial, middle, and deep. The deep layer tends to be the strongest and thickest component. After gastrulation, the ligament develops from somites present at each sequential spinal level that are derived from the mesodermal layer. The primary role of the ligament is to limit hyperflexion, and it provides the greatest strength in limiting flexion movements. The various pathological processes affecting the supraspinous ligament ultimately alter a patient's movement and stability and can subsequently become a source of pain.

References

1. Vaccaro A. 6 spinal embryology and anatomy of the pediatric and adult spine. In: Vaccaro AR, Fehlings MG, Dvorak MF, editors. Spine and spinal cord trauma. Stuttgart: Georg Thieme Verlag; 2011.
2. Bakkum BW, Bachop WE. Development of the spine and spinal cord. In: Clinical anatomy of the spine, spinal cord, and ANS; 2014. p. 541–65. https://doi.org/10.1016/B978-0-323-07954-9.00012-8.
3. Gilbert S. Developmental biology. 6th ed. Sunderland: Sinauer Associates; 2000.
4. Choudhri A. Pediatric neuroradiology. Stuttgart: Georg Thieme Verlag; 2017.
5. Scaal M. Early development of the vertebral column. Semin Cell Dev Biol. 2016;49:83–91. https://doi.org/10.1016/j.semcdb.2015.11.003.
6. Misawa H, Ohtsuka K, Nakata K, Kinoshita H. Embryological study of the spinal ligaments in human fetuses. J Spinal Disord. 1994;7:495–8.
7. Stern CD, Piatkowska AM. Multiple roles of timing in somite formation. Semin Cell Dev Biol. 2015;42:134–9.
8. Catala M. Embryology of the spine and spinal cord. In: Pediatric neuroradiology. Berlin Heidelberg, Berlin, Heidelberg: Springer; 2015. p. 1–53.
9. Heylings DJ. Supraspinous and interspinous ligaments of the human lumbar spine. J Anat. 1978;125:127–31.
10. Butt AM, Gill C, Demerdash A, et al. A comprehensive review of the sub-axial ligaments of the vertebral column: part I anatomy and function. Childs Nerv Syst. 2015;31:1037–59.
11. Butt AM, Gill C, Demerdash A, et al. A comprehensive review of the sub-axial ligaments of the vertebral column: part II histology and embryology. Childs Nerv Syst. 2015;31:1061–6.
12. Rissanen PM. The surgical anatomy and pathology of the supraspinous and interspinous ligaments of the lumbar spine with special reference to ligament ruptures. Acta Orthop Scand Suppl. 1960;46:1–100. https://doi.org/10.3109/ort.1960.31.suppl-46.01.
13. Johnson GM, Zhang M. Regional differences within the human supraspinous and interspinous ligaments: a sheet plastination study. Eur Spine J. 2002;11:382–8. https://doi.org/10.1007/s00586-001-0378-2.
14. Robertson D, Willardson R, Parajuli D, et al. The lumbar supraspinous ligament demonstrates increased material stiffness and strength on its ventral aspect. J Mech Behav Biomed Mater. 2013;17:34–43. https://doi.org/10.1016/j.jmbbm.2012.07.009.
15. Anderson B, Shahidi B. The impact of spine pathology on posterior ligamentous complex structure and function. Curr Rev Musculoskelet Med. 2023;16:616–26. https://doi.org/10.1007/s12178-023-09873-9.
16. Widmer J, Cornaz F, Scheibler G, et al. Biomechanical contribution of spinal structures to stability of the lumbar spine—novel biomechanical insights. Spine J. 2020;20:1705–16. https://doi.org/10.1016/j.spinee.2020.05.541.
17. Anderson AL, McIff TE, Asher MA, et al. The effect of posterior thoracic spine anatomical structures on motion segment flexion stiffness. Spine (Phila Pa 1976). 2009;34:441–6. https://doi.org/10.1097/BRS.0b013e318198c62d.
18. Gillespie KA, Dickey JP. Biomechanical role of lumbar spine ligaments in flexion and extension: determination using a parallel linkage robot and a porcine model. Spine (Phila Pa 1976). 2004;29:1208–16. https://doi.org/10.1097/00007632-200406010-00010.
19. Wu C-C, Jin H-M, Yan Y-Z, et al. Biomechanical role of the thoracolumbar ligaments of the posterior ligamentous complex: a finite element study. World Neurosurg. 2018;112:e125–33. https://doi.org/10.1016/j.wneu.2017.12.171.
20. Cornaz F, Widmer J, Farshad-Amacker NA, et al. Intervertebral disc degeneration relates to biomechanical changes of spinal ligaments. Spine J. 2021;21:1399–407. https://doi.org/10.1016/j.spinee.2021.04.016.

21. Iorio JA, Jakoi AM, Singla A. Biomechanics of degenerative spinal disorders. Asian Spine J. 2016;10:377. https://doi.org/10.4184/asj.2016.10.2.377.
22. Pizones J, Izquierdo E, Sánchez-Mariscal F, et al. Sequential damage assessment of the different components of the posterior ligamentous complex after magnetic resonance imaging interpretation. Spine (Phila Pa 1976). 2012;37:E662–7. https://doi.org/10.1097/BRS.0b013e3182422b2b.
23. Pizones J, Zúñiga L, Sánchez-Mariscal F, et al. MRI study of post-traumatic incompetence of posterior ligamentous complex: importance of the supraspinous ligament. Prospective study of 74 traumatic fractures. Eur Spine J. 2012;21:2222–31. https://doi.org/10.1007/s00586-012-2403-z.
24. Vordemvenne T, Hartensuer R, Löhrer L, et al. Is there a way to diagnose spinal instability in acute burst fractures by performing ultrasound? Eur Spine J. 2009;18:964–71. https://doi.org/10.1007/s00586-009-1009-6.
25. Wenker K, Quint J. Ankylosing spondylitis. Treasure Island: StatPearls; 2023.
26. Zhang Y, Hu X, Zhang C, et al. Suppression subtractive hybridization reveals differentially expressed genes in supraspinous ligaments of patients with ankylosing spondylitis. Mol Med Rep. 2015;11:4482–8. https://doi.org/10.3892/mmr.2015.3272.
27. Mine T, Kawai S. Ultrastructural observations on the ossification of the supraspinous ligament. Spine (Phila Pa 1976). 1995;20:297–302. https://doi.org/10.1097/00007632-199502000-00007.
28. Mori K, Yoshii T, Hirai T, et al. Prevalence and distribution of ossification of the supra/interspinous ligaments in symptomatic patients with cervical ossification of the posterior longitudinal ligament of the spine: a CT-based multicenter cross-sectional study. BMC Musculoskelet Disord. 2016;17:492. https://doi.org/10.1186/s12891-016-1350-y.

14 The Nuchal Ligament

R. Shane Tubbs and Joe Iwanaga

14.1 Introduction

The nuchal ligament is a triangular-shaped ligament with the upper border attaching to the external occipital protuberance of the skull, extending inferoposteriorly to the spinous process of C7. The nuchal ligament has been described in various ways in the anatomical literature, ranging from a strong band to merely a thin fibrous tissue or an intermuscular septum. Others have argued that the term nuchal ligament should be dropped as it is no more than an interlacing network of tendons originating from the posterior neck. Recent studies have shown that the nuchal ligament is a cranial extension of the supraspinous ligament, functioning as an anatomical division of the muscle in the posterior neck into left and right compartments. Functionally, the nuchal ligaments reduce the downward traction on the neck and prevent excessive flexion of the cervical spine.

R. S. Tubbs (✉)
Department of Anatomical Sciences,
St. George's University, Grenada, USA
e-mail: rtubbs@tulane.edu

J. Iwanaga
Department of Neurosurgery, Tulane Center for Clinical Neurosciences, Tulane University School of Medicine, New Orleans, LA, USA

14.2 Anatomy

The nuchal ligament is located at the bottom of the skull, spanning from the base of the external occipital protuberance to the spinous process of the seventh cervical vertebra (Fig. 14.1). The seventh cervical vertebra's spinous process is usually the largest protruding vertebra in the spinal column. The nuchal ligament is covered with multiple layers of cervical fascia, which are thin layers of tissue. In addition to the fascia, the trapezius mus-

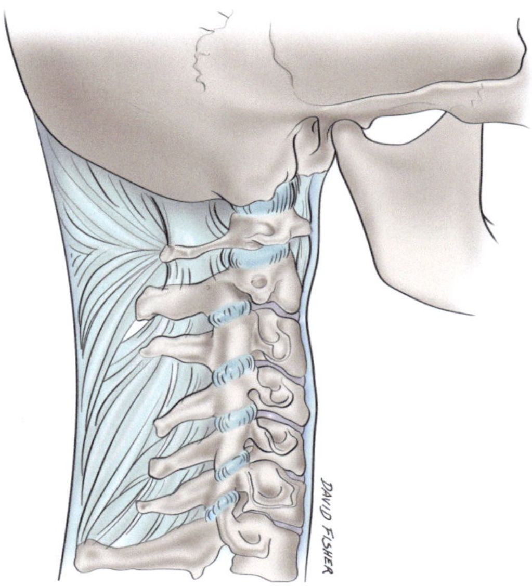

Fig. 14.1 Schematic drawing indicating the nuchal ligament (NL) from a lateral view

M. Turgut et al. (eds.), *Ligaments of the Vertebral Column*,
https://doi.org/10.1007/978-3-032-09070-6_14

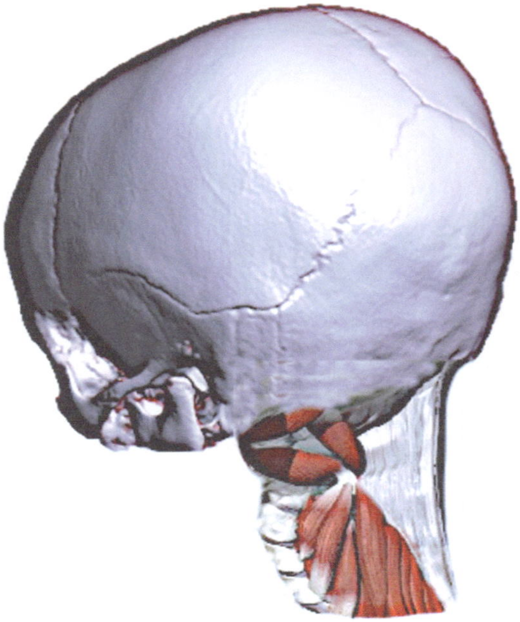

Fig. 14.2 Schematic drawing of the NL and its relationship to regional muscles of the posterior cervical spine. Posterolateral view

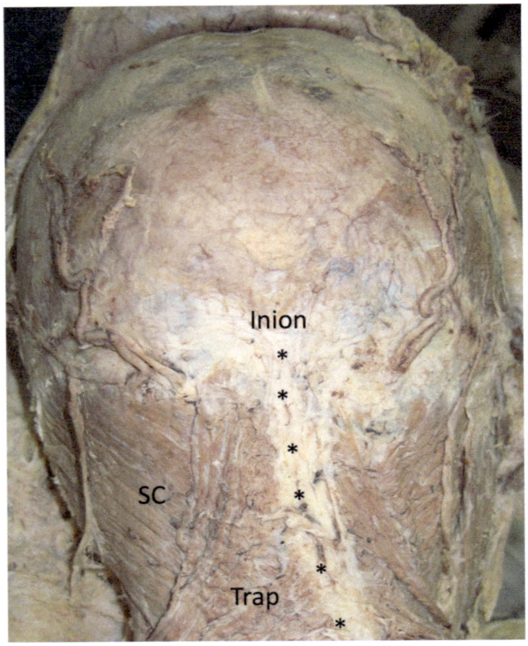

Fig. 14.3 Cadaveric dissection of the occiput and posterior neck, noting the midline NL (*) attached onto the inion superiorly Note some of the superficial muscles attaching to it such as the trapezius (trap) and splenius capitis (SC)

cle aponeurosis attaches to the nuchal ligament. The nuchal ligament is composed of two portions, a lamellar and a funicular portion. The lamellar portion consists of two layers separated by loose fatty connective tissue. The loose connective tissue inserts into the medial side of the bifid spinous process of the cervical vertebra. The funicular portion of the nuchal ligament is a posterior fibrous portion, which interlocks with the layers of the lamellar portion [8]. The nuchal ligament serves as an attachment site for several muscles, including the upper trapezius and deeper muscles of the posterior cervical spine (Figs. 14.2 and 14.3). There is considerable debate regarding the precise attachment sites of these muscles and their relationship to the nuchal ligament. This ligament has been described as a strong ligament in various anatomical literature. The ligament has been known to play a role in counteracting flexion of the head and stabilizing the head and the cervical spine. In addition, the ligament has been said to be well-positioned to provide a leverage advantage, as it attaches farther away from the axis of rotation in the neck than its muscular counterparts.

Although many consider the nuchal ligament noteworthy, others have a different opinion of this piece of thin fibrous cartilage. Some literature does not refer to it as a ligament at all, but as a purely fibrous membrane septum of the neck. Some believe that the nuchal ligament is simply a continuation of the thoracic supraspinous ligament. The nuchal ligament has been described as a septum that separates the right and left posterior muscles of neck and has also proven to be a reliable landmark for ensuring the midline of the cervical spine during surgery.

Because of many conflicting views of the nuchal ligament, a study was conducted by Mercer and Bogduk [9] to reevaluate the anatomy of the nuchal ligament. When studying the nuchal ligament on ten cadavers, it was found that this ligament displayed two distinct parts: the posterior raphe and a midline septum. As previously thought, it was confirmed that the nuchal ligament does not have tendinous fibers coming off the cervical vertebrae. These fibers only appeared at the C7 vertebra. The posterior raphe part of the ligament was confirmed not to be a ligament at all, as it was found not to connect bone to bone. However, the posterior raphe portion was composed of flattened, collagenous tissue in the coronal plane. This portion of the ligament was freely movable between its attachment sites of the external occipital protuberance and the tip of the seventh cervical vertebra. The midline portion of the dissected nuchal ligament consisted of fascia containing fat and vessels. This portion covered the raphe section posteriorly and became continuous with the splenius capitis and the upper trapezius fascia (Fig. 14.4). Anteriorly, the midline portion covered the vertebral column of the cervical spine. The nuchal ligament ensemble formed its attachments because of tendons in the surrounding muscles of the trapezius, splenius capitis, and the rhomboid minor [9].

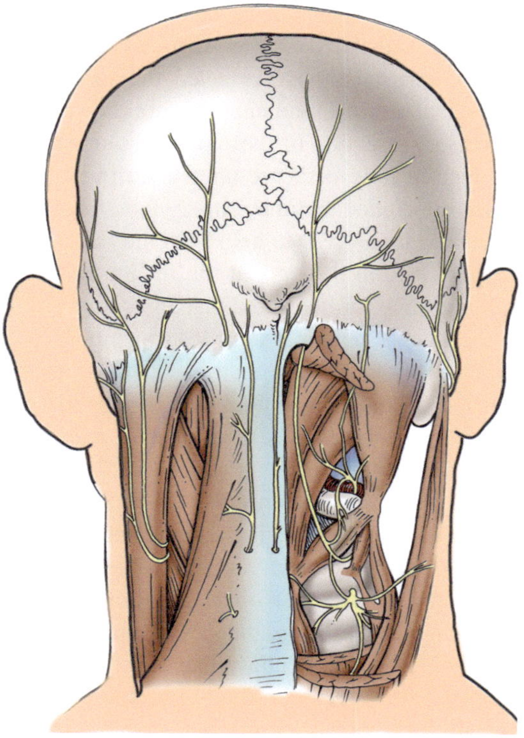

Fig. 14.4 Posterior view of the NL and adjacent upper trapezius. Note the midline NL being pierced by the third occipital nerves (posterior rami of C3)

Another cadaveric dissection study by Dean and Mitchell [3] was performed to elucidate the relationship between the nuchal ligament and the spinal dura mater, observing continuity between the two structures. This continuity was seen at the atlanto-occipital interspace and is believed that it could have biomechanical significance [3].

14.3 Biomechanics

The nuchal ligament in humans is much smaller compared to the similar anatomical structure in animals [4]. This is attributed to the vertical neck positioning in humans as the weight of the skull is evenly distributed along the upper vertebral column, thereby preventing the stretch and extension of the nuchal ligament observed in these animals. To better explain this phenomenon, a heavy weight load at the end of a long stick held vertically tends to be more stable when compared to the same weight held at the end of the same stick held horizontally. Fielding et al. (1976) further explained that a small force is required to maintain equilibrium in the vertical position, resulting in less tension being exerted on the lamellar portion of the nuchal ligament. This vertebral stabilization of the human neck has led to a decrease in the importance of the nuchal ligament in humans. The nuchal ligament, as previously stated, is made up of an even mixture of collagen and elastin, unlike that of ungulates, which consists mainly of elastic fiber (Fielding et al. 1976). It is therefore expected that the human nuchal ligament should be of reduced tensile strength. This was precisely what was observed in the elastic analysis studies by Fielding et al. (1976), with the human nuchal ligament noted to be approximately 70 to 80% stronger, more uniform, but less elastic when compared to quadrupeds (Fielding et al. 1976). Most authors have concluded that this ligament in humans has little importance in terms of stability and is essentially a midline intermuscular septum.

Sequentially staged dissection of the posterior cervical ligaments (namely the supraspinous, the infraspinous, nuchal, and ligamenta flava) by Takeshita et al. [13] demonstrated that removal of the nuchal ligament decreased the tangent stiffness of the cervical spine by 27% and an increase of 28% in cervical flexion range [13]. This study complements the findings of Fielding et al. (1976) and underscores the significance of the nuchal ligament in stabilizing cervical motion and maintaining head balance.

14.4 Imaging

The nuchal ligament can be visualized using various imaging techniques. Since the nuchal ligament plays a crucial role in neck stabilization and prevents neck hyperextension, most imaging modalities are employed when there is an indication of injury to the ligament. The most common imaging techniques used to diagnose ligament injuries are magnetic resonance imaging (MRI) and ultrasound [6]. Ligaments appear as echogenic structures on ultrasound and tend to exhibit anisotropy due to their structural uniformity. The echogenicity of a ligament is at maximum visibility when the ultrasound beam is oriented perpendicularly to the ligament fascicles [6]. Ultrasound, however, needs an acoustic shadow for proper ligament visibility, and sound waves are unable to penetrate through bony surfaces. This is where MRI is preferred, as it provides a clear view of the ligament and intra-articular tissues with higher spatial resolution compared to ultrasound [6].

Trauma, ossification, and calcification associated with the cervical spine, along with injury to the nuchal ligament, have prompted evaluation of the neck region with computed tomography (CT). In a retrospective study by Wang et al. [15], 372 patients with cervical spondylosis were evaluated using lateral plain radiographs and CTs for evidence of nuchal ligament ossification. Of the 372 patients evaluated, 185 had ossification of the nuchal ligaments, corresponding to an incidence of 49.7%. Wang et al. [15] used a two-dimensional sagittal plane reconstruction for their radiographic studies. They observed that 75.7% of the 185 patients had nuchal ligament ossification around the C4–C5 region and 81.1% in the C5–C6 region.

14.5 Clinical Relevance

As the exact anatomy of the nuchal ligament is debated, many researchers have overlooked its exact function, with some suggesting it has no clinical significance. The nuchal ligament is the most posterior structure of the cervical spine. With the largest movement arm being the sagittal rotation arm, it is thought to function in limiting excessive flexion. It is also thought to play a role in postsurgical kyphosis and whiplash. A study by Takeshita et al. [13] compared the nuchal ligament's role in restraining cervical spine flexion to other posterior ligaments in the cervical spine. The posterior ligaments were removed from 12 cadavers. The cervical spines were tested in three ways: the first with the cervical spine fully intact, the second with the entire nuchal ligament resected, and the third with the supraspinous, interspinous, and yellow ligaments resected. Each condition was tested under a load to evaluate the response. The study found that resecting the nuchal ligament increased the range of motion in flexion and also decreased stiffness. With multiple posterior ligaments resected, the researchers found that although the range of motion was also increased, resection of these other ligaments did not significantly decrease tangent stiffness [13]. It was concluded that the primary function of the nuchal ligament was to help with the balance of cervical flexion throughout the flexion range of motion. They further stated that any compromise to the nuchal ligament may lead to progressive kyphosis or localized junctional deformity and that the nuchal ligament should be treated with care and preserved when possible to maximize cervical flexion [13].

The nuchal ligament limits neck flexion at the cervical spine [13] and is predominantly injured in flexion injuries or surgical procedures. A grading scale has been established to grade nuchal ligament injuries. By grading the nuchal ligament injuries, researchers believe that there is a correlation to the severity of spinal injuries since the nuchal ligament is connected to the cervical spine. A study by Izadi et al. [7] described the implementation of this grading system. Thirty patients with traumatic cervical spinal injuries were obtained with an abnormal signal to the nuchal ligament. These injuries included soft tissue edema, ligament strains, and spine fractures. The grading system of the injuries was outlined as follows: grade I represents an edematous signal around the nuchal ligament, grade II represents intrinsic edema or a sprain of the fibers of the nuchal ligament, grade III represents a partial tear of the fibers, and grade IV represents a complete tear through the ligament. In this study of 30 patients, 5 had a grade I injury, 12 had a grade II injury, 7 had a grade III injury, and 6 had a grade IV injury. By implementing this simple grading system to assess the severity of damage to the nuchal ligament, the authors believed it could predict the severity of a spinal injury [7]. No further studies have been conducted to confirm the correlation between the grading system and the severity of cervical spine injuries.

In a study by O'Connell et al. [11], three patients with a history of automobile trauma were studied as they all developed soft tissue tumors between the nuchal ligament and deep cervical fascia. Two of the patients' "tumors" were described as painful, with thickening of the nuchal ligament in the areas of the tumor. Each of the three patients' fibrocartilage nodules was removed and classified as a nuchal fibrocartilaginous pseudotumor, as they did not exhibit any mitotic activity. The ligament tissue was degenerated in the areas of the tumors, as expected. Following a three to six-month follow-up, all the patients showed complete recovery and were currently asymptomatic. These pseudotumors were linked to the trauma of the nuchal ligament and soft tissue injury previously experienced by the patients. It is therefore important for doctors to carefully distinguish the pseudo tissue from other "cartilage matrix-producing, soft tissue-reactive lesions and neoplasms" [11].

Cools et al. [2] demonstrated the use of a nuchal ligament graft for duraplasty after decompression in children with Chiari malformation type I in their retrospective study. Nuchal ligament graft was used in 25 patients, with only one patient developing a cerebrospinal fluid leak (CSF) post-surgery. Of the 16 patients with symptomatic Chiari malformation, 14 experienced symptom improvement after surgery. Cools et al. [2] concluded that the rate of CSF leak postoperatively was comparable to that of other traditional methods using autologous and artificial grafts. However, further studies with a larger patient sample size may be needed to validate their findings correctly.

14.6 Ossification in the Nuchal Ligament

One pathology involving the nuchal ligament is ossification, commonly referred to as ONL (ossification of the nuchal ligament). ONL is predominantly seen in Asian patients, in which a soft tissue forms behind the spinous processes of the cervical spine. The ONL has previously been diagnosed as "calcareous bursitis, calcinosis circumscripta ligamenti nuchae, heterotopic development of the secondary nucleus of the spinous process of C6, and myositis ossificans circumscripta" [14]. Ossification typically occurs when a sesamoid bone forms from the substitution of calcified fibrocartilage. This sesamoid bone that forms resembles those found in other areas of the body. ONL formation may be secondary to trauma to the nuchal ligament or because of a chronic overload of the nuchal ligament. The study performed by Tsai et al. [14] investigated the correlation between the size of the ONL and neck symptoms, cervical active range of motion, lordotic curve, and cervical neural foramen stenosis. The study concluded that ONL may lead to stiffness in the flexion and extension range of motion, display degenerative changes in the spine, and exacerbate cervical neural foramen stenosis. However, no significant findings were discovered correlating ONL to cervical lordotic curve [14].

An alternative study by Paraskevas et al. [12] evaluated cases of sesamoid ossicles appearing in the nuchal ligament. These ossicles were small, round, nodular bones that could be housed in joints of the upper and lower limbs. These ossifications are typically asymptomatic; however, they do increase the individual's risk of injury.

Paraskevas et al. [12] followed two patients with ossifications in the nuchal ligament. The first case was one of a 55-year-old male who experienced chronic pain in the cervical spine and numbness in the upper limb. An X-ray revealed two ossifications in the nuchal ligament at the spinous processes of C4 and C5, with smooth borders of the ossifications. The proximal ossicle had an ovoid shape, and the distal ossicle was round. Clinically, it was observed that the patient experienced tenderness in the middle and lower third of the cervical spine, as well as a decreased range of motion in the cervical spine. The pain was shown to be cervical spondylosis at the C4 and C5 cervical vertebrae. The second patient was a 64-year-old female who was experiencing chronic pain in the cervical spine for 14 months. Similarly, she experienced a decreased range of motion of the cervical spine and tenderness. The ossicles found on her radiographs were near the spinous processes, and her neck pain was also linked to cervical spondylosis. Overall, in many cases, sesamoid ossicles in the nuchal ligament can go undetected unless imaging is performed. The origin of ossicle formation in the ligamentous or tendinous area is widely unknown. Ossification in the nuchal ligament may be misdiagnosed as "myositis ossificans circumscripta, nuchal fibrocartilaginous pseudotumor, calcinosis circumscripta, Clay-shoveler's fracture, neoplasms, and diseases with concomitant calcification deposition" [12].

There also seems to be a relationship between nuchal ligament calcification and obstructive sleep apnea (OSA). In a study by Ando et al. [1], 80 patients clinically diagnosed with OSA underwent cephalometric imaging examination to visualize and investigate the nuchal ligament for any evidence of calcification. The results showed that nuchal ligament calcification was present in 46.3% of these patients, and there was a positive correlation between calcification and the severity of OSA. The study also indicated that the prevalence of nuchal ligament calcification was much higher in patients with OSA when compared to previous studies with non-OSA individuals. Ando et al. [1] further suggested that the calcification might be attributed to the compensatory change in head position in OSA patients, along with increased weight, as these two mechanisms increase stress on the cervical spine.

14.7 Relevance in Other Species

The nuchal ligament is not exclusive to humans. Numerous studies have been conducted to elucidate the anatomy of the nuchal ligament in animals. An interesting study evaluated the head and neck positions of sport horses and their impact on the nuchal ligament [10]. This study looked at five fetal cadavers and six different head positions. In a horse, the nuchal ligament plays a role in locomotion using head and neck movement. It is thought that the nuchal ligament of a horse accounts for over half the oscillatory work when walking, and about one third when trotting and cantering. The six various positions in this study varied based on head and neck angles. The results showed that for the head and neck positions that required more active muscle support, the nuchal ligament was stretched. When the head position was over-bent and overworked, the nuchal ligament appeared to be stretched unevenly and was unable to function as an integrated unit. When the head was elevated and the nuchal ligament was not engaged, there was no stress or damage to the ligament. The nuchal ligament in horses is most effective when it is in a position that allows it to take some of the load off the neck and thorax. There was a greater risk of damage to the ligament and other muscles when the head was in a strained position [10].

The nuchal ligament was studied not only in horses but also in sheep fetuses. In the study by Fukuda et al., the morphogenesis of the nuchal ligament was assessed for the presence of elastic fibers. The study used light microscopy, transmission electron microscopy, and immunohistochemical methods to detect the elastic composition of the nuchal ligament in seven sheep fetuses and four postnatal sheep. The nuchal ligament tissue was evaluated using different histochemical stains. Fukuda et al. [5] observed that at higher maturity stages of development, the fetal tissue stained less. In the early stages of development, the elastic fibers contained a large number of myofibrils and relatively little amorphous material. In the later stages of development, the elastic fibers contained a small amount of fibrils but mature amorphous material. The study concluded that the microfibrils contained elastin, a crucial biomolecule that confers stretching properties. The microfibrils are likely sites where elastin is deposited during fetal development; however, the nature of the complex interaction between these two molecules remains unclear.

14.8 Conclusion

In conclusion, there is a lot of debate about the structure and function of the nuchal ligament. Further research is needed to create a unified understanding of the anatomy of the nuchal ligament and its clinical significance.

References

1. Ando E, Shigeta Y, Nejima J, Yamanaka H, Hirai S, Ogawa T, Clark GT, Enciso R. Assessment of the calcification of the nuchal ligament and osteophytes of the cervical spine in obstructive sleep apnoea subjects and snorers. J Oral Rehab. 2015;43(2):96–102. https://doi.org/10.1111/joor.12354.
2. Cools MJ, Quinsey CS, Elton SW. Chiari decompression outcomes using ligamentum nuchae harvest and duraplasty in pediatric patients with Chiari malformation type I. J Neurosurg Pediatr. 2018:1–5. https://doi.org/10.3171/2018.1.peds17670.
3. Dean NA, Mitchell BS. Anatomic relation between the nuchal ligament (ligamentum nuchae) and the spinal dura mater in the craniocervical region. Clin Anat. 2002;15(3):182–5. https://doi.org/10.1002/ca.10001.
4. Fielding JW, Burstein AH, Frankel VH. The nuchal ligament. Spine 1:3–14, 1976.
5. Fukuda Y, Ferrans VJ, Crystal RG. Development of elastic fibers of nuchal ligament, aorta, and lung of fetal and postnatal sheep: an ultrastructural and electron microscopic immunohistochemical study. Am J Anat. 1984;170(4):597–629.
6. Hodgson RJ, Oconnor PJ, Grainger AJ. Tendon and ligament imaging. Br J Radiol. 2012;85(1016):1157–72. https://doi.org/10.1259/bjr/34786470.
7. Izadi K, Go J, Kim M, Kim P, Law M. Grading of nuchal ligament injuries in cervical trauma patients with flexion injuries. American Society of Spine Radiology, 2012 lecture; 2012.
8. Kadri PA, Al-Mefty O. Anatomy of the nuchal ligament and its surgical applications. Neurosurg. 2007;301:4. https://doi.org/10.1227/01.neu.0000303985.65117.ea.
9. Mercer S, Bogduk N. Clinical anatomy of ligamentum nuchae. Clin Anat. 2003;16(6):484–93. https://doi.org/10.1002/ca.10121.
10. Nestadt C, Lusi M, Davies H. Effect of different head and neck positions on nuchal ligament dimensions in fetal foals. J Equine Vet Sci. 2015;35(2):153–60. https://doi.org/10.1016/j.jevs.2014.12.013.
11. O'Connell J, Janzen D, Hughes T. Nuchal fibrocartilaginous pseudotumor: a distinctive soft-tissue lesion associated with prior neck injury. Am J Surg Pathol. 1997;21(7):836–40.
12. Paraskevas G, Raikos A, Martoglou S, Ioannidis O. Sesamoid ossicles within the nuchal ligament. J Radiol Case Rep. 2011;5(8):22–9. https://doi.org/10.3941/jrcr.v5i8.708.
13. Takeshita K, Peterson E, Bylski-Austrow D, Crawford A, Nakamura K. The nuchal ligament restrains cervical spine flexion. Spine. 2004;29(18):388–93. https://doi.org/10.1097/01.brs.0000138309.11926.72.
14. Tsai YL, Weng MC, Chen TW, Hsieh YL, Chen CS, Huang MH. Correlation between the ossification of nuchal ligament and clinical cervical disorders. Kaohsiung J Med Sci. 2012;28(10):538–44. https://doi.org/10.1016/j.kjms.2012.04.016.
15. Wang H, Zou F, Jiang J, Lu F, Chen W, Ma X, Xia X, Wang L. Analysis of radiography findings of ossification of nuchal ligament of cervical spine in patients with cervical spondylosis. Spine. 2014;39(1). https://doi.org/10.1097/brs.0000000000000037.

15 Intertransverse Ligaments

Yuqiang Wang, Yao Zhao, and Yilin Liu

15.1 Introduction

The intertransverse ligaments (ITLs) connect adjacent transverse processes of the vertebrae. Their arrangement is multidirectional, and they can vary in form: typically membranous in the lumbar spine, cord-like in the thoracic spine, and often absent in the cervical spine. The ITL contributes to spinal stability by reinforcing the intervertebral bodies and limiting excessive forward flexion, thereby helping to prevent acute injuries to surrounding tendons and ligaments [1]. Although it receives less research attention than other key ligaments such as the anterior longitudinal ligament, posterior longitudinal ligament, and ligamentum flavum, it is crucial for maintaining overall spinal stability [2]. Therefore, it is important for healthcare professionals to recognize and emphasize its significance.

15.2 Anatomy

The primary function of the ITL is to enhance spinal stability and prevent excessive forward flexion, functions that are directly linked to its anatomical characteristics [3]. The morphology and role of the ITL differ among the regions of the spine. In the cervical region, it is composed of several irregular, discrete fibers. Although thin and fragile, it still helps limit cervical rotation and lateral bending [4]. In the thoracic region, it is a rounded, cord-like structure that is closely integrated with the deep muscles of the back (Fig. 15.1). In the lumbar region, it is thinner and typically membranous (Fig. 15.2). Notably, the lumbar ITL is thinner in the upper lumbar spine and becomes progressively thicker caudally. It also contributes to the formation of the iliolumbar ligament (Fig. 15.2), particularly between the fifth lumbar vertebra (L5) and the sacrum (S1), where the ITL merges with the iliolumbar ligament.

Y. Wang · Y. Zhao · Y. Liu (✉)
Department of the Orthopaedic Surgery, The First Affiliated Hospital of Zhengzhou University, Zhengzhou, China
e-mail: liu212381@126.com

M. Turgut et al. (eds.), *Ligaments of the Vertebral Column*,
https://doi.org/10.1007/978-3-032-09070-6_15

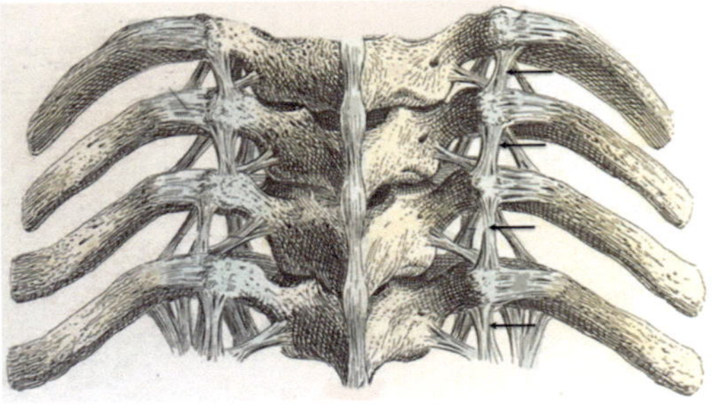

Fig. 15.1 Drawings illustrating the intertransverse ligament (ITL) (arrows) in the upper thoracic spine

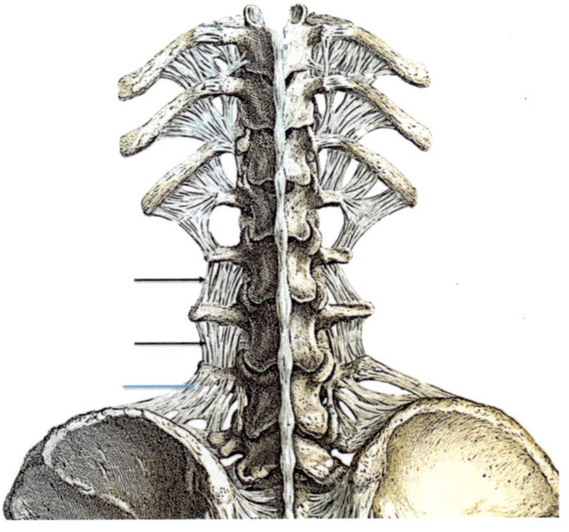

Fig. 15.2 Drawings illustrating the ITL (black arrows) in the lumbar spine. Note the lowest lumbar ITL contributing to the iliolumbar ligament (blue arrow)

15.3 Common Related Diseases

The ITL is vital for maintaining spinal stability by connecting the transverse processes of adjacent vertebrae [5]. Various diseases and conditions can affect it, leading to clinical manifestations. Degeneration or injury of the ITL is often associated with degenerative spinal disorders such as lumbar spinal stenosis and degenerative disc disease [1]. Abnormal tension or injury to it can disrupt normal spinal alignment, potentially contributing to conditions such as scoliosis or spondylolisthesis. Additionally, lumbar strain and chronic lower back pain can be linked to overuse or injury of the ITL [6].

Common forms of ITL injury include sprains, tears, and ruptures. Although there is no specific grading system for ITL injuries, they can be assessed by general ligament injury grading systems, which classify injuries on the basis of severity [7]:

First-degree injury (mild): Tiny tears or strains in the ligament, often without significant structural damage. Patients can experience mild discomfort or pain, but the ligament largely retains its functionality.

Second-degree injury (moderate): A partial tear of the ligament that results in notable pain and dysfunction. There can be swelling and bruising, and the patient's physical activities are often limited.

Third-degree injury (severe): A complete tear or rupture of the ligament, leading to significant loss of function and severe pain. In most cases, medical intervention is required, including possible surgical treatment and long-term rehabilitation.

15.4 Etiology and Pathology

Research on the etiology and pathology of ITL injuries is limited, and such injuries are typically associated with specific trauma or chronic strain. Common contributing factors include:

Occupational factors: Occupations that involve frequent bending, twisting, or heavy lifting, such as construction work and manual labor, can increase the likelihood of ITL injuries. Long-term chronic injury or inflammation can lead to fibrosis of the ligament, characterized by thickening and stiffening. This can further restrict the spine's range of motion and lead to chronic pain.

Sports injuries: Trauma or overuse commonly causes ITL injuries. Typical causes include car accidents, falls, and sports-related injuries, which can cause localized pain, stiffness, and limited movement. High-impact sports or physical activities such as weightlifting and wrestling also heighten the risk of ITL injury.

In more severe cases, external traumas such as spinal injuries due to accidents can injure the ITL significantly.

Age-related factors: As the body ages, the ITL can degenerate, resulting in decreased elasticity and strength. This degeneration heightens the risk of injury and compromises spinal stability, making the spine more susceptible to further injury. Age-related vertebral slippage can place abnormal stress on the ligaments, stretching them and contributing to ligament damage.

Acute or chronic inflammation: The ITL can become inflamed because of either acute trauma or chronic strain. This inflammation often results in pain, swelling, and stiffness. Chronic inflammation, if left untreated, can contribute to fibrosis and further impair ligament function.

15.5 Clinical Presentation

Injury to the ITL can result in a variety of symptoms depending on its severity and location. Common clinical manifestations include:

Localized pain and stiffness: Patients can experience localized pain and stiffness following injury, particularly in the neck or lower back. This discomfort is often exacerbated by movement.

Restricted movement: The patient's range of motion can be significantly reduced due to pain and stiffness, which impacts daily activities and overall mobility.

Nerve compression symptoms: If the injury leads to ligament hyperplasia (excessive tissue growth) or hypertrophy (thickening), it can compress nearby nerves. This can result in radiating pain, numbness, or weakness in the affected limbs [8].

Spinal instability: Severe ITL injury can lead to spinal instability, which increases the risk of further injury to the vertebrae and surrounding tissues.

Chronic pain: If untreated, ITL injuries can lead to persistent chronic pain and long-term complications, including joint degeneration and reduced spinal function.

15.6 Imaging Examination

Evaluation of ITL injuries primarily relies on imaging techniques such as X-ray, CT, and MRI. Each modality offers its own advantages for assessing ITL-related conditions:

X-ray: Since the ITL is composed mainly of soft tissue, it is difficult to visualize its details directly on X-ray. However, X-rays can be useful for assessing vertebral alignment and detecting fractures, which can indicate indirect effects of ligament injury, such as vertebral displacement or abnormal curvature.

Computed tomography (CT): CT scans provide detailed images of the bony structures, making them effective in detecting subtle vertebral changes or fractures that may be associated with ITL injury. CT has limited value for visualizing soft tissues, but it can sometimes reveal calcification of the ligament or other structural abnormalities, offering indirect signs of ITL pathology.

Magnetic resonance imaging (MRI): MRI is the best imaging modality for evaluating the ITL directly. It allows for the clear visualization of soft tissue structures, including ligaments, muscles, and intervertebral discs. MRI is particularly useful for assessing the integrity of the ITL, detecting tears, inflammation, or other lesions that are not always visible with other imaging methods.

15.7 Treatments

The primary treatment options for ITL injuries include:

15.7.1 Conservative Treatments, Including the Following

Rest: It is crucial to avoid activities that could aggravate the injury, allowing the ligament to heal properly.

Ice therapy: Applying ice for 15–20 min at a time, 3–4 times a day, during the first 24–48 h post-injury can help minimize pain and swelling.

Medications: Nonsteroidal anti-inflammatory drugs (NSAIDs) such as ibuprofen or naproxen can be used to reduce pain and inflammation.

Physical therapy: Once the acute phase has passed, physical therapy can be initiated. This can include the application of heat packs, ultrasound treatments, and specific stretching and strengthening exercises aimed at restoring function and fortifying the ligament.

15.8 Clinical Applications

The ITL has several important clinical applications, particularly in spinal positioning during imaging and interventions. Specific applications include:

Imaging: The ITL serves as an anatomical landmark for identifying and locating the transverse processes of adjacent vertebrae in imaging studies such as X-rays, CT scans, and MRI. This is crucial for assessing spinal stability and detecting potential pathological changes [9]. The ITL is an important reference point during ultrasound-guided nerve blocks and pain management procedures [10]. By identifying the location of the ITL accurately, physicians can enhance the precision and safety of injections and other interventions [11].

Surgical localization: In spinal surgery, the ITL aids surgeons in pinpointing the surgical site, particularly during procedures such as discectomy or vertebral fusion [12]. Accurate identification of the ITL allows for more precise operations and minimizes injury to surrounding tissues.

15.9 Conclusions

In summary, the ITL connects the transverse processes of adjacent vertebrae. Further studies are needed to better elucidate its anatomy and function.

References

1. Cornaz F, Widmer J, Farshad-Amacker NA, Spirig JM, Snedeker JG, Farshad M. Intervertebral disc degeneration relates to biomechanical changes of spinal ligaments. Spine J. 2021;21(8):1399–407.
2. Cornaz F, Widmer J, Farshad-Amacker NA, Spirig JM, Snedeker JG, Farshad M. Biomechanical contributions of spinal structures with different degrees of disc degeneration. Spine (Phila Pa 1976). 2021;46(16):E869–77.
3. Farajpour H, Jamshidi N. Effects of different angles of the traction table on lumbar spine ligaments: a finite element study. Clin Orthop Surg. 2017;9(4):480–8.
4. Johnson RM, Crelin ES, White AA 3rd, Panjabi MM, Southwick WO. Some new observations on the functional anatomy of the lower cervical spine. Clin Orthop Relat Res. 1975;111:192–200.
5. Zhang L, Zhang Q, Zhang Y, et al. The effect of concave-side intertransverse ligament laxity on the stress of AIS lumbar spine based on finite element method. Bioengineering (Basel). 2022;9(12):724.
6. Chazal J, Tanguy A, Bourges M, et al. Biomechanical properties of spinal ligaments and a histological study of the supraspinal ligament in traction. J Biomech. 1985;18(3):167–76.
7. Kalenak A, Morehouse CA. Knee stability and knee ligament injuries. JAMA. 1975;234(11):1143–5.
8. Song J, Lee JB, Suh JK. Clinicopathological considerations in patients with lumbosacral extraforaminal stenosis. J Clin Neurosci. 2009;16(5):650–4.
9. Widmer J, Cornaz F, Scheibler G, Spirig JM, Snedeker JG, Farshad M. Biomechanical contribution of spinal structures to stability of the lumbar spine-novel biomechanical insights. Spine J. 2020;20(10):1705–16.
10. Senthelal S, Dydyk AM, Mesfin FB. Ablative nerve block. In: StatPearls. Treasure Island: StatPearls Publishing; 2024.
11. Karmakar MK, Sivakumar RK, Sheah K, Pangthipampai P, Lönnqvist PA. The retro superior costotransverse ligament space as a new target for ultrasound-guided intertransverse process block: a report of 2 cases. A A Pract. 2022;16(7):e01610.
12. Greiner-Perth R, Böhm H, Allam Y. A new technique for the treatment of lumbar far lateral disc herniation: technical note and preliminary results. Eur Spine J. 2003;12(3):320–4.

The Midline Interlaminar Ligament 16

Joe Iwanaga

16.1 Introduction

The ligamentum flavum is a well-established paired ligament connecting adjacent laminae along the posterior aspect of the vertebral canal. It was traditionally described as comprising left and right components that can either fuse or remain distinct in the midline. However, in 2019, a separate, unpaired vertical ligament was observed in the midline, distinctly anterior to the interspinous ligament and separate from the ligamenta flava. This structure, named the midline interlaminar ligament (MIL), was first described by Simonds et al. in cadaveric dissections of the lumbar spine [6]. Subsequent investigations have explored its anatomical distribution beyond the lumbar region and studied its biomechanical properties. The MIL is now recognized as a discrete anatomical entity with potential implications for spinal stability, pain, and surgical access.

16.2 Anatomical Characteristics and Distribution

The original description by Simonds et al. was based on 24 vertebral levels from 10 fresh cadaveric specimens and focused exclusively on the lumbar spine. They found the MIL in approximately 76.5% of the lumbar intervertebral levels they dissected. It appeared as a thin, vertical ligament occupying the midline plane, slightly anterior to the ligamenta flava and posterior to the vertebral canal. It ran from the inferior lamina of one vertebra to the superior lamina of the vertebra below, near the midline gap (MLG) if it was present (Figs. 16.1 and 16.2). In view of its location, the MIL could be associated with the MLG, which has been previously studied [2–4]. Lirk et al. [3] found an MLG at L1, L2, L3, L4, and L5 in 22.2%,11.4%,11.1%, 9.3%, 0%, respectively. Zarzur [7] failed to find any MLG in 10 lumbar vertebral levels. The incidence of the lumbar MIL seems much higher than that of the lumbar MLG. However, no study mentioned the MIL until Simonds et al. [6] identified it. The

J. Iwanaga (✉)
Department of Neurosurgery, Clinical Neuroscience Research Center, Tulane University School of Medicine, New Orleans, LA, USA

Department of Neurology, Clinical Neuroscience Research Center, Tulane University School of Medicine, New Orleans, LA, USA

Department of Structural & Cellular Biology, Tulane University School of Medicine, New Orleans, LA, USA

Department of Neurosurgery and Ochsner Neuroscience Institute, Ochsner Health System, New Orleans, LA, USA

Dental and Oral Medical Center, Kurume University School of Medicine, Fukuoka, Japan

Division of Gross and Clinical Anatomy, Department of Anatomy, Kurume University School of Medicine, Fukuoka, Japan
e-mail: jiwanaga@tulane.edu

M. Turgut et al. (eds.), *Ligaments of the Vertebral Column*,
https://doi.org/10.1007/978-3-032-09070-6_16

ligament's mean length was approximately 9 mm and its width was close to 5 mm.

A subsequent study by Millhuff et al. [5] using 31 embalmed cadavers expanded the anatomical scope to include the cervical and thoracic spine. Their findings revealed that MILs were most prevalent in the lumbar spine, where they were found in 63.4% of the levels examined. The prevalence was much lower in the thoracic region (5.9%), and the cervical spine showed only a single instance (0.5%) at the C2–C3 level. Interestingly, the MIL was more often present in the thoracolumbar junction (T10–L1) than in other thoracic segments, suggesting a regional gradient toward the lumbar spine consistent with increasing mechanical demands. In this later study, MILs in the lumbar region were significantly longer (mean 16.4 mm) but narrower (mean 1.2 mm) than those observed in the initial study, possibly reflecting differences in sample preparation, population, or anatomical definitions.

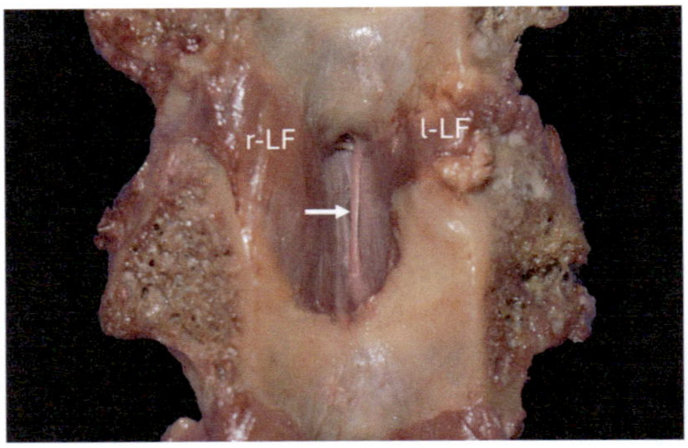

Fig. 16.1 Anterior view of the midline interlaminar ligament (MIL) in the lumbar spine (arrow). *LF* ligamentum flavum

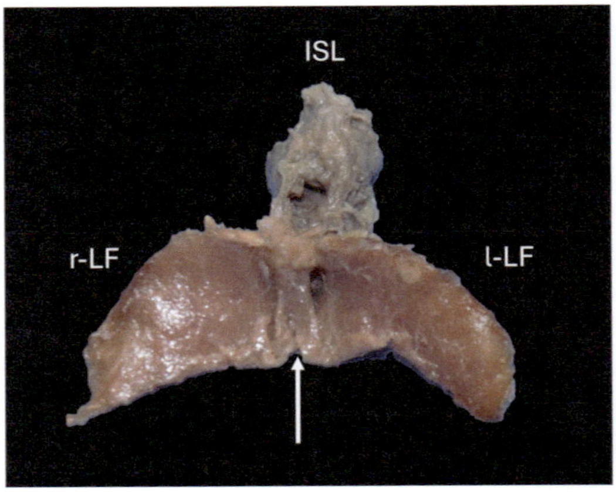

Fig. 16.2 Anterosuperior view of the MIL in the lumbar spine (arrow). *LF* ligamentum flavum, *ISL* interspinous ligament

16.3 Biomechanical and Histological Features

Biomechanical analyses indicate that the MIL has properties distinct from those of the more robust ligamentum flavum. Simonds et al. reported that a mean force of approximately 12.3 N was needed to cause failure, indicating roughly half the tensile strength of the adjacent ligamentum flavum (Fig. 16.3) [1]. In the Millhuff et al. study, the elastic modulus—reflecting tissue stiffness—averaged 39.8 MPa in lumbar MILs and was slightly higher (46.8 MPa) in thoracic MILs, though the difference was not statistically significant. Toughness, defined as the energy

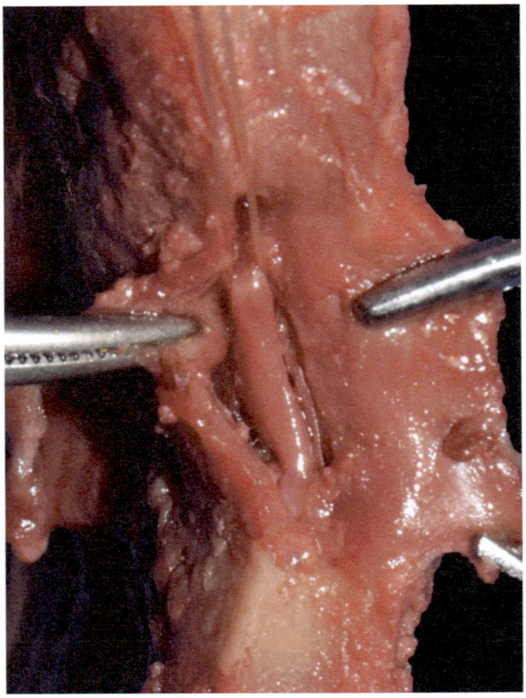

Fig. 16.3 Tensile strength test of the MIL

required to cause ligament rupture, was similarly comparable across regions but consistently lower in the MIL than the ligamentum flavum.

Histologically, the MIL contains fewer elastic fibers than the ligamentum flavum, suggesting less elastic recoil during spinal movement. However, it has a markedly higher concentration of nerve fibers, suggesting a possible function in proprioception or nociception. Bielschowsky staining revealed numerous neural elements (Fig. 16.4), while Verhoeff's stain highlighted the MIL's lower elastic fiber density (Fig. 16.5). The

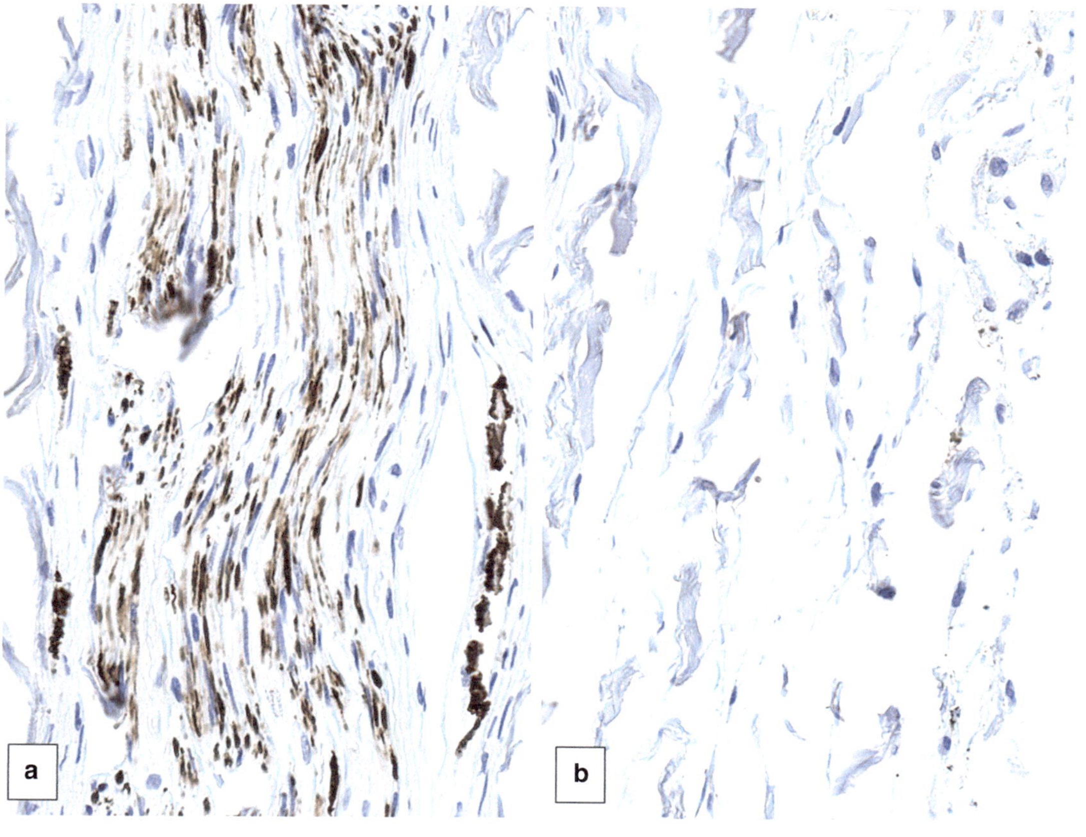

Fig. 16.4 Bielschowsky's silver stain revealing a greater concentration of nerve fibers (shown in brown) in the MIL (**a**) than the ligamentum flavum (LF) (**b**)

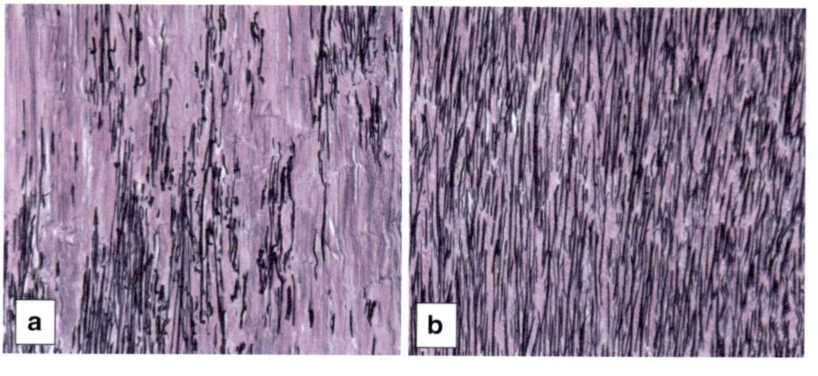

Fig. 16.5 Verhoff's elastic stain highlights a lower concentration of elastic fibers (black) in the MIL (**a**) than in the LF (**b**)

high neural density implies a possible role in sensory feedback mechanisms, especially in relation to posture, extension control, and potentially low back pain.

16.4 Functional and Clinical Relevance

The observed behavior of the MIL during spinal motion elucidates its function. In cadaveric motion testing, the MIL was taut during spinal extension and lax in flexion, suggesting a role in limiting hyperextension. This is consistent with the hypothesis that it acts as a posterior stabilizer, complementing the action of facet joints and other posterior ligaments. Although its tensile strength is modest, its orientation and placement could allow it to resist excessive posterior laminar displacement during motion.

Clinically, the MIL is relevant in procedures such as lumbar puncture or epidural anesthesia. When it is present, it could be inadvertently penetrated during midline needle insertion, possibly contributing to increased resistance or altered tactile feedback. Furthermore, its rich neural content suggests possible involvement in low back pain, particularly in settings of ligamentous injury or strain. Given the high prevalence of the MIL in the lumbar spine, its potential role in proprioceptive dysfunction and low back pain warrants further investigation.

16.5 Limitations and Future Directions

Both studies acknowledge the limitations inherent to cadaveric research, including the advanced age of specimens and potential alterations due to embalming. The prevalence and morphology of the MIL in younger individuals remain unknown. Also, the variations in MIL dimensions and presence across spinal levels suggest it could atrophy, or be developmentally absent, in some individuals. Future research should focus on characterizing the MIL in vivo using imaging or surgical observation, exploring its ontogeny, and investigating its sensory and functional significance using neurophysiological approaches. Longitudinal studies correlating MIL integrity with back pain or hyperextension injuries could also clarify its clinical importance.

16.6 Conclusion

The MIL is an anatomically distinct, vertically oriented ligament found primarily in the lumbar spine. Its biomechanical properties and neural characteristics suggest roles in extension stabilization and sensory feedback. Future research should include detailed neurohistological profiling, investigation of structural alterations in degenerative spine disease, and intraoperative imaging correlations to elucidate its clinical relevance.

References

1. Bogduk N. Clinical anatomy of the lumbar spine and sacrum. 3rd ed. New York: Churchill Livingston; 1997.
2. Lirk P, Kolbitsch C, Putz G, Colvin J, Colvin HP, Lorenz I, Keller C, Kirchmair L, Rieder J, Moriggl B. Cervical and high thoracic ligamentum flavum frequently fails to fuse in the midline. Anesthesiology. 2003;99:1387–90.
3. Lirk P, Moriggl B, Colvin J, Keller C, Kirchmair L, Rieder J, Kolbitsch C. The incidence of lumbar ligamentum flavum midline gaps. Anesth Analg. 2004;98:1178–80.
4. Lirk P, Colvin J, Steger B, Colvin HP, Keller C, Rieder J, Kolbitsch C, Moriggl B. Incidence of lower thoracic ligamentum flavum midline gaps. Br J Anaesth. 2005;94:852–5.
5. Millhuff A, Haddad H, Draper MS, Motzko M, Glueck E, Holland B, Wright B. The midline interlaminar ligament of the spine: an anatomical study. Clin Anat. 2023;36:618–23. https://doi.org/10.1002/ca.24003.
6. Simonds E, Iwanaga J, Ishak B, Reina MA, Oskouian RJ, Tubbs RS. Discovery of a new ligament of the lumbar spine: the midline interlaminar ligament. Spine J. 2020;20:1134–7. https://doi.org/10.1016/j.spinee.2019.12.003.
7. Zarzur E. Anatomic studies of the human ligamentum flavum. Anesth Analg. 1984;63:499–502.

17 Capsular Ligaments of the Spine

R. Shane Tubbs and Joe Iwanaga

17.1 Introduction

17.1.1 Anatomy

The facet capsular ligament fully encases the facet joint by covering the joint in a rostral to caudal direction with a non-uniform thickness [1] (Figs. 17.1, 17.2, 17.3, and 17.4). The lumbar facet capsule has been reported to be approximately 2.0 mm thick in the posterior region while being as much as 3.2 mm thick in the anterior region [1]. The superior and inferior regions of the capsule have been reported to be approximately 2.4 mm thick [1]. *Gray's Anatomy* identifies three distinct types of intracapsular structures: adipose tissue fat pads (anterosuperior, postero-inferior or a combination of the two), fibroadipose meniscoids (located at the superior or inferior pole or at both poles of the capsule), and connective tissue rims (either anterior or posterior or both) [2]. While the fat pads of the facet capsules are similar to those found in many other joint capsules, the connective tissue rims of the zygapophysial joint are representative of the capsular ligament [2]. Each joint is surrounded by a thin, loose capsular ligament, which attaches to the margins of the articular processes of adjacent vertebrae [3, 4]. The average length of the capsular ligament in the lumbar spine in 24 individuals' capsular ligaments was measured to be 16.4 mm (±2.9) and an average cross-sectional area of 43.8 mm2 (±28.3) [5].

R. S. Tubbs (✉)
Tulane University School of Medicine,
New Orleans, LA, USA
e-mail: rtubbs@tulane.edu

J. Iwanaga
Department of Neurosurgery, Tulane Center for
Clinical Neurosciences, Tulane University School of
Medicine, New Orleans, LA, USA

M. Turgut et al. (eds.), *Ligaments of the Vertebral Column*,
https://doi.org/10.1007/978-3-032-09070-6_17

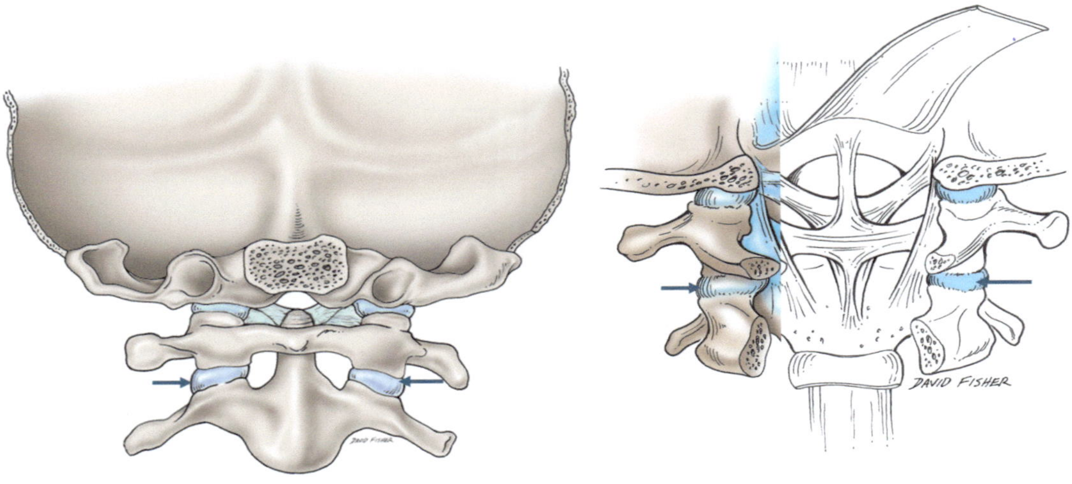

Fig. 17.1 Schematic drawings (left anterior view and right posterior view of the cervical facet capsules and their ligaments (arrows)

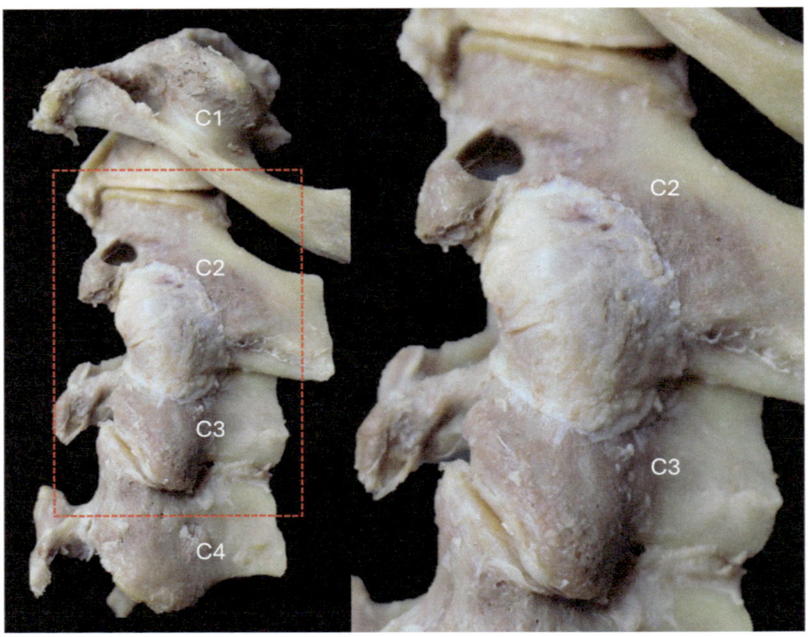

Fig. 17.2 Cadaveric dissections of the left C2/C3 cervical facet capsules and ligaments. The C3/C4 facet capsule and ligament have been removed for comparison

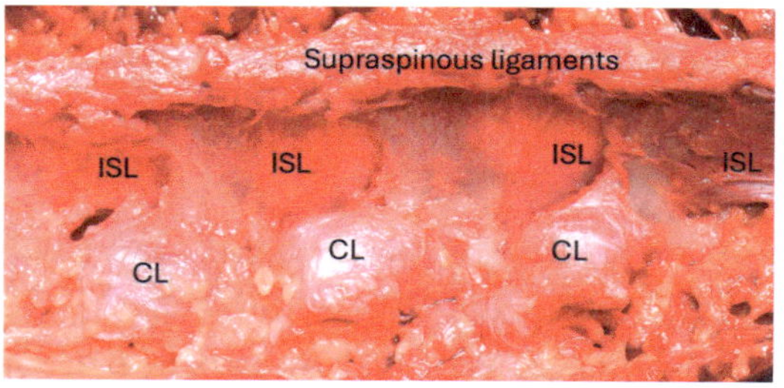

Fig. 17.3 Cadaveric dissection noting the lumbar capsular ligaments (CLs) (*) (Lateral view). *ISL* interspinous ligaments, *CL* capsular ligaments

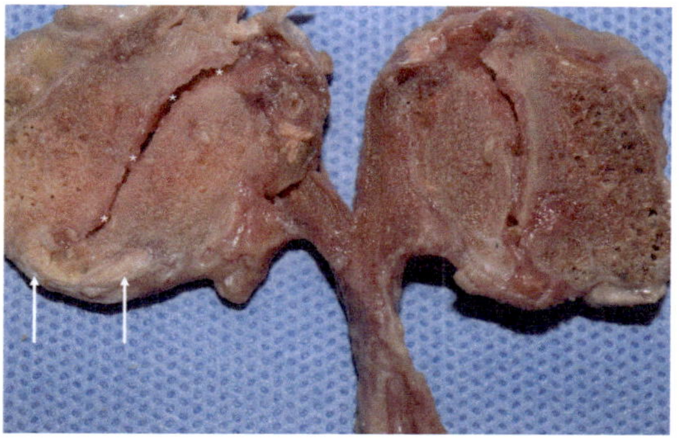

Fig. 17.4 Axial cut through the lumbar zygopophysial joints (*) and noting the left CL (arrows)

17.1.2 Function

Together with other accessory ligaments of the vertebral column, the capsular ligaments help stabilize the vertebral column and its joints. In the cervical region, the loose nature of this ligament allows for a wide range of movement [4]. However, in the sacral spine, the capsular ligament functions to prevent the lumbar vertebra from sliding anteriorly down the incline of the sacrum [4]. This is because the facets on S1 face posteromedial and interlock with the anterolateral facing inferior facets of the L5 vertebra [4].

17.1.3 Biomechanics

Due to the make-up of the facet capsular ligament, it can only provide mechanical resistance when the two adjacent vertebrae articulating in the zygapophysial joint undergo movement relative to one another [1]. The role of the ligament was demonstrated in studies using C3-C7 cadaveric spine segments subjected to 100 N of compression with either 2 nanometers (Nm) of sagittal bending or 5 Nm of axial torsion, before and after graded bilateral removal of the capsular ligament [1]. After removal of 50% of the facet capsule, axial rotation increased by 19% when torsion was applied while the vertical distance between the C4 and C6 spinous processes increased by 5% under flexion [1]. The extent of axial torsion and posterior displacement increased by 25% and 32%, respectively, after 75% of the facet capsule was removed [1]. The increases in the range of motion observed after capsular transection or removal support the hypothesis that the facet capsular ligament provides a substantial contribution to constraining vertebral motion, particularly flexion and lateral bending/torsion [1].

In 1999, Gudavalli and Triano used computer modeling to assess the lumbar spinal ligaments and found that the SSL carries the greatest load during flexion, followed by the LF, capsular ligament, intertransverse, and interspinous ligaments [6].

17.1.4 Imaging

The posterior ligamentous complexes, which include the interspinous ligament, ligamentum flavum, and the facet joint capsular ligaments, are not as well defined on MRI as the ALL or PLL [7, 8].

17.1.5 Clinical

Whiplash is the most common pathological process affecting the facet capsular ligament. There are also reported cases of ossification of the facet capsular ligaments [9].

References

1. Jaumard NV, Welch WC, Winkelstein BA. Spinal facet joint biomechanics and mechanotransduction in normal, injury and degenerative conditions. J Biomech Eng. 2011;133(7):071010.
2. Bannister LH, Berry MM, Collins P, Dyson M, Dussek JE, Ferguson MWJ, editors. Gray's Anatomy. 38th ed. New York: Churchill Livingston; 1996.
3. Dickman CA, Rosenthal DJ, Perin NI. Thoracoscopic spine surgery. New York: Thieme Medical Publishers; 1999.
4. Moore KL, Dalley AF, Agur AMR. Clinically oriented anatomy. 6th ed. Baltimore: Lippincott Williams & Wilkins; 2010.
5. Pintar FA, Yoganandan N, Myers T, Elhagediab A, Sances A Jr. Biomechanical properties of human lumbar spine ligaments. J Biomech. 1992;25(11):1351–6.
6. Gudavalli MR, Triano JJ. An analytical model of lumbar motion segment in flexion. J Manip Physiol Ther. 1999;22:201–8.
7. Heylings DJA. Supraspinous and interspinous ligaments of the human lumbar spine. J Anat. 1978;125(1):127–31.
8. Nachemson AL, Evans JH. Some mechanical properties of the third human lumbar interlaminar ligament (ligamentum flavum). J Biomech. 1968;1(3):211–20.
9. Kliewer MA, Gray L, Paver J, Richardson WD, Vogler JB, McElhaney JH, Myers BS. Acute spinal ligament disruption: MR imaging with anatomic correlation. J Magn Reson Imaging. 1993;3:855–61.

Part IV

The Craniocervical Ligaments

18 Atlanto-Occipital Ligaments

Dengpan Song and Fuyou Guo

18.1 Introduction

The atlanto-occipital ligaments are crucial structures in the craniovertebral junction, also known as the craniocervical junction (CCJ), and play a significant role in stabilizing the connection between the skull and the first cervical vertebra (atlas) [1]. This area is vital for various physiological functions, including head movement and cranial stability. The primary ligaments in this region include the anterior atlanto–occipital membrane (AAOM), posterior atlanto–occipital membrane (PAOM), and capsular joint ligaments, each contributing to the overall integrity and biomechanics of the atlanto–occipital joint [2].

The atlanto-occipital joint itself allows for flexion, extension, and limited lateral movement of the head, making these ligaments essential for maintaining proper alignment and preventing excessive motion that could lead to injury [3]. Their fibrous composition provides the necessary tensile strength, while their anatomical positioning ensures that they can effectively limit overextension and excessive translation of the atlas in relation to the occipital bone [4].

In clinical practice, understanding the anatomy and function of the atlanto-occipital ligaments is critical, particularly in the context of traumatic injuries, degenerative diseases, and surgical interventions involving the CCJ. Imaging examinations such as magnetic resonance imaging (MRI) and computed tomography (CT) play pivotal roles in evaluating ligament damage, aiding in the precise diagnosis of associated pathologies and guiding appropriate treatment (Figs. 18.1 and 18.2).

D. Song · F. Guo (✉)
Department of Neurosurgery, The First Affiliated Hospital of Zhengzhou University, Zhengzhou, Henan, China

International Joint Laboratory of Nervous System Malformations, Zhengzhou, Henan, China
e-mail: chyou666@hotmail.com

M. Turgut et al. (eds.), *Ligaments of the Vertebral Column*,
https://doi.org/10.1007/978-3-032-09070-6_18

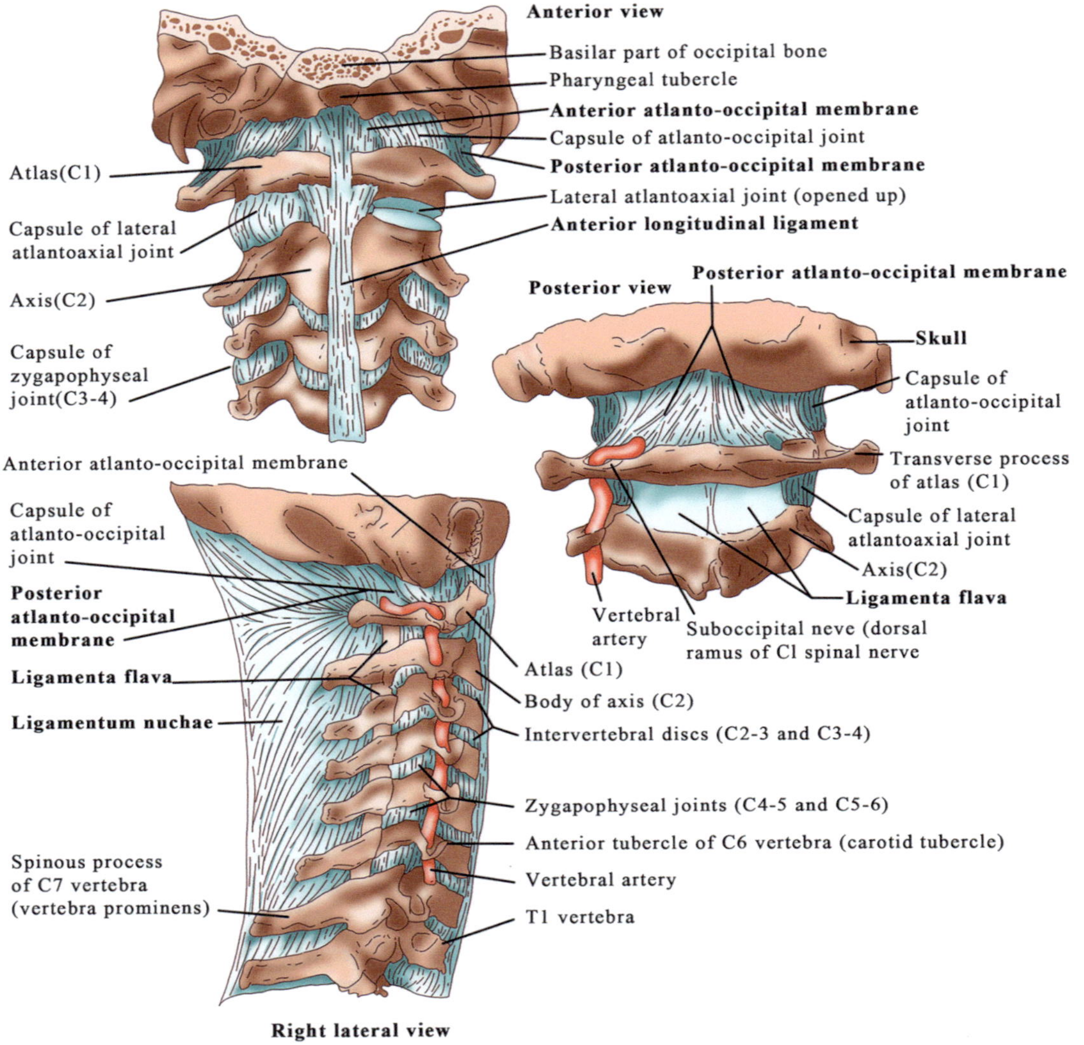

Fig. 18.1 Illustrative anatomy of the cervical spine: top left—anterior view with the prevertebral muscles removed depicting the anterior ligaments of the cranio-cervical junction (CCJ) and the upper subaxial cervical spine; top right—posterior view of the CCJ and relationship of the vertebral artery as it pierces the posterior atlanto-occipital membrane and overlying myofascia; and bottom left—lateral view of the cervical spine. (Offiah [2])

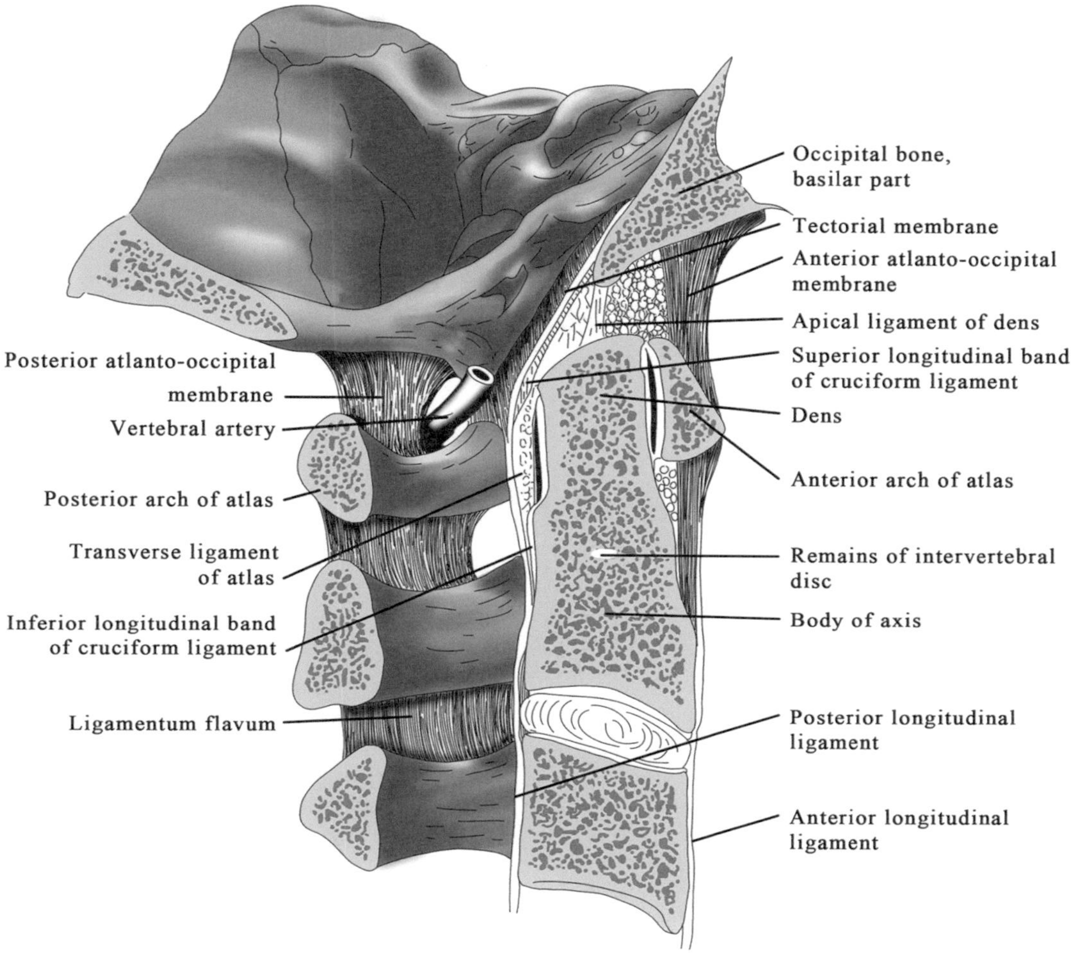

Fig. 18.2 Illustrative anatomy of the CCJ osseoligamentous structures: a right lateral view of sagittally sectioned CCJ in a median plane (i.e., viewed from right to left); b posterior view of the coronally sectioned CCJ; the tectorial membrane has been partly removed to expose deeper ligaments. (Offiah and Day [1])

18.2 Embryology and Development

The CCJ originates from the third embryonic layer, also known as the mesoderm, which forms between the ectoderm and the endoderm [5]. It appears in the third week of gestation and is divided into three regions. During gastrulation, cells from the embryonic plate condense and form the paraxial mesoderm on both sides of the notochord [1]. This mesoderm eventually separates into segmental clusters known as somites (42 pairs in humans), which differentiate into three parts: the external dermatome, the internal myotome, and the medial sclerotome. The sclerotome is located ventromedially and eventually develops into vertebrae, neural arches, ligaments, and membranes [1, 6] (Fig. 18.3).

The CCJ develops from four occipital somites and the first three cervical somites [1]. The first three occipital somites form the base of the occiput. The fourth occipital somite combines with the cranial part of the first cervical somite to form the sclerotome, which gives rise to the atlas, the precursor of the CCJ. It is divided into three parts: the lower occipital region, the vertebral body, and the neural arch. The cranial portion of the sclerotome in this axial region fuses with the

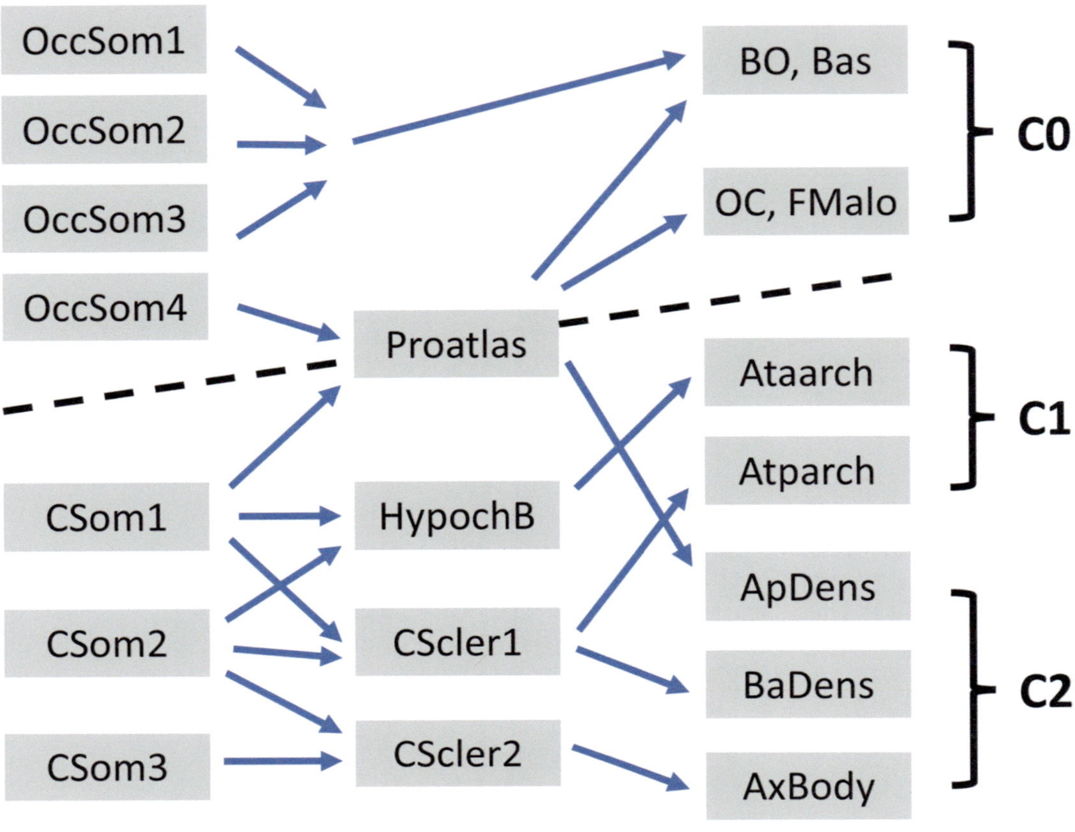

Fig. 18.3 Schematic of CCJ developmental segmentation and resegmentation during embryogenesis. Abbreviations: OccSom1 occipital somite 1; OccSom2—occipital somite 2; OccSom3—occipital somite 3; OccSom4—occipital somite 4; CSom1—cervical somite 1; CSom2—cervical somite 2; CSom3—cervical somite 3; CScler1—cervical sclerotome 1; CScler2—cervical sclerotome 2; BO—basiocciput; Bas basion; OC—occipital condyles; FMalp—anterolateral foramen magnum and opisthion; Ataarch—anterior arch of C1 vertebra (atlas); Atparch posterior arch of C1 vertebra (atlas); ApDens—apical segment of the dens; BaDens—basal segment of the dens; body of C2 vertebra (axis). The dashed black line denotes the embryological separation between the cranial skull base and the cervical spine during CCJ development. (Offiah and Day [1])

sclerotome portions of the first three occipital somites, forming the occipital base [5]. The lower portion of the fourth occipital somite forms the anterior tubercle of the atlas. The vertebral body of the atlas forms the apex cap of the odontoid process and the apical ligament. The neural arch of the atlas develops into the ventral part of the anterior arch and the dorsal part of the posterior arch. The ventral part forms the anterior margin of the foramen magnum and the occipital condyles, whereas the dorsal part forms the cruciform ligament, alar ligaments, the lateral masses of C1, and the upper part of the posterior arch of the atlas [5]. The caudal half of the fifth somite and the cranial half of the sixth somite combine to form the sclerotome of the first cervical vertebra. Similarly, the caudal half of the sixth somite and the cranial half of the seventh somite combine to form the sclerotome of the second cervical vertebra. Part of the first cervical sclerotome forms the base of the odontoid peg, whereas part of the second cervical sclerotome forms the body of the axis (C2). A significant characteristic of the first and second cervical sclerotomes, compared with the caudal sclerotomes, is that some parts do not transform into the annulus fibrosus or nucleus pulposus of intervertebral discs. The mesenchyme at these connection sites forms the upper dens synchondrosis between the apex of the odontoid peg and the dens base, as well as the lower dens synchondrosis between the dens base and the axis body (C2) [6, 7].

Two types of ligaments connect the components of the CCJ: local extensions of the spinal ligaments and specific to the CCJ, such as the apical ligament (tip of the dens), alar ligaments, and cruciform ligament [8]. The alar ligaments limit rotation of the upper cervical spine, whereas the transverse ligament of the atlas, the main component of the cruciform ligament, restricts flexion and anterior displacement of the atlas [9, 10]. Starting from the embryonic stage, namely, O'Rahilly stage 20 (with a crown–rump length of 20 mm), all the bones forming the CCJ, except for the odontoid process, are present as immature cartilage, and the occipital condyles have formed [11]. At this point, the transverse ligament of the atlas and the alar ligaments share a large amount of mesenchymal tissue with the future dens [11]. Additionally, the notochord passes through the future dens of the axis and reaches the midpoint of the anterior margin of the foramen magnum, developing the structure of the apical ligament [11]. Therefore, the apical ligament is generally considered a functional remnant of the notochord. From the latter half of this stage onward, the apical ligament, alar ligaments, and transverse ligament of the atlas begin to differentiate from the common mesenchymal mass shared with the dens of the axis and start to acquire a ligamentous structure. By O'Rahilly stage 21 (with a crown–rump length of 23 mm), the transverse ligament of the atlas, alar ligaments, and apical ligament begin to form distinct ligamentous structures [11].

Owing to the complexity of CCJ development, various CCJ abnormalities have been described. Congenital and developmental abnormalities and malformations affecting the CCJ complex may manifest as general or systemic diseases or specific structural abnormalities (Fig. 18.4).

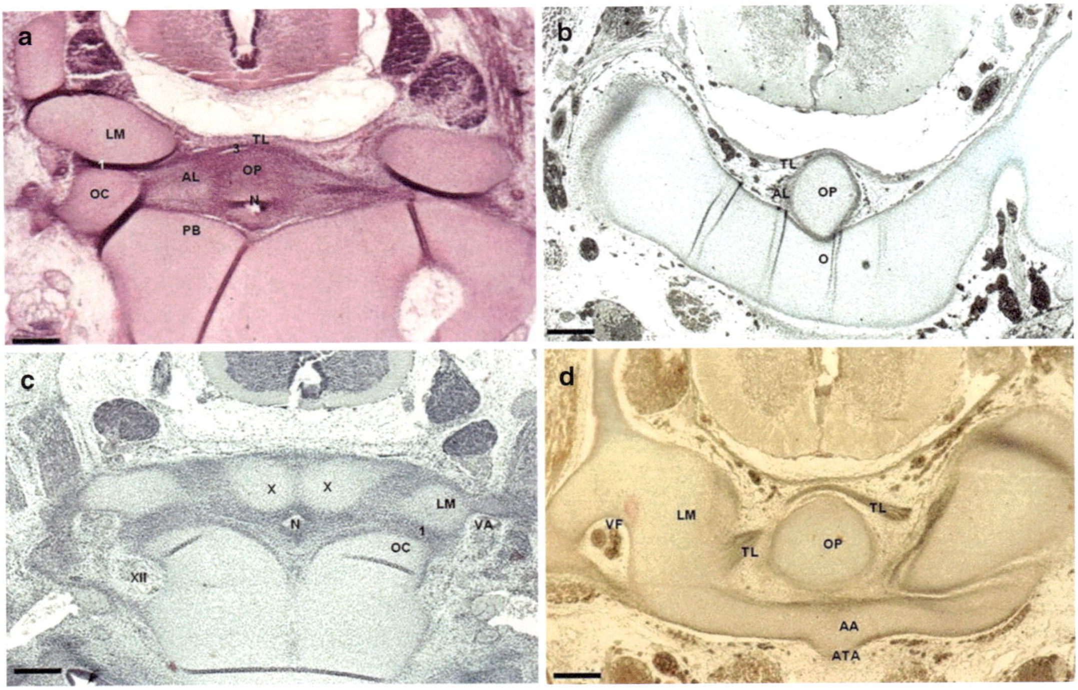

Fig. 18.4 (**a**). Human embryo: P.T.219 (crown–rump length 20 mm), O'Rahilly stage 20. Transverse section (10 mm thick). 1, articular interzone of the future atlanto-occipital joint; 3, transverse-odontoid joint; *AL* alar ligaments, *LM* lateral masses of the atlas, *N* notochord, *OC* occipital condyle, *OP* odontoid process, *PB* pars basioccipitalis, *TL* transverse atlantal ligament. Scale bar: 250 mm. (**b**). Human embryo: E.H.219 (crown–rump length 19 mm), O'Rahilly stage 20. 1, articular interzone of the future atlanto-occipital joint; XII, hypoglossal nerve, *LM* lateral mass of the atlas, *N* notochord, *OC* occipital condyle, *VA* vertebral artery, *X* axis. Scale bar: 250 mm. (**c**). Human embryo: P.E.28 (crown-rump length 23 mm), O'Rahilly stage 21. Transverse section (10 mm thick). *AL* alar ligaments, *O* occipital, *OP* odontoid process, *TL* transverse atlantal ligament. Scale bar: 250 mm. (**d**). Human embryo: P.E.28 (crown-rump length 23 mm), O'Rahilly stage 21. *AA* anterior arch of the atlas, *ATA* anterior tubercle of the atlas, *LM* lateral mass of the atlas, *OP* odontoid process, *TL* transverse atlantal ligament, *VF* vertebral foramen. Scale bar: 250 mm. (Hita-Contreras et al. [11])

18.3 Neuroanatomy, Biomechanics, Radiographic Features, and Pathological Changes

18.3.1 Superficial Anterior Atlanto-Occipital Ligament

18.3.1.1 Anatomy

The superficial anterior atlanto-occipital ligament (SAAOL) is the most common anterior ligament of the CCJ. Anatomy reveals the SAAOL as a slender, midline structure situated in front of the AAOM. This ligament extends from the basion of the clivus to the anterior tubercle of the C1 vertebra [3].

18.3.1.2 Biomechanics

This ligament becomes tight during hyperextension and relaxed during hyperflexion. Its tensile strength is relatively low compared with that of the alar and transverse ligaments. Therefore, the role of the CCJ is very limited and may play only a small role in the prevention of hyperextension injury [12].

18.3.1.3 Imaging Examination

MRI appearance:

T1-weighted imaging: The SAAOL appears as a thin, midline, cord-like, low-signal-intensity band due to its dense fibrous composition. It is typically located anterior to the atlanto-occipital joint, connecting from the anterior arch of the atlas to the basion. The SAAOL may blend with surrounding connective tissues, including muscles and other ligaments. In most cases, distinguishing the SAAOL from the AAOM through imaging alone is difficult.

T2-weighted imaging: Similar to T1-weighted images, SAAOL images have low signal intensity on T2-weighted images. Joint effusion in the atlanto-occipital region may present as high-intensity fluid, helping to delineate the ligament from surrounding structures.

Sagittal plane: In the sagittal view, the SAAOL can be seen as a thin, low-signal band extending from the anterior arch of the atlas to the occipital bone.

Axial plane: SAAOL is usually more challenging to visualize because of its thin profile and the depth at which it lies. It may appear as a low-signal band, but other adjacent structures may obscure it.

Coronal plane: The SAAOL may be difficult to isolate in the coronal view because of its anatomical position and relationship with other ligaments and membranes.

CT appearance:

CT imaging may not directly visualize the SAAOL because of its soft tissue composition, which is similar to that of other ligaments in this region. However, CT can be useful in assessing associated bony structural injuries, such as atlas and occipital bone fractures, to identify trauma or degenerative changes. Any calcifications or significant changes in the bony anatomy affecting SAAOL may be visible on CT.

18.3.1.4 Pathological Changes

Ligament thickening: In cases of trauma or chronic inflammatory conditions, the SAAOL may exhibit thickening, which can be seen as an increased area of low signal intensity on MRI.

Trauma: Injuries to the SAAOL, such as from whiplash or trauma, may result in partial tears. This can manifest as increased signal intensity in the surrounding tissues on T2-weighted MR images due to edema or hemorrhage.

18.3.2 Anterior Atlanto-Occipital Membrane

18.3.2.1 Anatomy

The AAOM is an elastic membrane structure that extends from the anterior margin of the foramen magnum of the occipital bone to the anterior arch of the atlas, connecting the two sides. It is located directly posterior to the longus capitis muscle and anterior to the ligament of Barkow. The AAOM also serves as the anterior wall of the supraodontoid space, which houses the alar, apical, and Barkow ligaments, as well as containing fat and veins [13] (Fig. 18.5).

18.3.2.2 Biomechanics

It is currently believed that the AAOM may function synergistically with the Barkow ligament to limit atlanto-occipital extension of the head. Additional studies revealed the biomechanical properties of this membrane, which is thought to play a marginal role in CCJ stability [4, 14].

18.3.2.3 Imaging

MRI appearance:

T1-weighted imaging: The AAOM is best depicted on an MRI for sagittal and coronal imaging as a fan-shaped, low-signal-intensity ligament extending out from the midline along the anterior arch of C1 to attach to the anterior clivus [3]. However, it is very difficult to visualize in the majority of cases because it is surrounded and partly intermingled with fat [4].

T2-weighted imaging: The AAOM continues to appear as a low-signal-intensity structure in T2-weighted images. Joint effusion or fluid in the atlanto-occipital joint may present as high signal intensity in T2-weighted sequences.

Sagittal plane: In the sagittal view, the AAOM is observed as a thin vertical structure connecting the anterior arch of the atlas and the anterior foramen magnum. Its low signal intensity can be distinguished from that of adjacent cerebrospinal fluid (CSF).

Axial plane: On axial MRI images, the AAOM is visible as a low-signal-intensity structure positioned anterior to the joint space between the atlas and the occipital bone.

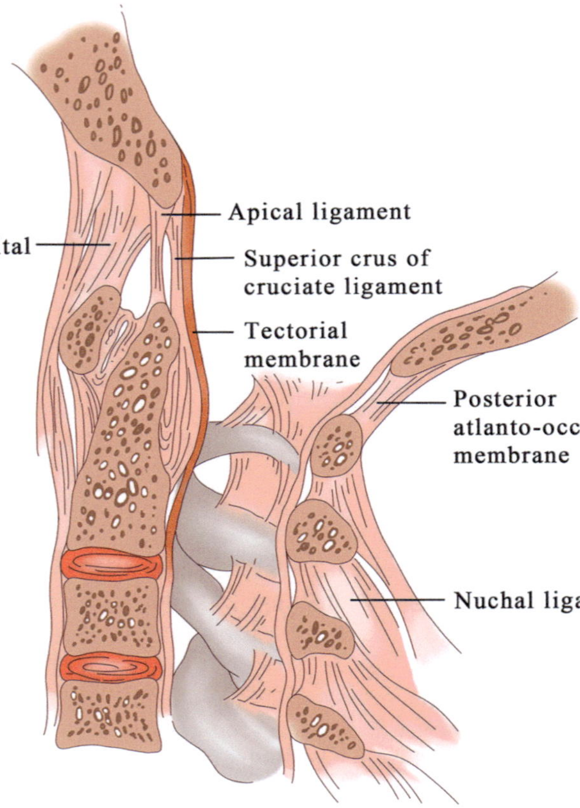

Fig. 18.5 Sagittal drawing of the neck and cranial base depicting the various specialized ligaments of the CCJ region. (Tubbs et al. [4])

Coronal plane: In the coronal view, the AAOM may be visualized as a horizontal band connecting the atlas to the occipital bone, but it is often difficult to isolate it from other surrounding anterior soft tissue structures on this plane.

CT appearance:

CT imaging does not typically visualize the AAOM directly because of its soft tissue composition. However, CT can be useful in detecting bony abnormalities in the atlas or occipital bone that may affect the membrane or indicate trauma in this region. Calcifications or degenerative changes in the membrane may occasionally be observed on CT, although this is rare.

18.3.2.4 Pathological Changes

Ligament thickening: In cases of trauma, chronic degeneration, or inflammatory conditions, the AAOM may thicken. This may be seen on an MRI as a slightly increased low-intensity signal structure. Surrounding joint effusion or edema may also be noted.

Trauma: Injuries to the AAOM, such as from whiplash or atlanto-occipital dislocation, may lead to partial or complete tears of the membrane. This can manifest as abnormally increased signal intensity around the ligament on a T2-weighted MRI due to edema or hemorrhage. Disruption of the normal low-signal-intensity band on imaging may indicate damage.

18.3.3 Atlanto-Occipital Capsular Ligament

18.3.3.1 Anatomy

The bony articulation between the occipital condyles and lateral masses of C1 constitutes the condylar-C1 joint. This joint is a synovial joint comprising the convex articular surface of the bilateral occipital condyle with the concave articular surfaces of the lateral masses of C1. The morphology of the joint is analogous to a teacup resting on a saucer. It allows approximately 25° of flexion/extension and 5° of rotation [4].

18.3.3.2 Biomechanics

The primary role of the capsular joint ligaments is to ensure the correct axial rotation of the upper cervical spine [15].

18.3.3.3 Imaging

MRI appearance:

T1-weighted imaging: The atlanto-occipital capsular ligament (AOCL) appears as a low-signal-intensity structure due to its fibrous nature. It is located around the atlanto-occipital joint, connecting the occipital bone and the atlas. It may blend with the surrounding joint capsule and is typically visible owing to the contrast between the ligament and the adjacent CSF or fat in the region. The joint space should measure <2 mm and be symmetric with respect to the contralateral side [3].

T2-weighted imaging: On a T2-weighted MRI, the AOCL continues to appear as a low-signal-intensity structure. The surrounding joint capsule and the articular cartilage within the atlanto-occipital joint may be highlighted, with the AOCL forming part of this complex. Fluid within the joint space appears as a high-signal-intensity area, offering contrast against the lower signal intensity of the AOCL and capsule.

Sagittal plane: The AOCL can be visualized on sagittal images as part of the joint capsule connecting the occipital condyles to the atlas. It runs vertically along the posterior aspect of the joint, with the ligament's attachment to the occipital condyles and the atlas being visible. The ligament and surrounding capsule appear as thin bands of low signal intensity around the joint.

Axial plane: On axial views, the AOCL is observed in the lateral regions of the atlanto-occipital joint space around the occipital condyles and superior articular facets of the atlas. It is visualized as part of the joint capsule, forming a low-signal-intensity rim around the joint space.

Coronal plane: The coronal plane may also provide visualization of the AOCL as it runs between the occipital condyles and the superior facets of the atlas, appearing as thin, linear, low-signal-intensity structures on either side of the midline.

CT appearance:

CT imaging typically does not provide detailed visualization of soft tissue structures such as the AOCL, but bony structures surrounding the ligament, such as the occipital condyles and the superior articular facets of the atlas, are well visualized. Joint space abnormalities, such as narrowing or osteoarthritic changes, can be indirectly assessed, but the ligament itself cannot be distinctly visualized on CT.

18.3.3.4 Pathological Changes

Capsular thickening: In conditions such as osteoarthritis or inflammatory joint diseases, the AOCL may undergo thickening or calcification, which could result in a restriction of motion or increased stiffness at the atlanto-occipital joint. MRI can detect these changes as a thickened, low-intensity ligament with possible associated joint effusion or inflammation within the joint space.

Joint effusion: In cases of trauma or inflammation, fluid may accumulate in the atlanto-occipital joint space, which may be observed on a T2-weighted MRI as high-signal-intensity effusion surrounding the AOCL and joint capsule.

Trauma: Traumatic injuries involving the AOCL, such as whiplash or atlanto-occipital dislocation, can lead to tearing or sprain of the ligament. On an MRI, this might manifest as increased signal intensity (edema or hemorrhage) within or around the ligament, as well as joint instability.

18.3.4 Posterior Atlanto-Occipital Membrane

18.3.4.1 Anatomy

The PAOM is a broad, thin and fan-shaped midline ligament that runs between the posterior C1 arch and the posterior margin of the foramen magnum and attaches the posterior arch of the atlas inferiorly to the posterior rim of the foramen magnum superiorly [3, 4]. It is continuous with the posterior atlanto-axial membrane and then the ligamentum flavum inferiorly, which is the superior extension of the ligamentum flavum at the C1 level [16]. The PAOM, together with the AAOM, extends laterally to the atlanto-occipital capsula. On each side of the membrane, it fuses laterally with the atlanto–occipital joint capsules [17]. The superior extension of the membrane fuses directly with the occipital dura, similar to the tectorial membrane with the retro-clival dura [16, 18]. The PAOM is located behind the rectus capitis posterior minor muscle and in front of the dura mater, forming a connection or crossing with it [19, 20]. This connective tissue bridge has been found in 67–100% of cadaver specimens and is considered a normal anatomical structure [17, 19]. The PAOM is actually composed of the deep fascia of the rectus capitis posterior minor muscle and the vertebral vascular sheath [18]. The PAOM tends to be laterally oriented, but the middle portion is often opaque because of the increased amount of vascularity and connective tissue. Nash et al. reported that the PAOM was fused with the spinal dura mater antero-inferiorly rather than attached directly to the posterior arch of the atlas. Importantly, the vertebral arteries (VAs) pierce the PAOM and then the dura mater to enter the posterior fossa [21, 22].

18.3.4.2 Biomechanics

The PAOM helps prevent hyperflexion and impingement of the atlas on the cervicomedullary junction and likely plays a major role in stabilizing the posterior CCJ [23].

18.3.4.3 Imaging

MRI appearance:

T1-weighted imaging: The PAOM is a broad but thin, low-signal-intensity structure due to its fibrous nature, running between the posterior arch of the atlas and the occipital bone that continues seamlessly as the ligamentum flavum inferior to C1 [3]. It may not always be distinctly visible because of its thinness and close association with surrounding structures.

T2-weighted imaging: On a T2-weighted MRI, the PAOM appears as a low-signal-intensity membrane in contrast to the adjacent CSF, which appears as a high-signal-intensity fluid, offering better delineation of the membrane. The PAOM is observed along the posterior aspect of the CCJ, extending from the posterior margin of the foramen magnum to the posterior arch of the atlas (C1).

Sagittal plane: The PAOM is best observed on sagittal images. It runs horizontally from the occipital bone to the posterior arch of the atlas. The membrane is thin and low in signal intensity and is situated anterior to the spinal cord and posterior to the subarachnoid space. The membrane's relationship to the spinal cord and subarachnoid space can be visualized, with the membrane acting as a barrier to posterior displacement of the cord at this junction.

Axial plane: On axial views, the PAOM appears as a thin band spanning the posterior margin of the foramen magnum and the atlas's posterior arch. The structure may be difficult to distinguish.

CT appearance:

Bone window: The PAOM itself is not directly visible on CT because it is a soft tissue structure, but CT can be useful for assessing any bony abnormalities associated with the CCJ, such as bony hypertrophy or posterior atlanto-occipital joint degeneration, which could affect the membrane.

18.3.4.4 Pathological Changes

Calcification: Although rare, calcification or ossification of the PAOM may be observed on CT scans as linear hyperdense regions. These are typically associated with degenerative changes or trauma and may limit the flexibility of the CCJ.

Hypertrophy or ossification: With degenerative conditions or following trauma, the PAOM may undergo hypertrophy or, in rare cases, ossification. This can lead to spinal canal narrowing, compressing the spinal cord or dural sac. On CT, this manifests as linear hyperdensities in the region of the membrane.

Trauma: The PAOM may be injured during trauma, such as whiplash injuries. Injuries may result in a thickened membrane or tearing, which can be caused by increased motion at the CCJ. On an MRI, there may be increased T2 signal intensity surrounding the membrane or at its attachment points, indicating edema or hemorrhage.

18.3.5 Cruciform Ligaments (Including Transverse Ligaments)

18.3.5.1 Anatomy

The cruciform ligament is a cross-shaped ligament-centered posterior to the dens that consists of a superior and inferior longitudinal band and a bilateral transverse band [3]. The superior longitudinal band ascends from the center of the ligament between the apical ligament anteriorly and the tectorial membrane posteriorly to the base of the foramen magnum. The inferior longitudinal band descends from the center of the ligament to be inserted on the posterior body of C2 [3]. The horizontal part of the cruciform ligament of the atlas is the transverse ligament of the atlas and is one of the most important ligaments in the body. It is the largest, strongest, and thickest craniocervical ligament (mean height/thickness 6–7 mm) [10]. The transverse ligament maintains stability at the CCJ by locking the odontoid process anteriorly against the posterior aspect of the anterior arch of C-1, and it divides the ring of the atlas into 2 compartments: the anterior compartment houses the odontoid process, and the posterior compartment contains primarily the spinal cord and spinal accessory nerves. The transverse ligament runs posterior to the odontoid process of C-2 and attaches to the lateral tubercles of the atlas bilaterally. The synovial capsule is located between the odontoid process and the transverse ligament. The ligament also has a smooth fibrocartilaginous surface to allow the odontoid process to glide against it [6]. The tectorial membrane, epidural fat, and dura mater are located dorsal to the transverse ligament [10]. The transverse ligament appears to exist in 2 distinct layers. The superficial layer is posterior to the alar ligaments and is hidden by the inferior margin. When the superficial layer is removed and the alar ligaments reflex superiorly, the fibers of the deep layer and their attachments can be observed [24]. It passes the dens 5 mm below the origin of the apical and alar ligaments; its length is 21.9 mm, and its thickness at the midportion is 2.5 mm [23]. The transverse ligament tubercles had a mean width and height of 5 and 6 mm, respectively. The intertubercular distance ranged from 14 mm to 16.5 mm (mean 15.2 mm) [4] (Fig. 18.6).

18.3.5.2 Biomechanics

The cruciform ligament of the atlas stabilizes the odontoid process within the ring of the atlas and plays an important role in maintaining the integrity of the atlanto-axial joint. It primarily restricts flexion movement of the atlanto-axial joint and prevents excessive anterior slipping of the atlas. After the cruciform ligament of the atlas (especially the transverse ligament of the atlas) ruptures, the range of motion of the atlanto-occipital joint can remain relatively normal, whereas the range of flexion, lateral bending, and axial rotation of the atlanto-axial joint increases to varying degrees, with the most noticeable increase being in flexion. Rupture of the cruciform ligament of the atlas inevitably leads to anterior atlanto-axial dislocation, and there is potential for rotational instability at this segment.

18.3.5.3 Imaging

MRI appearance:

Axial plane: In the axial plane, the transverse ligament of the atlas is primarily visible at the level of the mid-to-upper portion of the odontoid process. It appears as a strip of fibrous bundles with a low T2 signal and is attached to the medial tubercles of the left and right lateral masses of the atlas. Anterior to the central part of the ligament is a thin layer of articular cartilage, forming the posterior atlanto-odontoid joint with the posterior aspect of the odontoid process. Posterior to the cruciform ligament lies the tectorial membrane. The central portion of the transverse ligament is tightly adhered to the tectorial membrane, while the lateral edges are separated from it. Edema or disruption of the ligament, in cases of injury, may

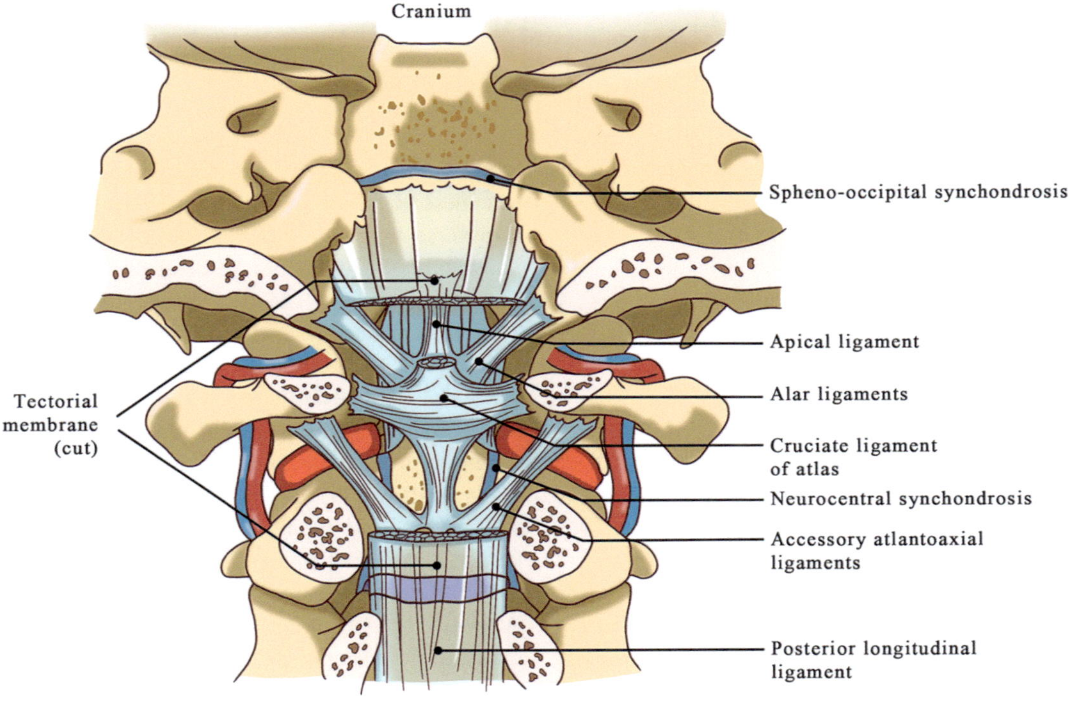

Fig. 18.6 Coronal, anterior illustration demonstrating the ligaments of the CCJ, including the tectorial membrane (cut), cruciate ligament, alar ligament, apical ligament, and posterior longitudinal ligament. (Fiester et al. [3])

result in increased signal intensity on T2-weighted images, reflecting damage or inflammation.

Coronal plane: The transverse ligament of the atlas is located at the level of the mid-posterior odontoid process and anterior to the dura mater; it is located above the body of the axis and is attached to the medial sides of the left and right lateral masses of the atlas, where it appears as a strip. The alar ligaments, running obliquely upward and outward, are visible superior to the transverse ligament. The superior and inferior longitudinal bands are thinner and more delicate; the superior band is closely adhered to the tectorial membrane and dura mater, making it difficult to distinguish, whereas the inferior band has a small amount of fat signal separating it from the tectorial membrane, allowing for partial clear visualization. T2-weighted or fat-suppressed MRI images may provide better contrast, with the ligament clearly delineated against the surrounding soft tissues.

Sagittal plane: The superior longitudinal band runs from the transverse ligament upward to the clivus (part of the occipital bone at the base of the skull). It appears as a thin, low-signal-intensity line extending from the transverse ligament to the anterior margin of the foramen magnum. It is often difficult to distinguish from the surrounding tectorial membrane and dura mater. The inferior longitudinal band runs from the transverse ligament downward to the body of C2. This band is visualized as a low-signal-intensity structure extending from the transverse ligament to the posterior aspect of the C2 body. The superior band can be challenging to differentiate from surrounding structures such as the posterior longitudinal ligament or the tectorial membrane.

CT appearance:

Bone window: The transverse ligament itself is not directly visible on CT because of its soft-tissue composition. However, CT bone windows can be helpful in assessing the bony structures that the ligament attaches to, including the lateral masses of C1 and the dens of C2. Bony avulsions of the transverse ligament's attachment sites, particularly in cases of trauma, can be seen as small bone fragments or irregularities in the lateral masses of C1.

18.3.5.4 Pathological Changes

Ossification or calcification: Although rare, ossification or calcification of the transverse ligament can be seen as linear or nodular hyperdensities on CT scans, particularly in cases of chronic degenerative conditions or trauma.

Injury: Injury to the transverse ligament can result in partial or complete rupture. Increased T2 signal intensity within the ligament or surrounding tissues indicates edema or hemorrhage. Atlanto-axial subluxation, where the atlas (C1) moves anteriorly relative to the axis (C2), may be observed, particularly on flexion–extension imaging.

Atlanto-axial instability: Injury to the transverse ligament can lead to atlanto-axial instability, resulting in excessive motion between C1 and C2. This may manifest as widening of the atlanto-dental interval on lateral radiographs or sagittal CT/MRI (typically >2.5 mm in adults), especially in dynamic studies (e.g., flexion–extension). Increased signals on a T2-weighted MRI around the ligament indicate injury or chronic degeneration. In some cases, however, an MRI does not permit accurate identification of the cruciate ligament because the anterior atlantal space is usually filled with soft tissue coalescing with the ligament. To differentiate between cruciate ligaments with no, mild, moderate, or severe lesions (grades 0–3), Krakanes et al. proposed a neuroradiological grading system [25].

18.3.6 Alar Ligaments

18.3.6.1 Anatomy

The alar ligaments are a pair of ligaments originating from the posterior surface of the upper third of the odontoid process. They extend obliquely outward and attach to the medial aspect of the ipsilateral occipital condyle. The ligaments are symmetrical on both sides, resembling butterfly wings. The ligaments run from the posterolateral aspect of the odontoid process, laterally forming an angle ranging from 125° to 210° with a mean angle of 154° [26]. The mean length and diameter of the alar ligament are 8.8 and 7.3 mm, respectively, and the shape is tubular, elliptical or rectangular [27, 28]. The cross-sectional shape of the alar ligament can be round, ovoid, or winglike [29]. The ligament is narrow at its origin compared with its width at the insertion, thus giving each ligament a "V" shape. The alar ligament attaches the axis to the base of the skull. In terms of histological characteristics, the alar ligaments are composed primarily of collagen fibers, which run parallel to the long axis of the ligament. As a result, alar ligaments exhibit high stiffness and low elasticity in their mechanical properties, making them prone to injury (Fig. 18.7).

18.3.6.2 Biomechanics

The alar ligaments are major stabilizers of the CCJ and help hold the dens upright and in close conjunction with the skull base and anterior C1 arch [3]. They are the main restraints to axial rotation in the upper cervical spine and act to limit axial rotation and lateral bending on the contralateral side [4]. They are the only ligaments, with the exception of the transverse ligament, that are strong enough to stabilize the CCJ and prevent anterior displacement of the atlas. If the transverse ligament ruptures, the alar ligaments become responsible for preventing atlantal subluxation [4]. Cadaveric dissections have shown that transaction of alar ligaments causes an increase in flexion–extension, lateral bending, and especially rotation movements between the occiput and the atlas and between the atlas and the axis [30]. The increase in rotation motion could generate a rotatory atlanto-axial instability that manifests as an increase in the C1-2 range of motion (ROM), predominantly through an increase in the neutral zone; however, the elastic zone and flexibility do not change significantly. The neutral zone and ROM are also increased during lateral bending and flexion-extension movements [31, 32]. The rotation to the right is limited by the left alar ligament and vice versa; the inferior part of the alar ligament is generally

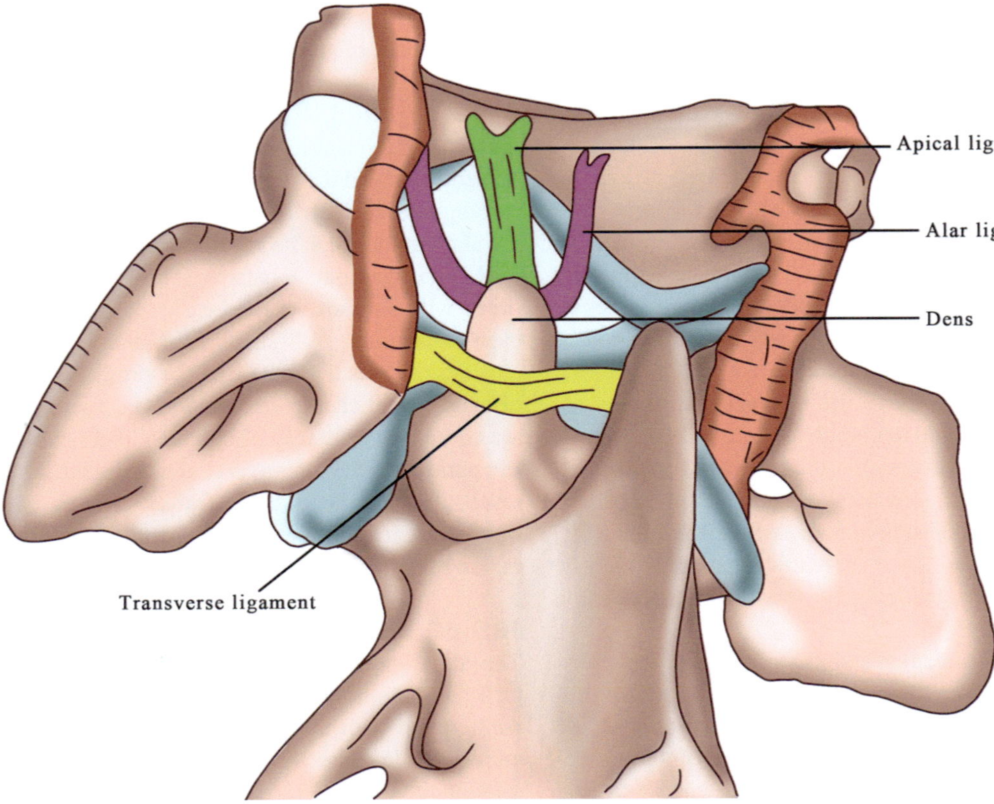

Fig. 18.7 Alar ligaments (pink), apical ligament (green) and transverse ligament (yellow). (Fiester et al. [3])

stretched first [9]. The alar ligament limits the axial rotation on the contralateral side to approximately 90°. Damage to this ligament results in further axial rotation, which can result in compression or damage to the VA or the spinal accessory nerves [33, 34]. Alar ligament injury often occurs in motor vehicle collisions and is believed to be a cause of whiplash-associated disorders [33, 34]. During flexion and extension movements of the cervical–occipital region, the alar ligaments are particularly susceptible to injury when subjected to axial rotational forces. The ligament on the side that is taut in the horizontal direction is more likely to be injured than the contralateral ligament, which is more relaxed [35]. Research by Kaale et al. [36] indicated that anteroposterior impacts are more likely to damage the alar ligaments than posterolateral impacts are and that the location of the injury is related to the rate of rotation. At higher rates (50°/s, 100°/s, 400°/s), damage occurs within the ligament itself, whereas at lower rates (4°/s), injuries are more common at the ligament's bony attachment sites. After injury to the alar ligaments, the range of motion in various directions at the atlanto-occipital joint remains relatively normal; however, the ranges of lateral bending and rotation at the atlanto-axial joint increase significantly, leading to instability in axial rotation. It is generally believed that the coordinated action of the bilateral alar ligaments is essential for effectively limiting excessive axial rotation at the atlanto-axial joint [37].

18.3.6.3 Imaging

MRI appearance:

Sagittal plane: The alar ligament was best viewed in the coronal and sagittal planes and appeared as a thin hypointense T2 band extending from the superolateral dens to the medial surface of the occipital condyles. In the axial plane, the alar ligament appears at the level of the upper odontoid process and below the occipital condyles, presenting as a fan-shaped fiber bundle attached between the posterior aspect of the odontoid tip and the medial margin of the occipital condyle [38]. The surrounding structures, such as the dens, occipital bone, and soft tissue, may help localize the general area where the alar ligaments attach.

Coronal plane: In the coronal plane, the alar ligament is visible in sections through the posterior aspect of the odontoid process and the occipital condyle, appearing as a long, obliquely upward fiber bundle attached between the posterior aspect of the odontoid tip and the medial margin of the occipital condyle. The surrounding alar ligament is composed of adipose tissue [38]. The alar ligaments show, in the majority of patients, a low MRI signal intensity (hypointense ligament); however, approximately one-fifth of healthy subjects show a hyperintense signal [29, 34]. The variation in fiber compaction may explain these differences because fat and connective tissue interposed between fibers have higher proton density than do the fibers themselves [5]. Fat-suppressed sequences can improve visualization by reducing the signal from surrounding fat and increasing contrast between the ligament and adjacent structures. The oblique, upward course of the alar ligaments from the dens to the occipital condyles can be clearly observed on high-resolution coronal images.

Axial plane: On axial images through the upper dens, the alar ligaments appear as paired, symmetrical low-signal bands extending laterally from the dens toward the occipital condyles. These ligaments are typically observed just below the level of the foramen magnum. T2-weighted sequences can demonstrate their location, with the surrounding venous plexus and fat helping to provide contrast.

CT appearance:

Bone window: On standard CT scans, the alar ligaments are not typically visible owing to the limited soft-tissue contrast of CT. However, the bony attachments of the alar ligaments at the occipital condyles and the dens may help infer their location. Ossification or calcification of the alar ligaments, although rare, may present as linear or nodular hyperdensities extending from the dens to the occipital condyles. These findings are most often related to degenerative changes or chronic injury (Fig. 18.8).

18.3.6.4 Pathological Changes

Injury: Alar ligament tears or sprains can occur due to trauma, particularly in cases of high-velocity flexion–extension injuries. On MRI, ligament injury may manifest as increased signal intensity within the ligament on T2-weighted images, indicating edema or tearing. Discontinuity of the ligament fibers may be observed in more severe injuries, particularly on high-resolution T2-weighted or proton-density sequences. Traumatic alar ligament injuries occur particularly in the lateral half near the condylar insertion, indicating that this transitional zone represents the weakest point and the predominant site of injury. The high prevalence of asymmetry and structural alterations of the alar ligament in asymptomatic individuals complicates the use of MRI scans to identify causes of neck pain in symptomatic individuals [34, 39].

Instability: Atlanto-occipital or atlanto-axial instability due to alar ligament damage can sometimes be inferred from abnormal motion of the upper cervical spine on dynamic imaging (e.g., flexion–extension views) or by direct MRI evidence of ligamentous injury. In cases of ligamentous instability, one might observe widening of the lateral atlanto-dental interval by imaging studies.

18.3.7 Transverse Occipital Ligament

18.3.7.1 Anatomy

The transverse occipital ligament (TOL) is a small accessory ligament of the CCJ that is located posterosuperior to the alar ligaments and odontoid process [4]. It attaches to the inner aspect of the occipital condyles, posterosuperior to the alar ligament, superior to the transverse ligament, and extends horizontally across the foramen magnum [40]. Tubbs et al. [40] identi-

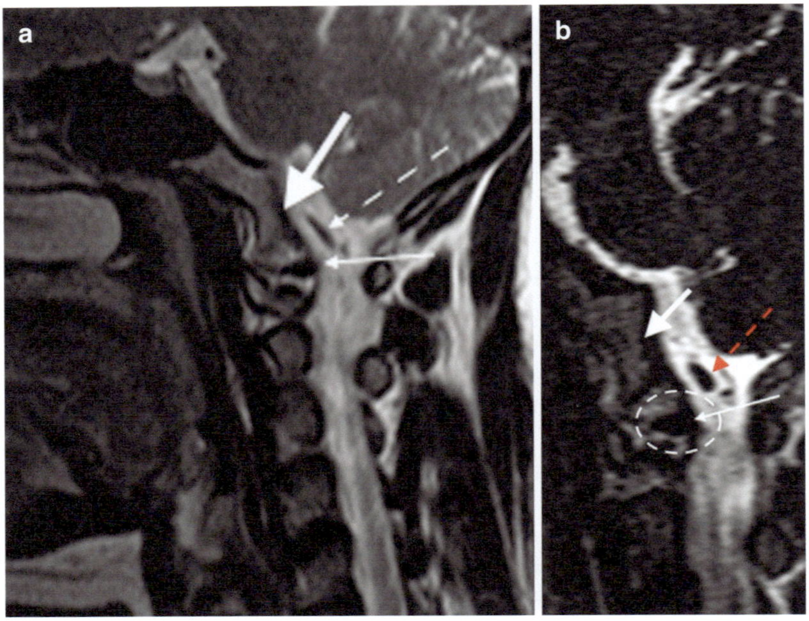

Fig. 18.8 (**a**). Right parasagittal T2-weighted image of the cervical spine focusing on the CCJ shows the right alar ligament (long thin white arrow) between its attachments to the dens and the right occipital condyle—the right vertebral artery flow void (broken long thin white arrow) and the right basiocciput (thick white arrow); (**b**). right parasagittal multiplanar reconstructed T2 SPACE image of the CCJ showing the right alar ligament (long thin white arrow) between its attachments to the dens and the right occipital condyle, the right vertebral artery flow void (broken red arrow) and the right basiocciput (thick white arrow). (Offiah [2])

fied the TOL in 7 (77.8%) of 9 human cadavers. The mean width, length, and thickness of the ligament were 3.4, 19.4, and 1.3 mm, respectively. However, Ackerman and Cooper reported TOLs in only 2 bodies (8.3%) of 24 and reported that TOLs were attached to both the odontoid process and the alar ligaments. Dvorak et al. [9] reported that TOL is present in only approximately 10% of the population. The discrepancies in the occurrence of the TOL in the samples could be due to the proximity and similar morphology to the alar ligament. Clinically, TOL may be encountered during transoral odontoidectomy [4].

18.3.7.2 Biomechanics

The TOL is thought to have functions similar to those of the alar ligaments in helping to stabilize the CCJ. The TOL represents the uppermost fibers of the alar ligament that sometimes cross the midline [4]. However, Tubbs et al. [40] did not consistently find a connection between the TOL and the odontoid process or alar ligaments. When attached to the alar ligament, the possible functions of the TOL include providing additional support in stabilizing lateral bending, flexion, and axial rotation of the head. The TOL may also prevent posterior displacement of the apical ossicles of the odontoid process, as the transverse ligament ends inferior to the apex of the odontoid process [40].

18.3.7.3 Imaging

MRI appearance:

Sagittal plane: The transverse occipital ligament is generally a low-signal-intensity structure on both T1- and T2-weighted MRI images, similar to most ligaments. It can be difficult to distinguish from surrounding soft tissues clearly because of its small size, but it lies in close proximity to the tectorial membrane and other stabilizing ligaments of the atlanto-occipital joint.

Axial plane: On axial images, the TOL may appear as a thin, linear band extending across the posterior region of the atlanto-occipital joint. However, it may blend with nearby soft tissues, making its visualization challenging.

Coronal plane: The coronal plane might offer a more detailed view of the horizontal orientation of the TOL, particularly in the posterior atlanto-occipital region. However, given its size, it may still be difficult to differentiate from nearby ligaments, such as the atlanto-occipital membrane. Like in the sagittal view, high-resolution imaging is necessary for optimal visualization.

CT appearance:

Soft-tissue window: On standard CT imaging, the transverse occipital ligament, like other soft-tissue structures, is not typically well visualized unless there is calcification or ossification. Surrounding bony landmarks, such as the occipital bone and the atlas, can help infer its location.

Bone window: If there is ossification or calcification of the ligament (which is rare), it may appear as a linear hyperdense structure on a CT bone window. This might be observed in cases of degenerative changes or trauma to the CCJ.

18.3.7.4 Pathological Changes

Injury: Injuries to the TOL are rarely isolated and often occur in conjunction with other ligaments, such as the alar or transverse ligaments. MRI can detect ligamentous injury through increased signal intensity or discontinuity, but injuries specifically involving the TOL are seldom reported.

Degeneration: Degenerative changes in the TOL are not commonly documented, but when they are present, they may involve ossification or calcification, which can be detected via CT imaging.

18.3.8 Lateral Atlanto-Occipital Ligament

18.3.8.1 Anatomy

The lateral atlanto-occipital (LAO) ligament runs just lateral to the AAOM, is attached to the anterolateral aspect of the transverse process of the atlas, and is inserted into the jugular process of the occipital bone [41]. This ligament runs immediately posterior to the rectus capitis lateralis muscle and has fibers that extend in the opposite direction to the muscle (that is, the muscle runs laterally to the medial muscle, and the ligament runs medially to the lateral muscle). Additionally, the LAO ligament is related posteriorly to the VA and anteriorly to the jugular vein as it exits the jugular foramen [41]. The LAO ligament was present bilaterally. The mean length, width, and thickness of this ligament were 22, 5, and 2 mm, respectively. Surgically, the LAO ligament may be encountered during lateral approaches to the CCJ, as rectus capitis lateralis can be identified via this landmark [41, 42] (Fig. 18.9, Table 18.1).

18.3.8.2 Biomechanics

The ligament plays a role in limiting lateral flexion of the head. When the LAO ligament was transected in cadavers, Tubbs et al. [41] reported an increase in lateral flexion of the contralateral side of 3–5°. Additionally, the LAO ligament may play a small role in limiting axial rotation of the atlanto-occipital joint. Tubbs et al. [41] noted tautness of the LAO ligament on contralateral rotation of the head on the atlas.

18.3.8.3 Imaging

MRI appearance:

The LAOL typically appears as a thin, elongated structure on coronal and axial MRI scans. It is situated laterally between the atlas (C1) and the occipital bone, providing stability to the atlanto-occipital joint. On T1-weighted MRI images, the ligament may show low to intermediate signal intensity, whereas on T2-weighted MRI images, it maintains a low signal because of the dense collagen fibers.

CT appearance:

On CT scans, the LAO ligament is not directly visualized as a soft tissue structure but can be inferred from the osseous landmarks of the atlas and occipital bone. It appears as a continuity between the lateral masses of the atlas and the occipital condyles, with any bony changes or calcifications potentially impacting its integrity.

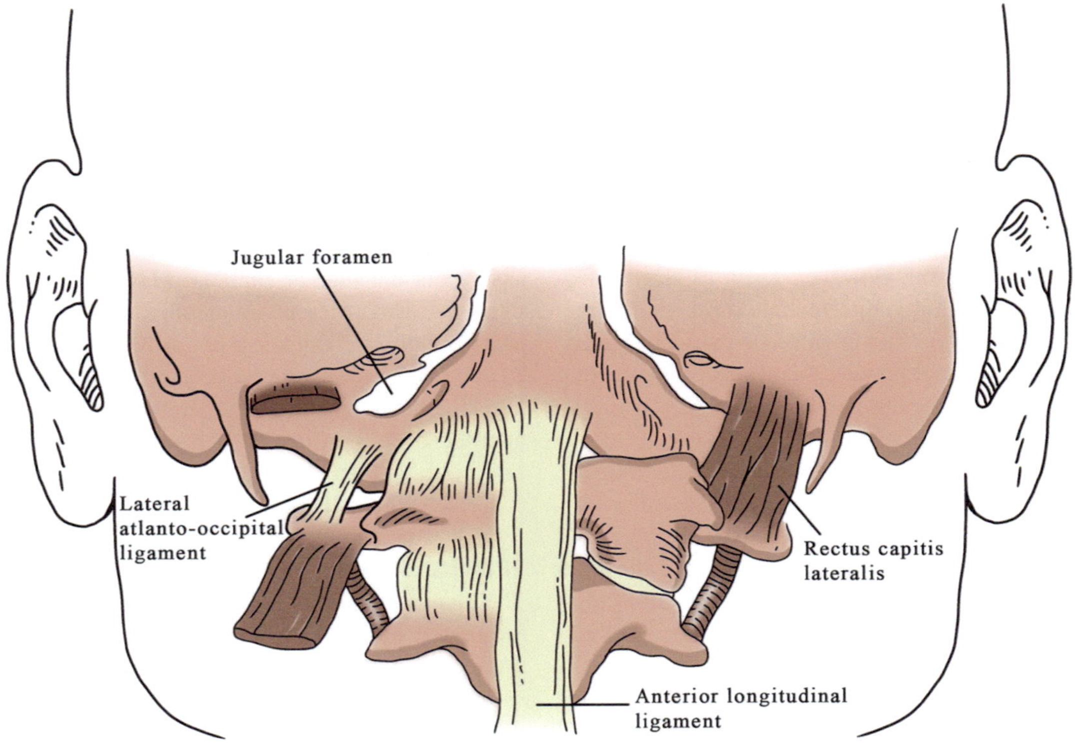

Fig. 18.9 Schematic view of the jugular foramen, lateral atlanto-occipital ligament, anterior longitudinal ligament and rectus capitis lateralis. (Tubbs et al. [41])

Table 18.1 Results of measurements of the lateral atlanto-occipital ligament*

Characteristic	Value
Angle	20°–32° (mean 26°)
Length	1.5–3 cm (mean 2.2 cm)
Width	0.35–0.75 cm (mean 0.5 cm)
Thickness	1.0–3.5 mm (mean 2.0 mm)
Tensile force	30.4–44.1°N (mean 37.5°N)
Lateral Xexion	5°–10° (mean 8°)

*The data given in this table was taken from Tubbs et al. [41]

Angle = deviation from midline from the origin to the insertion of the LAO; lateral Xexion = the degree of motion in lateral Xexion, where maximal tautness of the LAO was observed. *LAO* lateral atlanto-occipital

18.3.8.4 Pathological Changes

Pathological conditions, such as ligamentous injuries or degenerative changes, may not be directly visualized but can lead to instability in the atlanto-occipital region. MRI can help identify associated edema or inflammatory changes in the surrounding soft tissues, indicating possible ligamentous injury.

18.3.9 Barkow Ligaments

18.3.9.1 Anatomy

Barkow ligament was found to be a horizontal band attached to the anteromedial aspect of the occipital condyles anterior to the attachment of the alar ligaments. The Barkow ligament was located just anterior to the superior aspect of the dens, with fibers traveling anterior to the alar ligaments but with no connection to these structures. Tubbs et al. [43] reported that the ligament was present in 12 (92.3%) of 13 cadavers, observing an attachment between the Barkow ligament and the AAOM at the midline in 9 specimens (75%). The mean length, width, and thickness were found to be 2.5, 4, and 3.5 mm, respectively. They also reported that the mean tensile strength

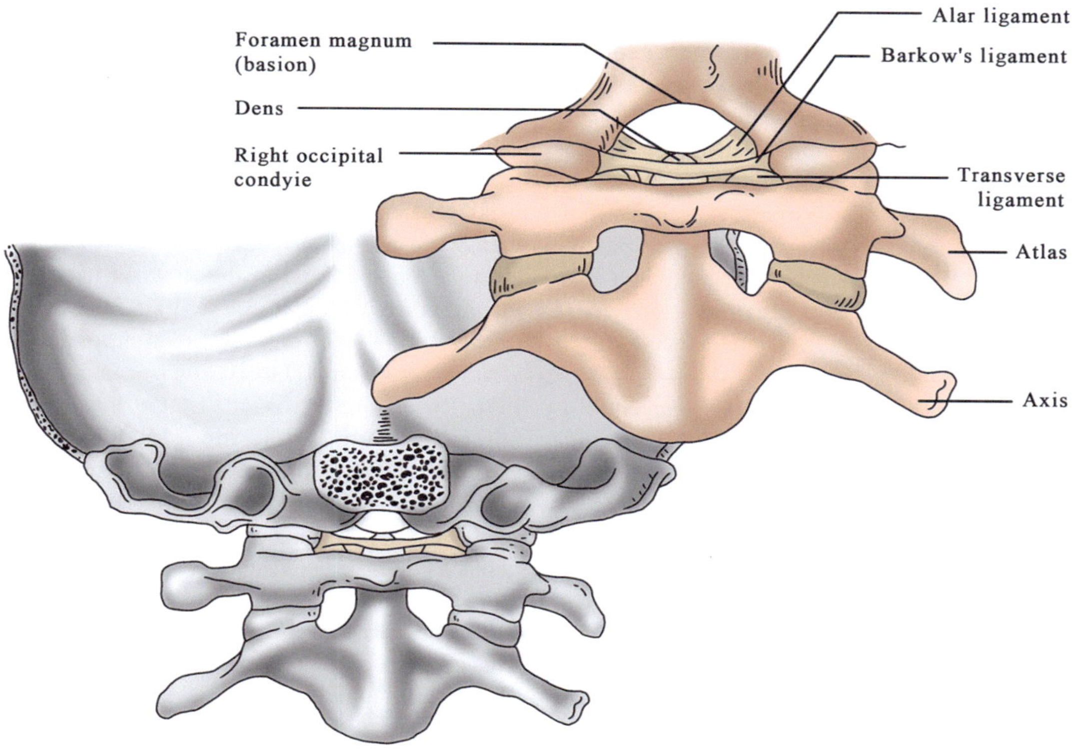

Fig. 18.10 Schematic drawing of the bones and ligaments that bind the anterior CCJ. Note the position of the Barkow ligament. For reference, observe the alar ligament and its more posterior attachment onto the dens. (Tubbs et al. [43])

was 28 N, and the ligament was found to be smaller than the transverse ligament but had a similar course [4, 43]. The Barkow ligament may be encountered in anterior transoral procedures, which require resection of lesions along the anterior CCJ. This ligament can be encountered just anterior to the dens and may be a sentinel structure to the surgeon, alerting the surgeon to the nearby presence of the dens and alar ligaments [43] (Fig. 18.10).

18.3.9.2 Biomechanics

The Barkow ligament may function to support the CCJ, limiting extension of the atlanto-occipital joint, and may assist the transverse ligament in containing the odontoid process. Tubbs et al. [43] noted that the only movement that caused tautness of the Barkow ligament was extension of the atlanto-occipital joint. As the head was extended, the Barkow ligament was stretched against the odontoid process; therefore, resistance to this movement was provided. Interestingly, the transverse ligament must be intact for the Barkow ligament to function properly. The ligament may inhibit lateral displacement of a unilateral occipital condyle fracture [4, 43].

18.3.9.3 Imaging

MRI appearance:

Sagittal plane: The Barkow ligament may appear as a low-signal-intensity structure on both T1- and T2-weighted MRI images. Its visualization on an MRI can be challenging because of its small size and the proximity of other soft tissues and ligaments at the CCJ. It is typically found anterior to the tectorial membrane and may appear as part of the connective tissue structures that form the anterior wall of the atlanto-occipital region.

Axial plane: In axial sections, the Barkow ligament can be visualized in conjunction with the AAOM. It may not be as distinctly visible because of the overlap with surrounding connective tissues and nearby vasculature. Fat suppression techniques for MRIs can sometimes help delineate the ligament more clearly if there is surrounding inflammation or edema.

Coronal plane: The coronal view offers limited utility for directly visualizing the Barkow ligament. However, some portions of the ligament may be visible in the region of the AAOM or its attachments to the occipital bone.

CT appearance:

Owing to the soft tissue of the ligament, it is not well visualized via standard CT imaging unless there is ossification or calcification. However, the bony landmarks to which the Barkow ligament attaches—such as the occipital bone and the anterior arch of the atlas—can be well demonstrated, helping to infer its location.

18.3.9.4 Pathological Changes

Ligamentous injuries in the CCJ may involve the Barkow ligament, particularly in cases of hyperflexion, hyperextension, or rotational trauma. MRI can reveal disruption of the ligament through abnormal signal intensity or discontinuity, but injuries to this specific ligament are rarely isolated and often occur in conjunction with other ligaments, such as the transverse or alar ligaments. Degenerative changes in the Barkow ligament, such as calcification or ossification, may be observed in CT but are not as common as changes in the more prominent ligaments, such as the tectorial membrane or alar ligaments. These changes are typically incidental findings without significant clinical impact unless they contribute to instability.

18.3.10 Apical Ligaments

18.3.10.1 Anatomy

The apical ligament, also known as the middle odontoid ligament or suspensory ligament, extends from the tip of the dens to the anterior margin of the foramen magnum and is situated between the AAOM and cruciform ligament [44, 45]. The ligament runs in the triangular area between the left and right alar ligaments, known as the supraodontoid space (apical cave), which is filled with connective tissue, fat, and a small venous plexus [13, 45]. Studies have shown that the apical ligament, the superior longitudinal band of the cruciform ligament, the tectorial membrane, and the dura mater are tightly adhered at the anterior margin of the foramen magnum, making them difficult to separate. Its length ranges from 3 to 11 mm (mean 7.5 mm), and its width ranges from 1.5 to 10 mm (mean 5.1 mm) [45]. Reports have shown that the ligament is missing in nearly 20% of cases [45]. It is considered a vestigial structure, representing a tiny notochordal remnant with surrounding elastic fibers, and behaves analogously to a rudimentary nucleus pulposus between the basion and C2 [3].

18.3.10.2 Biomechanics

The apical ligament is generally considered a vestigial structure that offers no added stability to the CCJ area [45].

18.3.10.3 Imaging

MRI appearance:

Sagittal plane: The ligament appears as a thin, midline T2 hypointense band extending between the base and tip of the dens or anterior atlanto-axial joint space. It is outlined by a small fat pad in the supradental recess [3]. The ligament may be obscured by surrounding connective tissues, fat, or vascular structures, making it difficult to differentiate from adjacent structures.

Axial plane: The apical ligament may be seen in the midline at the level of the upper dens. It is surrounded by connective tissue, fat, and small veins, making its direct visualization more challenging, especially in routine imaging.

Coronal plane: The apical ligament is visible at the level of the odontoid tip and appears as a slender, elongated structure. It attaches at both ends to the tip of the odontoid process and the anterior midline margin of the foramen magnum. The coronal view is not typically the best plane for evaluating this ligament, and it is usually seen only incidentally.

CT appearance:

The apical ligament is not easily visible via standard CT imaging because of the lack of contrast between soft tissues, but its bony attachments to the dens and the occipital bone can be visualized. CT can be useful if there is calcification or ossification of the ligament, which might appear as a thin, linear hyperdense structure along the ligament's course.

18.3.10.4 Pathological Changes

Injury: Injuries to the apical ligament are rare because of its small size and limited functional significance. However, trauma that affects the CCJ (such as hyperflexion or hyperextension injuries) could result in damage to the apical ligament, often in combination with other ligaments such as the alar ligaments or the transverse ligament. However, damage to this ligament alone is rarely of clinical concern because of its minor stabilizing role.

18.3.11 Tectorial Membranes

18.3.11.1 Anatomy

The tectorial membrane is a longitudinal fibrous band that covers the posterior surface of the cruciform ligament of the atlas. It is relatively thin but broad and strong, representing the upward continuation of the posterior longitudinal ligament. It originates from the posterior aspect of the body of the axis (C2) and attaches superiorly to the anterior margin of the foramen magnum at the base of the occiput, as well as to the medial surfaces of the atlanto-occipital joints. The dura mater is located posterior to the tectorial membrane. The tectorial membrane is composed of 2–3 distinct layers that run through the length of the ligament and then fuse together at the posterior longitudinal ligament. The outermost layer is the widest and attaches as far laterally as the hypoglossal canals. The second layer is relatively thick and runs from the clivus to the body of the axis. A small bursa is often present between the 2 layers of the odontoid process. The third layer is the deepest and discontinuous, as it attaches to the clivus above and then becomes frayed in the area above the odontoid apex. Nerves and vessels often run between the different layers of the tectorial membrane [13]. The mean length, width, and thickness of this membrane were 6, 3, and 1 mm, respectively (Table 18.2).

Table 18.2 Summary of tectorial membrane dimensions*

Characteristic	Value
Length of thectorial membrane	5.0–7.5 cm (mean 6.0 cm)
Width of tectorial membrane in the cervical region	2.0–3.3 cm (mean 3.0 cm)
Width of tectorial membrane at the skull base	2.0–3.5 cm (mean 2.5 cm)
Thickness of tectorial membrane	0.5–1.2 mm (mean 1.0 mm)

*The data given in this table was taken from Tubbs et al. [46]

18.3.11.2 Biomechanics

The biomechanical role of the tectorial membrane in the CCJ area is controversial. The main function of the tectorial membrane is generally believed to be to limit physiological flexion and excessive extension of the atlanto-axial joint. Its rupture can lead to increased flexion and extension movements in the atlanto-axial joint, resulting in potential instability at this segment. Research by Kaale et al. indicated that tectorial membrane injuries occur during extreme hyperextension and hyperflexion movements of the CCJ region and are frequently associated with whiplash injuries, particularly from rear-end impacts. Krakenes et al. [25] reported that, with isolated sectioning of the tectorial membrane, instability was observed only during flexion. A study conducted by Tubbs et al. [46] revealed that the tectorial membrane did not directly inhibit cervical flexion but rather prevented the odontoid process from impinging into the cervical canal. They reported that flexion of the CCJ made the tectorial membrane fully taut at 15° and that extension made the tectorial membrane fully taut at 20°. The tensile strength of this ligament was found to be 76 N. The tectorial membrane could not be taut with any lateral flexion or axial rotation of the joint [4].

18.3.11.3 Imaging

MRI appearance:

Sagittal plane: The tectorial membrane appears in the plane between the bilateral occipital condyles. In the mid-sagittal plane, passing through the dens, the tectorial membrane originates from the posterior aspect of the body of the axis (C2) and continues downward as the posterior longitudinal ligament. It ascends posterior to the cruciform ligament of the atlas and attaches to the base of the clivus in the occipital bone, appearing as a slender, low-signal structure. This plane clearly demonstrates the course and adjacent structures of the tectorial membrane, making it an ideal plane for visualization. In this plane, the tectorial membrane is closely adhered to the apical ligament, the superior longitudinal band of the cruciform ligament, and the dura mater at the anterior midline margin of the foramen magnum, making them difficult to distinguish.

Axial plane: The tectorial membrane appears as a transverse low-signal band extending between the occiput and the posterior aspect of the C2 vertebra in the axial plane. It is often difficult to differentiate from the surrounding dura mater and adjacent ligaments in this plane. It lies posterior to the dens and adjacent to the transverse ligament, and the central part of the tectorial membrane may blend with the dura mater and the cruciform ligament, making clear demarcation challenging.

Coronal plane: The tectorial membrane is generally not well visualized in the coronal plane, and this view is not typically used for its evaluation.

CT appearance:

On CT, the tectorial membrane is not easily visualized because of the limited contrast resolution for soft tissues. However, the bony attachments of the tectorial membrane to the clivus and the C2 body can be identified. Calcification or ossification of the tectorial membrane is rare but, when present, may be seen as hyperdense (bright) areas on CT.

18.3.11.4 Pathological Changes

Trauma, such as hyperextension or hyperflexion (e.g., whiplash injuries), may lead to partial or complete disruption of the tectorial membrane, resulting in instability of the atlanto-axial joint. MRI can detect the disruption of the tectorial membrane, seen as discontinuity or abnormal signal intensity in the ligament. Disruption or rupture of the tectorial membrane may lead to increased flexion–extension motion in the atlanto-axial joint and potential instability at the CCJ. Degenerative changes can sometimes lead to calcification or ossification of the tectorial membrane, which may be observed on CT scans but is less commonly observed on MRI. These changes may be asymptomatic or related to chronic neck pain or stiffness.

18.3.12 Nuchal Ligaments

18.3.12.1 Anatomy

The nuchal ligament is the cephalic extension of the supraspinous ligament extending from the C-7 spinous process to the incision of the occipital bone. With the shorter spinous processes of the cervical vertebrae and the lordotic curve of the cervical spine, this ligament forms a midline septation dividing the posterior neck muscles on the left and right sides. Moreover, some of these muscles attach medially to this structure [4].

18.3.12.2 Biomechanics

The nuchal ligament restricts hyperflexion of the cervical spine. Interestingly, some studies have reported a greater concentration of proprioceptive fibers in this structure and have suggested that it may play a role in maintaining proper alignment of the cervical spine [4].

18.3.12.3 Imaging

MRI appearance:

Sagittal plane: The nuchal ligament typically appears as a midline, elongated, low-signal (dark) structure on T1- and T2-weighted images. It spans from the occiput to the spinous processes of the cervical vertebrae (C7). Owing to its dense collagen fibers, it has low signal intensity, which contrasts with the higher signal intensity of the surrounding soft tissues and muscles.

Axial plane: In cross-sections, it appears as a narrow band of low signal, running along the posterior neck and anchored between the cervical spinous processes and the posterior muscles.

Coronal plane: Less frequently used for visualizing the nuchal ligament, it may be seen as a thin, vertical band running through the posterior midline of the cervical region.

CT appearance:

The nuchal ligament is often not distinctly visualized on CT because it blends with the surrounding soft tissues. However, in cases of calcification or ossification (which can occur with aging or degenerative changes), the ligament may appear as a linear hyperdense structure along the midline of the neck.

X-ray:

When calcified, it may present as a linear opacity along the posterior aspect of the cervical spine.

18.3.12.4 Pathological Changes

Degenerative changes such as calcification or ossification of the nuchal ligament are more common in older individuals and may be associated with conditions such as diffuse idiopathic skeletal hyperostosis. Trauma to the neck may cause disruption or strain of the nuchal ligament, although this is not easily detected on imaging unless it is associated with other cervical injuries.

In conclusion, the atlanto-occipital ligaments play crucial roles in stabilizing the CCJ, contributing to the range of motion and biomechanical balance of the upper cervical spine. These ligaments, including the SAAOL, AAOM, atlanto-occipital capsular ligament, PAOM, cruciform ligament, alar ligament, transverse occipital ligament, lateral atlanto-occipital ligament, Barkow ligament, apical ligament, and nuchal ligament, have distinct embryological origins and developmental pathways that define their anatomical and functional characteristics. Understanding the neuroanatomy, biomechanics, and radiographic features of these ligaments is essential for diagnosing pathological changes and providing appropriate clinical management for patients with disorders affecting the CCJ. Advanced imaging examinations, such as MRI and CT, are pivotal in evaluating these structural abnormalities, particularly in cases of trauma, congenital malformations, or degenerative conditions (Tables 18.3, 18.4, and 18.5).

Table 18.3 Ligaments of the CCJ and their respective attachments and functions published via the UCSF Surgical Neuroanatomy Collection [47]*

Location	Name	Insertions	Function
Posterior	Transverse ligaments	Connects the anterior surface of odontoid process with the posterior surface of the atlas' anterior arch	Acts as the main stabalizer for the atlanto-axial joint and allows for rotation around this joint
	Alar ligament	Connects the lateral sides of the odontoid process with the base of the skull	Acts as a stabalizer for the atlanto-axial joint and prevents excessive rotation around the joint
	Transverse occipital ligament	Located superior to the bottom of the alar ligament and attaches to the inner walls of the atlas' occipital condyles	Provides support to flexion and rotation of the head
	Barkow ligament	Connects to the anterior aspects of the occipital condyles and wraps around the posterior edge of the odontoid process	Minimizes extension of the Atlanto-axial joint
	Apical ligament	Attaches the odontoid process to the basion of the foramen magnum	Provides minimal stabalization to the atlanto-axial joint
	Tectorial membrane	Composed of three layers that run from the clivius to the body of the axis and connect laterally to the hypoglossal canals	Limits extension at atlanto-occipital joint and flexion at the atlanto-axial joint
	Posterior atlanto-occipital membrane	Connects the inferior edge of the atlas' posterior arch with the posterior edge of the foramen magnum	Minimal stability of the cranio-cervical junction
	Accessory atlanto-axial ligament	Attaches to the dorsal surface of the Axis body and travels upward and inserts posteriorly into the transverse ligament	Limits the axial rotation of the head
	Anterior atlanto-occipital membrane	Attaches to the superior edge of the atlas' anterior arch and connects to the anterior edge of the foramen magnum	Limits the extension of the atlanto-occipital joint
Anterior	Anterior atlanto-axial membrane	Connects the inferior surface of the atlas' anterior arch with the superior anterior surface of the Axis' body	Limits the extension of the atlanto-axial joint
	Lateral atlanto-occipital membrane	Connects the lateral surface of the atlas' transverse process with the jugular of the occipital bone	Limits the lateral flexion of the head

*The data given in this table was taken from Vigo et al. [47]

Table 18.4 Summary of mean values and statistical results of ligament morphometric measurements [48]*

	Normal population (n = 93)					Chiari malformation population (n = 25)					Statistics
Radiological variable	Mean	SD	Median	Minimum	Maximum	Mean	SD	Median	Minimum	Maximum	*P*
L1	23.0[a]	3.6	23.0	12.1	31.4	21.3[a]	2.5	21.4	17.2	24.9	0.027[a]
L2	10.7[b]	2.0	10.4	5.1	15.4	8.8[a]	3.8	8.9	1.1	16.6	0.007[a]
W1	1.59	0.49	1.50	0.80	3.40	1.73	0.46	1.70	1.00	2.90	0.200
W2	1.39	0.43	1.40	0.60	3.40	1.60	0.48	1.60	1.00	2.50	0.089
W3	1.48	0.42	1.50	0.79	2.60	1.33	0.45	1.25	0.60	2.20	0.207
W4	1.58	0.36	1.50	0.80	2.60	1.58	0.37	1.60	1.00	2.20	0.946
R1	15.43[a]	4.44	15.12	7.38	28.50	13.03[a]	3.59	12.46	8.55	22.80	0.019[a]
R2	8.25[a]	2.51	7.77	3.41	20.29	6.12[a]	3.40	6.17	0.61	13.18	0.006[a]

*The data given in this table was taken from Karaaslan et al. [48]

[a]Denotes a statistically significant difference in these parameters between groups. *SD* standard deviation, *L1* transverse ligament length, *L2* alar ligament length, *W*1 transverse ligament width, *W*2 alar ligament width, *W*3 posterior atlanto-occipital membrane width, *W*4 anterior atlanto-occipital membrane width, *R*1 transverse ligament length/width ratio, *R*2 alar ligament length/width ratio

Table 18.5 Anatomically discernible ligaments related to the CCJ and MRI discernibility as discrete ligamentous structures and their relative contributions to the stability of the CCJ (in isolation)*

Anatomical ligaments of the craniocervical junction	MRI-discernible	Stability contribution
Stability contribution	+	++
Alar ligament	+	++
Cruciform (cruciate) ligament—transverse	+	++
Cruciform (cruciate) ligament—longitudinal	+/–	+/–
Apical ligament	+/–	+/–
Barkow ligament	+/–	+
Atlanto-occipital capsular ligament	+	+
Atlanto-axial capsular ligament	+	+
Anterior atlanto-occipital membrane	+	+
Posterior atlanto-occipital membrane	+	+
Anterior atlanto-axial membrane	+	+
Nuchal ligament (ligamentum nuchae)	+	+
Lateral atlanto-occipital ligament	–	–
Accessory atlanto-axial ligament	–	–
Transverse occipital ligament	–	–

*The data given in this table was taken from Offiah and Day [1]

References

1. Offiah CE, Day E. The craniocervical junction: embryology, anatomy, biomechanics and imaging in blunt trauma. Insights Imaging. 2017;8:29–47.
2. Offiah CE. Craniocervical junction and cervical spine anatomy. Neuroimaging Clin N Am. 2022;32:875–88.
3. Fiester P, Rao D, Soule E, Orallo P, Rahmathulla G. Anatomic, functional, and radiographic review of the ligaments of the craniocervical junction. J Craniovertebr Junction Spine. 2021;12:4–9.
4. Tubbs RS, Hallock JD, Radcliff V, Naftel RP, Mortazavi M, Shoja MM, Loukas M, Cohen-Gadol AA. Ligaments of the craniocervical junction. J Neurosurg Spine. 2011;14:697–709.
5. Debernardi A, D'Aliberti G, Talamonti G, Villa F, Piparo M, Collice M. The craniovertebral junction area and the role of the ligaments and membranes. Neurosurgery. 2015;76(Suppl 1):S22–32.
6. Menezes AH. Craniocervical developmental anatomy and its implications. Childs Nerv Syst. 2008;24:1109–22.
7. Pang D, Thompson DN. Embryology and bony malformations of the craniovertebral junction. Childs Nerv Syst. 2011;27:523–64.
8. Raybaud C. Anatomy and development of the craniovertebral junction. Neurol Sci. 2011;32(Suppl 3):S267–70.
9. Dvorak J, Schneider E, Saldinger P, Rahn B. Biomechanics of the craniocervical region: the alar and transverse ligaments. J Orthop Res. 1988;6:452–61.
10. Dickman CA, Mamourian A, Sonntag VK, Drayer BP. Magnetic resonance imaging of the transverse atlantal ligament for the evaluation of atlantoaxial instability. J Neurosurg. 1991;75:221–7.
11. Hita-Contreras F, Roda O, Martinez-Amat A, Cruz-Diaz D, Merida-Velasco JA, Sanchez-Montesinos I. Embryonic and early fetal period development and morphogenesis of human craniovertebral junction. Clin Anat. 2014;27:337–45.
12. Nidecker AE, Shen PY. Magnetic resonance imaging of the Craniovertebral junction ligaments: Normal anatomy and traumatic injury. J Neurol Surg B Skull Base. 2016;77:388–95.
13. Haffajee MR, Thompson C, Govender S. The supra-odontoid space or "apical cave" at the craniocervical junction: a microdissection study. Clin Anat. 2008;21:405–15.
14. Harris MB, Duval MJ, Davis JJ, Bernini PM. Anatomical and roentgenographic features of atlantooccipital instability. J Spinal Disord. 1993;6:5–10.
15. Crisco JR, Oda T, Panjabi MM, Bueff HU, Dvorak J, Grob D. Transections of the C1-C2 joint capsular ligaments in the cadaveric spine. Spine (Phila Pa 1976). 1991;16:S474–9.
16. Tubbs RS, Wellons JR, Blount JP, Oakes WJ. Posterior atlantooccipital membrane for duraplasty. J Neurosurg. 2002;97:266–8.
17. Zumpano MP, Hartwell S, Jagos CS. Soft tissue connection between rectus capitus posterior minor and the posterior atlanto-occipital membrane: a cadaveric study. Clin Anat. 2006;19:522–7.

18. Nash L, Nicholson H, Lee AS, Johnson GM, Zhang M. Configuration of the connective tissue in the posterior atlanto-occipital interspace: a sheet plastination and confocal microscopy study. Spine (Phila Pa 1976). 2005;30:1359–66.
19. Hack GD, Koritzer RT, Robinson WL, Hallgren RC, Greenman PE. Anatomic relation between the rectus capitis posterior minor muscle and the dura mater. Spine (Phila Pa 1976). 1995;20:2484–6.
20. Thompson VP. Anatomical research lives! Nat Med. 1995;1:297–8.
21. Akar Z, Kafadar AM, Tanriover N, Dashti RS, Islak C, Kocer N, Kuday C. Rotational compression of the vertebral artery at the point of dural penetration: case report. J Neurosurg. 2000;93:300–3.
22. Tubbs RS, Ammar K, Liechty P, Wellons JR, Blount JP, Salter EG, Oakes WJ. The marginal sinus. J Neurosurg. 2006;104:429–31.
23. Krakenes J, Kaale BR, Moen G, Nordli H, Gilhus NE, Rorvik J. MRI of the tectorial and posterior atlanto-occipital membranes in the late stage of whiplash injury. Neuroradiology. 2003;45:585–91.
24. Panjabi MM, Oda T, Crisco JR, Oxland TR, Katz L, Nolte LP. Experimental study of atlas injuries. I. Biomechanical analysis of their mechanisms and fracture patterns. Spine (Phila Pa 1976). 1991;16:S460–5.
25. Krakenes J, Kaale BR, Nordli H, Moen G, Rorvik J, Gilhus NE. MR analysis of the transverse ligament in the late stage of whiplash injury. Acta Radiol. 2003;44:637–44.
26. Krauss WE, Bledsoe JM, Clarke MJ, Nottmeier EW, Pichelmann MA. Rheumatoid arthritis of the craniovertebral junction. Neurosurgery. 2010;66:83–95.
27. Farley FA, Gebarski SS, Garton HL. Tectorial membrane injuries in children. J Spinal Disord Tech. 2005;18:136–8.
28. Panjabi MM, Oxland TR, Parks EH. Quantitative anatomy of cervical spine ligaments. Part I. Upper cervical spine. J Spinal Disord. 1991;4:270–6.
29. Krakenes J, Kaale BR, Rorvik J, Gilhus NE. MRI assessment of normal ligamentous structures in the craniovertebral junction. Neuroradiology. 2001;43:1089–97.
30. Lopez AJ, Scheer JK, Leibl KE, Smith ZA, Dlouhy BJ, Dahdaleh NS. Anatomy and biomechanics of the craniovertebral junction. Neurosurg Focus. 2015;38:E2.
31. Panjabi M, Dvorak J, Crisco JR, Oda T, Hilibrand A, Grob D. Flexion, extension, and lateral bending of the upper cervical spine in response to alar ligament transections. J Spinal Disord. 1991;4:157–67.
32. Panjabi M, Dvorak J, Crisco JR, Oda T, Wang P, Grob D. Effects of alar ligament transection on upper cervical spine rotation. J Orthop Res. 1991;9:584–93.
33. Derrick LJ, Chesworth BM. Post-motor vehicle accident alar ligament laxity. J Orthop Sports Phys Ther. 1992;16:6–11.
34. Pfirrmann CW, Binkert CA, Zanetti M, Boos N, Hodler J. MR morphology of alar ligaments and occipitoatlantoaxial joints: study in 50 asymptomatic subjects. Radiology. 2001;218:133–7.
35. Kaale BR, Krakenes J, Albrektsen G, Wester K. Whiplash-associated disorders impairment rating: neck disability index score according to severity of MRI findings of ligaments and membranes in the upper cervical spine. J Neurotrauma. 2005;22:466–75.
36. Kaale BR, Krakenes J, Albrektsen G, Wester K. Head position and impact direction in whiplash injuries: associations with MRI-verified lesions of ligaments and membranes in the upper cervical spine. J Neurotrauma. 2005;22:1294–302.
37. Werne S. Studies in spontaneous atlas dislocation. Acta Orthop Scand Suppl. 1957;23:1–150.
38. Tubbs RS, Salter EG, Oakes WJ. The accessory atlantoaxial ligament. Neurosurgery. 2004;55(400–402):402–4.
39. Ishak B, Glinski AV, Dupont G, Lachkar S, Yilmaz E, Iwanaga J, Unterberg A, Oskouian R, Tubbs RS, Chapman JR. Update on the biomechanics of the Craniocervical junction, part II: alar ligament. Global Spine J. 2021;11:1064–9.
40. Tubbs RS, Griessenauer CJ, McDaniel JG, Burns AM, Kumbla A, Cohen-Gadol AA. The transverse occipital ligament: anatomy and potential functional significance. Neurosurgery. 2010;66(1–3):3.
41. Tubbs RS, Stetler W, Shoja MM, Loukas M, Hansasuta A, Liechty P, Acakpo-Satchivi L, Wellons JC, Blount JP, Salter EG, Oakes WJ. The lateral atlantooccipital ligament. Surg Radiol Anat. 2007;29:219–23.
42. Parkinson D. The posterior cranial fossa: microsurgical anatomy and surgical approaches. Neurosurgery. 2001;48:1196.
43. Tubbs RS, Dixon J, Loukas M, Shoja MM, Cohen-Gadol AA. Ligament of Barkow of the craniocervical junction: its anatomy and potential clinical and functional significance. J Neurosurg Spine. 2010;12:619–22.
44. de Oliveira E, Rhoton AJ, Peace D. Microsurgical anatomy of the region of the foramen magnum. Surg Neurol. 1985;24:293–352.
45. Tubbs RS, Grabb P, Spooner A, Wilson W, Oakes WJ. The apical ligament: anatomy and functional significance. J Neurosurg. 2000;92:197–200.
46. Tubbs RS, Kelly DR, Humphrey ER, Chua GD, Shoja MM, Salter EG, Acakpo-Satchivi L, Wellons JR, Blount JP, Oakes WJ. The tectorial membrane: anatomical, biomechanical, and histological analysis. Clin Anat. 2007;20:382–6.
47. Vigo V, Hirpara A, Yassin M, Wang M, Chou D, De Bonis P, Abla A, Rodriguez RR. Immersive surgical anatomy of the Craniocervical junction. Cureus. 2020;12:e10364.
48. Karaaslan B, Borcek AO, Ucar M, Aykol S. Can the Etiopathogenesis of Chiari malformation be Craniocervical junction stabilization difference? Morphometric analysis of Craniocervical junction ligaments. World Neurosurg. 2019;128:e1096–101.

Atlanto-Axial Ligaments

19

Mengzhao Feng and Fuyou Guo

19.1 Introduction

The ligamentous system of the atlanto-axial joint is a complex array of connective tissue structures located at the cranio-cervical junction. It originates during embryo development and strengthens progressively as the fetus matures. These ligaments consist mainly of collagen and elastin fibers, exhibiting exceptional toughness and elasticity, which are crucial for the physiological movements of the cervical spine [1, 2].

The ligaments are strategically located around the atlanto-axial joint, which is the articulation between the atlas (C1) and axis (C2) vertebrae (Fig. 19.1). There are several of them: the transverse ligament of the atlas, apical ligament, alar ligaments, cruciform ligament of the atlas, and accessory atlanto-axial ligament [3, 4]. Their collagen fibers provide tensile strength, and their elastin fibers confer elasticity [5]. The precise

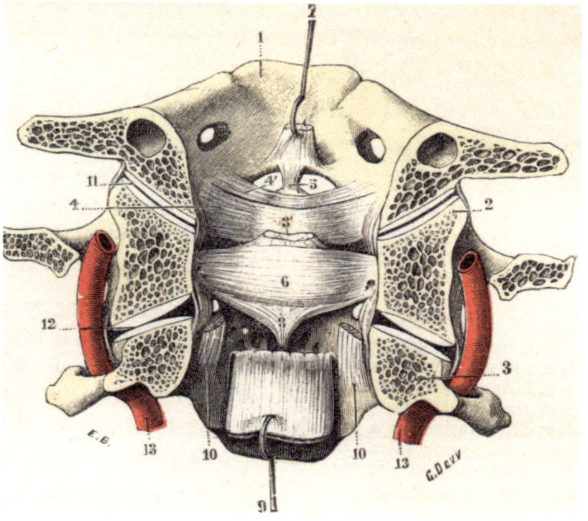

Fig. 19.1 Schematic drawing of the ligaments of the craniocervical junction. (After Testut). The apical ligament (5) and cruciform ligament (3 and 6) are illustrated. Also note the accessory atlanto-axial ligament (10) and alar ligaments located between the apical and cruciform ligaments. The relationship of the vertebral arteries (red) are shown

M. Feng · F. Guo (✉)
Department of Neurosurgery, The First Affiliated Hospital of Zhengzhou University, Zhengzhou, Henan, China

International Joint Laboratory of Nervous System Malformations, Zhengzhou, Henan, China
e-mail: chyou666@hotmail.com

M. Turgut et al. (eds.), *Ligaments of the Vertebral Column*,
https://doi.org/10.1007/978-3-032-09070-6_19

arrangement of these fibers contributes to the ability of ligaments to resist deformation under load and return to their original shape after the stress is removed [6].

Ligaments are crucial for stabilizing the odontoid process of the axis and preventing excessive movement, which could compromise the spinal cord [7]. They restrict the range of motion of the head and neck, particularly rotation, to protect neural structures from injury. Dysfunction or injury to the ligaments of the atlanto-axial joint can result in a spectrum of clinical manifestations, ranging from minor instability to severe neurological deficits [8]. Therefore, the integrity of these ligaments is critical for the overall health and function of the cranio-cervical junction [9]. Understanding the definitions and roles of these ligaments is essential for clinicians to diagnose, treat, and manage conditions affecting the upper cervical spine.

19.2 Atlanto-Axial Ligament Anatomy

19.2.1 Apical Ligament

The apical ligament is a slender, fibrous structure that lies deep within the transverse ligament of the atlas. It originates from the tip of the odontoid process, a bony projection from the axis vertebra, and inserts into the anterior edge of the foramen magnum, a large opening at the base of the skull (Fig. 19.1).

Functionally, the apical ligament acts as a check ligament, resisting posterior displacement of the odontoid process. The apical ligament may also be involved in fine-tuning the rotational movements of the head to ensure smooth and controlled rotation.

19.2.2 Alar Ligaments

The alar ligament (AL) are a strong, cord-like ligaments that arise from the lateral aspect of the odontoid process (Fig. 19.1). They extend laterally and upward, attaching to the medial surfaces of the occipital condyles, which are bony prominences on the skull that articulate with the atlas [10, 11].

These ligaments are crucial for limiting the rotational movement of the head and atlas along the axis [12]. They provide a stabilizing force that prevents excessive rotation, which can lead to instability and potentially to spinal cord injury [13]. The AL are particularly important during rotational movements of the neck such as turning the head to look over the shoulder.

19.2.3 Transverse Ligament of Atlas

The transverse ligament of atlas is a broad, strong ligament positioned posteriorly to the odontoid process. It connects the lateral masses of the atlas and effectively forms a bony ligamentous ring around the odontoid process (Figs. 19.1, 19.2, 19.3, and 19.4) [14].

Its primary function is to stabilize the odontoid process against the anterior arch of the atlas [15], preventing it from being displaced posteriorly into the spinal canal, which would pose a serious risk to the spinal cord. The TLA is considered one of the most important ligaments of the upper cervical spine because of its role in preventing atlanto-axial instability and potential spinal cord injury [16].

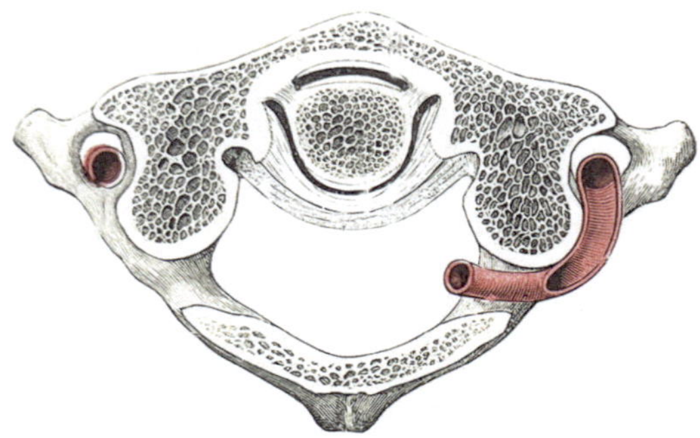

Fig. 19.2 Schematic drawing of the transverse atlantal ligament. Also note the vertebral arteries (red). (After Testut)

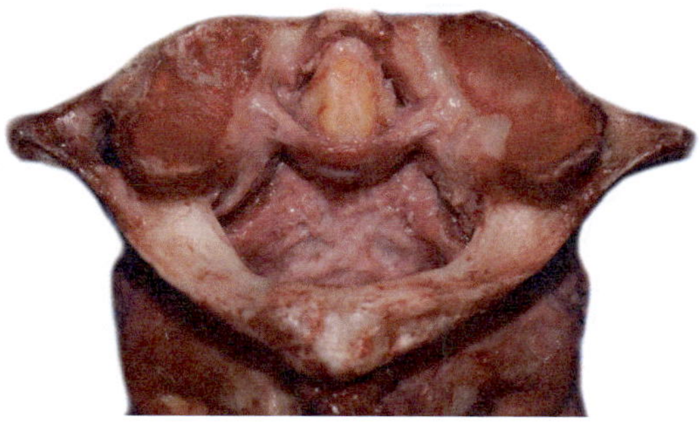

Fig. 19.3 Articulated cadaveric C1 and C 2 vertebrae with intact transverse ligament

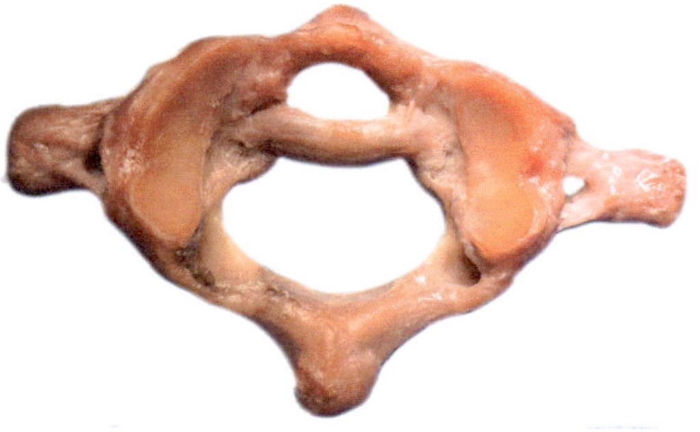

Fig. 19.4 Disarticulated C1 noting the intact transverse ligament in a cadaveric specimen

19.2.4 Cruciform Ligament of Atlas

The cruciform ligament of atlas (CLA) is a complex structure that includes both the transverse ligament and longitudinal fibers that extend from it. The term "cruciform" refers to the cross shape formed by these fibers. The CLA enhances the stability of the TLA by reinforcing the ligamentous ring around the odontoid process. This contributes to the overall rigidity of the atlanto-axial joint, ensuring that the joint can withstand forces generated during head movement.

19.2.5 Accessory Atlanto-Axial Ligament

The accessory atlanto-axial ligament (AAL) originates from the lateral masses of the atlas and slopes downward and medially, attaching to the posterior aspect of the axis vertebra (Fig. 19.1).

It limits the rotational movement of the atlas along the axis, which stabilizes the joint further. It is particularly important in controlling the range of motion during neck flexion and extension.

19.2.6 Tectorial Membrane

The tectorial membrane is a broad, strong ligament located within the spinal canal. It covers the odontoid process and other ligaments in the region, and provides additional support and stability to the atlanto-axial joint (Fig. 19.1). It extends from the foramen magnum to the upper cervical vertebrae and contributes to the overall structural integrity of the spinal column. Each of these ligaments makes its own distinctive contribution to the stability and function of the atlanto-axial joint, ensuring that the head moves freely while delicate neural structures within the spinal canal are protected.

Owing to their strategic positioning and structural properties, these ligaments are critical in the biomechanics of the cranio-cervical junction. They ensure that the head can move with agility while simultaneously protecting the spinal cord and other neural structures from injury.

19.3 Blood Supply to the Atlanto-Axial Ligaments

19.3.1 Vertebral Artery

The vertebral artery (VA) is a major supplier of blood to the atlanto-axial ligaments. It ascends through the transverse foramina of the cervical vertebrae and enters the skull through the foramen magnum (Figs. 19.1 and 19.2). As it ascends, several branches are formed.

Muscular branches: These supply the muscles surrounding the atlanto-axial joint, which indirectly support the ligaments.

Meningeal branches: These supply the meninges, which in turn provide a vascular supply to the adjacent ligaments.

Spinal branches: These penetrate the spinal canal and supply it with branches reaching the ligaments.

19.3.2 Occipital Artery

The occpital artery (OA) arises from the external carotid artery and has several branches that extend into the muscles and ligaments of the posterior neck.

Muscular branches: These supply the muscles around the cranio-cervical junction, indirectly supporting the ligaments.

Meningeal branches: These supply the meninges and ligaments associated with the occipital bone and atlas.

19.3.3 Deep Cervical Artery

The deep cervical artery (DCA), a branch of the subclavian artery, supplies blood to the deep muscles and ligaments of the neck.

Muscular branches: These supply the deep muscles of the neck, which are critical for the stability of the cervical spine and indirectly support the ligaments.

19.3.4 Ligament-Specific Blood Supply

Each ligament of the atlanto-axial joint receives a specific blood supply from its surrounding arterial network.

Apical ligament: receives blood from branches of the VA and OA.

AL: supplied by branches of the VA and DCA.

TLA: primarily supplied by the VA, with contributions from the DCA.

CLA: receives blood from branches of the transverse ligament and the surrounding muscular branches.

AAL: supplied by the DCA and branches from the VA.

Tectorial membrane: receives blood from the VA and DCA.

The vascular supply to the ligaments of the atlanto-axial joint is complex and critical for maintaining cranio-cervical junction stability. The VA, OA, and DCA are pivotal in nourishing the ligaments and ensuring their structural integrity and function. Disruptions of this vascular network can have significant clinical implications, highlighting the importance of understanding and preserving the blood supply in both clinical practice and surgical interventions.

19.4 Physiological Functions of the Atlanto-Axial Ligaments

19.4.1 Stabilization of the Odontoid Process

The odontoid process, also known as the dens, is a distinct bony projection that rises superiorly from the body of the axis (C2) vertebra. It is pivotal in the atlanto-axial joint, which connects the atlas (C1) and the axis (C2). The odontoid process articulates with the anterior arch of the atlas, forming a crucial atlanto-axial joint [17]. The TLA is a broad, strong ligament located directly posterior to the odontoid process. It connects the lateral masses of the atlas and effectively creates a bony and ligamentous ring encircling the odontoid process. This ring is critical for maintaining the position of the odontoid process and preventing movement in an unsafe direction. A primary function of the TLA is to prevent posterior displacement of the odontoid process, which can compress the spinal cord if it moves posteriorly, leading to serious neurological complications, including paralysis. The TLA acts as a barrier, ensuring that the odontoid process remains in its proper anterior position relative to the spinal cord.

The TLA is the main ligament responsible for stabilizing the odontoid process, but it works in conjunction with others such as the alar ligament (AL) and apical ligament [18]. The AL extends from the odontoid process to the occipital condyles and helps limit rotational movement, further stabilizing the odontoid process [19]. The apical ligament connects the tip of the odontoid process to the anterior edge of the foramen magnum and provides additional support and stability [20].

The integrity of the TLA is crucial for the health of the upper cervical spine. Injuries or disruptions to it can lead to instability of the atlanto-axial joint, potentially resulting in displacement of the odontoid process and spinal cord compression [21]. This can manifest clinically as neck pain, limited neck movement, and neurological symptoms such as weakness or numbness in the limbs.

In cases of trauma such as whiplash or cervical spine fractures, the TLA can be injured, leading to instability and an increased risk of odontoid process displacement [22–24]. The TLA can be eroded in degenerative conditions such as rheumatoid arthritis, compromising its ability to stabilize the odontoid process [25, 26]. In both scenarios, the potential for spinal cord compression and neurological injury is increased. In some cases, surgical intervention is necessary to repair or reinforce the TLA, particularly if there is severe instability or following trauma [27]. Understanding the anatomy and function of the TLA is essential for surgeons to manage conditions affecting the atlanto-axial joint effectively and to prevent further complications.

In pathological conditions such as aging, the TLA often calcifies naturally. A retrospective cross-sectional study showed that the prevalence of TLA calcification in asymptomatic healthy individuals is 3.5%, increasing significantly with advancing age [28, 29]. This study categorized calcified lesions into two types: type 1 presents as thin calcifications measuring less than 2 mm, and type 2 is characterized by thicker curvilinear lesions exceeding 2 mm. Notably, there were annual morphological changes in these calcified lesions, 14% of cases showing enlargement of the lesion and 16% demonstrating a decrease or disappearance.

Calcification of the TLA has been traditionally implicated in conditions that cause acute neck pain and stiffness, commonly referred to as the crowned dens syndrome [30, 31]. However, it is important to recognize that such calcifications in asymptomatic individuals could indicate age-related degenerative change rather than an active inflammatory process [32]. The implications of TLA calcification extend beyond anatomical alterations that can lead to spinal cord compression and consequent neurological deficits. The propensity of type 2 calcifications to increase over time suggests an increased risk of spinal cord impingement with age.

Considering these findings, it is imperative that clinicians monitor the cervical spine health of aging patients, particularly for signs of TLA calcification or its progression. Early detection and appropriate intervention are necessary to prevent the potential neurological complications associated with spinal cord compression. The natural course of TLA calcification underscores the importance of understanding the degenerative processes that affect the cranio-cervical junction and the need for timely clinical intervention to mitigate the risk of neurological compromise.

19.4.2 Restriction of Excessive Movement

The AL are key to limiting rotational movements of the head [33]. They extend from the odontoid process to the occipital condyles and ensure that the head does not rotate beyond safe limits; they are crucial for limiting the rotational movement of the head on the neck [34]. When the head is turned from side to side, the ALs act as restraints, preventing the head from rotating beyond a certain limit [35]. This is vital for maintaining the stability of the cranio-cervical junction and protecting the spinal cord.

As the head rotates, the ALs become taut and provide a counterforce to resist further rotation. This tension in them acts as a brake, limiting the extent of head rotation and preventing the odontoid process from moving too far laterally, which could potentially cause instability or injury [36].

In conjunction with other ligaments and neck structures, the AL functions to provide comprehensive stability. For instance, the TLA and apical ligament also contribute to the overall stability of the odontoid process, but the AL specifically targets rotational movements.

Injuries to the ALs can result in excessive head rotation, leading to instability at the atlanto-axial joint [37]. This can cause neck pain, headaches, and dizziness [38]. In severe cases, it can also lead to spinal cord compression and neurological deficits, highlighting the importance of these ligaments in maintaining the structural integrity of the neck [39]. In traumatic conditions such as whiplash or sports injuries, the ALs can be stretched or torn, leading to a condition known as atlanto-axial rotatory subluxation. This condition is characterized by abnormal rotation of the atlas along the axis, which can cause neurological symptoms if the spinal cord is compromised [40]. If the ALs are severely injured or have been surgically removed, the head can be prone to excessive rotation [41]. Surgical interventions such as fusion procedures can then be required to stabilize the joint and prevent further damage, limiting movement and providing additional support. The AL are essential for everyday activities that involve turning the head such as driving, looking over the shoulders, or simply interacting with the environment. Their role in limiting rotation helps ensure that these movements are performed safely and without causing injury.

19.4.3 Support During Head Movement

The apical ligament and AAL provide support during flexion and extension of the head. The apical ligament connects the tip of the odontoid process to the anterior edge of the foramen magnum, helping stabilize the head during forward movement [42].

During forward flexion of the head (nodding), the apical ligament becomes taut, providing a stabilizing force that helps maintain the position of the odontoid process. This prevents the odontoid process from moving excessively anteriorly, potentially compressing the spinal cord or other neural structures. When the head is extended backward, the apical ligament relaxes to accommodate the movement, but it still provides a degree of support and restraint, preventing the odontoid process from moving too far posteriorly and ensuring that the head does not hyperextend.

The AAL is another ligament that provides head support during movement. It originates from the lateral masses of the atlas (C1), slopes downward and medially, and attaches to the posterior aspect of the vertebral axis (C2). It helps limit the rotational movement of the atlas on the axis, providing additional stability. The apical ligament and AAL work in conjunction with other ligaments such as the TLA and AL to provide comprehensive support to the head and neck [43]. While the TLA primarily stabilizes the odontoid process posteriorly, the apical ligament and AAL contribute to anterior and lateral stability.

Injuries to the apical ligament or AAL can result in instability of the cranio-cervical junction, leading to symptoms such as neck pain, limited head movement, and neurological symptoms if the spinal cord or nerve roots are compromised. Understanding the role of these ligaments is crucial for the diagnosis and treatment of conditions affecting the upper cervical spine. In cases of trauma such as falls or motor vehicle accidents, the apical ligament and AAL can be stretched or torn, leading to instability of the odontoid process. This can result in atlanto-axial instability, which can be serious and potentially life-threatening if not properly managed [44]. The apical ligament and AAL are essential for everyday activities that involve head movements, such as looking up at the sky, nodding in agreement, or turning the head to look over the shoulder. Their role in providing support and stability ensures that these movements can be performed safely without causing injuries.

19.4.4 Protection of Neural Structures

The CLA and tectorial membrane provide protective barriers around the spinal cord, preventing the odontoid process from moving backward and injuring the spinal cord during neck movement.

The CLA and tectorial membrane work together to prevent the odontoid process from moving backward. This is particularly important during neck movements such as flexion, when the odontoid process could be driven backward into the spinal cord if not restrained. By maintaining the position of the odontoid process, these ligaments reduce the risk of spinal cord injury and ensure that neural structures within the spinal canal are protected.

The biomechanical properties of the CLA and tectorial membrane are crucial for their protective functions. They must be sufficiently strong and flexible to withstand the forces generated during neck movements and still provide the necessary restraint on the odontoid process. The elasticity of the ligaments allows them to stretch slightly during movement, accommodating the range of motion while still providing support and protection.

Injury to the CLA or tectorial membrane can lead to instability of the atlanto-axial joint, potentially resulting in spinal cord compression and neurological symptoms. This can manifest as neck pain, limited neck movement, weakness, or numbness of the limbs [45]. In severe cases such as traumatic injuries or pathological processes such as tumors or infections, the protective barrier provided by these ligaments can be compromised, leading to serious neurological consequences.

In the event of trauma such as a high-speed car accident or fall, the forces applied to the neck can strain or tear the CLA and tectorial membrane. This can result in atlanto-axial instability and an increased risk of spinal cord injury [46]. The integrity of these ligaments can be compromised in degenerative diseases or inflammatory conditions, leading to laxity and a reduced ability to protect the spinal cord. During surgical procedures involving the upper cervical spine such as spinal fusion or decompression, the integrity of the CLA and tectorial membrane must be carefully preserved to maintain the protective barrier around the spinal cord [47]. Surgical reinforcement of these ligaments is sometimes necessary to restore stability and protect the spinal cord, particularly in cases of severe instability or traumatic injuries [27].

19.4.5 Maintenance of Cranio-Cervical Alignment

Integrity of the atlanto-axial ligaments is essential for keeping the skull aligned with the cervical spine [48]. In particular, the TLA ensures that the atlas (C1) and axis (C2) vertebrae maintain their proper relationship, which is critical for the overall stability of the cervical spine.

The TLA is a broad, strong ligament that connects the lateral masses of the atlas and forms a ring around the odontoid axis. It is critical for maintaining alignment of the atlas and axis vertebrae. It prevents the odontoid process from moving posteriorly, which could otherwise lead to misalignment and potential compression of the spinal cord. The alar ligaments arise from the lateral aspects of the odontoid process and are attached to the medial aspects of the occipital condyle. They limit rotational movements of the head, ensuring that the skull remains aligned with the cervical spine during such movements [49].

The apical ligament connects the tip of the odontoid process to the anterior edge of the foramen magnum. It helps stabilize the odontoid process during flexion and extension of the head and contributes to maintaining cranio-cervical alignment. The accessory atlanto-axial ligament originates from the lateral masses of the atlas and attaches to the posterior aspect of the axis vertebra. It provides additional stability and limits rotational movement, contributing further to maintaining cranio-cervical alignment. Proper alignment between the skull and cervical spine is essential for the normal functioning of the neck and for protecting the spinal cord and nerve roots. Misalignment can lead to a variety of symptoms including neck pain, headaches, and neurological symptoms such as numbness or weakness of the arms [50].

Injuries or pathological conditions that affect atlanto-axial ligament integrity can lead to cranio-cervical malalignment. This can result in conditions such as atlanto-axial instability or dislocation, which can be serious and potentially life-threatening if the spinal cord is compromised. In such cases, conservative management with immobilization or surgical intervention can be needed to restore stability and alignment. In cases of trauma such as whiplash or high-impact accidents, the atlanto-axial ligaments can be stretched or torn, leading to malalignment of the skull and the cervical spine [51]. This can result in a range of symptoms requiring immediate medical attention and intervention. The atlanto-axial ligaments are crucial in everyday activities involving head and neck movement. They allow for a wide range of motion while ensuring that the skull remains properly aligned with the cervical spine and protecting the spinal cord and nerve roots from injury.

The integrity of the atlanto-axial ligaments, particularly the TLA, is fundamental for maintaining the proper alignment of the skull with the cervical spine. This alignment is critical for overall stability of the cervical spine, normal functioning of the neck, and protection of the spinal cord and nerve roots. Significant clinical manifestations can result if it is disrupted, and medical intervention can be needed to restore stability and prevent further complications.

19.5 Atlanto-Axial Ligamentous Developmental Malformations

Atlanto-axial ligamentous developmental malformations (ALDM) encompass a spectrum of congenital disorders that can significantly affect the structural and functional integrity of the upper cervical spine. These anomalies specifically target ligamentous structures at the crucial junction between the skull and spinal column, involving the occipital bone and the atlas (C1) and axis (C2) vertebrae. The effect of these anomalies extends beyond local biomechanical issues, often leading to a cascade of neurological symptoms resulting from instability, and potentially to spinal cord compression in this critical region [52].

FBN1, located on chromosome 15q21.1, encodes fibrillin-1, a key component of extracellular microfibrils. Fibrillin-1 is essential for the structural integrity of the connective tissues. Mutations in *FBN1* have been implicated in various connective tissue disorders including Marfan syndrome. In the context of ALDM, *FBN1* mutations can result in the weakening of crucial ligaments around the atlanto-axial joint such as the TLA, AL, and apical ligament. This can lead to atlanto-axial dislocation (AAD) and basilar invagination (BI) [53].

The prevalence of *FBN1*-related disorders, including ALDM, is estimated at one in 5000 individuals. Atlanto-axial ligamentous developmental malformations can be inherited in an autosomal dominant manner, with variable expressivity and reduced penetrance. Familial clustering of ALDM has been reported [53]. This condition can also occur sporadically owing to de novo mutations.

In a previous study, DNA sequence variants in *FBN1* were identified in 39 of 50 cases (78%) with developmental cervical-vertebral joint anomalies [54]. Exons 25, 26, 27, and 28 exhibited variable patterns of DNA bands in single-stranded conformation polymorphisms, which, upon sequencing, yielded DNA sequence variations in the intronic region of the *FBN1* gene at rates of 14, 14, 6, and 44%, respectively. These findings suggest that *FBN1* mutations are significant genetic factors contributing to ALDM.

19.5.1 Clinical Features of Atlanto-Axial Ligamentous Developmental Malformation

Craniovertebral junction anomalies: Weakening or malformation of these ligaments owing to *FBN1* mutations can predispose individuals to

AAD, a condition in which the atlas (C1) and axis (C2) vertebrae are no longer properly aligned. This dislocation can lead to spinal instability, spinal cord compression, and consequent neurological deficits [55, 56]. Moreover, when AAD coexists with basilar invagination (BI), the odontoid process of the axis vertebra is drawn upward into the foramen magnum, which can exacerbate the compression of neural structures and lead to a myriad of neurological symptoms.

Neurological manifestations: Patients often present with a range of neurological symptoms depending on the type of malformation. Common signs include limb weakness, dizziness, sensory disturbances, ataxia, nystagmus, unsteady gait, paralysis, epileptic seizures, and incontinence [57].

Syringomyelia: Co-occurrence with developmental anomalies of the atlanto-axial ligaments, presenting with symptoms such as separation of pain and temperature sensations in the cervical and thoracic regions and muscle atrophy or deformity in the limb.

Cerebrospinal fluid (CSF) Circulation Abnormalities: Most patients complain of occipital headaches that are heavy, pressing, or pulsating, and are exacerbated by physical exertion, Valsalva maneuvers, or sudden changes in posture.

Ocular symptoms: A significant proportion of patients experience symptoms such as retro-orbital pain, visual floaters, photophobia, blurred vision, diplopia, and visual field loss.

Aural symptoms: Symptoms such as dizziness, balance disorders, tinnitus, aural pressure, hearing loss, and auditory hypersensitivity are common.

19.5.2 Impact of Atlanto-Axial Ligamentous Developmental Malformation

Compression of neural structures: Compression of the brainstem, cerebellum, and spinal cord owing to abnormal development and instability in the cranio-cervical junction.

Spinal cord injury: Manifestations include limb weakness, spasticity, sensory hyperesthesia or disturbances, and proprioceptive deficits.

Quality of life: Chronic occipital pain and discomfort owing to abnormal CSF circulation can significantly affect daily activities and quality of life [32]. If chronic, symptoms such as pain and motor deficits can lead to significant disability and reduced functionality. Moreover, the psychological effect of living with uncertainty and the fear of potential neurological deterioration can be no less challenging.

19.5.3 Diagnosis of Atlanto-Axial Ligamentous Developmental Malformations

Diagnostic imaging is indispensable for evaluating ALDM [58]. Imaging by radiography, CT, and MRI provides detailed visualization of the bony structures and soft tissues, allowing malformations, instability, and neural compression to be identified accurately [59–61]. These imaging studies are crucial not only for diagnosis but also for surgical planning, as they inform the selection of the most appropriate intervention and help in anticipating potential challenges during surgery [62].

19.5.4 Surgical Intervention of Atlanto-Axial Ligamentous Developmental Malformation

Surgical intervention is often warranted for patients with ALDM, particularly when conservative treatment fails to alleviate symptoms or when there is a risk of neurological deterioration. Surgical objectives include stabilizing the cranio-cervical junction, decompressing neural structures, and preventing further instability [63, 64]. However, these surgeries are technically demanding and carry inherent risks owing to the proximity of vital structures such as the spinal cord and the vertebral artery. Meticulous preoperative assessment and postoperative care are crucial for optimizing outcomes and minimizing complications.

19.6 Conclusion

The atlanto-axial joint, a pivotal component of the cranio-cervical junction, is subject to a complex interplay of biomechanical forces that enable a wide range of head and neck movements essential for daily functioning to be made. This chapter provides an in-depth analysis of the critical role of the atlanto-axial ligaments in maintaining the stability and mobility of this region while also safeguarding the underlying neural structures from potential injury.

The anatomical intricacies of the atlanto-axial ligaments—the transverse ligament of the atlas, apical ligament, alar ligament, cruciform ligament of the atlas, and accessory atlanto-axial ligament—are described in detail. Each of these ligaments makes its distinctive contribution to the stability and function of the atlanto-axial joint, highlighting the importance of their structural integrity for the overall health and function of the cranio-cervical junction.

The clinical implications of these ligaments have been extensively discussed, emphasizing their indispensable role in preventing excessive movements that could lead to spinal cord compromise. The critical contribution of the vascular network to the health of these ligaments, including the vertebral, occipital, and deep cervical arteries, has also been emphasized. Disruptions of this vascular network can have significant clinical implications, underscoring the importance of understanding and preserving the blood supply in clinical practice and surgical interventions.

The effect of developmental malformations, such as those associated with *FBN1* mutations, on the integrity and function of these ligaments has been explored. These malformations can potentially lead to neurological symptoms and spinal cord compression, highlighting the need for advanced imaging techniques such as radiography, CT, and MRI in the diagnostic process. These imaging modalities are vital for visualizing bony structures and soft tissues so that malformations, instabilities, and neural compression can be identified.

This chapter also discusses surgical interventions for atlanto-axial ligamentous developmental anomalies. The complexities and risks associated with such procedures have been emphasized along with the importance of meticulous preoperative planning and postoperative care. The role of surgical stabilization in managing conditions affecting the upper cervical spine has been highlighted, particularly in cases of severe instability or subsequent trauma.

The physiological functions of the atlanto-axial ligaments have been discussed, including stabilization of the odontoid process, restriction of excessive movement, support during head movement, protection of neural structures, and maintenance of cranio-cervical alignment. These functions are crucial for the normal functioning of the neck and for protecting the spinal cord and nerve roots. Any disruption of the integrity of these ligaments can lead to various symptoms and immediate medical attention and intervention can be required.

The conclusion of this chapter underscores the importance of a comprehensive understanding of the atlanto-axial ligaments for the diagnosis, treatment, and management of conditions affecting the upper cervical spine. The intricate balance between stability and mobility at the cranio-cervical junction is maintained through the coordinated action of these ligaments, and any disruption of this balance can have significant clinical consequences.

In pathological conditions such as aging, the potential for degenerative changes in the ligaments, such as calcification of the transverse ligament, has been discussed. Calcification can lead to spinal cord compression and subsequent neurological deficits, making routine check-ups of the cervical spine important, particularly for aged patients.

This chapter highlights the importance of understanding the biomechanics of the cranio-cervical junction during trauma. Injuries to the atlanto-axial ligaments can result in instability, leading to symptoms such as neck pain, limited cranial movement, and neurological symptoms if the spinal cord or nerve roots are compromised. The value of advanced imaging in the diagnosis and surgical planning of these conditions has been emphasized.

In conclusion, the atlanto-axial ligaments are vital for the stability and function of the craniocervical junction. Their integrity is essential for the normal movement of the cranium and neck and for protecting delicate neural structures within the spinal canal. Any compromise of these ligaments resulting from developmental malformations, degenerative processes, or traumatic injuries can have significant clinical implications. This chapter has provided a thorough overview of the anatomy, physiology, and clinical relevance of the atlanto-axial ligaments, presenting a foundation for further research and clinical advancements in the management of conditions affecting this critical region of the spine.

References

1. Goel A. Atlantoaxial instability: evolving understanding. Acta Neurochir Suppl. 2019;125:59–62.
2. Wittig TM, Ziegeler K, Kreutzinger V, Golchev M, Ponsel S, Diekhoff T, Ulas ST. Dual-energy computed tomography collagen density mapping of the Cranio-cervical ligaments-a retrospective feasibility study. Diagnostics (Basel). 2022;12(12):2966.
3. Charbonneau L, Watanabe K, Chaalala C, Bojanowski MW, Lavigne P, Labidi M. Anatomy of the craniocervical junction – a review. Neurochirurgie. 2024;70(3):101511.
4. Tubbs RS, Salter EG, Oakes WJ. The accessory atlantoaxial ligament. Neurosurgery. 2004;55(2):400–2.
5. Beyer B, Feipel V, Dugailly PM. Biomechanics of the upper cervical spine ligaments in axial rotation and flexion-extension: considerations into the clinical framework. J Craniovertebr Junction Spine. 2020;11(3):217–25.
6. Zheng N, Chi YY, Yang XH, Wang NX, Li YL, Ge YY, Zhang LX, Liu TY, Yuan XY, Yu SB, Sui HJ. Orientation and property of fibers of the myodural bridge in humans. Spine J. 2018;18(6):1081–7.
7. Oakes PC, Sardi JP, Iwanaga J, Topale N, Oskouian RJ, Tubbs RS. Translation of Hecker's 1922 "the occipital-atlanto-axial ligament system": a study in comparative anatomy. Clin Anat. 2017;30(3):322–9.
8. Hu D, Yang X, Wang J. Traumatic posterior atlanto-axial dislocation without fracture of odontoid process: a case report and systematic analysis of 19 cases. J Orthop Trauma. 2015;29(9):e342–5.
9. Martin MD, Bruner HJ, Maiman DJ. Anatomic and biomechanical considerations of the craniovertebral junction. Neurosurgery. 2010;66(3 Suppl):2–6.
10. Osmotherly PG, Folbigg SL, Symonds JT. Normal range of movement during rotation stress testing for the alar ligaments: an observational study. J Manip Physiol Ther. 2022;45(2):137–43.
11. Roy S, Hol PK, Laerum LT, Tillung T. Pitfalls of magnetic resonance imaging of alar ligament. Neuroradiology. 2004;46(5):392–8.
12. Takizawa N, Nomura A, Fujita Y. Rare cause of nuchal pain: calcification of the alar ligament. J Rheumatol. 2016;43(1):177–8.
13. Scholz M, Kandziora F, Hildebrand F, Kobbe P. Verletzungen der oberen Halswirbelsäule: update zu Diagnostik und management [Injuries of the upper cervical spine: update on diagnostics and management]. Unfallchirurg. 2017;120(8):683–700.
14. Ishak B, Dupont G, Lachkar S, Yilmaz E, Glinski AV, Altafulla J, Kikuta S, Iwanaga J, Chapman JR, Oskouian R, Tubbs RS. Update on the biomechanics of the Craniocervical junction-part I: transverse Atlantal ligament in the elderly. Global Spine J. 2021;11(2):180–6.
15. Ott N, Harland A, Scaal M, König J, Bredow J, Eysel P, Müller LP, Meyer C. The role of the transversal ligament on the atlantoaxial complex – bending forces at C1/2 flexion limits in the elderly. Clin Biomech (Bristol, Avon). 2021;84:105329.
16. Zhang P, Jin G, Sun Z, Jiang J, Liu Q. An in vitro biomechanical study of the ectopic functional reconstruction of the transverse ligament of atlas. World Neurosurg. 2023;172:e220–4.
17. Jain N, Verma R, Garga UC, Baruah BP, Jain SK, Bhaskar SN. CT and MR imaging of odontoid abnormalities: a pictorial review. Indian J Radiol Imaging. 2016;26(1):108–19.
18. Iwanaga J, Sardi J, Voin V, Chapman JR, Oskouian RJ, Tubbs RS. Anatomy of alar ligament part I: Morphometrics and variants. World Neurosurg. 2017;107:1001–6.
19. Sardi JP, Iwanaga J, Voin V, Schmidt C, Loukas M, Chapman JR, Oskouian RJ, Tubbs RS. The alar ligaments: a cadaveric and radiologic comparison study. World Neurosurg. 2018;110:517–20.
20. Menezes AH, Traynelis VC. Anatomy and biomechanics of normal craniovertebral junction (a) and biomechanics of stabilization (b). Childs Nerv Syst. 2008;24(10):1091–100.
21. Shen K, Deng Z, Yang J, Liu C, Zhang R. Novel posterior artificial atlanto-odontoid joint for atlantoaxial instability: a biomechanical study. J Neurosurg Spine. 2018;28(5):459–66.
22. Meyer C, Eysel P, Stein G. Traumatic atlantoaxial and fracture-related dislocation. Biomed Res Int. 2019;2019:5297950.
23. Kim SK, Chang DG, Park JB, Seo HY, Kim YH. Traumatic atlanto-axial rotatory subluxation and dens fracture with subaxial SCIWORA of Brown-Sequard syndrome: a case report. Medicine (Baltimore). 2021;100(16):e25588.
24. Fiester P, Orallo P, Soule E, Rao D, Tavanaiepour D. Utility of anterior Atlantodens interval widening on cervical spine CT for assessing transverse Atlantal ligament injury. Global Spine J. 2023;13(8):2319–26.

25. Sharif K, Sharif A, Jumah F, Oskouian R, Tubbs RS. Rheumatoid arthritis in review: clinical, anatomical, cellular and molecular points of view. Clin Anat. 2018;31(2):216–23.
26. Wasserman BR, Moskovich R, Razi AE. Rheumatoid arthritis of the cervical spine – clinical considerations. Bull NYU Hosp Jt Dis. 2011;69(2):136–48.
27. Riascos R, Bonfante E, Cotes C, Guirguis M, Hakimelahi R, West C. Imaging of Atlanto-occipital and atlantoaxial traumatic injuries: what the radiologist needs to know. Radiographics. 2015;35(7):2121–34.
28. Anno M, Oshima Y, Taniguchi Y, Matsubayashi Y, Kato S, Soma K, Oka H, Hayashi N, Tanaka S. Prevalence and natural course of transverse ligament of the atlas calcification in asymptomatic healthy individuals. Spine (Phila Pa 1976). 2018;43(24):e1469–73.
29. Rothschild B. Alar and transverse ligament calcification and crown dens. J Rheumatol. 2016;43(6):1251.
30. Oka A, Okazaki K, Takeno A, Kumanomido S, Kusunoki R, Sato S, Ishihara S, Kinoshita Y, Nishina M. Crowned dens syndrome: report of three cases and a review of the literature. J Emerg Med. 2015;49(1):e9–e13.
31. Godfrin-Valnet M, Godfrin G, Godard J, Prati C, Toussirot E, Michel F, Wendling D. Eighteen cases of crowned dens syndrome: presentation and diagnosis. Neurochirurgie. 2013;59(3):115–20.
32. Fortin JD. Precision diagnostic disc injections. Pain Physician. 2000;3(3):271–88.
33. Missori P, Marruzzo D, Peschillo S, Domenicucci M. Clinical remarks on acute post-traumatic atlanto-axial rotatory subluxation in pediatric-aged patients. World Neurosurg. 2014;82(5):e645–8.
34. Sardi JP, Iwanaga J, Schmidt C, Rustagi T, Chapman JR, Oskouian RJ, Tubbs RS. Anatomy of the alar ligament: part II: variations of its attachment onto the dens. World Neurosurg. 2017;107:1007–11.
35. Iwanaga J, Sardi JP, Laws T, Chapman JR, Oskouian RJ, Tubbs RS. Anatomy of alar ligament part III: biomechanical study. World Neurosurg. 2017;107:1012–5.
36. Ng C, Dominguez JF, Feldstein E, Houten JK, Spirollari E, Gandhi CD, Cole CD, Kinon MD. Does alar ligament injury predict conservative treatment failure of atlantoaxial rotatory subluxation in adults: case report and review of the literature. Spinal Cord Ser Cases. 2021;7(1):103.
37. Wong ST, Ernest K, Fan G, Zovickian J, Pang D. Isolated unilateral rupture of the alar ligament. J Neurosurg Pediatr. 2014;13(5):541–7.
38. Steilen D, Hauser R, Woldin B, Sawyer S. Chronic neck pain: making the connection between capsular ligament laxity and cervical instability. Open Orthop J. 2014;8:326–45.
39. Henderson FC Sr, Rosenbaum R, Narayanan M, Koby M, Tuchman K, Rowe PC, Francomano C. Atlanto-axial rotary instability (fielding type 1): characteristic clinical and radiological findings, and treatment outcomes following alignment, fusion, and stabilization. Neurosurg Rev. 2021;44(3):1553–68.
40. Pang D. Atlantoaxial rotatory fixation. Neurosurgery. 2010;66(3 Suppl):161–83.
41. Wölfle-Roos J. Atlasblockade und Lig.-alare-Läsion – unterschätzt oder übertrieben? [Atlas block and alar ligament lesion-underestimated or overrated?]. Schmerz. 2024;38(5):352–8.
42. Jain AK, Tawari M, Rathore L, Sahana D, Mishra H, Kumar S, Sahu RK. An experience with Goel-harms C1-C2 fixation for type II odontoid fractures. J Craniovertebr Junction Spine. 2022;13(2):175–81.
43. Ishak B, Glinski AV, Dupont G, Lachkar S, Yilmaz E, Iwanaga J, Unterberg A, Oskouian R, Tubbs RS, Chapman JR. Update on the biomechanics of the Craniocervical junction, part II: alar ligament. Global Spine J. 2021;11(7):1064–9.
44. Barbeito A, Guerri-Guttenberg RA. Inestabilidad cervical en el paciente quirúrgico [Cervical spine instability in the surgical patient]. Rev Esp Anestesiol Reanim. 2014;61(3):140–9.
45. Kinon MD, Nasser R, Nakhla J, Desai R, Moreno JR, Yassari R, Bagley CA. Atlantoaxial rotatory subluxation: a review for the Pediatric emergency physician. Pediatr Emerg Care. 2016;32(10):710–6.
46. Cardoso AC, Fontes RB, Tan LA, Rhoton AL Jr, Roh SW, Fessler RG. Biomechanical effects of the transcondylar approach on the craniovertebral junction. Clin Anat. 2015;28(5):683–9.
47. Lvov IS, Grin' AA, Nekrasov MA, Kordonskiy AY, Sytnik AV. Metody ventral'noĭ dekompressii u patsientov s atlanto-aksial'nymi dislokatsiiami travmaticheskogo i netravmaticheskogo geneza [Ventral decompression techniques in patients with traumatic and non-traumatic atlanto-axial dislocations]. Zh Vopr Neirokhir Im N N Burdenko. 2018;82(1):33–40.
48. Reber K, Bürki A, Vizcaino Reves N, Stoffel M, Gendron K, Ferguson SJ, Forterre F. Biomechanical evaluation of the stabilizing function of the atlantoaxial ligaments under shear loading: a canine cadaveric study. Vet Surg. 2013;42(8):918–23.
49. Osmotherly PG, Rivett DA, Mercer SR. Revisiting the clinical anatomy of the alar ligaments. Eur Spine J. 2013;22(1):60–4.
50. Hong S, Kim GU. Traumatic posterior dislocation of atlanto-axial joint with anterior arch fracture in the patient of atlanto-occipital assimilation: a case report. Int J Surg Case Rep. 2024;114:109133.
51. Kaale BR, McArthur TJ, Barbosa MH, Freeman MD. Post-traumatic Atlanto-axial instability: a combined clinical and radiological approach for the diagnosis of pathological rotational movement in the upper cervical spine. J Clin Med. 2023;12(4):1469.
52. Goel A, Vutha R, Shah A. Evolving concepts of Craniovertebral and spinal instability. Adv Tech Stand Neurosurg. 2023;46:125–47.
53. Koppe D, Markart M, Ertel W. Die atlantoaxiale Dislokation [Dislocation of the atlantoaxial joint]. Unfallchirurg. 2014;117(6):568–71.
54. Chauhan AK, Chandra PS, Goyal N, Chowdhury MR, Banerjee J, Tripathi M, Kabra M. Weak ligaments and sloping joints: a new hypothesis for development of

congenital atlantoaxial dislocation and basilar invagination. Neurospine. 2020;17(4):843–56.
55. Bouaré F, Lmejjati M, Mpando D. Spontaneous atlanto-axial dislocation and trisomy 21: causal factors and management. Pan Afr Med J. 2019;33:3.
56. Haque S, Bilal Shafi BB, Kaleem M. Imaging of torticollis in children. Radiographics. 2012;32(2):557–71.
57. Menezes AH, Dlouhy BJ. Database review of 514 patients with Os Odontoideum. Detailed analysis of 258 surgically treated (1978-2019). Adv Tech Stand Neurosurg. 2024;53:217–34.
58. Charrow J, Alden TD, Breathnach CA, Frawley GP, Hendriksz CJ, Link B, Mackenzie WG, Manara R, Offiah AC, Solano ML, Theroux M. Diagnostic evaluation, monitoring, and perioperative management of spinal cord compression in patients with Morquio syndrome. Mol Genet Metab. 2015;114(1):11–8.
59. Liao S, Jung MK, Hörnig L, Grützner PA, Kreinest M. Injuries of the upper cervical spine-how can instability be identified? Int Orthop. 2020;44(7):1239–53.
60. Bray KY, Platt SR, Kent M, Olby NJ, Early PJ, Mariani CL, Muñana KR, Holmes SP. Magnetic resonance imaging characteristics of atlanto-axial subluxation in 42 dogs: analysis of joint cavity size, subluxation distance, and craniocervical junction anomalies. Open Vet J. 2023;13(9):1091–8.
61. Mańczak M, Gasik R. Cervical spine instability in the course of rheumatoid arthritis – imaging methods. Reumatologia. 2017;55(4):201–7.
62. Du JY, Aichmair A, Kueper J, Wright T, Lebl DR. Biomechanical analysis of screw constructs for atlantoaxial fixation in cadavers: a systematic review and meta-analysis. J Neurosurg Spine. 2015;22(2):151–61.
63. Steinmetz MP, Mroz TE, Benzel EC. Craniovertebral junction: biomechanical considerations. Neurosurgery. 2010;66(3 Suppl):7–12.
64. Yanni DS, Perin NI. Fixation of the axis. Neurosurgery. 2010;66(3 Suppl):147–52.

Part V

The Costovertebral Ligaments

Costotransverse and Costovertebral Joints

20

Aishwarya Gilkes and R. Shane Tubbs

20.1 Introduction

Though rarely discussed, the ligaments of the spine are prominent structures. Their clinical importance is being increasingly recognized. From being a potential cause of chronic back pain to improving surgical outcomes, it is vital to consider them during clinical practice. This chapter will discuss the costotransverse and costovertebral joints, which are found at the two regions of contact between the ribs and the thoracic vertebrae. They are primarily responsible for stabilizing the ribs during everyday movements of the thoracic cage. Throughout this chapter, we will explore the anatomy, function, pathology, and clinical relevance of these joints.

20.2 Anatomy

The ribs articulate with the thoracic vertebrae at two points: where the head of the rib meets the body of the numerically corresponding thoracic vertebra, known as the "costovertebral joint", and where the tubercle of the rib meets the transverse process of the corresponding vertebra [1].

The costovertebral joints are arthrodial joints that connect the heads of the ribs with the bodies of the thoracic vertebrae. Ribs 2–9 are typical ribs, and their heads articulate with their corresponding vertebra and the vertebra above. They articulate via the superior and inferior articulating facets or costal demifacets on the heads of the ribs. The superior rib demifacet articulates with the lower facet of the vertebral body above, while the inferior rib facet articulates with the upper costal facet of its corresponding vertebra. Each joint is a plane synovial joint, and the rib facets span an intervertebral disc.

While all the other ribs articulate with the numerically identical vertebra and the vertebra above, the first rib articulates only with the first thoracic vertebra, and ribs 10–12 articulate only with their corresponding vertebrae [1].

The costovertebral joint has two ligaments: the intra-articular ligament and the radiate ligament. The former is a short horizontal ligament made of flat bands arising from the crest between the demifacets on the heads of the ribs within the synovial joint and attaching to the intervertebral discs. These bands, therefore, divide the synovial joints into two. Since the first, tenth, eleventh, and twelfth ribs articulate only with their corresponding vertebrae, they have no intra-articular ligaments, so they have only one joint [2].

A. Gilkes
Rutgers Health, Newark Beth Israel Medical Center, Boston, MA, USA

R. S. Tubbs (✉)
Tulane University School of Medicine, New Orleans, LA, USA
e-mail: rtubbs@tulane.edu

M. Turgut et al. (eds.), *Ligaments of the Vertebral Column*,
https://doi.org/10.1007/978-3-032-09070-6_20

The radiate ligament (Fig. 20.1) is composed of three flat fasciculi—superior, inferior, and lateral bundles—originating beyond the articular surface of the anterior part of the head of the rib. The superior fasciculus inserts into the body of the vertebra above, and the inferior fasciculus inserts into the body of the vertebra below. Short, intermediate fibers run horizontally to the intervertebral disc [3].

The radiate ligament for the first rib does not divide into three fasciculi; instead, its fibers are attached to the body of the eighth cervical and the first thoracic vertebrae. The tenth, eleventh, and twelfth ribs have no triradiate attachments either. However, the fibers of the ligaments attach to the vertebra above and to the vertebra with which the rib articulates [3].

The costotransverse joint is the point of articulation between the facet of the costal tubercle of the neck of the rib and the transverse processes of the corresponding vertebra. The eleventh and twelfth ribs lack this articulation. The joint is reinforced by three ligaments: costotransverse, superior costotransverse, and lateral costotransverse.

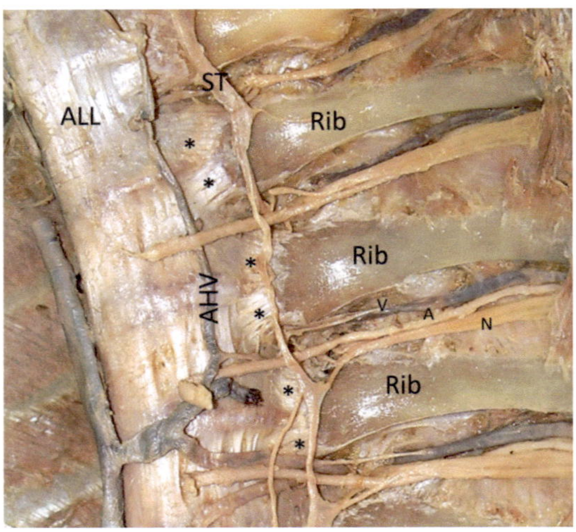

Fig. 20.1 Cadaveric dissection of the posteromedial left thoracic wall noting the radiate ligaments (*). Note the adjacent ribs and interval intercostal vein (v), artery (a), and nerve (n). The sympathetic trunk (ST), anterior longitudinal ligament (ALL) are accessory hemiazygos vein (AHV) are also shown

The costotransverse ligament comprises sheets of connective tissue that fill the costotransverse foramen between the posterior aspects of the necks of the ribs and the transverse processes of the adjacent vertebrae. It is absent in the eleventh and twelfth ribs [4].

The superior costotransverse ligaments (Figs. 20.2 and 20.3) are strong fibrous bands. They attach the neck of the rib to the inferior border of the transverse process of the thoracic vertebra above. They are made of two layers, anterior and posterior.

The anterior layer originates from the crest of the neck of the rib and inserts into the inferior border of the transverse process above, then blends laterally with the internal intercostal membrane. The posterior layer originates posteriorly at the neck of the rib and extends superiorly, inserting into the inferior border of the transverse process of the vertebra above. It blends

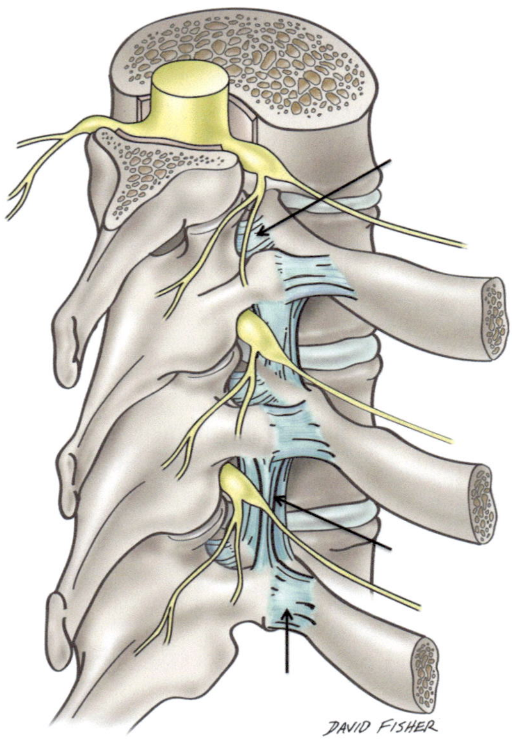

Fig. 20.2 Schematic drawing noting various ligaments of the costovertebral joints: the costotransverse ligament (upper arrow), superior costotransverse (middle arrow) and lateral costotransverse ligament (lower arrow)

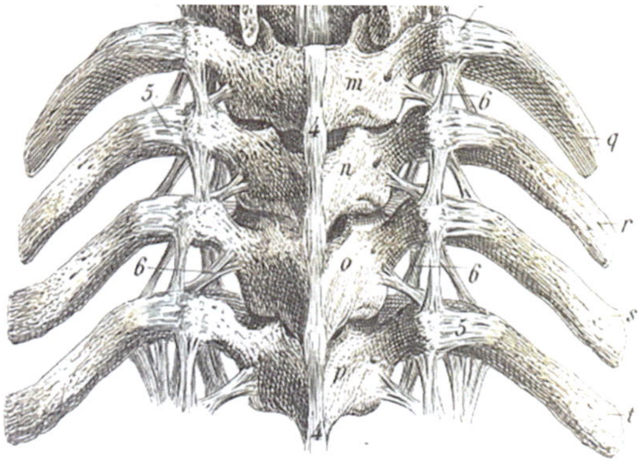

Fig. 20.3 Posterior depiction of many of the larger and smaller costovertebral ligaments. Note the lateral costotransverse ligament (5), superior costotransverse ligament (6), and adjacent vertebrae (m-p), ribs (q-t), and the supraspinous ligament (4). From Bock's Hand-Atlas der Anatomie des Menschen (Verlag der Rengerschen Buchhandlung, Berlin, 1860)

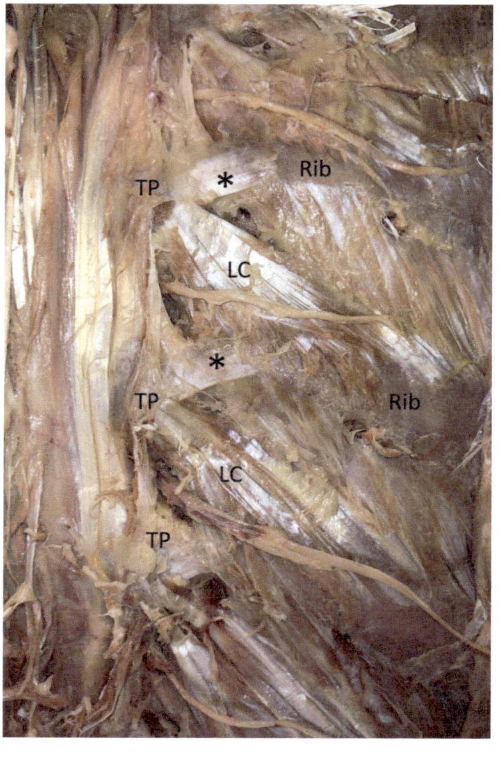

Fig. 20.4 Cadaveric dissection of the right costotransverse junction (posterior view). The midline is to the left. Note the lateral costotransverse ligaments (*), levator costarum muscle (LC) and transverse processes (TPs) of the thoracic vertebrae. The dorsal rami of this region are shown but not labeled

with the external intercostal muscles laterally. The first rib has no superior costotransverse ligament, and the twelfth rib has a lumbosacral ligament that attaches its shaft to the transverse process of the first lumbar vertebra [5].

The lateral costotransverse ligaments (Fig. 20.4) are made of short, thick fibers. They join the rough, non-articular parts of the costal tubercles to the apices of the transverse processes of the thoracic vertebrae [6].

20.3 Function

The costovertebral joint and costovertebral ligaments play a pivotal role in thoracic stabilization, load-bearing, mobility, protection, and chest wall movement, while also contributing significantly to respiratory effort. The thoracic architecture allows motion in all planes [1]. The costotransverse joints are composed of oval-shaped facets with a major axis. From vertebrae T1 to T5, the major axis is vertical; at the joint facets of the lower vertebrae, T6 to T10, it is horizontal and slightly inclined anteriorly and downward. This enables the first five ribs to move on a sagittal plane and the lower five on a transverse plane [7].

In flexion-extension, the range of motion begins at four degrees at T1 and increases incrementally to 12 degrees at T12. Lateral twisting typically allows for six to seven degrees of rotation per vertebral segment. The range of rotation is inverse to that of flexion: T1 rotates nine degrees, and there is an incremental decrease to two degrees at T12. Rib-joint stiffness is greatest at T2 and weakest at T10 [1].

The thoracic skeleton is important in load bearing, providing 30–40% of thoracic spine stiffness. The costovertebral complex also serves as scaffolding for the musculature of the thoracic spine and shoulder. The above motions and loads stress the costovertebral attachments at both the vertebral body and the transverse process. Fortunately, the strong costovertebral and costotransverse ligaments stabilize these joints and add flexibility [1].

The costovertebral complex is mandatory for the respiratory movement of the chest wall. The major muscle groups that insert onto the ribs, determining the movements of the costotransverse joints, are the respiratory muscles: the internal and external intercostals, scalenes, sternocleidomastoid, and serratus anterior and posterior. Activation of these muscles causes motions on the sagittal plane of the ribs, which can affect the costotransverse joints directly [7]. The range of motion at any individual thoracic joint is small, but the frequency of movement of these joints is great.

The main muscles inserted on the spinous processes of the thoracic vertebrae include the trapezius and rhomboid. They allow motion in the axial plane opposite to the predominant plane of the more cranial costotransverse joints. The muscles of the intermediate plane, the nuchal muscles (the semispinalis of the head, neck, and back) that extend and rotate the vertebral column, are inserted on the transverse processes, stressing the joint mainly in the sagittal plane. Considering the main activity of these muscles, it appears evident that repeated movements of the shoulder (especially flexion, external rotation, and abduction), of the head (especially flexion-extension and rotation), of the scapula (abduction and adduction), and the thoracic spine (torsion) can cause inflammation through overuse of the costotransverse joints [7].

The length of the transverse process also affects the costovertebral complex. As its length and concomitant costotransverse articular surface vary, the leverage it exerts on the costovertebral joint also varies. Movement of the thoracic wall a few millimeters anteriorly, cephalically, or laterally can increase thoracic volume by approximately one-half liter [1].

The costovertebral complex plays a crucial role in the biomechanics of chest wall movement. The costovertebral ligaments enable the actions of the costovertebral joints and intervertebral movement. These ligaments function to affix, stabilize, and allow some motion of the ribs on the thoracic vertebrae at the costovertebral joints. Thanks to their stabilization properties, they help with the load-bearing, protection, posture, and scaffolding roles provided by the thoracic skeleton. Moreover, they allow and limit the movement of the ribs at the transverse joint, enabling maximum expansion of the thoracic cavity as needed to meet respiratory demands. Lastly, their actions on the costovertebral and intervertebral complexes allow lateral bending and axial rotation [1].

20.4 Pathology

The cause of thoracic back pain in an individual is quite challenging to identify amidst many differential diagnoses. Many causes of thoracic back pain affect the components of the thoracic spine. While costotransverse and costovertebral pain are causes of thoracic back pain, they are often unrecognized [8]. Joint dysfunction, rib neck fractures, osteoarthritis, ankylosing spondylitis, and other spondyloarthritis conditions can all affect the costotransverse and costovertebral joints. Furthermore, other inflammatory and traumatic states can affect the costovertebral ligaments, most commonly straining of those ligaments [1].

Costovertebral strains result from injury to the ligaments, cartilage, or both when compression and torsional forces at the joint are greater than the joint can withstand. Many posterior rib fractures occur between the costovertebral and costotransverse joints and are thought to result from the strength of the costovertebral and costotransverse ligaments [1].

Osteoarthritis is a degenerative joint disease caused by the breakdown of articular cartilage and underlying erosion of the subchondral bone and synovium. It is thought to be caused by prolonged mechanical stress on the joint and a low-grade inflammatory process. Osteoarthritis of the costovertebral joints is quite common, and its presentation can range from asymptomatic to severely debilitating [1].

Spondyloarthritis is a collective term for chronic inflammatory diseases that involve the joints and the entheses; it includes ankylosing spondylitis, psoriatic arthritis, reactive arthritis, arthritis associated with inflammatory bowel disease, and undifferentiated spondyloarthritis. Ankylosing spondylitis primarily affects the axial skeleton by altering the biomechanical properties of the spine through an idiopathic, chronic inflammatory process, resulting in a brittle, minimally compliant spinal column. The involvement of the costovertebral and costotransverse joints renders the chest wall rigid, thereby preventing it from expanding fully during inspiration, resulting in a significant reduction in exercise capacity. Furthermore, the spinal ligaments, including the costovertebral and costotransverse, are ossified in ankylosing spondylitis, resulting in a fixed kyphotic thoracic spine. Lastly, an ankylosed, noncompliant rib cage can lead to a restrictive lung disease pattern [1].

20.5 Imaging

Traditionally, ligaments are best imaged using magnetic resonance imaging (or computed tomography. As the costotransverse and costovertebral joints are further investigated, various modalities are employed to examine spinal ligament pathologies and guide treatment for these conditions. Modalities used include ultrasound (US), single-photon enhanced computed tomography (SPECT), and technetium-99m-methylene diphosphonate (Tc-99m MDP) bone scintigraphy.

US has been used to identify joint inflammation in the costotransverse and costovertebral joints in patients with stinging pain in the paravertebral region [7].

High-density, linear, multifrequency probes scan along the long axis (transverse plane) and the rib's short axis (sagittal plane) to detect possible joint effusion and compare injured joints with adjacent uninjured joints. Lower-frequency probes are required for obese patients or those with increased muscle mass, as the joints lie deeper than they do in leaner individuals. The focus is placed on the joint plane, and tissue harmonic imaging is activated to enable the identification of possible fluid collections in the small joint capsules. The sagittal plane is especially useful for detecting possible joint effusion and inflammation. This scan enables the simultaneous comparison of two or three adjacent joints (depending on the probe length) to detect pathological differences. US evidence of effusion within the joints can be used as a sure sign of involvement of those structures [7].

US-guided intra-articular injections into the costotransverse and costovertebral joints have been used to relieve pain and have proven effective for treating appropriate cases of chronic thoracic back pain [9].

SPECT has also been used to detect and diagnose costovertebral joint arthropathy. It has been combined with appropriate treatment modalities, such as pain medication or radiofrequency ablation, to reduce thoracic back pain [8].

Tc-99m-MDP bone scintigraphy has been used in patients with ankylosing spondylitis. It has proved able to detect both costotransverse and costovertebral joint involvement. It has shown superior ability in detecting early changes related to ankylosing spondylitis before the development of bone changes that become visible on radiographs [10]. Furthermore, it can detect costotransverse joint inflammation [11].

20.6 Clinical/Surgical Applications

Knowledge of the anatomy of the costotransverse and costovertebral joints is clinically important and has surgical relevance. However, this information is becoming increasingly surgically relevant with the advent and implementation of less invasive procedures, such as the minimally invasive costotransversectomy, which uses only a single incision [12].

Further knowledge of these structures should improve the complication rate following lateral extracavitary approaches and costotransversectomies [13, 14].

Knowledge of the costotransverse and costovertebral joints is helpful in image-guided procedures for resection or radiofrequency ablation of these joints [8, 11, 15, 16].

Simply having knowledge of these joints and the possible pathologies that can occur in these regions creates another significant differential diagnosis, which could benefit patients with chronic thoracic back pain immensely through diagnosis and treatment.

References

1. Saker E, Graham RA, Nicholas R, et al. Ligaments of the costovertebral joints including biomechanics, innervation, and clinical applications: a comprehensive review with application to approaches to the thoracic spine. Cureus. 2016;8(11) https://doi.org/10.7759/cureus.63958.
2. Interarticular ligament of head of rib (left): Complete anatomy. https://www.elsevier.com/resources/anatomy/connective-tissue/connective-tissue-of-thorax/interarticular-ligament-of-head-of-rib-left/19171
3. Radiate ligament of head of rib. https://www.elsevier.com/resources/anatomy/connective-tissue/connective-tissue-of-thorax/radiate-ligament-of-head-of-rib/24714
4. Costotransverse ligament (right). https://www.elsevier.com/resources/anatomy/connective-tissue/connective-tissue-of-thorax/costotransverse-ligament-right/20522
5. Superior costotransverse ligament. https://www.elsevier.com/resources/anatomy/connective-tissue/connective-tissue-of-thorax/superior-costotransverse-ligament/24165
6. Lateral costotransverse ligament. https://www.elsevier.com/resources/anatomy/connective-tissue/connective-tissue-of-thorax/lateral-costotransverse-ligament/17229
7. Del Chiaro A, Ciampi B, Franzoni F, et al. Inflammatory disease if the costotransverse joints: US evaluation in 15 symptomatic patients. J Ultrasound. 2022;25:167–75. https://doi.org/10.1007/s40477-021-00589-5.
8. Ko BW, Park SJ, Kim KW. Single-photon emission-computed tomography in detection of costovertebral joint injury after cervical spine surgery: a case report. Int J Pain. 2022;13(1):36–40. https://doi.org/10.56718/ijp.21-005.
9. Yoon KB, Kim SH, Park SJ, et al. Clinical effectiveness of ultrasound-guided costotransverse joint injection in thoracic back pain patients. Korean J Pain. 2016;29(3):197–201. https://doi.org/10.3344/kjp.2016.29.3.197.
10. Collie DA, Smith GW, Merrick MV. 99mTc-MDP scintigraphy in ankylosing spondylitis. Clin Radiol. 1993;48(6):392–7. https://doi.org/10.1016/s0009-9260(05)81107-9.
11. De Biase G, Gassie K, Abode-Iyamah K, et al. Image-guided right T10 costotransverse joint resection for costotransversitis: operative technique and nuances: 2-dimensional operative video. Oper Nerorsurg (Hagerstown). 2021;21(36):e254. https://doi.org/10.1093/ons/opab118.
12. Zairi F, Nzokou A, Sunna T, et al. Minimally invasive costotransversectomy for the resection of large thoracic dumbbell tumors. Br J Neurosurg. 2016;31(2):179–83. https://doi.org/10.1080/02688697.2016.1233317.
13. Lubelski D, Abdullah KG, Steinmetz MP, et al. Lateral extracavitary, costotransversectomy, and transthoracic thoracotomy approaches to the thoracic spine review of techniques and complications. J Spinal Disord Tech. 2013;26(4):222–32. https://doi.org/10.1097/BSD.0b013e31823f3139.
14. Spallone A, Visocchi M, Greco F, et al. Costotransversectomy in the surgical treatment of medic lateral thoracic disk herniations: long-term results and recent minimally invasive technical adjuncts. In: Visocchi M, editor. The funnel: from the skull base to the sacrum. Acts Neurochirurgica supplement, vol. 135. Cham: Springer; 2023. p. 375–83. https://doi.org/10.1007/978-3-031-36084-8_57.
15. Patel J, Eaves AM, Deschler E, et al. Radiofrequency ablation of the costotransverse joint in a case of chronic thoracic back pain. Cureus. 2024;16(7):e63958. https://doi.org/10.7759/cureus.63958.
16. Pontes JPM, Ferreira-Pinto PH, Pestana da Costa LFN, et al. Resection arthroplasty for isolated costotransverse joint osteoarthritis: a case report and literature review. Surg Neurol Int. 2022;13:62. https://doi.org/10.25259/SNI_88_2022.

21 The Lumbocostal Ligament

Joe Iwanaga and R. Shane Tubbs

21.1 Introduction

21.1.1 Anatomy

The lumbocostal ligament (called "vertebrocostal ligament" or "ligament of Henle") (Fig. 21.1) has been underrepresented in the medical literature and joins the twelfth rib to the lumbar spine. Moreover, descriptions of this ligament have varied. For example, some sources state that this fibrous band arises from the transverse process of the first lumbar vertebra, and others report that it originates from the transverse processes of the first and second lumbar vertebrae [1, 5]. The formation of the ligament begins from the costal processes of the lumbar vertebrae. Here, reinforced fiber strands radiate in a fan-shaped configuration into the middle layer of the thoracolumbar fascia, forming at the upper end the lumbocostal ligament [6]. Along the same path as the ligament is the quadratus lumborum muscle, which lies lateral and posterior to the psoas major muscle [7]. This flat muscle inserts onto the lower border of the twelfth rib, fixing it in place to assist the action of the diaphragm in inspiration.

21.1.2 Clinical Relevance

The lumbocostal ligament is near the superior lumbar triangle (also known as "Grynfelt's triangle") [2, 6]. This region, believed to arise when the serratus posterior inferior is poorly developed [6], is supported by the thoracolumbar fascia from the internal abdominal oblique muscle and the transversus abdominis and is covered by the latissimus dorsi [2]. The triangle is bound laterally by the posterior border of the internal abdominal oblique, medially by the quadratus lumborum, and superiorly by the twelfth rib and the lumbocostal ligament [2]. The superior lumbar triangle represents the peritoneal opening of the musculo-aponeurotic tunnel and constitutes a weak area in the posterior abdominal wall, making it a potential space for herniation [2, 6]. Theoretically,

J. Iwanaga
Tulane University School of Medicine, New Orleans, LA, USA

R. S. Tubbs (✉)
Department of Neurosurgery, Tulane Center for Clinical Neurosciences, Tulane University School of Medicine, New Orleans, LA, USA
e-mail: rtubbs@tulane.edu

M. Turgut et al. (eds.), *Ligaments of the Vertebral Column*,
https://doi.org/10.1007/978-3-032-09070-6_21

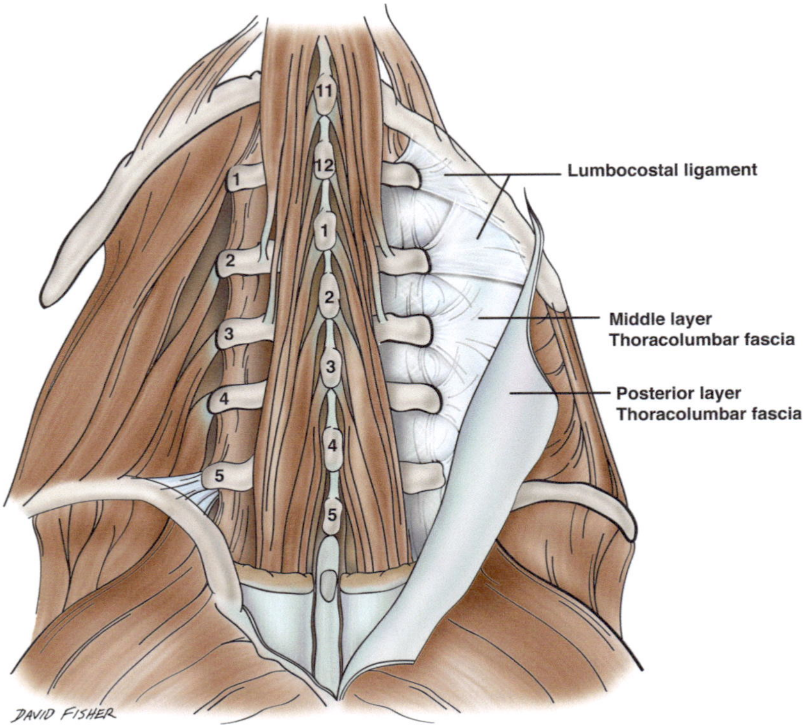

Fig. 21.1 Schematic view of the posterior lower back. Note the right lumbocostal ligament and its relationships to regional bony anatomy and fascial layers

larger lumbocostal ligaments might decrease the chances of herniation in this area, although future studies would need to demonstrate this.

21.1.3 Surgery

Approaches to the retroperitoneal space often use an oblique lumbar incision that begins at the lateral margin of the erector spinae muscle located at the level of the twelfth rib. Next, the latissimus dorsi and the external abdominal oblique aponeurosis are divided. As the surgeon proceeds layer by layer, the lumbocostal ligament will also be divided [4]. This ligament can also be used as a landmark in the muscle-sparing lumbar incision approach to the kidney [4]. Additionally, the lumbocostal ligament is involved in the dissection of a flap from the transversus abdominis and thoracolumbar fascia when a nephropexy technique is utilized to cover the surface of the kidney [3]. With a better understanding of this ligament, its size and relationships to the subcostal nerve and adjacent dorsal rami may be visualized on preoperative magnetic resonance imaging, helping to tailor various approaches to this region more effectively.

In an anatomical study, Saker et al. [8] identified a lumbocostal ligament in all cadaveric specimens. The ligament was posterior to the quadratus lumborum muscle on all sides. The mean length of the ligament was 3 cm. The overall shape of the ligaments ranged from short, narrow bands to large, rhomboidal sheets. Inferiorly, the lumbocostal ligament blended with the middle layer of the thoracolumbar fascia on all sides. The ligament attached to the transverse processes of L1 on 25% of sides and onto the transverse processes of L1 and L2 on 75% of sides. The ligament became taut with rib elevation and was lax with rib depression. Vetter and colleagues [9] reported a case where the subcostal nerve (T12) pierced the lumbocostal ligament.

Finally, Elsharkawy et al. [10], also in a cadaveric study, found that injection of anesthetic was blocked cranially by the lumbocostal ligament with posterolateral quadratus lumborum block approaches.

21.2 Conclusion

Although infrequently reported in the literature, the lumbocostal ligament can have implications both clinically and surgically. Therefore, knowledge of its anatomy can be important.

References

1. Benzel EC. Spine surgery: techniques, complication avoidance, and management. Philadelphia: Saunders (Elsevier); 2012.
2. Guillem P, Czarnecki E, Duval G, Bounoua F, Fontaine C. Lumbar hernia: anatomical route assessed by computed tomography. Surg Radiol Anat. 2002;24(1):53–6.
3. Larionova TA. Nephropexy using a transverse musculofascial flap and the indications for it. Urol Nefrol. 1992;3:7–11.
4. Lierse W. Applied anatomy of the pelvis. Berlin: Springer-Verlag; 1987.
5. MacLennan GT. Hinman's atlas of urosurgical anatomy. Philadelphia: Saunders (Elsevier); 2012.
6. Rickenbacher J, Landolt AM, Theile K. Applied anatomy of the Back. Berlin: Springer-Verlag; 1982.
7. Thorek P. Anatomy in surgery. New York: Springer-Verlag; 1985.
8. Saker E, Tardieu GG, Alonso F, Chung BS, Fisahn C, Loukas M, Tubbs RS. The forgotten lumbocostal ligament: anatomical study with application to thoracolumbar surgery. Cureus. 2016;8(12):e925.
9. Vetter M, Iwanaga J, Tubbs RS. Piercing of the lumbocostal ligament by the subcostal nerve: a previously unreported case. Cureus. 2017;9(11):e1825.
10. Elsharkawy H, Bajracharya GR, El-Boghdadly K, Drake RL, Mariano ER. Comparing two posterior quadratus lumborum block approaches with low thoracic erector spinae plane block: an anatomic study. Reg Anesth Pain Med. 2019; https://doi.org/10.1136/rapm-2018-100147.

Part VI

The Sacroiliac Ligaments

22 Ligaments of the Sacrum

Joe Iwanaga and R. Shane Tubbs

22.1 Introduction

The sacroiliac joint is a diarthrodial synovial joint [1] located within the pelvis between the sacrum and ilium. Its primary functions are shock absorption and torque conversion, as well as pelvic stabilization. It also offsets the load of the trunk on the lower limbs [1]. The basis of kinematic support between the pelvis and vertebral column from the sacroiliac joint lies mainly in the structure of the surrounding ligaments and fascia, and in the involvement of the gluteus maximus and piriformis muscles and the long head of the biceps femoris [2]. The posterior weight-bearing sacroiliac complex provides most of the structural stability to the pelvic ring, owing largely to its physical structure. The posterior sacroiliac joint ligaments are arranged to form a suspension bridge [3].

Anatomically, the sacroiliac joint is described as a symphysis, with synovial characteristics confined to the distal portion of the iliac side [4].

J. Iwanaga
Department of Neurosurgery, Tulane Center for Clinical Neurosciences, Tulane University School of Medicine, New Orleans, LA, USA

R. S. Tubbs (✉)
Tulane University School of Medicine, New Orleans, LA, USA
e-mail: rtubbs@tulane.edu

22.2 Anatomy of the Sacroiliac Joint

Like most joints, the sacroiliac joint begins development around the tenth week of embryonic life [5, 6]. At this stage, a cavity begins to form in a primitive area space, which develops fully into the sacroiliac joint by the eighth month of gestation [7]. The sacroiliac joint undergoes postnatal structural changes as children begin walking. Intra-articular ridges and depressions develop secondary to an adaptation to gravitational stress through it [7]. In the adult, the joint ultimately assumes an L-shape, which enables it to provide solid stabilization.

The sacroiliac joint has been classified anatomically as a symphysis with some characteristics of a synovial joint exclusive to the distal cartilaginous portion at the iliac side [2]. Histologically, the joint surfaces are lined with hyaline cartilage, with some thinning on the cartilage of the ileum, which is described as fibrocartilaginous [7].

The sacroiliac joint can be visualized distinctly by guided radiography. This technique allowed earlier researchers to compare male and female pelves at different stages of life. Male and female pelves are quite similar during intrauterine and pre-pubertal development, and the characteristic though slight sex differences do not become evident before adolescence [6]. Between the ages of 12 and 14 years, the sacroiliac

M. Turgut et al. (eds.), *Ligaments of the Vertebral Column*,
https://doi.org/10.1007/978-3-032-09070-6_22

ligaments in males begin to strengthen while those in females become more mobile, a phenotypic feature that allows the female pelvis to facilitate and tolerate childbirth [8]. Notwithstanding this sexual dysmorphism, each sacroiliac joint is characteristically 1–2 mm wide [9].

As indicated earlier, the sacroiliac joint attaches the spine to the pelvis and absorbs forces because of its ligamentous stabilization. The structure, thickness, and orientation of said ligaments allow the sacroiliac joint to compensate for a difference in orientation between a more convex ilium promontory at S2 and a sacrum that is significantly concave [9].

The sacroiliac joint should be viewed as a continuous ligamentous stocking based on the interconnections of the various regional ligaments and fascial structures, as outlined in the literature [7]. Conceptually, the continuity of this ligamentous stocking provides a unitary function to the lumbosacral pelvic region. In fact, this abstract description of the sacroiliac joint indicates that the ligamentous stocking is the primary support of the osseous elements, not only within the sacroiliac joint but by extension in the entire lumbosacral pelvic region [7]. It is anchored through the thoracolumbar fascia of the back and the hamstring to the sacrotuberous ligament complex of the pelvis [7].

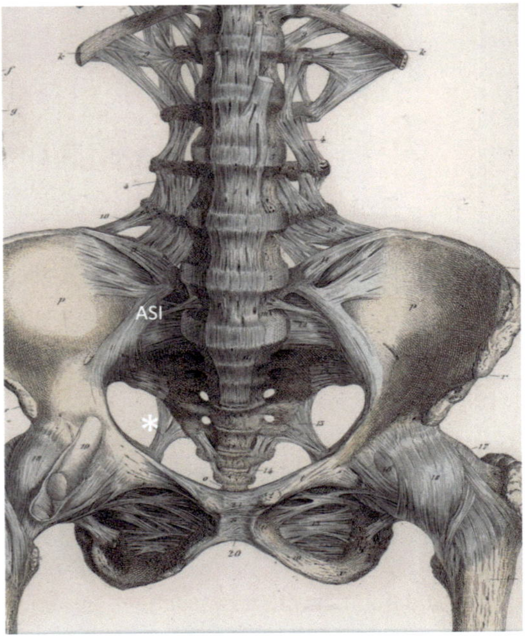

Fig. 22.1 Anterior view of the pelvis and lower lumbar spine. Note the anterior sacroiliac ligament (ASI) and sacrospinous ligament (*). (After Bock)

22.3 Ligamentous Anatomy

22.3.1 Anterior Sacroiliac Ligament

On the anterior aspect of the sacroiliac joint lies the anterior sacroiliac ligament (Fig. 22.1), an anteroinferior capsular thickening [10]. Its long transverse fibers extend from the base and lateral part of the sacrum to the medial margin of the auricular surface of the ilium [11]. Its superior part represents the extension of the iliolumbar ligament. At its caudal border, it blends with the cranial fibers of the sacrospinous ligament [7]. Considered to contain thin and weak fibers overall, the anterior sacroiliac ligament is well developed near the arcuate line and the posterior inferior iliac spine, where it connects the third sacral segment to the ilium [10]. Pelvic fractures involving anterior sacroiliac ligaments (B-fractures, "open book fractures") are considered rotationally unstable but vertically stable. In these cases, the posterior ligamental arch is at least partially intact, hence the vertical stability.

22.3.2 Interosseous Sacroiliac Ligament

The vast interosseous sacroiliac ligament (Fig. 22.2) is considered the strongest of the sacroiliac joint-supporting ligaments [7]. It encloses the axial joint, fills the spaces posterior and cephalad to the synovial portion of the joint, and provides multi-directional structural stability [7]. It also has the most extensive bony origin and volume of all sacroiliac joint ligaments in both sexes [12], though it is larger in females. In contrast, the anterior and posterior sacroiliac ligaments are larger in males [7].

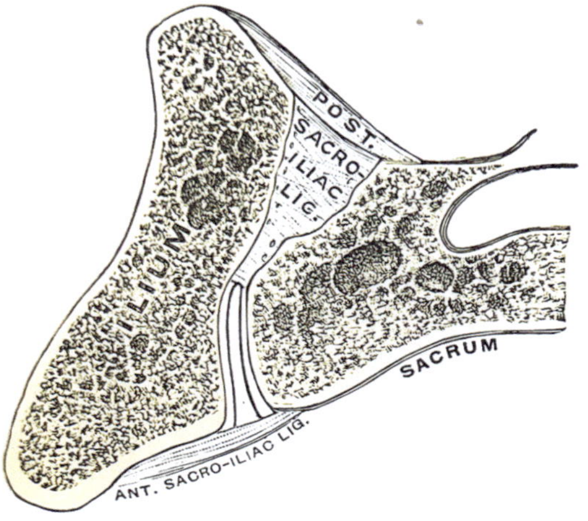

Fig. 22.2 Superior view of the axially sectioned pelvis noting the sacroiliac joint and surrounding ligaments. Note the interosseous, anterior and posterior sacroiliac ligaments (after Testut)

The interosseous sacroiliac ligament is located between the ilium and sacrum and maintains a funnel-shaped complex orientation, its apex being connected to the sacrum [7]. Since it is difficult to establish the border between the fibrous apparatus and cartilage, its anatomical coordinates cannot be confirmed more precisely. It is contained within the joint space, while the appropriately named "posterior sacroiliac ligament" covers the posterior surface of the joint facet [9]. The interosseous sacroiliac ligament lies deep to the posterior sacroiliac ligament [11].

22.3.3 Long Posterior Sacroiliac Ligament

The long posterior sacroiliac ligament (Fig. 22.3) is more superficial, and its fibers are oriented vertically [11]. It has proximal and distal regions of osseous attachment [11, 13], between which is its middle portion containing a confluence of three layers: the erector spinae aponeurosis, the "deep fascial layer," and the gluteal aponeurosis [13, 14]. Beneath the "deep fascial layer" sits a collection of adipose and loose connective tissue that contains lateral branches of the posterior sacral rami [15].

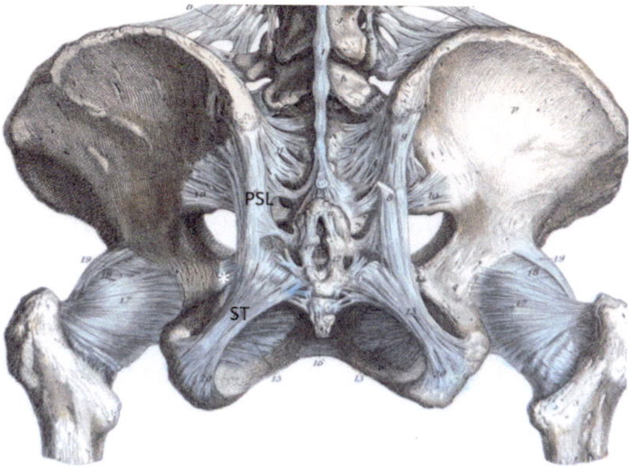

Fig. 22.3 Posterior view of the ligaments surrounding the sacroiliac joint. Note the posterior sacroiliac ligament (PSL) and sacrotuberous ligament (ST). Also note the sacrospinous ligament (*). (After Bock)

22.3.4 Short Posterior Sacroiliac Ligaments

Little is known about the features and characteristics of the posterior sacroiliac joint ligaments [16]. The short posterior sacroiliac ligaments originate from the posterior tuberosity of the ilium and terminate on the lateral part of the sacrum. Innervation is supplied by fine branches from the posterior rami of the spinal nerves [16]. The fibers of the short posterior ligaments run more horizontally and represent the deeper part. Their location enables posterior flaring or diastasis of the joint to be prevented [11].

22.3.5 Iliolumbar Ligament

The iliolumbar ligament (Fig. 22.3) is also anatomically important for establishing the structure of the sacroiliac joint. In some individuals, it begins at the transverse processes of L4 and L5 [17]. The structural heterogeneity of this ligament is worth mentioning [7]. It is attached to the pelvis by two main ligaments and extends to the sacroiliac joint capsule. It is highly variable but consists mainly of anterior and posterior aspects [10]. According to Pool-Goudzwaard et al., it restricts the sagittal movement of the sacroiliac joint [17, 18].

22.3.6 Sacrotuberous Ligament

The sacrotuberous ligament (Fig. 22.3) is considered crucial in the kinematic chain, as it directly supports the transmission of force and load transfer from the spine and sacrum to the lower limbs. It is almost vertically oriented with a broad base to the posterior superior iliac spine, the posterior sacroiliac ligaments, the lateral sacral crest, and the lateral margins of the lower sacrum/upper coccyx. It attaches to the medial margin of the ischial tuberosity. The superficial fibers are continuous with the tendon of the biceps femoris [10, 11]. Along with the sacrospinous ligament, it anchors the sacrum to the ischium and prevents upward tilt [11]. It is tensed during nutation and also subjected to increased tension by the biceps femoris and/or gluteus maximus muscles [7].

It has been showed that simulated biceps femoris muscle force influenced tension in the sacrotuberous ligament [2, 19]. The gross anatomy was studied in 50 formalin-fixed cadavers; all specimens had a sacrotuberous ligament with a ligamentous part, while 87% also exhibited a membranous (falciform) segment [19]. The falciform segment extended towards the ischioanal fossa and was further divided into three subcategories by the characteristics of its extensions [19]. Type I falciform extensions had processes that tracked along the ischial ramus, terminating at the obturator fascia. Type II had processes that tracked along the ischial ramus, joined the obturator fascia, and continued to the ischionanal fossa. The type III subgroup had no falciform extensions [19].

22.3.7 Sacrospinous Ligament

The sacrospinous ligament (Figs. 22.1 and 22.3) is a relatively thin, triangular ligament that converges on the ischial spine and extends to the lateral margins of the sacrum and coccyx anterior to the sacrotuberous ligament, with which it blends in part [10, 11]. It converts the sciatic notches into foramina [10, 20]. Sacrospinous ligament fixation is an important technique for treating pelvic organ prolapse. It enables the vagina to be brought to a level above the levator ani muscle by suspending it from the sacrospinous ligament [21, 22].

22.3.8 Sacrococcygeal Ligaments

Minor ligaments that attach the sacrum to the coccyx include the lateral sacrococcygeal, posterior, and anterior sacrococcygeal ligaments (Figs. 22.1 and 22.3).

22.4 Function

The ligaments of the sacroiliac joint are the anterior, posterior, interosseous, sacrotuberous and sacrospinous. The iliolumbar ligaments are also anatomically and clinically important for sacroiliac joint stability. Since the sacroiliac joint is a weight-bearing joint, it functions mainly in absorbing multi-directional forces, a characteristic more evident when all of the ligaments are intact and show no degenerative pathology [23, 24]. As a unit, the joint facilitates nutation and counternutation of the pelvis around the femoral head [25].

In 460 BCE, Hippocrates proposed that the sacroiliac joint was mobile only during pregnancy. However, studies beginning in the eighteenth century revealed that sacroiliac joints are capable of mobility in both males and females [7, 25].

The sacroiliac joint is essential for transferring loads effectively between the spine and legs [26, 27]. In a study of 13 fresh-frozen cadaver pelves, the researchers cut each pelvis and measured the effects of incisions in individual sacroiliac joint ligaments on its stability [28]. They concluded that although ligament size and the mode by which force is loaded onto the pelvis are relevant factors, the principal determinant of sacroiliac joint stability is directly correlated to ligamentous patency [28].

The posterior and anterior sacroiliac ligaments influence the forward and lateral resistance of the sacrum [16]. The posterior layer of the thoracolumbar fascia, erector spinae, and part of the sacrotuberous ligament lie in close anatomical proximity to the posterior sacroiliac ligament [7]. The long posterior sacroiliac ligament connects the sacrum to the posterior superior iliac spine. It can slacken owing to increased tension in the latissimus dorsi or the gluteus maximus muscle [7], and disruption of it destabilizes the entire sacroiliac joint. Moreover, its patency is the basis for the classification of sacroiliac joint fractures [28].

The anterior and posterior ligaments provide approximately 30% inhibition of sacral gliding, as quantified following the application of various loads to cadaveric pelvic specimens [16]. This finding supported the assumption that the interosseous, sacrospinous, and sacrotuberous ligaments also confer mechanical stability on the sacroiliac joint.

The smooth and planar articular surfaces of the sacroiliac joint are present from birth and early childhood and permit movement in all directions, the primary restraint on motion being the strong interosseous sacroiliac ligament [25]. Histologically, this ligament consists of fibrocartilage and is divided into posterior and anterior portions [29]. Connected to the posterior and anterior sacroiliac transverse ligaments, it is important for increasing joint stability via force closure [7, 18]. Although the evidence is inconclusive, current kinematic studies appear to show the axis of sacroiliac joint rotation near or/and within the boundaries of the interosseous ligament [30, 31]. Given its bony origin and its sheer volume compared to other reinforcing ligaments, the interosseous ligament is a major contributor to multi-directional structural stability, irrespective of sex [12].

Studies of embalmed specimens indicate that the sacrotuberous ligament (Fig. 22.3) is important in the kinematic chain between the pelvis and vertebral column [7]. Its main part connects the sacrum to the ischial tuberosity [7]. Mechanical loading of it restricts nutation of the sacrum, coupled with the influence of the long head of the biceps and gluteus maximus, which attach to the sacrotuberous ligaments [7].

The main function of the sacrospinous ligament (Figs. 22.1 and 22.3) is to prevent rotation of the ilium past the sacrum, and many investigations have revealed that laxity of this ligament and the sacrotuberous ligament allows such revolution [7]. However, the general conclusion is that the sacrotuberous and sacrospinous ligaments contribute little to overall pelvic stability [28].

22.5 Sacroiliac Joint Pain and Disease

Non-specific back pain is a common cause of morbidity [32]. Lower back pain is limited to the regions below the lower margins of the 12th rib and the gluteal fold and occurs in 60–80% of people during their lifetime [32]. It is often due to sacroiliac joint instability [16, 27]. Sacroiliac joint pain is reputed to be a source of lower back pain, with a worldwide prevalence reported to range from 0.4% to 35% [33]. The risk of lower back pain in pregnant populations is 89% [33]. In chronic back pain populations, patients whose symptoms failed to centralize after three or more positive provocation sacroiliac joint tests have a 77% chance of having sacroiliac joint pain.

Instability of the sacroiliac joint due to loosening or injury of the sacroiliac ligaments most commonly follows trauma or inflammation and is a cause of sacroiliac joint pain [27]. Pain is also reportedly caused by minor movements that result in collisions between the complementary ridges and grooves of the sacroiliac joint [7].

Several authors have indicated a gender difference in the misalignment of the sacroiliac joint. Gender-related differences in sacroiliac joint pain could suggest a higher rate of sacroiliac joint misalignment in young females [7]. Among patients aged 10–20 years presenting with lower back pain secondary to sacroiliac joint misalignment, 77% were female [34].

There is a gender difference in the position of the center of gravity, which is more anterior in men [7, 35]. This indicates a longer lever arm in men than in women, resulting in higher loads on the joints. Therefore, since higher loads are usually placed on the joints in males, the male sacroiliac joint often becomes stronger, with more restricted mobility [7].

The long posterior sacroiliac ligament (Fig. 22.3) was subjected to tensile stress during physiological loading of the sacroiliac joint [15]. The surrounding soft tissue structures, such as the ipsilateral erector spinae aponeurosis and the sacrotuberous ligament, were subjected to similar forces. The findings indicated that compression of the penetrating lateral branches of the sacral rami in the long posterior sacroiliac ligament during states of tension could generate low back pain [15]. However, the study also considered the possibility that although pain in the long posterior sacroiliac ligament area can originate from the ligament itself, these ligaments commonly contain sensory receptors, so it can also be generated indirectly by irritation of neurovascular bundles that penetrate the ligament. Overall, the study concluded that the S2, S3 lateral branches of the posterior sacral plexus penetrate and possibly innervate the long posterior sacroiliac ligament, and consequently provide an anatomical basis for the long posterior sacroiliac ligament potentially acting as a pain generator [35].

The iliolumbar ligament (Figs. 22.1 and 22.2) has been described as a possible source of pain because it can be strained by flexion of L5 [36]. Slouched standing postures occur in everyday activities such as washing dishes, brushing teeth, and vacuuming. Over time, such positions can cause low back pain. Patients suffering from acute low back pain often present with pain at the site of the iliolumbar ligament. The effects of simulated muscle tension on this ligament and the L5-S1 intervertebral disc angle were measured in embalmed specimens [36] by sensors attached to the anterior band of each iliolumbar ligament halfway between the transverse process of L5 and the ilium. The study revealed forward rotation of L5 with respect to the sacrum when the rectus abdominis was strained. This suggests that strain on the iliolumbar ligament caused by spinal flexion may contribute to acute lower back pain in situations involving minor axial spinal load.

22.6 Treatment of Sacroiliac Joint Pain

Low back pain is due to SI joint dysfunction in up to 35% [33, 37, 38], and in response to the disease burden and the hope for improved outcomes, significant efforts have been made to elucidate and treat its various etiologies. Medical management has proved effective in treating sacroiliac joint pain, including specific lumbopelvic stabilization training and corticosteroid injections into the intra-articular space [33]. Another treatment proposed for sacroiliac ligament and joint pain is bipolar radiofrequency ablation. This could work as a long-lasting treatment for patients with sacroiliac dysfunction who report temporary pain relief with local anesthetic injection into the joint [39].

In one study, nine subjects with sacroiliac joint pain were treated with a series of radiofrequency lesioning adjacent to the lateral posterior foraminal aperture, plus conventional monopolar lesioning at the L5 posterior ramus [40]. Each subject was contacted every month for 12 months to rate their current pain level after the procedure. Eight of the nine subjects were satisfied with the procedure [40]. The researchers concluded that radiofrequency sensory ablation of the sacroiliac joint using bipolar strip lesions is a technically uncomplicated and low-risk procedure; its effects on pain, disability, and satisfaction are promising [40].

In the past, surgeons were reluctant to consider the sacroiliac joint as a pain generator. However, increasing attention has recently been given to this topic, and numerous studies have demonstrated that the sacroiliac joint is innervated and mobile. If it becomes arthritic over time, this can result in low back pain [38, 41–43].

Long-term responses from medical treatments of chronic sacroiliac joint dysfunction are very limited. Thus, surgical management with sacroiliac joint fusion has been used, and many authors recommend the following to assess surgical candidacy for a sacroiliac joint fusion: consistent pain coming from the sacroiliac joint with a positive Fortin finger sign [44], at least three positive provocative examination maneuvers [45], and a positive reduction of pain in response to sacroiliac joint injections. Two approaches to sacroiliac joint fusion have been published, posterior and lateral transiliac, which the most recent published series have utilized. Open sacroiliac joint fusion has been performed since the 1920s but is no longer the preferred approach due to its invasiveness and lengthy recovery periods [46]. In contrast, minimally invasive sacroiliac joint fusion has been reported recently. MIS sacroiliac joint fusion is technically less morbid and associated with less blood loss, shorter operative time, reduced hospital length of stay, and fewer operative complications than open fusion [45–48]. Across multiple studies and implant manufacturers, MIS sacroiliac joint fusion provides rapid and sustained significant improvement in pain, disability, and quality of life scores, with a significant decrease in opioid use in most patients [45–48]. However, further research on these techniques is recommended.

22.7 Conclusion

The sacroiliac ligaments connect the sacrum and ilium in the pelvic region, and their primary function is to stabilize and support the sacroiliac joint in combination with the strength and support of the surrounding muscles. Common injuries and complaints associated with sacroiliac ligament pathology can manifest as sacroiliac joint pain or lower back pain. Treatments for these complaints most commonly include bipolar radiofrequency ablation and corticosteroid injections. Sacroiliac joint fusion provides a clinically significant improvement in pain and disability scores. Clinicians should evaluate and examine the sacroiliac joint in their differential diagnosis for low back pain and consider sacroiliac joint fusion surgery with the right patient selection when medical options are otherwise limited.

References

1. Hansen HC, McKenzie-Brown AM, Cohen SP, Swicegood JR, Colson JD, Manchikanti L. Sacroiliac joint interventions: a systematic review. Pain Physician. 2007;1:165–84.
2. Vleeming A, Wingerden J, Snijders C, Stoeckart R, Stijnen T. Load application to the sacrotuberous ligament; influences on sacroiliac joint mechanics. Clin Biomech. 1989:204–9.
3. Tile M. Pelvic ring fractures: should they be fixed? J Bone Joint Surg Br. 1988;1:1–12.
4. Puhakka KB, Melsen F, Jurik AG, Boel LW, Vesterby A, Egund N. MR imaging of the normal sacroiliac joint with correlation to histology. Skeletal Radiol. 2004;1:15–28.
5. Brolinson PG, Kozar AJ, Cibor G. Sacroiliac joint dysfunction in athletes. Curr Sports Med Rep. 2003;1:47–56.
6. Solonen KA. The sacroiliac joint in the light of anatomical, roentgenological and clinical studies. Acta Orthop Scand. 1957;Suppl:1–127.
7. Vleeming A, Schuenke MD, Masi AT, Carreiro JE, Danneels L, Willard FH. The sacroiliac joint: an overview of its anatomy, function and potential clinical implications. J Anat. 2012;6:537–67.
8. Dechow E, Davies RK, Carr AJ, Thompson PW. A randomized, double-blind, placebo-controlled trial of sclerosing injections in patients with chronic low back pain. Rheumatology (Oxford). 1999;12:1255–9.
9. Foley BS, Buschbacher RM. Sacroiliac joint pain: anatomy, biomechanics, diagnosis, and treatment. Am J Phys Med Rehabil. 2006;12:997–1006.
10. Standring S. Gray's Anatomy. Elsevier; 2016.
11. Bogduk N. Clinical anatomy of the lumbar spine and sacrum. London: Churchill Livingstone; 1997.
12. Steinke H, Hammer N, Slowik V, Stadler J, Josten C, Böhme J, et al. Novel insights into the sacroiliac joint ligaments. Spine (Phila Pa 1976). 2010;3:257–63.
13. Vleeming A, Pool-Goudzwaard AL, Hammudoghlu D, Stoeckart R, Snijders CJ, Mens JM. The function of the long dorsal sacroiliac ligament: its implication for understanding low back pain. Spine (Phila Pa 1976). 1996;5:556–62.
14. McGrath C, Nicholson H, Hurst P. The long posterior sacroiliac ligament: a histological study of morphological relations in the posterior sacroiliac region. Joint Bone Spine. 2009;1:57–62.
15. McGrath MC, Zhang M. Lateral branches of dorsal sacral nerve plexus and the long posterior sacroiliac ligament. Surg Radiol Anat. 2005;4:327–30.
16. Wang M, Dumas GA. Mechanical behavior of the female sacroiliac joint and influence of the anterior

and posterior sacroiliac ligaments under sagittal loads. Clin Biomech (Bristol, Avon). 1998;4-5:293–9.
17. Pool-Goudzwaard A, Hoek van Dijke G, Mulder P, Spoor C, Snijders C, Stoeckart R. The iliolumbar ligament: its influence on stability of the sacroiliac joint. Clin Biomech (Bristol, Avon). 2003;2:99–105.
18. Pool-Goudzwaard AL, Kleinrensink GJ, Snijders CJ, Entius C, Stoeckart R. The sacroiliac part of the iliolumbar ligament. J Anat Pt. 2001;4:457–63.
19. Loukas M, Louis RG, Hallner B, Gupta AA, White D. Anatomical and surgical considerations of the sacrotuberous ligament and its relevance in pudendal nerve entrapment syndrome. Surg Radiol Anat. 2006;2:163–9.
20. Doty J, Rengachary S. Surgical disorders of the sacrum. New York: Thieme Medical Publishers, Inc; 1994.
21. Ağaçayak E, Yaman Tunç S, İçen MS, Başaranoğlu S, Fındık FM, Sak S, et al. Should we add unilateral sacrospinous ligament fixation to vaginal hysterectomy in management of stage 3 and stage 4 pelvic organ prolapse? Turk J Obstet Gynecol. 2015;3:144–50.
22. Tseng LH, Chen I, Chang SD, Lee CL. Modern role of sacrospinous ligament fixation for pelvic organ prolapse surgery – a systemic review. Taiwan J Obstet Gynecol. 2013;3:311–7.
23. DonTigny RL. Function and pathomechanics of the sacroiliac joint. A review. Phys Ther. 1985;1:35–44.
24. Eichenseer PH, Sybert DR, Cotton JR. A finite element analysis of sacroiliac joint ligaments in response to different loading conditions. Spine (Phila Pa 1976). 2011;22:E1446–52.
25. Rosatelli AL, Agur AM, Chhaya S. Anatomy of the interosseous region of the sacroiliac joint. J Orthop Sports Phys Ther. 2006;4:200–8.
26. Slipman CW, Whyte WS, Chow DW, Chou L, Lenrow D, Ellen M. Sacroiliac joint syndrome. Pain Physician. 2001;2:143–52.
27. Kim YH, Yao Z, Kim K, Park WM. Quantitative investigation of ligament strains during physical tests for sacroiliac joint pain using finite element analysis. Man Ther. 2014;3:235–41.
28. Vrahas MS, Wilson SC, Cummings PD, Paul EM. Comparison of fixation methods for preventing pelvic ring expansion. Orthopedics. 1998;3:285–9.
29. Ehara S, et al. The accessory sacroiliac joint: a common anatomic variant. AJR Am J Roentgenol. 1988;4:857–9.
30. Egund N, Olsson TH, Schmid H, Selvik G. Movements in the sacroiliac joints demonstrated with roentgen stereophotogrammetry. Acta Radiol Diagn (Stockh). 1978;5:833–46.
31. Sturesson B, Uden A, Vleeming A. A radiostereometric analysis of the movements of the sacroiliac joints in the reciprocal straddle position. Spine (Phila Pa 1976). 2000;2:214–7.
32. Taxter AJ, Chauvin NA, Weiss PF. Diagnosis and treatment of low back pain in the pediatric population. Phys Sportsmed. 2014;1:94–104.
33. Laslett M. Evidence-based diagnosis and treatment of the painful sacroiliac joint. J Man Manip Ther. 2008;3:142–52.
34. Stoev I, Powers AK, Puglisi JA, Munro R, Leonard JR. Sacroiliac joint pain in the pediatric population. J Neurosurg Pediatr. 2012;6:602–7.
35. Bellamy N, Park W, Rooney PJ. What do we know about the sacroiliac joint? Semin Arthritis Rheum. 1983;3:282–313.
36. Snijders CJ, Hermans PF, Niesing R, Spoor CW, Stoeckart R. The influence of slouching and lumbar support on iliolumbar ligaments, intervertebral discs and sacroiliac joints. Clin Biomech (Bristol, Avon). 2004;4:323–9.
37. Schwarzer AC, Aprill CN, Bogduk N. The sacroiliac joint in chronic low back pain. Spine (Phila Pa 1976). 1995;20(1):31–7.
38. Sembrano JN, Polly DW Jr. How often is low back pain not coming from the back? Spine (Phila Pa 1976). 2009;34(1):E27–32.
39. Pino CA, Hoeft MA, Hofsess C, Rathmell JP. Morphologic analysis of bipolar radiofrequency lesions: implications for treatment of the sacroiliac joint. Reg Anesth Pain Med. 2005;4:335–8.
40. Burnham RS, Yasui Y. An alternate method of radiofrequency neurotomy of the sacroiliac joint: a pilot study of the effect on pain, function, and satisfaction. Reg Anesth Pain Med. 2007;1:12–9.
41. Vilensky JA, O'Connor BL, Fortin JD, et al. Histologic analysis of neural elements in the human sacroiliac joint. Spine (Phila Pa 1976). 2002;27(11):1202–7.
42. Sturesson B, Uden A, Vleeming A. A radiostereometric analysis of movements of the sacroiliac joints during the standing hip flexion test. Spine (Phila Pa 1976). 2000;25(3):364–8.
43. Szadek KM, Hoogland PV, Zuurmond WW, de Lange JJ, Perez RS. Nociceptive nerve fibers in the sacroiliac joint in humans. Reg Anesth Pain Med. 2008;33(1):36–43.
44. Fortin JD, Falco FJ. The Fortin finger test: an indicator of sacroiliac pain. Am J Orthop (Belle Mead NJ). 1997;26(7):477–80.
45. Vleeming A, Van Wingerden JP, Dijkstra PF, Stoeckart R, Snijders CJ, Stijnen T. Mobility in the sacroiliac joints in the elderly: a kinematic and radiological study. Clin Biomech (Bristol, Avon). 1992;7(3):170–6.
46. Sachs D, Capobianco R. One year successful outcomes for novel sacroiliac joint arthrodesis system. Ann Surg Innov Res. 2012;6(1):13.
47. Lorio MP, Polly DW Jr, Ninkovic I, Ledonio CG, Hallas K, Andersson G. Utilization of minimally invasive surgical approach for sacroiliac joint fusion in surgeon population of ISASS and SMISS membership. Open Orthop J. 2014;8:1–6.
48. Polly DW, Swofford J, Whang PG, et al. Two-year outcomes from a randomized controlled trial of minimally invasive sacroiliac joint fusion vs. non-surgical management for sacroiliac joint dysfunction. Int J Spine Surg. 2016;10:8.

Part VII

Other Ligaments

Anterior Dural (Hofmann's) Ligaments

23

Brianna L. Hines and R. Shane Tubbs

23.1 Introduction

The anterior dural ligaments, commonly referred to as Hofmann's ligaments (HL), are fibrous bands tethering the anterior dura to the spinal canal [1]. First observed by Meckel in 1817 and Humphry in 1858, these ligaments were defined in 1898 by the eponymous Max Hofmann as membranous structures connecting the anterior dura to the posterior longitudinal ligament (PLL) [2, 3]. Trolard had reported the presence of these ligaments in the lumbosacral area in 1888, so the ligaments are sometimes referred to as Trolard's ligament [3, 4]. There is a paucity of literature regarding HL and their presence is not always documented in cadaveric studies [5]; in some cases, authors report dural adhesions caused by disc herniation or aging [6–8], which are likely HL [9, 10]. Additional confusion is likely due to the variety of alternate names for HL: authors have referred to HL as the ventral or anterior meningovertebral ligaments [9–13], anterior durovertebral ligaments [14], anterior ligaments of the dura mater [15], anterior sacrodural ligaments [16], and median sagittal septum [17, 18].

B. L. Hines (✉)
Tulane University School of Medicine, New Orleans, LA, USA
e-mail: bhines@tulane.edu

R. S. Tubbs
Department of Structural and Cellular Biology, Tulane University School of Medicine, New Orleans, LA, USA

Department of Neurosurgery, Tulane University School of Medicine, New Orleans, LA, USA

Department of Neurosurgery, Ochsner Health System, New Orleans, LA, USA

Department of Neurosurgery and Ochsner Neuroscience Institute, Ochsner Health System, New Orleans, LA, USA

Department of Anatomical Sciences, St. George's University, West Indies, Grenada

23.2 Anatomic Description

Regardless of nomenclature, HL continue to be defined as fibrous bands connecting the anterior dura and spinal canal (Figs. 23.1 and 23.2), though the criteria have expanded from Hofman's original terms to include ligaments attaching to periosteum or intervertebral disc (IVD), in addition to those attaching to the PLL [5, 11, 17–19]. HL maintain a tight adherence between the PLL and dura, and at some levels the two even fuse [20–23]. Spencer classified HL by attachment site and established three categories: medial, lateral, and radicular [12, 18]. Medial ligaments connect the anterior dura to the PLL and are the thickest [12, 17, 18]. Lateral ligaments attach anterolateral dura to lateral PLL or adjacent periosteum and are less sturdy [12, 17, 18]. Thinnest of all, radicular ligaments span from the dural sleeve of the proximal spinal nerve to the spinal

M. Turgut et al. (eds.), *Ligaments of the Vertebral Column*,
https://doi.org/10.1007/978-3-032-09070-6_23

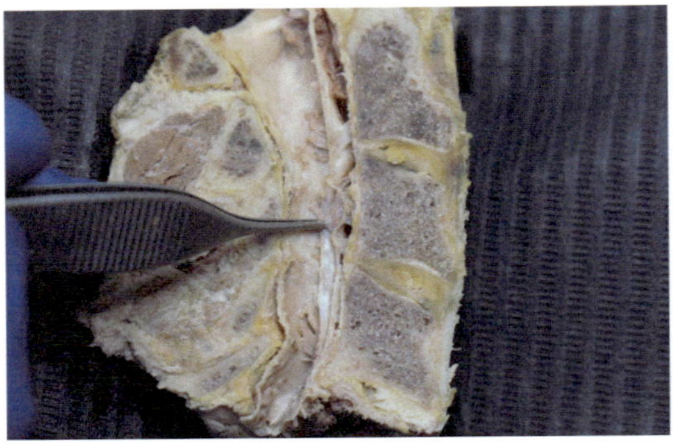

Fig. 23.1 Sagittal cadaveric section noting Hoffmann's ligaments (HL) in the upper cervical spine just posterior to the odontoid process

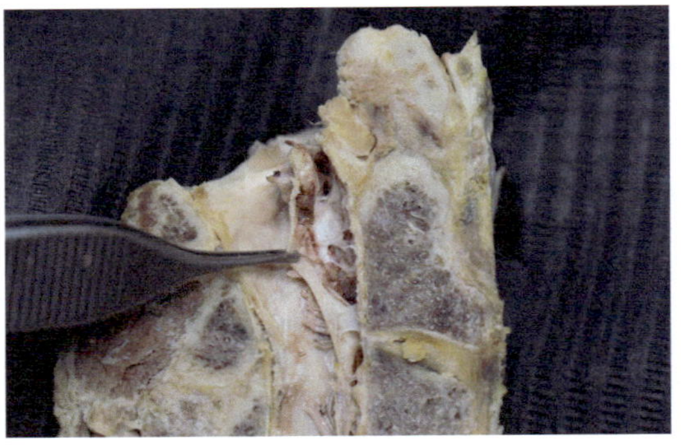

Fig. 23.2 Sagittal cadaveric section noting HL in the upper cervical spine just posterior to the C3 vertebra

bone, attaching at the vertebral body, pedicle, or IVD at the level of the foramen [12, 17, 18]. Radicular are the shortest of all the subgroups, with a mean length of 14.9 mm compared to 26.2 mm and 26.9 mm for medial and lateral groups, respectively [12]. These delicate ligaments attaching to the exiting nerve root sleeve were not recognized by Hofmann but have since been described by several authors [12, 17, 18]. Spencer's categorization system has been criticized as an oversimplification of the myriad attachment configurations [23]; nonetheless, most authors have adopted its use [12, 17, 18].

In cadaveric studies, the vast majority of cadavers are found to have some HL, though there is a great deal of variation in their quantity and vertebral location [11, 12, 16, 18, 23]. Early reports failed to identify HL in the thoracic region [9] but they have since been identified at levels spanning C7-L5 [23]. It is debated which region contains the most HL, with one study reporting the most ligaments in the lower thoracic region [23] while other studies found the lower lumbar region to contain more [14, 17, 24]. Generally a HL is restricted to a single vertebral level but in some cases it spans several levels [23]. A given vertebral level can have multiple HL; five is the most that has been reported [1, 23]. They are inconsistently symmetrical: some authors note that HL tend to develop in pairs of right- and left-sided ligaments at a given vertebral level [18, 25], while other studies found no such tendency [11, 23].

23.3 Morphology and Histological Structure

HL do not have a uniform appearance and may resemble fine fibrous bands, narrow trabeculae, or wide sheets of connective tissue [9, 18, 22]. In the thoracic and upper lumbar area the ligaments are typically thin and wispy, with weak attachments [10, 17, 23]. Cervical ligaments tend to be thicker with more tensile strength [14]. Lumbosacral ligaments are the most robust of all and have the greatest resistance to stretch [9, 10, 12, 14, 17, 18, 23]. In some cases ligaments in the lower lumbar region condense to form long sheets that can insert over several levels and may be 7–8 mm wide [9, 18, 23]. Ligament length also varies greatly, ranging from 0.5–28.8 mm [23], but there is no consensus on a relationship between length and anatomic region [12, 23, 25]. Authors also disagree on the orientation of the ligaments: some assert that HL always angle cranially towards the dura [25], while others report heterogeneous orientation [4, 9, 23]. Wadhwani et al. describe a caudocranial orientation from dura to PLL in the upper thoracic and cervical regions, which switches to a craniocaudal orientation in the lumbar region [23]. The turning point occurs at T8/T9, where the angle is orthogonal [23].

HL are composed of fibrous connective tissue bundles mixed with type 1 collagen and a small amount of elastic fibers [1, 10, 11].

Surrounding these bundles are venous plexuses, fat, and areolar tissue [10, 11]. At either end of the ligament, its tissue merges with the outer layer of the attachment site. Therefore HL tissue mixes with the external fibroelastic layer of the dura on one end, and on the other, it becomes continuous with either the osteofibrous wall of the vertebral wall or the outer PLL [9, 11]. Sometimes HL fibers will continue through the PLL into the vertebral endosteum [9]. Where the ligament comes into contact with the spinal nerve laterally, its fibers mix with those of the epineurium [11]. Some authors have observed vascular structures traveling within HL [11]. Dural tissue removed from their attachments to HL at L4/L5 has been shown to contain disrupted neurovascular bundles, leading authors to speculate that HL contain branches of the sinuvertebral nerve [24].

23.4 Embryological Formation

It is believed that HL develop from connective tissue progenitors in the epidural space, though their precise origin is uncertain [5, 19, 22]. There is limited literature regarding their formation [5, 22]. Some studies of the fetal epidural space have found it to be filled with undifferentiated mesenchyme [22, 26], while other authors have identified fibrocytes and adipocytes as early inhabitants in this space [19]. Kimmell et al. speculate that as these cells differentiate they develop distinct layers surrounding the spinal cord [19]. With vertebral growth the layers become disrupted, resulting in discontinuous connections that become the epidural ligaments [19].

Serial fetal anatomical studies have provided some insights into the timeline of HL formation. Munkasci et al. saw the earliest appearance of HL in a 50 mm CRL fetus [5, 27], which correlates well with studies done by Geers and Hamid, who reported identifying early versions of HL at 11 weeks and 13 weeks, respectively [1, 11]. However, Hamid et al. found that these early precursors were supplemented by fibrous HL at 21 weeks, and by 39 weeks the thinner bands had disappeared [1]. Regardless of the exact timeline, most authors agree that from early weeks of development a weak HL precursor is present that is more flexible in order to grow with the changing fetus [1, 11, 23]. The development of the flexion curve and difference in growth rates between the vertebral column and the dura could explain the variation in HL orientations [1, 11, 24, 25]. Once the spine is more fully formed, HL can thicken and become stronger, allowing for greater stability after birth when spinal mobility increases [5, 23].

23.5 Function

HL are predominantly ascribed stabilizing and protective functions [9, 14, 16, 19, 23]. Observations that the dural sac maintains its position in cadavers rather than collapsing, which would be expected without the supportive pressure of cerebrospinal fluid (CSF), lend support to a structural function [5, 28]. HL provide a firm attachment to the spinal canal that steadies the cord and aligns it with movements of the vertebral column, particularly flexion and lateral inclination [9, 14, 16]. The fibrous structure of the ligaments anchors the dural sac to the canal, and a small amount of elastic fibers allow for minimal movements [19]. The variable presence of HL explains differences in spinal mobility between individuals and between vertebral segments [23]. The denser ligaments of the lumbosacral region are likely necessary to counteract the tension of lordosis on the dural conus [9, 24]. In the context of a stabilization function, the change in orientation observed by Wadhwani et al. would make sense as in upper regions of the spine they limit inferior movement of the cord, and in lower regions they limit superior movement [23]. At the T8/T9 level, where rotational movement is greatest, the orthogonal angle would allow freedom of movement [23].

In addition to the thecal sac, HL provide anchoring and protection to the exiting spinal nerves [18, 23]. Radicular HL prevent trauma to the nerve from spinal motion, especially extension [23]. Fixation of the nerve neutralizes excessive movements within the canal and resists posterior or medial displacement [23]. By maintaining a consistent distribution of peridural fat, HL can provide further neuronal protection [10]. Furthermore, HL may help in absorbing and redistributing shock after spinal trauma, mitigating damage to peridural neurovascular structures [16].

23.6 Imaging

The delicate nature of HL makes them difficult to visualize on imaging, but researchers have been able to do so in some cases, having greater success on magnetic resonance imaging (MRI) than computed tomography (CT) [10, 29]. In cases where MRI is contraindicated, CT myelography may improve visualization [17]. The ligaments appear as a thin line with similar density on CT to the IVD and dura [9, 29]. The medial HL are typically clearer than lateral, possibly because they are more firmly condensed by the pressure of surrounding peridural fat, while laterally there may be less fat due to displacement by the internal venous plexus [9, 17]. The presence of surrounding fat also aids in the visualization of the ligaments by providing contrast [9, 17].

Some pathologic states cause the appearance of HL to become more obvious. Ossification or calcification of HL can make them more evident on imaging [9, 30]. Sometimes, a bony spur is visible at the midpoint of the vertebral body on CT, which may demarcate HL insertion points where traction spurs formed due to pressure from surrounding dilated veins [9]. In cases of lumbar epidural lipomatosis, the shape of the dural sac can become deformed, and varying insertion patterns of the anterior and posterior dural ligaments may be inferred by the spiculations of the dural contour [11]. The contour of HL becomes very evident when they are surrounded by carcinomatous vertebral metastases because the disease classically spares the ligaments, resulting in the "draped curtain sign" [31].

23.7 Clinical and Surgical Considerations

HL are an important consideration when performing interventions in the epidural space. While the posterior dural ligaments may be more relevant to a posterior approach, the anterior dural ligaments can also affect the posterior epidural space. Differing HL configurations determine how the epidural space is partitioned. If adjacent spinal segments have HL existing in parallel, this can create a localized space between them [11]. The presence of both a medial and a lateral HL at one level divides the anterior epidural space into subcompartments [12]. One is found between the two HL and communicates through fenestrations with the contralateral space [12]. Because there are no superior or inferior boundaries, this space may continue for the length of the spinal canal. The lateral subcompartment communicates freely with the posterior epidural space, but it is bound in the longitudinal plane by nerve roots and radicular HL [12]. This partitioning of the epidural space can cause uneven distribution of injected drugs that affects their pharmacokinetics [5, 11, 20]. Variations in the epidural space may also affect catheter introduction and positioning [11].

Awareness of HL may help prevent complications during spine surgery. While the posterior dural ligaments are more often a source of concern, caution should be taken to avoid HL as well, especially when the lateral or anterior epidural space is accessed. Excessive manipulation of the ligaments could result in dural tear due to the ligaments' strong attachments, or hemorrhage in cases where the ligaments have venous attachments [11, 32, 33]. Krystkiewicz et al. advise transecting HL after visualization during corpectomy and oncology cases where the PLL is intact and the anterior dura is adherent to the tumor [12]. During microdiscectomy for disc herniation, transecting HL is often necessary in order to access the anterior epidural space and remove disc fragments [12].

23.8 Pathology

It is widely believed that HL play an underacknowledged role in the pathogenesis of radiculopathy [13, 18, 20, 22, 25]. Radicular HL hold the spinal nerves tightly against the periosteum, allowing even a small disc bulge to cause neuronal compression [18]. Disc protrusion can also cause neuronal harm indirectly by acting on an HL, which transmits the force to the spinal nerve [5, 22, 32]. The tension induced on the nerve can harm it directly or compromise its microvascularization and potentially cause ischemic pain [22]. Ventral compression can produce pain due to HL holding the nerve anteriorly despite adequate space to move posteriorly in the canal [13, 18, 22, 25]. These mechanisms could explain both cases of asymptomatic disc protrusion as well as why some patients suffer from radiculopathy without radiographic evidence of foraminal compression [13, 18, 22, 25]. HL involvement in disc protrusion could explain why the severity of symptoms often does not correlate with imaging, as well as variability in patient response to physical maneuvers [16–18, 22, 24]. The HL may also transmit compressive force from the nerve root to the PLL, periosteum, or annulus fibrosus, all of which are well innervated by the sinuvertebral nerve [22]. Increased density of HL in the lumbosacral area where disc bulge is common may contribute to the high incidence of symptomatic protrusions in this region [17].

Beyond protrusion, HL can be involved in disc herniation and extrusion as limiting structures to migration. An extruded disc may be shown on imaging, displacing HL and dura to the contralateral side [9]. HL confine migrated disk fragments to the anterior epidural space and prevent movement from one side to the other [9, 10, 12, 29]. As the thickest ligaments, medial HL provide the strongest barrier to disk migration, while lateral HL are more likely to be violated, allowing for migration from the subarticular to the foraminal zone [12]. Only a few cases of migration of sequestered material in the posterolateral direction have been reported, and it is postulated that in these cases the HL or another barrier to migration must have perforated [34, 35]. Theoretically, HL would also deter the movement of other materials, such as granulomatous tissue or hematoma [10]. Whether HL can prevent the spread of infection is unknown and may be an area for future investigation, as posterior epidural abscesses are more common than anterior [5].

Additional pathologies involving HL concern the calcification of these ligaments. Some authors theorize that calcification of the dural ligaments could affect mobility and possibly injure the dural sac or nerve roots [9, 17]. In a study of patients with type 1 CSF leaks and spiculated spinal lesions, Takai et al. found that the lesions were connected to the PLL and generally were fibrotic or calcified, with no discogenic or degenerative osteophytic tissue on histological analysis [30]. Based on this evidence they speculated that HL can become calcified and prone to cause tears in the ventral dura mater with spinal movement. The higher incidence of dural tears at the cervicothoracic or thoracolumbar junctions may be explained by greater displacement of the dural sac in these regions due to differences in flexibility between spinal regions [30]. The cause of ligament calcification is unclear, but it is likely related to repetitive movements and individual predisposition [9]. On CT, calcified HL were visualized as high-density lesions indistinguishable from osteophytic spurs, ossified PLL, or calcified disc herniation [30].

23.9 Future Directions

Further study of HL can bring more widespread recognition of this commonly found ligament and elucidate its role in pathology. Authors have shown it is possible to visualize HL on imaging, so with practice clinicians may be able to identify the ligament more often and gain a better knowledge of its anatomical configuration before intervention in the region. Recent findings of calcified HL in association with CSF leaks should be investigated further, as well as their role in other spinal pathologies. Other studies have provided insights into the appearance of the dural sac in different disease processes based on whether they involve the PLL or dural ligaments [29, 36, 37];

further research determining which diseases of the anterior epidural space violate HL could help clinicians formulate a diagnosis for pathologies involving the anterior epidural space, which can present similarly.

23.10 Conclusion

HL are normal anatomic structures with a high degree of variation in their quantity and location. They play an important role in stabilizing the anterior dura to the PLL or spinal canal and help align the cord with vertebral movements to prevent injury. HL may be involved in the pathogenesis of radiculopathy and disc herniation, and could explain cases where clinical presentation does not align with what is seen on imaging. Further research is needed to explore the role of HL in other spinal pathologies, including type 1 CSF leaks, anterior epidural abscesses, and neoplasms. HL are sometimes visible on imaging and can be helpful in diagnosing pathologies. Awareness of their presence and firm dural attachments can help avoid surgical complications. The influence of HL on epidural interventions merits further investigation.

References

1. Hamid MF-BC, Delmas V, Plaisant O. The human lumbar anterior epidural space: morphological comparison in adult and fetal specimens. Surg Radiol Anat. 2002;24(3):194–200. https://doi.org/10.1007/s00276-002-0041-6.
2. Hofmann M. Die Befestigung der Dura mater im Wirbelkanal. Arch Anat Entwicklungsgesch. 1898:403–12.
3. Newell RLM. The spinal epidural space. Clin Anat. 1999;12(5):375–9. https://doi.org/10.1002/(sici)1098-2353(1999)12:5%3C375::aid-ca7%3E3.0.co;2-6.
4. Trolard P. Recherches sur l'anatomie des meninges spinales, des nerfs sacre et du filum terminal dans le canal sacré. Arch Physiol. 1888;2(198)
5. Tardieu GG, FC, Loukas M, Moisi M, Chapman J, Oskouian RJ, Tubbs RS (2016) The epidural ligaments (of Hofmann): a comprehensive review of the literature. Cureus 8(9). https://doi.org/10.7759/cureus.779.
6. Blikra G. Intradural herniated lumbar disc. J Neurosurg. 1969;31(6):676–9. https://doi.org/10.3171/jns.1969.31.6.0676.
7. MacMillan J, SJ, Kambin P (1991) Routes and incidence of communication of lumbar discs with surrounding neural structures. Spine 16(2):167–171.
8. Teng P, PC (1964) Intrathecal dislocation of lumbar intervertebral disc. Neurochirurgia 7(2). https://doi.org/10.1055/s-0028-1095409.
9. Scapinelli R. Anatomical and radiologic studies on the lumbosacral meningo-vertebral ligaments of humans. J Spinal Disord. 1990;3(1):6–15.
10. Scapinelli R. The meningovertebral ligaments as a barrier to the side-to-side migration of extruded lumbar disc herniations. Acta Orthop Belg. 1992;58(4):436–41.
11. Geers C, LF, Behets C, Malghem J, Cosnard G, Lengelé BG. Polygonal deformation of the Dural sac in lumbar epidural lipomatosis: anatomic explanation by the presence of Meningovertebral ligaments. AJNR Am J Neuroradiol. 2003;24(7):1276–82.
12. Krystkiewicz K, Maślanka M, Skadorwa T, Ciszek B, Tosik M, Furtak J. Meningovertebral ligaments could be a barrier for migration of a herniated intervertebral disc: an anatomical study. Front Surg. 2022;9 https://doi.org/10.3389/fsurg.2022.969244.
13. Santos JLM, Kalhorn SP. Anatomy of the posterolateral spinal epidural ligaments. Surg Neurol Int. 2021;12(33) https://doi.org/10.25259/SNI_894_2020.
14. Sakka L, Gabrillargues J, Coll G. Anatomy of the spinal meninges. Oper Neurosurg. 2016;12(2):168–88. https://doi.org/10.1227/NEU.0000000000001048.
15. Plaisant O, Sarrazin JL, Cosnard G, Schill H, Gillot C. The lumbar anterior epidural cavity: the posterior longitudinal ligament, the anterior ligaments of the dura mater and the anterior internal vertebral venous plexus. Acta Anat. 1996;155(4) https://doi.org/10.1159/000147816.
16. Barbaix E, Girardin MD, Hoppner JP, Van Roy P, Clarijs JP. Anterior sacrodural attachments – Trolard's ligaments revisited. Man Ther. 1996;1(2) https://doi.org/10.1054/math.1996.0255.
17. Bashline SD, Bilott JR, Ellis JP. Meningovertebral ligaments and their putative significance in low back pain. J Manip Physiol Ther. 1996;19(9):592–6.
18. Spencer DL, Irwin GS, Miller JA. Anatomy and significance of fixation of the lumbosacral nerve roots in sciatica. Spine. 1983;8(6):672–9. https://doi.org/10.1097/00007632-198309000-00014.
19. Kimmell KT, Dayoub H, Shakir H, Sincoff EH. Spinal dural attachments to the vertebral column: an anatomic report and review of the literature. Surg Neurol Int. 2011;2(1) https://doi.org/10.4103/2152-7806.82990.
20. Hogan QH. Lumbar epidural anatomy. A new look by cryomicrotome section. Anesthesiology. 1991;75(5) https://doi.org/10.1097/00000542-199111000-00007.
21. Hogan QH. Epidural anatomy: new observations. Can J Anaesth. 1998;45(5 Pt 2) https://doi.org/10.1007/BF03019206.

22. van Dun PLS, Girardin MRG. Embryological study of the spinal dura and its attachment into the vertebral canal. Int J Osteopath Med. 2006;9(3):85–93. https://doi.org/10.1016/j.ijosm.2006.07.002.
23. Wadhwani S, Loughenbury P, Soames R. The anterior dural (Hofmann) ligaments. Spine. 2004;29(6) https://doi.org/10.1097/01.brs.0000115129.59484.24.
24. Parke WW, Watanabe R. Adhesions of the ventral lumbar dura. An adjunct source of discogenic pain? Spine. 1990;15(4):300–3. https://doi.org/10.1097/00007632-199004000-00010.
25. Wiltse LL. Anatomy of the extradural compartments of the lumbar spinal canal. Peridural membrane and circumneural sheath. Radiol Clin North Am. 2000;38(6):1177–206. https://doi.org/10.1016/s0033-8389(08)70003-4.
26. Beaujeux R, Wolfram-Gabel R, Kehrli P, Fabre M, Dietemann JL, Maitrot D, Bourjat P. Posterior lumbar epidural fat as a functional structure? Histologic specificities. Spine. 1997;22(11):1264–8. https://doi.org/10.1097/00007632-199706010-00021.
27. Munkácsi I. The epidural ligaments during fetal development. Acta Morphol Hung. 1990;38(3–4):189–97.
28. Parkin IG, Harrison GR. The topographical anatomy of the lumbar epidural space. J Anat. 1985;141:211–7.
29. Schellinger D, Manz HJ, Vidic B, Patronas NJ, Deveikis JP, Muraki AS, Abdullah DC. Disk fragment migration. Radiology. 1990;175(3) https://doi.org/10.1148/radiology.175.3.2343133.
30. Takai K, Endo T, Komori T. Calcified Hofmann's ligaments as the cause of spinal cerebrospinal fluid leaks associated with spinal ventral dural tears. J Neurosurg Spine. 2024;42(1) https://doi.org/10.3171/2024.7.SPINE24480.
31. Shah LM, Salzman KL. Imaging of spinal metastatic disease. Int J Surg Oncol. 2011;2011(1) https://doi.org/10.1155/2011/769753.
32. Chen R, Shi B, Zheng X, Zhou Z, Jin A, Ding Z, LV H, Zhang H. Anatomic study and clinical significance of the dorsal Meningovertebral ligaments of the thoracic dura mater. Spine. 2015;40(10):692–8. https://doi.org/10.1097/BRS.0000000000000860.
33. Lee HG, Kang MS, Kim SY, Cho KC, Na YC, Cho JM, Jin BH. Dural injury in unilateral Biportal endoscopic spinal surgery. Glob Spine J. 2020;11(6) https://doi.org/10.1177/2192568220941446.
34. Mraja HM, Kaya O, Mammadov T, Karadereler S, Hamzaoglu A. Anterior-to-posterior epidural migration of a lumbar disc herniation at L1-L2: a case report. Cureus. 2022;14(8) https://doi.org/10.7759/cureus.27568.
35. Mobbs RJ, Steel TR. Migration of lumbar disc herniation: an unusual case. J Clin Neurosci. 2007;14(6):581–4. https://doi.org/10.1016/j.jocn.2006.04.002.
36. Kim DH, Rosenblum JK, Panghaal VS, Freeman KD, Lui YW. Differentiating neoplastic from nonneoplastic processes in the anterior extradural space. Radiology. 2011;260(3) https://doi.org/10.1148/radiol.11102287.
37. Strauss SB, Gordon SR, Burns J, Bello JA, Slasky SE. Differentiation between tuberculous and pyogenic spondylodiscitis: the role of the anterior Meningovertebral ligament in patients with anterior epidural abscess. AJNR Am J Neuroradiol. 2020;41(2):364–8. https://doi.org/10.3174/ajnr.A6370.

The Peridural (Epidural) Membrane

24

Brianna L. Hines and R. Shane Tubbs

24.1 Introduction

The peridural membrane (PDM) is also known as the epidural membrane. According to Bridge [1], von Luschka [2] was the first to note the presence of a cellulo-elastic membrane separating dura from periosteum in 1850. Early authors continued to describe a membrane surrounding the dura, most notably Fick in 1904 [3] and Frykholm in 1951 [4]. However, it was not until 1975 that Dommisse accurately described the membrane and named it [5–8]. Dommisse's nomenclature has been widely adopted by authors, though the PDM has also often been referred to as the epidural membrane [1, 4, 9–11]. Some studies accurately describe the PDM but fail to label it as such: alternate terms used that correspond to the PDM have included endorachis [12], lateral membrane [13, 14], and fibrous fatty cellular complex [15]. A few authors have challenged the existence of a PDM, claiming instead that the sheath of tissue outside the dura is periosteum [16, 17], a superficial layer of the posterior longitudinal ligament (PLL) [10], or an outer layer of the dura mater [18]. In support of the PDM's presence and contradiction to these theories, many researchers have found evidence of a PDM in human and non-human studies [1, 8, 11, 19]; some believe that there is only the PDM and no periosteum within the SC [7, 8]. In Dommisse's original description, the author advised that the PDM is often mislabeled as the outer layer of dura [6–8].

B. L. Hines (✉)
Tulane University School of Medicine, New Orleans, LA, USA
e-mail: bhines@tulane.edu

R. S. Tubbs
Department of Structural and Cellular Biology, Tulane University School of Medicine, New Orleans, LA, USA

Department of Neurosurgery, Tulane University School of Medicine, New Orleans, LA, USA

Department of Neurosurgery, Ochsner Health System, New Orleans, LA, USA

Department of Neurosurgery and Ochsner Neuroscience Institute, Ochsner Health System, New Orleans, LA, USA

Department of Anatomical Sciences, St. George's University, West Indies, Grenada

24.2 Anatomic Description

The PDM is a continuous, fibrous sheath that surrounds the dura, separating it from the walls of the vertebral canal (VC) (Figs. 24.1 and 24.2) [8, 19, 20]. The only interruptions in the structure are perineural evaginations that occur at the neural foramina where the PDM extends to cover the exiting spinal nerves [8, 15, 20]. The PDM has numerous attachments to both the dura and the VC, including epidural ligaments, fibrous attachments, lymphatic vessels, arteries, and veins [19,

M. Turgut et al. (eds.), *Ligaments of the Vertebral Column*,
https://doi.org/10.1007/978-3-032-09070-6_24

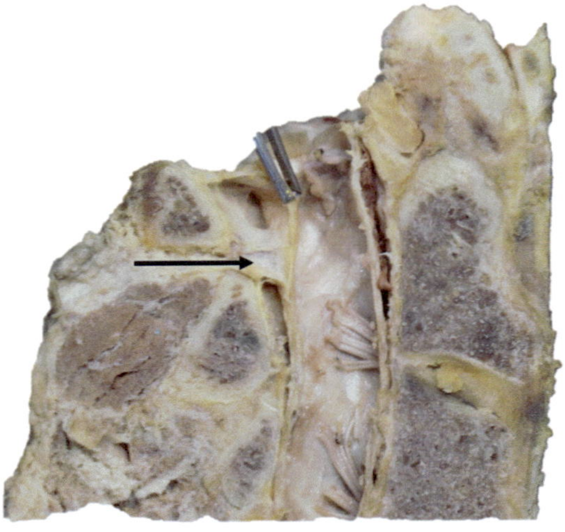

Fig. 24.1 Sagittal section of the upper cervical spine with the spinal cord removed. The posterior spinal dura mater is displaced anteriorly, revealing the peridural membrane (PDM) (arrow)

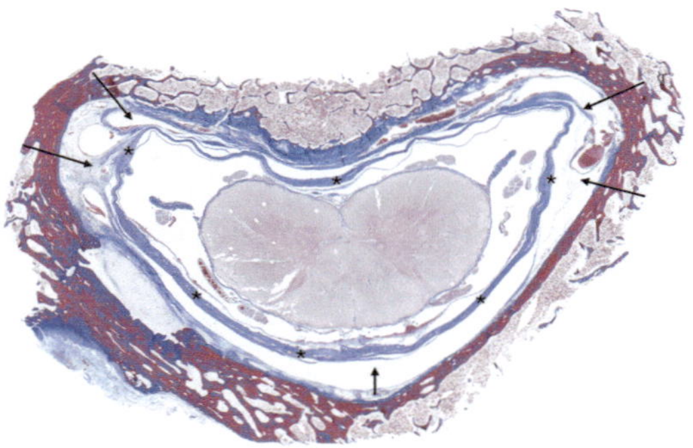

Fig. 24.2 Axial histological section through the cervical spine. The spinal cord is visible in the center of the image, surrounded by the dura mater (*). Note the components of the PDM (arrows) (Masson's trichrome)

20]. At some points, the membrane directly contacts the VC walls, but it is always separated from the dura by the epidural space [19]. The PDM has a close relationship with Batson's plexus. Recent studies have found that the veins of the plexus run within the membrane [6, 19], but historical views state that the plexus lies on the membrane and frequently penetrates it [7, 8, 21]. A third subset of studies portrays the plexus lying anteriorly to the membrane with no direct contact between the structures [4, 13, 22].

The segments of the PDM can be examined in three broad categories: anterior, posterior, and lateral/perineural [4, 15, 19]. Anteriorly, the PDM forms the boundary of the anterior epidural space, which exists between the PDM and dura [8, 21]. The space anterior to the PDM can be referred to as the premembranous space [7, 8]. Here, the PDM is in close contact with the PLL: some authors claim that the structures are adjacent but remain separate [8, 21], but further studies have shown the fibers of the PDM are continuous with both the superficial and deep layers of PLL [19, 20, 23]. In these studies, the PLL appears as a thick band of tissue within the PDM, covered posteriorly by a thin layer of PDM [19, 20, 23]. The PDM also blends with the periosteum of the vertebral body as well as the anterior longitudinal ligament at the anterior margin of the intervertebral foramen [10, 21].

The posterior PDM is more delicate compared to the anterior membrane [19]. The structure still contains fibrous tissue, fat, and veins, but is thin, translucent, and easily ruptured [19]. The more fragile nature of the posterior PDM may relate to the smaller size of the posterior epidural venous plexus compared to the anterior [19]. The posterior PDM thickens on its lateral edges, where it harbors some of the larger veins of the plexus [19]. It appears to blend with the periosteal lining of the neural arch [8].

Laterally, the PDM covers the VC walls and extends into the neural foramen [4, 8, 15, 19, 20]. In the lateral recess, the PDM contains the veins that form the lateral margin of the anterior epidural venous plexus [19]. The PDM covering the lateral pedicles is very thin; the epidural fat covering it lends the membrane support and is continuous with the fat in the neural foramen and posterior epidural space [19, 20]. Moving further laterally, in the infrapedicular region, the PDM thickens where it envelopes the anastomosing veins connecting to the epidural venous plexuses and sub-pedicular transforaminal veins

[19]. The PDM evagination into the neural foramen forms a cone-shaped cuff around the exiting spinal nerve and perineural fat and veins [19]. The PDM here is thicker than that of the pedicular region, with an extraforaminal portion of varying length [19, 20]. This extension of the PDM may be referred to as perineural [19, 20], periradicular [4], epiradicular [9, 11], or circumneural [8].

As it travels through the neural foramen, the perineural PDM maintains a distance from the periosteum, thus creating two pockets of space between the perineural PDM and the pedicle [19, 20]. These compartments are referred to as the suprapedicular and infrapedicular compartments [20]. Posteriorly, the compartment is bordered by the facet joint; anteriorly, it is bound by the intervertebral disc, and medially, part of the supradicular PDM partitions the space from the spinal canal [20]. There is communication between the compartments and the epidural space exterior to the PDM [23]. Within the infra- and suprapedicular compartments, there is often an intraforaminal ligament, connective tissue, vessels, and nerves [19]. It is thought that these nerve branches may be offshoots from the primary posterior ramus of the exiting spinal nerve [19].

24.3 Morphology

The consistency and continuity of the PDM have been debated by authors [5]. Dommisse's original observations revealed a thick membrane with two layers [5, 6]. Similarly, Loughenbury, Wadhwani, and Soames [21] found the membrane to be "well-developed." Wiltse et al. [7] describe the membrane as thinner than periosteum, but about one-quarter the toughness of dura. Meanwhile, Frykholm [4] also found the membrane to be double-layered, but still delicate and extremely thin, though its thickness varied between anterior and posterior segments. Multiple other authors have described the membrane as thin, delicate, or translucent [1, 5, 9, 13, 14, 24]. One study estimated the thickness of the PDM to be less than 1 mm [14]. Bosscher et al. [19] propose that the PDM has both thick and thin segments, which can be classified based on region: the thin membrane is found in the posterior, pedicular, infrapedicular, and distal perineural regions. Thick segments include the anterior, suprapedicular, and proximal perineural PDM [19].

The continuous nature of the membrane is validated by most authors [15, 17, 19, 21, 24]. However, some studies describe a structure anatomically similar to the PDM except that it is "lacy" and "incomplete" [5, 10, 11, 22]. A possible explanation for these findings is that these reports are describing a different structure, which Loughenbury, Wadhwani, and Soames [21] term the "superficial membrane of the PLL." Their study observed variable existence of a lacy, incomplete membrane in addition to the consistent presence of a continuous PDM [21]. It is possible that reports documenting a PDM with interruptions may, in fact, be describing this structure [5].

24.4 Histological Structure

The connective tissue composing the PDM is a mix of areolar, fibrous, and adipose tissues containing well-developed systems of arteries, veins, and lymphatics [19, 23, 25]. The exact tissue composition of the PDM varies between cadavers and between vertebral levels [19, 23]. Plaisant et al. [15] found evidence of collagen fibers within the membrane, which they described as a fibrous, fatty, cellular complex containing numerous vessels. The intima of the PDM is composed of one or two cell layers containing mostly fibroblasts and endothelium-like cells with occasional histiocytes [19, 23]. Within the intima, there are crypt-like indentations that increase the functional surface area of the PDM [19, 23]. A subintima of areolar connective tissue is usually present [23]. In some regions, the PDM becomes continuous with the adventitia of enclosed blood and lymph vessels [19, 23]. Enclosed vessels are often irregularly shaped with thickening of the tunica muscularis [19, 23]. The tunica muscularis of enclosed vessels, as well as the adventitia of the PDM, contains CD44, CD55, and HAS2+ cells, suggesting a role in hyaluronan production, lubrication, and inflammatory mediation [23].

The histological structure differs between the regions of the PDM, in keeping with the macroscopic variations noted [19]. Anterior segments are generally thicker with more fibrous tissue to accommodate large vessels, while posterior segments contain thinner PDM that is more suitable for the smaller vessels it envelops [23]. Thin PDM is primarily composed of loose connective and adipose tissue, often supported by epidural fat [19, 23]. Medially, the intima of the anterior PDM segments is continuous with the intima and subintima of the posterior PLL surface, so that the PLL may appear to be a dense collection of fibrous tissue within the PDM [19, 23].

The PDM has been shown to contain nerve fibers and endings in both human [1, 2, 19, 23, 25] and non-human studies [26]. Density, diameter, and myelination of fibers vary throughout the PDM, with fibers being larger and more numerous in anterior segments [19, 25]. Nerve fiber density has a negative correlation with the density of inflammatory cells present [19]. The presence of nerve fibers on staining may also change in response to membrane physiological activity [19]. These nerves likely have a nociceptive function as they have been shown to contain C-fibers and immunoreact to CGRP and substance P [25].

24.5 Embryology

Little is known about PDM development: most studies of vertebral embryology describe the formation of a VC lining, but the literature does not agree in all aspects of VC development [5]. Further complicating the situation, many of these studies do not use the term PDM [5]. Most agree that the VC lining shares the same mesodermal anlage as dura [5, 17, 22, 27–29]. von Lüdinghausen describes the development of an endorachis, which becomes the lining of the VC, from the same mesenchyme as the pia and arachnoid [5, 12]. Often, researchers compare the development of the spinal dura to that of the cranial. In the cranium, the dura is composed of an outer endosteal layer, which contains vessels and nerves and ends at the foramen magnum, and an inner meningeal layer that continues caudally as the spinal dura [26]. Sandwiched between these layers and separating them are the dural venous sinuses [17]. Researchers speculate that the spinal dura may also originate as a double-layered structure, with the epidural venous plexuses forming the epidural space [17, 26, 29]. In this case, the PDM, also a well-innervated and highly vascular structure, would correspond to the endosteal layer.

Van Dun and Girardin [17] referred to the common originator of the PDM, PLL, and dura mater as the "embryonic dura mater," based on the mesenchymal cells they found lining the posterior surface of the vertebral bodies and discs. In an 8-week embryo, they observed the stratification of these cells into three layers: an inner layer that gave rise to the dura mater, a middle layer adjacent to the vertebral body, and an outer layer that would become the perichondrium and the periosteal layer (PLL) [17]. This middle layer could conceivably become PDM. This timeframe correlates with studies observing the development of a well-formed epidural space at 8 weeks, which is caused by the division between the cell layers that give rise to the periosteum and dura [28–30]. Epidural space formation first begins cranially at around 6 weeks, developing caudally over time, in a lateral to anterior to posterior sequence [28, 30]. The epidural space contains vessels from inception [28, 30]; further development of venous channels occurs in the following weeks and may contribute to the separation of dura and perichondrium [24, 29]. For this reason, Newell [24] speculates that PDM may be of endothelial origin, positing that this mechanism of formation makes the PDM a modified venous sinus. Meanwhile, Rodionov and Asfandiyarov [28] do not specifically mention the PDM but differentiate the perimedullar mesenchyma into an inner layer of neural crest cells that give rise to the pia and arachnoid and an outer layer of somites, designated the "primary pavement of the vertebral canal," from which dura and periosteum develop. These authors further propose that the formation of the epidural space is primarily dictated by interactions between the spinal cord and the walls of the VC [28].

There is some evidence that the PDM develops later than these studies indicate. In a cadaveric study, Hayashi et al. [10] first observed a connective tissue membrane surrounding the dura at 14 weeks. At 13 weeks, the earliest time point they studied, Hamid et al. [16] observed a double-layered connective tissue containing vessels covering the vertebral walls. They believed this tissue to be periosteum rather than PDM based on the presence of osteoblasts, and failed to identify a PDM in any of their samples [16].

24.6 Function

Most researchers agree that the PDM plays a major role in supporting and protecting the dural sac. The multitude of attachments of the PDM anchors the spinal cord to the VC walls and interspinous ligaments [5]. By blending with the periosteum of the vertebral body, the PDM becomes continuous with the anterior longitudinal ligament, thereby forming complete circumferential support of the vertebral body [10, 21]. Because the PDM is a longitudinal structure, it is reasonable to infer that it provides support to the entire vertebral column [5]. The perineural PDM, along with the surrounding fat and veins, may provide stability and cushioning for exiting spinal nerves, acting as a counterforce to traction forces that displace them [4, 21]. The protection the PDM provides to the soft tissues of the VC may be especially important during development [10].

The PDM can also act as a protective barrier around the spinal cord [5]. The membrane limits the posterior migration of disk fragments, thereby protecting the cord from local compression [4, 8, 13, 14]. The presence of the PDM likely also impedes the posterior extension of a vertebral neoplasm, infection, or premembranous hematoma [5, 8]. Segregation of the epidural space from the vertebral body by the PDM could explain why vertebral infections rarely affect more than one level [8].

Recent studies have investigated additional roles of the PDM in maintaining the epidural space and mediating inflammation [23]. Immunohistochemical analysis has shown that multifunctional hyaluronan receptor CD44 and hyaluronic acid synthetase 2 marker HAS2 are present throughout the PDM as well as in the tunica muscularis of enveloped blood vessels [23]. The lining and sub-lining of the PDM are immunoreactive for fibroblast-like synoviocytes, which can secrete hyaluronan, a molecule commonly associated with providing lubrication and matrix structural support in joints [23, 31]. Additionally, an endoscopic study of spine surgery patients with persistent postoperative back pain revealed that after surgery, when the PDM is removed, the epidural space undergoes severe fibrosis and obliteration [32]. Based on this evidence, researchers believe that the PDM and/or its enclosed vessels are essential for lubricating the epidural space and maintaining tissue health [23]. The presence of CD44, which performs additional functions in mediating inflammation, as well as the inflammatory markers CD55 and CD68, indicates a role for the PDM in the immune response [23].

Of particular interest clinically, there is growing evidence for a nociceptive function of the PDM. As described earlier, nerve fibers embedded in the membrane have been demonstrated in several histological studies of the PDM [1, 2, 19, 23, 25, 33]. Many of these nerves can relay pain, as they contain C-fibers and are immunoreactive to CGRP and substance P [25]. During endoscopy, inflamed-appearing PDM is painful to the touch, while normal-appearing PDM is not sensitive [27].

24.7 Imaging

It is challenging to visualize the PDM on imaging due to its adherence to the VC; however, it can sometimes be identified as a delicate line that is more apparent on magnetic resonance imaging

(MRI) than on computed tomography (CT) [14, 34]. A greater amount of fat in the anterior epidural space clarifies the PDM, making it most obvious at the L5/S1 level and in obese patients [14]. In pathological states, the PDM may become more obvious. For example, spontaneous intracranial hypotension causes the PDM to bow posteriorly as cerebrospinal fluid moves from the dural sac to the epidural space; the enhancement of the fluid adjacent to the membrane can make the PDM more evident [34]. In these cases, CT myelography will show leaked contrast gathering in the epidural space where it is bound by the PDM; this collection may resemble a tubular pseudocyst [34]. In cases of a vertebral body neoplasm or infection spreading posteriorly, the PDM contains the disease, and the premembranous space may be seen to swell [14]. In advanced cases, the PDM typically remains intact but can be displaced posteriorly [14].

24.8 Clinical and Surgical Considerations

The PDM can be directly identified during epiduroscopy [5, 20, 27]. The membrane is visualized as a continuous sheath with a mottled exterior due to its vascular nature [20]. The spectrum of consistencies, ranging from well-developed, thick membranes to thin and translucent tissue, is evident on epiduroscopy [20]. In pathologic states, the membrane may become hyperemic and its veins dilated [20, 27]. Identification of an inflamed PDM can be helpful in forming a diagnosis. Cases of low back pain thought to be nonspecific or psychosomatic have been shown to have pain reproducible by touching a hyperemic pedicular PDM during epiduroscopy [20]. The procedure may also be performed therapeutically: mechanical disruption of the PDM using an endoscope has been successfully utilized to achieve sustained relief in patients with low back pain [19, 20, 35]. The exact mechanism of pain relief is unknown, but it may be due to the dissipation of inflammatory material or denervation of the sensitive peripheral nerve distribution (PDM) [20].

The impact of the PDM on other procedures in the epidural space is not well known and merits further research. Its structure likely impacts the neuraxial distribution of drugs injected into the epidural space [5]. For example, it is thought that the periradicular extensions of the PDM maintain the proximity of epidural anesthetics to the spinal nerve; therefore, the variation in length of these evaginations likely impacts the effectiveness of the drugs [8]. When performing radiculography, if sufficient contrast is injected, it can be visualized in the periradicular sheath; however, if the patient has undergone spine surgery, the space may be too fibrosed for contrast to be seen [8]. During discography, contrast may be seen in the premembranous space, resembling a hematoma, if the vertebral body is overfilled and leaking, or if the needle inadvertently punctures the PDM [8]. Similarly, if the vertebral body is overfilled during percutaneous vertebroplasty, cement may leak out into the premembranous space, where it is contained by the PDM [36]. This protective function of the PDM could prevent serious complications [5]. Clinicians should be mindful that PDM rupture can be caused by rough manipulation of the cannula during this procedure [36].

24.9 Pathologies

While the PDM generally restricts the movement of disc fragments and other foreign material, there are rare cases of violation. One case has been reported of posterolateral migration of a disk fragment, in which it is assumed that one of the barriers to migration, possibly the PDM, must have perforated [37]. In another instance, a sequestered disk fragment was found to have migrated underneath the PDM and PLL; intraoperatively, the PDM had to be cut to remove the fragment [8]. Migration anterior to the PDM is also seen in apophyseal avulsion fractures, which are more common in adolescents [8].

Researchers speculate that the PDM may be an unrecognized source of back pain for a large subset of patients [19, 27]. Bosscher et al. hypothesize that tissue breakdown products, formed from trauma or disc degeneration, may aggregate within the suprapedicular compartment created by the PDM over time, causing inflammation and sensitization of the membrane [19, 27]. If sensitization travels with the PDM or its vessels to affect the epidural space, this mechanism could explain the relief of low back pain achieved through epidural steroid injections [27]. Because it is well innervated, the PDM may also be involved in relaying nociceptive signals in cases of disc herniation or iatrogenic fibrosis [5]. Persistent back pain after spinal surgery may be due to severe epidural fibrosis that occurs without the lubrication provided by the PDM [20]. It is possible that some cases of successful laminectomy or discectomy achieve pain relief through removal of an inflamed PDM, more so than decompression [27].

24.10 Future Directions

The involvement of the PDM in spinal pathologies merits further investigation. Already, researchers have trialed a new procedure, percutaneous ablation and curettage and inferior foraminotomy, to directly denervate the sensitive tissues of the PDM and remove inflammatory material from the suprapedicular compartment [27]. Early studies have shown success in using this method to treat low back pain [27], but further evidence is needed. The role of the PDM and suprapedicular compartment in spinal disorders should be further studied, as this may lead to more accurate diagnoses and treatment options for patients with back pain. The PDM may also bring new clarity to spinal pathologies relating to its role in mediating the immune response and providing lubrication to the epidural space, both of which require further exploration.

Another area of uncertainty with potential clinical ramifications is the influence of the PDM on epidural drug distribution. Due to discrepancies in the anatomic description of the PDM in relation to the venous plexuses, it is unclear how pressure variations may affect fluid dynamics in the epidural space [19]. Furthermore, there is a paucity of literature regarding the embryological development of the PDM, which could provide insights into additional functions of the membrane [5]. Universally agreed-upon nomenclature and definitions regarding the PDM are developing over time. Future studies will benefit from the consistent use of these terms, enabling researchers to more clearly delineate the PDM's anatomy, embryology, and functions.

24.11 Conclusion

The PDM is a continuous connective tissue sheath surrounding the dura that is highly vascular and well-innervated. The membrane has both thick and thin areas composed of areolar, adipose, and fibrous tissues. Laterally, the circumneural PDM extends with the exiting spinal nerve out of the neural foramen. Anteriorly, PDM tissue merges with the PLL. The epidural space is formed between the dura and the PDM, while the space anterior to the PDM can be referred to as the premembranous space. The membrane can act as a barrier, keeping material in and out of the epidural space. Its multitude of connections to the vertebral walls allow it to provide support to the dural sac while maintaining distance between the dura and periosteum. The circumferential and longitudinal nature of the PDM enables stability for the entire spinal column. The development of the PDM is largely unknown, but it likely originates from the same anlage as the dura. It is thought that the venous sinuses play an important role in separating the PDM from the dura to form the epidural space. The exact timeline is debated, but the PDM may form as early as 9 weeks, and it probably plays a protective role for the spinal cord during development. New research is uncovering evidence that the PDM can be a source of back pain; further study is needed to better understand the clinical ramifications.

References

1. Bridge CJ. Innervation of spinal meninges and epidural structures. Anat Rec. 1959;133:553–63.
2. von Luschka H. Die Nerven des Menschlichen Wirbelkanales. Tübingen: H Laupp; 1850.

3. Fick R. Handbuch der Anatomie und Mechanik der Gelenke. Jena: Gustav Fisher; 1904.
4. Frykholm R. Cervical epidural structures, periradicular and epineurial sheaths. Acta Chir Scand. 1951;102(1):10–20.
5. Ansari S, Heavner JE, McConnell DJ, Azari H, Bosscher HA. The peridural membrane of the spinal canal: a critical review. Pain Pract. 2012;12:315–25. https://doi.org/10.1111/j.1533-2500.2011.00510.x.
6. Dommisse GF. The arteries and veins of the human spinal cord from birth. Edinburgh: Churchill Livingstone; 1975.
7. Wiltse LL, Fonseca AS, Amster J, Dimartino P, Ravessoud FA. Relationship of the dura, Hofmann's ligaments, Batson's plexus, and a fibrovascular membrane lying on the posterior surface of the vertebral bodies and attaching to the deep layer of the posterior longitudinal ligament. Spine. 1993;18(8):1030–43. https://doi.org/10.1097/00007632-199306150-00013.
8. Wiltse LL. Anatomy of the extradural compartments of the lumbar spinal canal. Peridural membrane and circumneural sheath. Radiol Clin North Am. 2000;38(6):1177–206. https://doi.org/10.1016/s0033-8389(08)70003-4.
9. Hasue M, KS, Sakuyama Y, Ito T. Anatomic study of the interrelation between lumbosacral nerve roots and their surrounding tissues. Spine. 1983;8(1):50–8. https://doi.org/10.1097/00007632-198301000-00010.
10. Hayashi K, Yabuki T, Kurokawa T, Seki H, Hogaki M, Minoura S. The anterior and the posterior longitudinal ligaments of the lower cervical spine. J Anat. 1977;124:633–6.
11. Kikuchi S. Anatomical and experimental studies of nerve root infiltration. J Japan Orthop Assoc. 1982;56:605.
12. von Lüdinghausen M. Ligaments and adipose tissue in the epidural space. Anat Anz. 1967;121:294–312.
13. Schellinger D, Manz HJ, Vidic B, Patronas NJ, Deveikis JP, Muraki AS, Abdullah DC. Disk fragment migration. Radiology. 1990;175(3) https://doi.org/10.1148/radiology.175.3.2343133.
14. Schellinger D. Patterns of anterior spinal canal involvement by neoplasms and infections. AJNR Am J Neuroradiol. 1996;17:953–9.
15. Plaisant O, Sarrazin JL, Cosnard G, Schill H, Gillot C. The lumbar anterior epidural cavity: the posterior longitudinal ligament, the anterior ligaments of the dura mater and the anterior internal vertebral venous plexus. Acta Anat. 1996;155(4) https://doi.org/10.1159/000147816.
16. Hamid M, Fallet-Bianco C, Delmas V, Plaisant O. The human lumbar anterior epidural space: morphological comparison in adult and fetal specimens. Surg Radiol Anat. 2002;24(3):194–200. https://doi.org/10.1007/s00276-002-0041-6.
17. van Dun PLS, Girardin MRG. Embryological study of the spinal dura and its attachment into the vertebral canal. Int J Osteopath Med. 2006;9(3):85–93. https://doi.org/10.1016/j.ijosm.2006.07.002.
18. Covino BG, Scott D. Handbook of epidural anaesthesia and analgesia. Orlando: Grune and Stratton; 1985.
19. Bosscher HA, Grozdanov P, Warraich II, MacDonald CC, Day MR. The anatomy of the peridural membrane of the human spine. Anat Rec. 2021;304(4) https://doi.org/10.1002/ar.24476.
20. Bosscher H. Lumbosacral epiduroscopy. In: Regional nerve blocks in anesthesia and pain therapy; 2022. https://doi.org/10.1007/978-3-030-88727-8_53.
21. Loughenbury PR, Wadhwani S, Soames RW. The posterior longitudinal ligament and peridural (epidural) membrane. Clin Anat. 2006;19(6) https://doi.org/10.1002/ca.20200.
22. Hogan Q. Lumbar epidural anatomy. A new look by cryomicrotome section. Anesthesiology. 1991;75(5) https://doi.org/10.1097/00000542-199111000-00007.
23. Bosscher HA, Grozdanov PN, Warraich II, MacDonald CC, Day MR. The peridural membrane of the spine has characteristics of synovium. Anat Rec. 2021;304(3):631–46. https://doi.org/10.1002/ar.24474.
24. Newell RLM. The spinal epidural space. Clin Anat. 1999;12(5) https://do.org/10.1002/(SICI)1098-2353(1999)12:5<375::AID-CA7>3.0.CO;2–6.
25. Bosscher HA, Heavner JE, Grozdanov P, Warraich IA, Mitchell S, Wachtel MS, Dertien J. The peridural membrane of the human spine is well innervated. Anat Rec. 2016;299(4) https://doi.org/10.1002/ar.23315.
26. Kumar R, BR, Dunsker SB, Keller JT (1996) Innervation of the spinal dura: myth or reality? Spine 21(1):18–25.
27. Bosscher HA, Heavner JE. Lumbosacral epiduroscopy findings predict treatment outcome. Pain Pract. 2014;14(6) https://doi.org/10.1111/papr.12112.
28. Rodionov AA, Asfandiyarov RI. Morphogenesis of the epidural space in humans during the embryonic and early fetal periods. Neurosci Behav Physiol. 2010;40:137–42.
29. Sensenig EC. The early development of the meninges of the spinal cord in human embryos. Contrib Embryol Carnegie Inst. 1951;34:147–57.
30. Patelska-Banaszewska W. The development of the epidural space in human embryos. Folia Morphol (Warsz). 2004;63(3):273–9.
31. Gupta RC, Lall R, Srivastava A, Sinha A. Hyaluronic acid: molecular mechanisms and therapeutic trajectory. Front Vet Sci. 2019;6 https://doi.org/10.3389/fvets.2019.00192.
32. Bosscher HA, Heavner JE. Incidence and severity of epidural fibrosis after back surgery: an endoscopic

study. Pain Pract. 2010;10(1):18–24. https://doi.org/10.1111/j.1533-2500.2009.00311.x.
33. Hovelacque A. Le nerf sinuvertebral. An Anat Pathol Med Chir. 1925;2:435–43.
34. Chen CJ, Lee T, Hsu HL, Tseng YC, Wong YC, Wang LJ. Spinal MR findings in spontaneous intracranial hypotension. Neuroradiology. 2002;44(12) https://doi.org/10.1007/s00234-002-0876-x.
35. Bosscher HA, Heavner JE. Treatment of common low back pain: a new approach to an old problem. Pain Pract. 2015;15(6) https://doi.org/10.1111/papr.12224.
36. Hostin R, Carr J, Gupta MC, Hazelwood S, Dublin A. Importance of the peridural membrane in percutaneous vertebroplasty. Clin Spine Surg. 2005;18(1) https://doi.org/10.1097/01.bsd.0000127704.83334.1a.
37. Mobbs RJ, Steel TR. Migration of lumbar disc herniation: an unusual case. J Clin Neurosci. 2007;14(6):581–4. https://doi.org/10.1016/j.jocn.2006.04.002.

The Denticulate Ligaments

25

Joe Iwanaga and R. Shane Tubbs

25.1 Introduction

The denticulate ligaments are bilateral lateral projections from the spinal cord to the inner aspect of the dura [5–7, 27] (Fig. 25.1). These structures are positioned between the anterior and posterior roots of the spinal nerves [5]. They were first reported in 1739 by the Swiss scientist Johann Jacob Huber [21], but there has been increasing controversy regarding their anatomical depiction (number, shape, attachments, and function). While limited, the histological findings regarding the denticulate ligaments are important for our understanding. They comprise collagen fibers arranged in longitudinal, transverse, and oblique positions [4]. The thickness of those fibers differs among spinal levels [5]. Clinically, the denticulate ligaments serve as landmarks for identifying the anterior and posterior rootlets of the spinal cord, the vertebral artery, and spinal accessory nerves at the foramen magnum [3, 5].

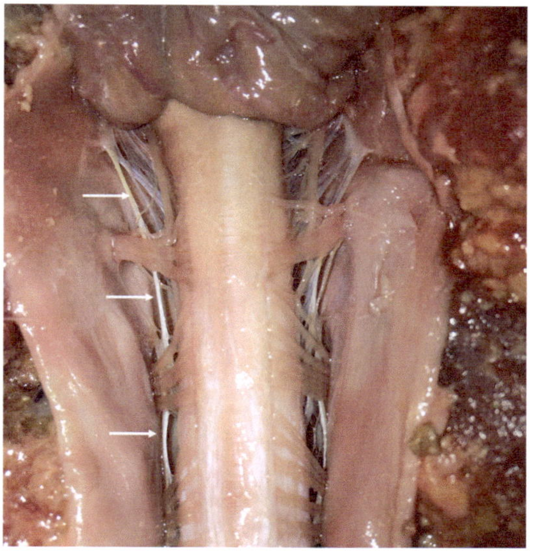

Fig. 25.1 Posterior view of an intradural cadaveric dissection of the craniocervical junction and upper cervical spinal cord. Note the denticulate ligaments (arrows). Upper cervical posterior rootlets are seen traveling posterior to these structures

25.2 Macroscopic Anatomy

The denticulate ligaments are described as 20–21 fibrous spinal projections that stabilize the spinal cord within the spinal canal [6]. Each denticulate ligament is covered by a leptomeningeal layer that continues with the arachnoid and pia mater of the spinal cord [1]. These ligaments consist of triangular pairs that extend from the lateral aspect

J. Iwanaga
Department of Neurosurgery, Tulane Center for Clinical Neurosciences, Tulane University School of Medicine, New Orleans, LA, USA

R. S. Tubbs (✉)
Tulane University School of Medicine, New Orleans, LA, USA
e-mail: rtubbs@tulane.edu

M. Turgut et al. (eds.), *Ligaments of the Vertebral Column*,
https://doi.org/10.1007/978-3-032-09070-6_25

of the spinal cord and attach to the inner aspect of the dura mater [12] (Figs. 25.2 and 25.3). Others report the denticulate ligaments as long bilateral ribbon-like ligamentous structures that suspend the spinal cord within the dural sac [16].

Ceylan et al. found that the denticulate ligaments were only present in the cervical and thoracic regions of the spine [6]. They described no denticulate ligaments in the lumbar or sacral levels. Their most significant observation was that each denticulate ligament was a single, narrow fibrous strip, ranging from the craniovertebral junction to T12 [6]. This is consistent with the finding of Tubbs et al.: the last denticulate ligament was present at the level of the conus medullaris between the spinal roots of the T12 and L1 nerves [27]. Each ligament comprised triangular extensions perpendicular to the vertebral column [6]. The base of each extension was projected from a narrow fibrous strip of the denticulate ligament in which the apex was attached to the dura mater.

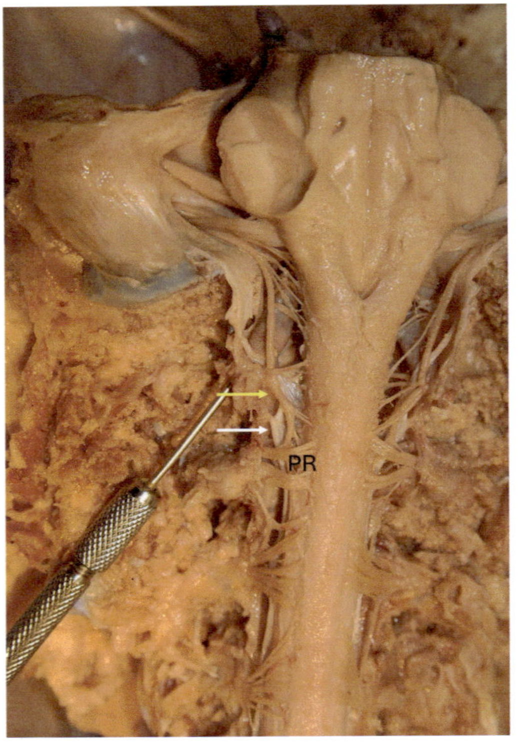

Fig. 25.2 Posterior view of the denticulate ligaments (white arrow). The cerebellum has been removed, and the upper cervical posterior rootlets (PR) are seen. Also, note the spinal part of the spinal accessory nerve (yellow arrow)

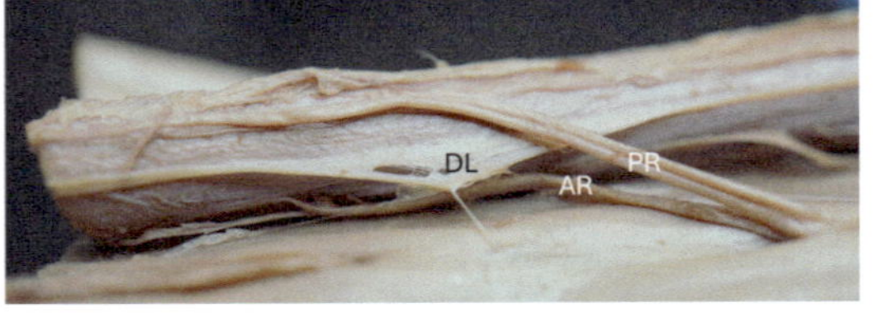

Fig. 25.3 Note the denticulate ligament (DL) ends in a prong-like portion that then inserts into the dura mater. Also note that this ligament is fenestrated. The ligament is shown here separating the posterior (PR) and anterior roots (AR) of a thoracic spinal nerve

The apex of each projection varied with the spinal region. Each apex in the cervical region was attached to the dura by a 3–5 mm long fibrous band or bands (single or double) (Fig. 25.3). In the upper thoracic region, no such fibrous bands were present as the apices of the extensions attached directly to the dura. The fibrous bands were also present in the lower thoracic region, but they were longer than those in the cervical region (21–26 mm) [6]. This is likely due to the varying motion capacities of different regions of the spinal column. The cervical and lower thoracic portions contain fibrous bands that attach to the dura, allowing mobility within their respective areas. However, the apices can connect directly to the dura due to the lack of mobility in the upper thoracic regions [6]. At both levels of the vertebral column, the apical attachments are positioned superomedially to the intervertebral foramen of the inferior vertebrae. As dissection progressed inferiorly, the distance from the dural attachment to the intervertebral foramen increased (10 mm at the cervical levels, 10–15 mm at the upper thoracic levels, and 15–20 mm at the T11 and T12 levels) [6].

Comparable literature supports Ceylan et al. in reporting that the denticulate ligaments in the cervical region are attached to the dura approximately 2 mm posteriorly and 3 mm cephalad to the nerve root foramen [26, 27]. Each denticulate ligament becomes closer to the intervertebral foramen caudal to its attachment than to the more cephalically placed denticulate ligament [26, 27].

25.3 Intracranial Denticulate Ligament

Uniquely, the intracranial denticulate ligament, the first or highest denticulate ligament, is often the largest of the denticulate ligaments [4]. Among the five cadavers examined by Ceylan et al., the mean length of the intracranial denticulate ligament was 12 mm, and the mean width was 8 mm [6]. This denticulate ligament was found to be attached laterally to the dura over the marginal sinus and just above the entrance of the vertebral artery as it pierced the dura. Through its course, the intracranial denticulate ligament was closely related to the spinal accessory nerve posteriorly and to the vertebral artery anteriorly [6]. Tubbs et al. [28] studied the intracranial denticulate ligament and found that on 20% of sides, the ligament is also attached to the adventitia of the vertebral artery. These authors found that the posterior spinal artery traveled posterior to this ligament in 93% of the sides, and following unilateral transection, rotation of the spinomedullary junction increased by approximately 25%.

25.4 Fetal Denticulate Ligaments

Elvan et al. [7] studied the denticulate ligaments during the fetal period. Denticulate ligaments were more prominent in the cervical and upper thoracic regions when the posterior roots were retracted medially. They ranged in number from 20 to 23, including five double denticulate ligament processes within the same interval.

In contrast, no denticulate ligament processes were present in 14 other intervals, where they were recorded as absent [7]. Elvan et al. thus established that denticulate ligament processes can present unilaterally or as double intervals within the same antenatal period [7]. As in previous studies [4, 8], they observed that the distance between the denticulate ligament processes increased, coursing inferiorly to the conus medullaris. This is believed to be because the vertebral bodies become larger from the cervical to lumbar sections of the vertebral column [5].

25.5 Histology

Few studies have investigated the histological nature of the denticulate ligaments. Elvan et al. analyzed ten histological denticulate ligament specimens and found that the denticulate ligaments were composed of collagen fibrous bundles. Histological examination revealed that the fibrous strip of the denticulate ligament consisted of longitudinal collagen fibers, while the triangular projection contained transverse and oblique collagen fibers [6, 14]. The fibrous strip portion was also attached to the spinal cord by loose connective tissue [6]. The denticulate ligaments penetrated the substance of the spinal cord at various cervical intervals to form a stronger attachment. The denticulate ligaments at the cervical spinal levels were thicker than those at thoracic levels [6]. Nicholas and Weller, using scanning electron microscopy, found that the denticulate ligaments consist of a collagenous core covered by a layer of leptomeningeal cells, continuous with the pia and arachnoid. These authors also demonstrated that the denticulate ligaments fuse with the subpial collagen of the spinal cord [18].

25.6 Pathology

Katarzyna et al. explored the properties of the denticulate ligaments in the cervical spine because of their higher incidence of injury, which is attributed to their high mobility [14]. Sawada et al. reported a meningioma arising from the denticulate ligament at the C1 level. No dural attachment was identified [23]. Meningiomas of the cervicomedullary junction are often classified based on their relationship to the denticulate ligament [4].

Within the myelomeningocele population, the upper denticulate ligaments are variable in length, thickened, and abnormally taut [11, 13]. The denticulate ligaments have been linked to the kinking of the medullary spinal junction in patients diagnosed with Chiari II malformation [6]. Bedford et al. proposed that the patient in their case report diagnosed with spondylosis had additional spinal cord injury due to hypertrophic denticulate ligaments [2]. The so-called Ginkgo leaf sign is seen in spinal meningiomas and is due to the interaction of the tumor with the denticulate ligament [15].

In 147 cases of spasmodic torticollis, Aksik found two cases where the spinal accessory nerve was compressed by a hypertrophied denticulate ligament. A case of cervical brachialgia from an abnormally attached denticulate ligament has been reported [12].

25.7 Anatomical Variations

There is little literature about variations of the denticulate ligaments. However, the ligaments are usually at the most lateral point of the spinal cord. Patel et al. reported an abnormal arrangement of the intracranial denticulate ligament around the posterior inferior cerebellar artery (PICA) [19]. In their case report, the right PICA, arising from the vertebral artery (VA), took an extremely lateral course toward the entrance of the VA into the posterior cranial fossa, where it turned around the lateral edge of the intracranial denticulate ligament and then reversed, traveling medially toward the brainstem. As the PICA was tethered to the intracranial denticulate ligament, there was slight compression against the floor of the posterior cranial fossa [14]. Notably, this denticulate ligament appeared duplicated into two slips, the horizontal portion connecting at the first cervical nerve distal to the turn of the PICA.

As mentioned above, in fetuses, Elvan et al. found an absence of the denticulate ligament at some levels and two ligaments at one spinal interval in others. Such variants have also been reported in adults [7]. The denticulate ligaments can be fenestrated [27], and one to three smaller prongs can be used to attach to the inner surface of the dura mater. The tips of the denticulate ligaments in the thoracic region can be heavier and more blunted [9]. These prongs can be longer in the cervical region.

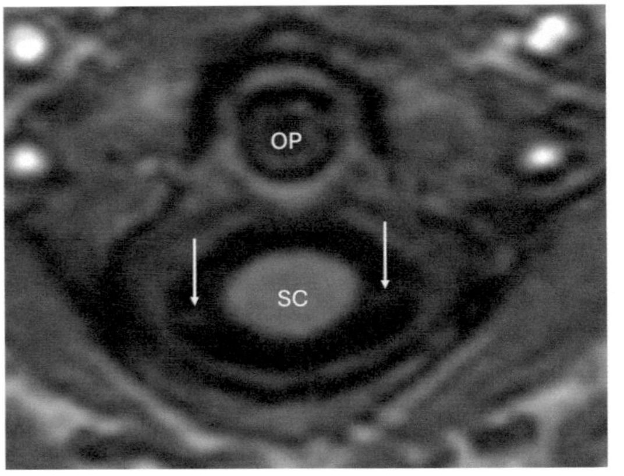

Fig. 25.4 Axial T1-weighted MRI through the cervical spine. Note the odontoid process (OP), spinal cord (SC), and adjacent denticulate ligaments (arrows)

25.8 Imaging

Although small, the denticulate ligaments can be visualized using various medical imaging tools. Historically, they were seen on myelography [9]. Today, they are readily seen on MRI, both 1.5 T and 3.0 T [25] (Fig. 25.4).

25.9 Biomechanics

The denticulate ligaments have been described as stabilizing or suspending the spinal cord within the vertebral canal (Fig. 25.5). Although the function is debatable, some have suggested that the ligaments restrict cranial-caudal motion, while others restrict anterior-posterior motion [10]. In human cadavers, Tubbs et al. found that the denticulate ligaments were stronger in the cervical region and decreased in strength as they moved caudally [27]. These authors also found that the denticulate ligaments became less resistant to anteriorly directed forces as the spinal cord coursed caudally. Inferior to T8, the spinal cord contacted the anterior spinal canal before

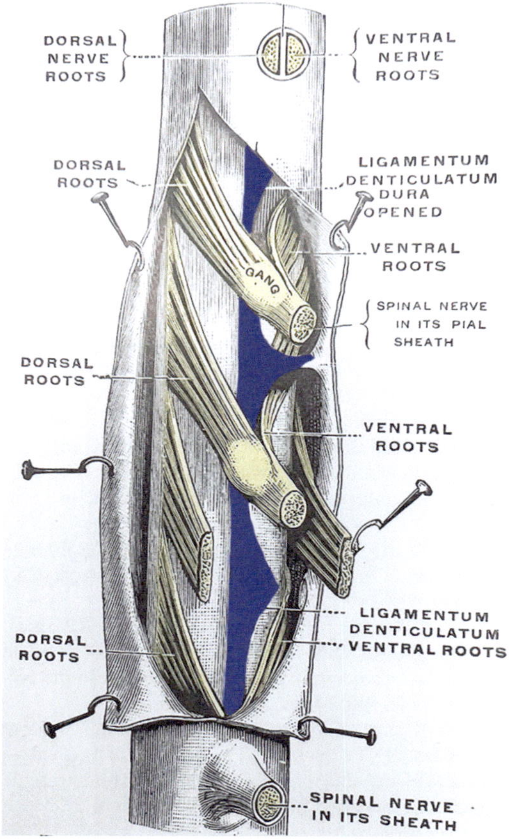

Fig. 25.5 Lateral view of the denticulate ligaments (blue) and their relationship to the spinal dura mater and surrounding nerve rootlets. (After Testut)

the denticulate ligaments became taut. They also compared the forces necessary to produce tautness in the denticulate ligaments with posterior distraction at different spinal cord levels; the denticulate ligament in the upper thoracic region seemed more resistant to the same posterior distraction [27]. When cranial and caudal stresses were compared, the denticulate ligaments tended to be more resistant to caudal stress owing to the decreased motion of the spinal cord (6–7 spinal segments caudally and 10–11 spinal segments cranially) once they were made taut [27]. In dogs, Tunturi concluded that the elasticity of the spinal cord and its investments was due primarily to the denticulate ligaments and pia [30].

In the cervical spines of pigs [30], Polak-Kraśna et al. found that the rupturing force of the denticulate ligament was 1.01+/−0.21 N [20].

25.10 Surgical Significance

The denticulate ligaments are significant landmarks for identifying spinal pathways during cordotomy, such as the dorsal root entry zone (DREZ), and serve as a barrier between the anterior and posterior compartments of the spinal canal [6]. In specific intramedullary or intradural extramedullary tumors, they provide a reliable landmark for identifying a midline entry point to the spinal cord despite any distortion caused by those tumors [6]. The denticulate ligaments are frequently cut for access to more anterior structures, and a suture can be placed through them to retract the spinal cord. One study suggested that sectioning the denticulate ligaments in the lower lumbar levels, superior to the conus medullaris, could yield better results when transecting the filum terminale in patients with a tethered spinal cord [6].

Although sectioning of denticulate ligaments to treat cervical spondylotic myelopathy was abandoned because they have little effect on stabilizing anteroposterior directional movements of the spinal cord [1], cutting the denticulate ligaments on the approach side allows surgeons to manipulate the spinal cord with minimal retraction and to release adhesions through the anterior dural defect [6]. The upper cervical denticulate ligaments, including the intracranial, are significant in isolating contributions, e.g., the nerve of McKenzie to the spinal accessory nerve for denervation of spasmodic torticollis [7]. Tubbs et al. [29] found that McKenzie's nerve was found in 70% of 30 cadaveric sides, and the highest denticulate ligament was pierced on 11 sides (52.4%). On three sides (14.3%), the nerve traveled through two prongs of the denticulate ligament. Bedford et al. reported that hypertrophic denticulate ligaments can compress the C2 root of the spinal accessory nerve [2].

Seichi et al. reported that in three patients diagnosed with myelomeningocele, temporary recovery was achieved by transecting the denticulate ligaments of the spinal cord in the lumbosacral region [24]. Lastly, arteries to the lateral spinal cord have been classified based on their relationship with the denticulate ligament, i.e., preligamentous or postligamentous [22]. Nagata et al. reported two patients with spasmodic torticollis who responded to microvascular decompression of the spinal accessory nerve as it was compressed between the C1 denticulate ligament and vertebral artery [17].

25.11 Conclusion

As the denticulate ligament can be an important landmark during spine and craniocervical procedures, its anatomy should be well known by spine surgeons.

References

1. Adeeb N, Mortazavi MM, Deep A, et al. The pia mater: a comprehensive review of the literature. Childs Nerv Syst. 2013;29(10):1803–10.
2. Bedford PD, Bosanquet FD, Russell WR. Degeneration of the spinal cord associated with cervical spondylosis. Lancet. 1952;2:55–9.
3. Bruneau M, George B. Classification system of foramen magnum meningiomas. J Craniovertebr Junction Spine. 2010;1:10–7.
4. Budohoski KP, Barone DG, Mediratta S, Ross MI, Kirollos RW, Santarius T, Trivedi RA. Far Lateral Approaches: C1 Meningioma with Vertebral Artery Involvement: 3-Dimensional Operative Video. Oper Neurosurg (Hagerstown). 2022;22(1):e48.
5. Carpenter MB. Core text of neuroanatomy. 3rd ed. Baltimore: Williams & Wilkins; 1991. p. 2–3.
6. Ceylan D, Tatarlı N, Abdullaev T, et al. The denticulate ligament: anatomical properties, functional and clinical significance. Acta Neurochir. 2012;154:1229–34.
7. Elvan Ö, Kayan G, Aktekin M. The anatomical features of denticulate ligament in human fetuses. Surg Radiol Anat. 2020;42(8):969–73.
8. Emery JL. Kinking of the medulla in children with acute cerebral oedema and hydrocephalus and its relationship to the dentate ligaments. J Neurol Neurosurg Psychiatry. 1967;30:267–75.
9. Epstein BS. An anatomic, myelographic and cinemyelographic study of the dentate ligaments. Am J Roentgenol Radium Therapy, Nucl Med. 1966 Nov;98(3):704–12.
10. Grostic JD. Dentate ligament- cord distortion hypothesis. Chiropractic Res J. 1988;1:47–55.
11. Gürer B, Canbay S, Bozkurt M, Cikla U, Hananya T, Okut H, Başkaya MK. Microsurgical anatomy of the denticulate ligaments and their relationship with the axilla of the spinal nerve roots. Clin Anat. 2014;27:733–7.
12. Hauge T. An Uncommon Attachment of the Dentate Ligament Causing Cervical Brachialgia. Acta Chir Scand. 118:189.
13. Heidari Pahlavian S, Yiallourou T, Tubbs RS, et al. The impact of spinal cord nerve roots and denticulate ligaments on cerebrospinal fluid dynamics in the cervical spine. PLoS One. 2014;9:e91888.
14. Polak-Kraśna K, Robak-Nawrocka S, Szotek S, Czyż M, Gheek D, Pezowicz C. The denticulate ligament—tensile characterisation and finite element micro-scale model of the structure stabilising spinal cord. J Mech Behav Biomed Mater. 2019;91:10–7.
15. Krishnan P. Gingko leaf sign: a classical imaging finding in spinal meningiomas. Asian J Neurosurg. 2023;18(1):228–9.
16. Moore KL. Clinically oriented anatomy. 2nd ed. Baltimore: Williams & Wilkins; 1992. p. 616–7.
17. Nagata K, Matsui T, Joshita H, Shigeno T, Asano T. Surgical treatment of spasmodic torticollis: effectiveness of microvascular decompression. No To Shinkei. 1989;41(1):97–102.
18. Nicholas DS, Weller RO. The fine anatomy of the human spinal meninges. A light and scanning electron microscopy study. J Neurosurg. 1988;69:276–82.
19. Patel A, Baudoin J, Chaiyamoon A, Cardona JJ, Carrera A, Reina F, Iwanaga J, Dumont AS, Tubbs RS. An unusual arrangement between the highest denticulate ligament and posterior inferior cerebellar artery. Anatomy & Cell Biology. 2023;56(3):394–7.
20. Polak-Kraśna K, Robak-Nawrocka S, Szotek S, Czyż M, Gheek D, Pezowicz CJ. The denticulate ligament – Tensile characterisation and finite element micro-scale model of the structure stabilising spinal cord. Mech Behav Biomed Mater. 2019;91:10–7.
21. Rengachary SS, Pelle D, Guthikonda M. Contributions of Johann Jacob Huber to the surface anatomy of the spinal cord and meninges. Neurosurgery. 2008;62:1370–3.

22. Rojas S, Ortega M, Rodríguez-Baeza A. Anatomical study of the pial arterial network in human spinal cords. Clin Anat. 2021;34(4):596–604.
23. Sawada M, Nakae T, Munemitsu T, et al. Spinal meningioma arising from the denticulate ligament. World Neurosurg. 2018;115:329–33.
24. Seichi A, Hoshino Y, Ikegawa S, et al. Cervical spinal cord atrophy associated with spina bifida. Paraplegia. 1993;31:262–4.
25. Seragioli R, Simao MN, Simao GN, et al. Assessment of the cervical spine denticulate ligament using MRI volumetric sequence: comparison between 1.5 tesla and 3.0 tesla. J Neuroradiol. 2018;45(2):147–51.
26. Stoltmann HF, Blackwood W. An anatomical study of the role of the dentate ligaments in the cervical spinal canal. J Neurosurg. 1966;24:43–6.
27. Tubbs RS, Salter G, Grabb PA, Oakes WJ. The denticulate ligament: anatomy and functional significance. J Neurosurg Spine. 2001;94:271–5.
28. Tubbs RS, Mortazavi MM, Loukas M, et al. The intracranial denticulate ligament: anatomical study with neurosurgical significance. J Neurosurg. 2011;114:454–7.
29. Tubbs RS, Salter G, Grabb PA, et al. The nerve of McKenzie: anatomic study with application to intradural rhizotomy for spasmodic torticollis. Br J Neurosurg. 2014;28:650–2.
30. Tunturi AR. Elasticity of the spinal cord, pia, and denticulate ligament in the dog. J Neurosurg. 1978;48:975–9.

Part VIII

Management of Common Clinical Problems Affecting the Spinal Ligaments

26 Ossification of Spinal Ligaments

Yilin Liu and Fuyou Guo

26.1 Introduction

Ossification of spinal ligaments (OSL) is a common clinical disease characterized by heterotopic ossification of the spinal ligament, which leads to the narrowing of spinal canal diameter, followed by spinal cord and/or nerve root lesions. It mainly includes ossification of the posterior longitudinal ligament (OPLL) and ossification of ligamentum flavum (OLF) [1]. OSL is an important cause of spinal stenosis and spinal cord compression [2]. Patients with OSL typically have neurological symptoms varying from simple discomfort to severe myelopathy, which will cause difficulty walking and wreak havoc on patients' daily lives [3]. Therefore, understanding the etiology and pathogenesis of OSL is of great clinical significance for the prevention and treatment.

Y. Liu
Department of Orthopaedic Surgery, The First Affiliated Hospital of Zhengzhou University, Zhengzhou, Henan, China

F. Guo (✉)
Department of Neurosurgery, The First Affiliated Hospital of Zhengzhou University, Zhengzhou, Henan, China

International Joint Laboratory of Nervous System Malformations, Zhengzhou, Henan, China
e-mail: chyou666@hotmail.com

26.2 Epidemiology

Patients with OSL are generally over 40 years old. The incidence of OPLL varies by ethnic group. The reported incidence of OPLL is 3% in Japan, 0.2% to 1.8% in China, 0.95% in South Korea, 0.12% in the United States, and 0.1% in Germany, respectively [4]. OLF is most commonly observed in the Asian population and occurs at an average age of 60 years [5]. The reported prevalence of thoracic OLF is diverse (3.8%–63.9%) [6]. OPLL usually occurs in the cervical spine, whereas OLF is found in the thoracic and lumbar spine [3]. OPLL and OLF can coexist in some patients [7].

26.3 Etiology and Risk Factors

26.3.1 Genetics

OPLL is a multifactorial and polygenic disease. Previous epidemiological studies have found a high incidence of OPLL within families, so genetic factors have been considered to play a role in OPLL development [8]. Koike et al. used the meta-analysis and conditional analysis to identify 14 genome-wide significant OPLL loci [9].

M. Turgut et al. (eds.), *Ligaments of the Vertebral Column*,
https://doi.org/10.1007/978-3-032-09070-6_26

26.3.2 Endocrine and Metabolic Factors

Some studies have demonstrated the relationship between OPLL and other endocrine and metabolic factors, such as type 2 diabetes [10], high body mass index [11], low inorganic phosphate, X-linked hypophosphatemic rickets [12] and increased C-reactive protein [13]. Obese individuals are also predisposed to OLF [14].

26.3.3 Mechanical Stress and Trauma

Heterotopic ossification of ligaments and tendons is triggered by trauma-caused tissue damage [15], and OSL is no exception. Repetitive tensile stress to the spinal ligaments is also a cause of OSL [16].

26.3.4 Inflammation and Immune Responses

Inflammation and immune responses also influence OSL. Tissue injury, as described previously, will trigger systematic inflammatory responses with the involvement of many immune cells, including monocytes and lymphocytes. Monocytes/macrophages can influence the development of heterotopic ossification [17], which suggests that immune responses also contribute to OSL.

26.4 Pathophysiology

Hypertrophy of ligament tissue and proliferation of chondrocytes are the first steps of ossification, followed by chondrocyte maturation and calcification. Then the entry of osteoblasts and the induction of blood vessels drive the process of ossification [18]. The expression of osteocalcin and collagen fibers in the matrix increased, while the expression of elastic fibers decreased. At the same time, the expressions of bone morphogenetic protein (BMP), transforming growth faction-β (TGF-β), osteopontin (OPN), and vascular endothelial growth factor (VEGF) increased. The activity of alkaline phosphatase (ALP) was enhanced. The mRNA expressions of Osterix and Runx2 in ossified ligament cells were significantly higher than in non-ossified cells [19–24].

26.5 Clinical Presentation

26.5.1 OPLL

OPLL is an ectopic ossification and (or) calcification of the posterior longitudinal ligament resulting in an excessive osteogenic state. Taking a careful medical history and a thorough physical examination are crucial for the diagnosis of OPLL [25]. Although 5% of patients were asymptomatic, careful inquiry may have revealed clinical symptoms including myelopathy and nerve root damage. Spinal cord damage is caused by compression of the spinal cord by OPLL, and the symptoms of spinal cord compression can be exacerbated when combined with cervical spinal stenosis. Patients with spinal cord lesions frequently present with balance issues and impairments in fine motor skills, such as difficulties with writing and buttoning clothes. Patients may require instrumental or wheelchair-assisted ambulation as the myelopathy develops. A positive Rhomberg sign and a positive tandem gait are early signs of gait or balance dysfunction. In addition, there may be tendon hyperreflexia or even clonus in the upper and lower limbs. Pathological reflexes such as the Hoffmann reflex suggest upper motor neuron damage. Scapular hyperreflexia may occur when spinal cord function is impaired above the C3 level. Rotation dyskinesia or rapid posterior and prerotation difficulties of the hand can be seen in myelopathy [26].

26.5.1.1 Ossification of the Posterior Longitudinal Ligament of the Cervical Spine (COPLL)

The main clinical manifestations of COPLL are cervical axial symptoms, radicular symptoms and spinal cord symptoms, which can have a long asymptomatic period due to the slow progression and insidious disease. COPLL is prone to secondary spinal stenosis in the cervical spine, and posterior vertebral body ossification may lead to a reduction in the lost diameter of the spinal canal, neurological dysfunction, and even paralysis [27]. The spinal cord and nerve roots are not only subjected to continuous static compression, but also to the "broken top" of ossified material in the moving cervical spine, which may lead to rapid aggravation of the spinal cord after minor trauma, and neurological function may not be restored even after surgical decompression.

26.5.1.2 Ossification of Posterior Longitudinal Ligament of Thoracic Spine (TOPLL)

TOPLL is not common in clinical practice, and its incidence is much lower than that of cervical posterior longitudinal ligament ossification COPLL [28, 29]. The incidence of clinical symptoms in patients with TOPLL is lower than that in patients with COPLL because of the stability of the thoracic spine compared with the cervical spine. TOPLL may be asymptomatic for a long period of time, but when detected, it is often progressively aggravated, resulting in severe spinal cord injury or even paralysis. The clinical manifestations of TOPLL are similar to those of cervical spondylosis and lumbar intervertebral disc herniation, and COPLL is often present at the same time, which makes it easy to be missed or misdiagnosed in clinical practice [30]. However, OPLL of the lower thoracic spine or thoracolumbar segment, due to the compression of the lumbar bulge and/or conus of the spinal cord, can be characterized by the damage of upper and lower motor neurons at the same time [31]. Due to the low mobility of the thoracic spine, dynamic factors are not critical in thoracic spinal cord lesions.

26.5.2 Thoracic Ossification of Ligamentum Flavum (TOLF)

The clinical presentation of TOLF is more complex. Patients mostly have symptoms of sensory and motor dysfunction below the injured level. In the early stage of the disease, thoracic back pain and lower limb numbness can be seen, and when the disease progresses, chest girdling sensation and spastic paralysis of the lower limbs can occur, and sphincter dysfunction and saddle sensory impairment can be found in patients with lumbar enlargement and spinal cord cones [32]. Typical symptoms of TOLF on physical examination include upper motor neuron damage of the lower limbs, such as hypesthesia or even loss of sensation, increased muscle tone, decreased muscle strength, hyperactive ciliary reflexes, and positive pathologic signs. It should be noted that when damage to the spinal cord cones is caused by TOLF segmental pathology, the clinical manifestations can be extensive lower motor neuron damage, such as loss of tendon reflexes, decreased muscle tone, or even mixed upper and lower motor neuron damage, such as sensory loss or even disappearance of both lower limbs [33].

26.5.3 Ossification of the Anterior Longitudinal Ligament (OALL) and Diffuse Idiopathic Skeletal Hyperostosis (DISH)

OALL of the cervical spine is a common but seldom symptomatic condition that occurs mainly in the elderly population. OALL usually does not require clinical intervention, but it can sometimes lead to airway obstruction and jeopardize patient safety. The anterior longitudinal ligament of the cervical spine may cause difficult tracheal intubation. Therefore, it is important for anesthesiologists to be aware that cervical OALL may lead to airway difficulties [34]. DISH is a rare idiopathic spinal disorder characterized by "form of flow" ossification of the anterior longitudinal ligament of the spine of unknown etiology [35]. DISH of the cervical spine can cause severe dysphagia, and ossification of the anterior longitudinal ligament can lead to spinal ankylosis [36].

26.6 Diagnosis

26.6.1 OPLL

Imaging is the primary diagnostic method for OPLL. Ossifications along the course of the PLL can be seen posterior to the vertebral body on lateral radiographs (Fig. 26.1). OPLL is morphologi-

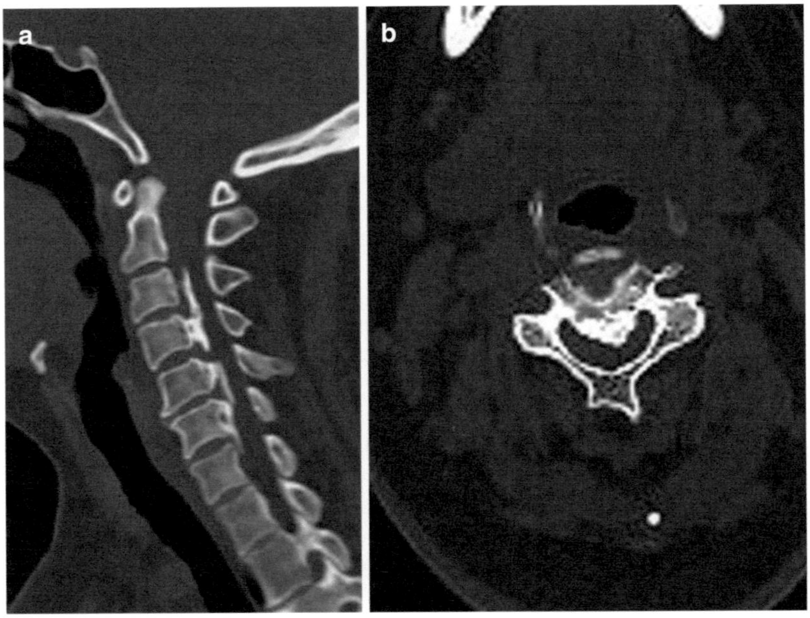

Fig. 26.1 CT spine images of a COPLL patient. (**a**) Sagittal CT demonstrating continuous OPLL from C3 to C6. (**b**) Axial CT of C4 vertebral body demonstrating a continuous OPLL

cally classified into four types: limited (confined to the space at the posterior margin of the intervertebral disc), segmental (noncontinuous ossification located posterior to the vertebral body), continuous (extension of the ossification across several vertebral bodies and the posterior margin of the disc), and mixed (a combination of segmental and continuous) [37]. In addition, OPLL is not always easy to visualize and diagnose on lateral radiographs, and computed tomography (CT) scanning can be the best imaging test for the diagnosis and evaluation of patients with suspected OPLL. Moreover, the use of 2D CT images has significantly improved the diagnostic rate of OPLL [37], as well as the ability to understand the ossification of the dural sac, and in severe cases, the "bilateral sign" can be observed, which suggests the possibility of dural sac defects [38]. In recent years, Takahisa Ogawa et al. [39] constructed a deep convolutional neural network to realize the diagnosis of OPLL based on radiographs with the rapid development of artificial intelligence.

26.6.2 OLF

Currently, CT and magnetic resonance imaging (MRI) examinations are used as the main imaging instruments for the diagnosis of OLF, and both are often used in combination for the diagnosis of TOLF (Fig. 26.2). The location and morphology of TOLF, and whether it is accompanied by dural ossification, can be demonstrated on the basis of CT (Fig. 26.3). Besides, OLF and hypertrophy of the ligamentum flavum can also be identified by CT. Although the display of the ossification pattern by MRI is not as distinct as that by CT, MRI demonstrates the signal changes of the pathologic segments and the spinal cord, and can detect the multiple segmental pathologies that are prone to be neglected by CT scanning [40, 41]. In both T1- and T2-weighted MRI images, the TOLF exhibits low signal and protrudes into the spinal canal in a spherical or beak-like pattern. Accordingly, the spinal cord compressed by TOLF may exhibit high signal, which is considered to represent edema, necrosis, or hemorrhage in acute spinal cord injuries, whereas the high signal in the spinal cord in chronic spinal cord compression represents neurally demyelinating lesions and the formation of microscopic cavities in the spinal cord [42].

26.6.3 DISH

DISH is a disease characterized by progressive ossification of ligaments throughout the body.

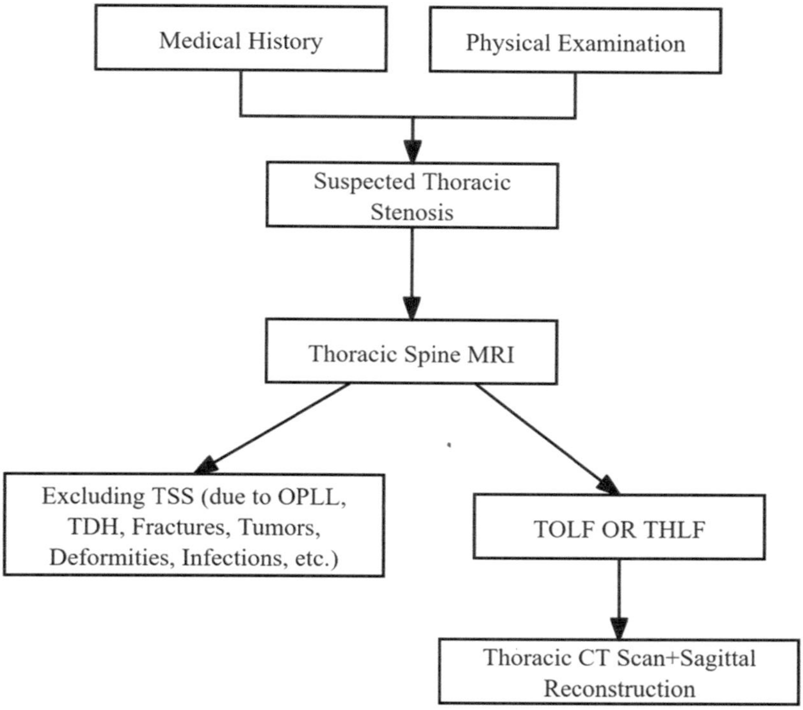

Fig. 26.2 Diagnostic flow chart

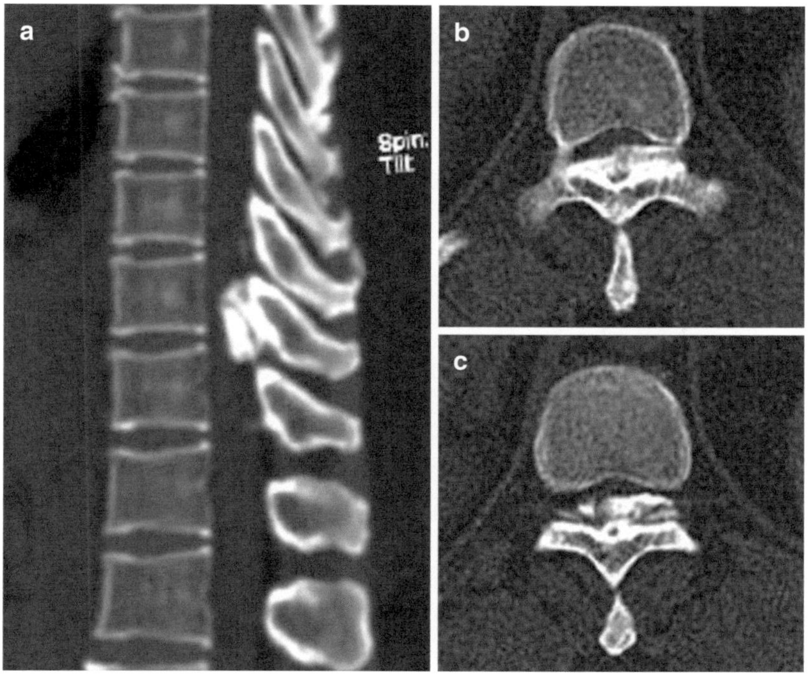

Fig. 26.3 CT spine images of a TOLF patient. (**a**) Sagittal CT demonstrating OLF. (**b**, **c**) Axial CT images showed the invasion of the spinal canal by OLF

Imaging manifestations include: (1) fluid ossification of the anterolateral aspect of at least 4 adjacent vertebrae, with smooth anterior edges of ossification, preferably on the right side of the vertebrae; (2) relative preservation of intervertebral disc height; and (3) no articular ankylosis of the sacroiliac joints. Diagnostic accuracy is improved with CT, which increases the number of DISH cases by approximately 25% [43] (Fig. 26.4).

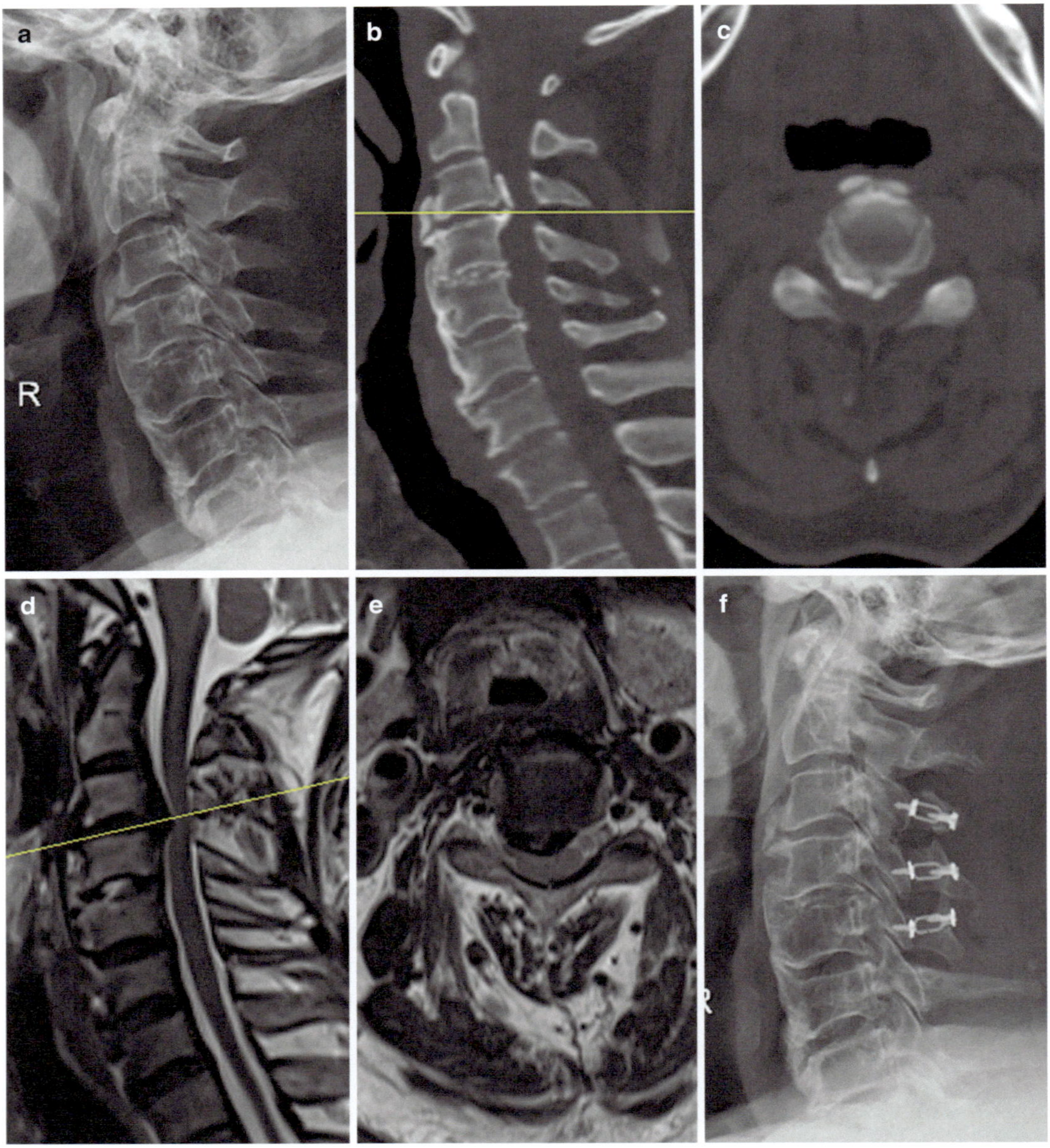

Fig. 26.4 X-ray, CT, and MRI spine images of the patients with DISH accompanied by COPLL. (**a**) Lateral radiographs showed the formation of continuous osteophytes at the anterior edges of multiple vertebrae. (**b**, **c**) Sagittal and axial CT images clearly showed osteophytes at the anterior and posterior edges of the vertebral bodies. (**d**, **e**) MRI images demonstrate significant compression of the spinal cord at the C3/4 level. (**f**) Postoperative X-ray of posterior cervical single-opening laminoplasty for C3 to C5

26.7 Differential Diagnosis

26.7.1 OPLL

To differentiate from OPLL are degenerative vertebral joint ankylosis, disc herniation with calcification, chordoma, DISH, ankylosing spondylitis, and dialysis-induced epidural calcification [44].

26.7.2 OLF

The early clinical symptoms of TOLF are likely to be confused with lumbar spine disorders such as lumbar spinal stenosis and lumbar disc herniation, as well as pathologies of the spinal cord itself, and are often comorbid with other spinal pathologies such as OPLL and disc herniation of the thoracic and lumbar regions [45].

26.8 Treatment

26.8.1 Cervical OPLL

26.8.1.1 Conservative Treatment

Asymptomatic patients with no obvious spinal cord compression or spinal cord degeneration on imaging can be treated symptomatically with cervical external fixation support, application of nonsteroidal anti-inflammatory drugs and neuroprotective drugs. However, conservative treatment is not effective in stopping the progression of cervical OPLL, so a close follow-up is needed for patients to pay attention to the progress of the disease [46].

26.8.1.2 Surgical Treatment

The purpose of cervical OPLL surgery is to relieve neuromedullary compression and restore the physiologic curvature and intervertebral height of the cervical spine. And the main surgical approaches are the anterior approach, posterior approach, and combined anterior and posterior approach (Fig. 26.5). Among them, anterior approach surgery is able to completely decompress the spinal nerves through direct disposal of the ossified material, and at the same time, it is more effective in reconstructing the physiological curvature of the cervical spine [47]. Current anterior approach surgery includes anterior cervical discectomy and fusion (ACDF), anterior cervical corpectomy and fusion (ACCF), Open bone window with Williams-Isu method, and anterior controllable antidisplacement and fusion (ACAF).

ACDF removes the disc only, causing little damage to the vertebral body, and can remodel the physiological curvature of the cervical spine by restoring the height of the intervertebral space, which is effective for patients with bridging cervical OPLL with <50% of canal encroachment, or patients with obvious cervical disc herniation. However, ACDF has the disadvantage of insufficient decompression, and complications such as dysphagia and adjacent spondylolisthesis may occur in the postoperative period. In recent years, with the birth of new techniques such as oblique cut posterior endplates, Zero-P fusion, and Hook spondylolisthesis fusion and their application to ACDF, such complications have been effectively controlled. Kahaer et al. [48] found that the Zero-P cage had a better surgical outcome and a lower incidence of postoperative complications than the traditional cage. Another study showed that the Zero-P fusion technique can achieve effective results in multiple-segmental ACDF and reduce the incidence of dysphagia and other complications [49] (Fig. 26.6).

Compared with ACDF, ACCF has a larger decompression range and adopts a surgical approach of subtotal resection of the vertebral body, which directly treats the ossified material, with obvious surgical effects. Studies have shown that ACCF is significantly better than ACDF in improving cervical spine dysfunction in patients with cervical OPLL. However, while expanding the decompression range, multiple segmental vertebral body resection tends to disrupt the sagittal balance of the cervical spine, and titanium mesh subsidence is also a problem that has been addressed in ACCF [50].

The ACAF technique was proposed by Prof. Jiangang Shi's team, in which the ossified material formed in the posterior longitudinal ligament

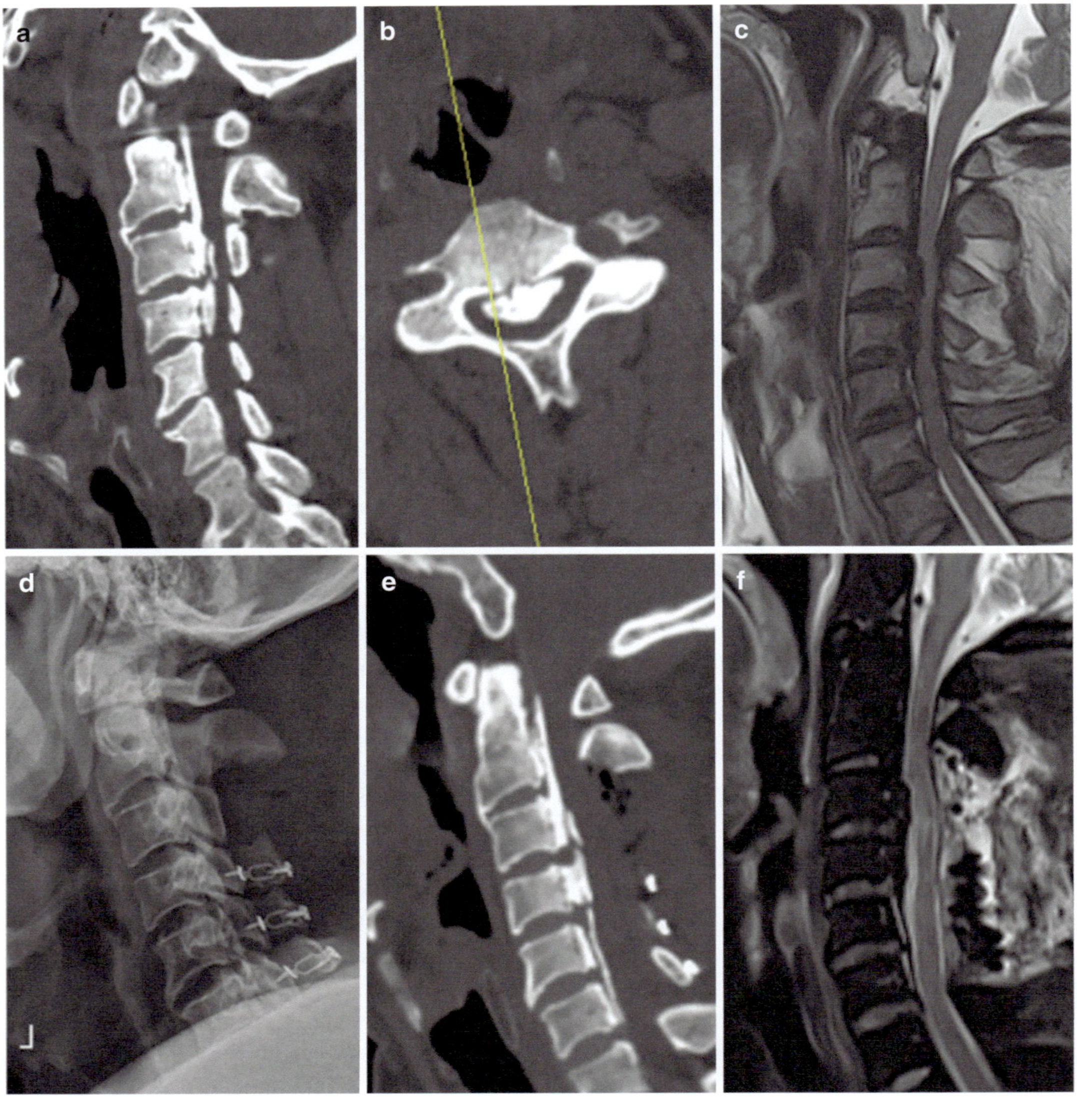

Fig. 26.5 Preoperative and postoperative images of patients with COPLL (C2-C5). (**a, b**) Sagittal and axial CT images showed ossification at the posterior of the vertebral bodies. (**c**) MRI images demonstrate significant compression of the spinal cord. (**d, e, f**) Postoperative X-ray, CT and MRI images of posterior laminoplasty of C4–6, laminectomy of C3, and subaxial decompression at C2

of the cervical spine is not treated, but the corresponding segmental vertebrae and the ossified material are moved anteriorly as a whole, thus relieving the compression of the spinal nerve roots [51]. The ACAF is a simple procedure, with a low incidence of spinal cord injury and cerebrospinal fluid leakage, and the results of many studies have shown that the effectiveness of the ACAF in the treatment of cervical spine OPLL surgery is favorable [52].

With regard to posterior surgery, indirect decompression of the spinal cord is accomplished by enlarging the effective volume of the spinal canal, which is suitable for patients with multiple-segmental cervical OPLL with a positive K-line. Single-door laminoplasty is favored by spine sur-

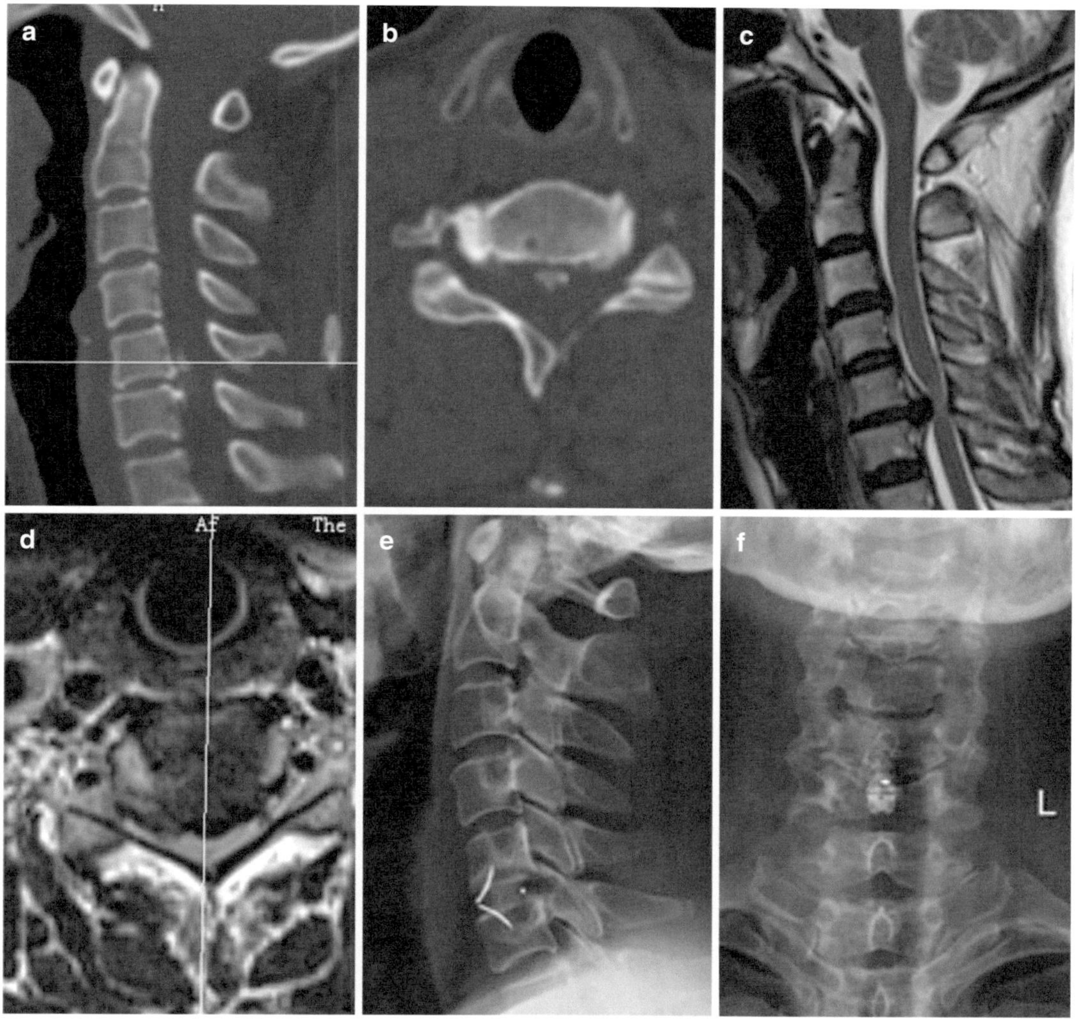

Fig. 26.6 ACDF using Zero-P system for treatment of focal COPLL. (**a, b**) CT images showed that ossification was confined to the posterior of the vertebral body or at the level of the intervertebral disc. (**c, d**) MRI showed compression of the spinal cord. (**e, f**) The anteroposterior and lateral X-rays were taken after ACDF

geons because of its low technical requirements, large decompression area, and high safety. However, the surgical exposure process requires the stripping of the posterior cervical musculoskeletal ligaments, which is likely to cause cervical instability and is not conducive to the patient's later recovery. In order to solve this problem, posterior cervical single-open-door laminoplasty has been modified by the addition of strong fixation of lateral pedicle screws, which can reestablish cervical spine stability. Some studies have shown that single-opening laminoplasty combined with lateral block screws can effectively rebuild the stability of the cervical spine and improve the axial cervical symptoms of patients [53].

Combined anterior and posterior surgery is a better option for patients with complex cervical OPLL with disc herniation, long segmental ossification of the posterior longitudinal ligament, severe sagittal stenosis of the spinal canal, and anterior and posterior compression of the spinal cord. Combined anterior and posterior surgery is needed to improve the condition of spinal canal stenosis, decompress the spinal canal indirectly through posterior surgery, and then directly process the ossified material using anterior surgery, so as to protect the spinal nerves from damage and reduce the risk of cerebrospinal fluid leakage [54].

26.8.2 TOPLL

Most patients with OPLL have no obvious symptoms, and once symptoms appear, they tend to worsen progressively and conservative treatment is ineffective; thus, surgical treatment is a more effective treatment method [55]. At present, TOPLL is mainly divided into direct decompression and indirect decompression. Direct decompression refers to the direct resection of the ossified posterior longitudinal ligament that compresses the spinal cord, and the surgical modalities include anterior cleavage of the sternum or clavicular approach decompression, lateral anterior approach decompression, posterior approach decompression of a 360° ring, and anterior-posterior combined approach decompression. Indirect decompression is achieved by indirectly enlarging the inner volume of the spinal canal to reduce spinal cord compression and expanding the spinal cord fluttering range to achieve the decompression effect, and the current surgical procedures include posterior wall resection with bone grafting and fusion, and posterior laminectomy [56].

26.8.2.1 Direct Anterior Decompression

Direct resection of the ossified posterior longitudinal ligament via an anterior approach has the effect of completely removing the lesions and achieving complete decompression, and is currently recognized as the first choice for the treatment of TOPLL [57]. The anterior approach is divided into the split sternal or clavicular approach and the extrapleural and extraperitoneal access for laminectomy, with the former being applicable to the upper thoracic spine (T1 ~ T3) and the latter mainly used for the middle and lower thoracic spine (T4 ~ T11) [58]. Anterior decompression can directly remove the ossified material, release the compression, adequately decompress, and maintain the existence of physiological kyphosis of the thoracic spine, so anterior decompression is a more reasonable and thorough way theoretically. Anterior decompression can achieve satisfactory surgical results, but the complexity of surgical access, high technical requirements, high trauma, and high incidence of postoperative complications make anterior decompression still unavailable for the treatment of long-segment OPLL.

26.8.2.2 Indirect Posterior Decompression

Posterior decompression involves resection of the posterior vertebral plate and the possibly ossified ligamentum flavum to make the space for the spinal cord to drift backward larger and to avoid compression of the spinal cord by the anterior ossified ligamentum flavum in order to achieve the effect of indirect decompression. However, because of the physiological characteristics of thoracic kyphosis, the space for the spinal cord in the thoracic segment to drift posteriorly is limited, and the anterior OPLL as the main source of compression is not resolved, so the effect of posterior decompression is often inadequate [59]. Currently, the most widely used posterior indirect decompression is simple posterior laminectomy and posterior decompression and fusion. Simple posterior laminectomy destabilizes the spine and carries a high risk of postoperative neurological dysfunction. Yamazaki et al. [60] reported two patients with neurological dysfunction after simple posterior laminectomy, who recovered their neurological function after remedial fixation and fusion. A multicenter retrospective study reported better surgical outcomes for those who underwent fixed fusion than those who did not when multiple surgical procedures were compared [61]. And posterior decompression surgery has a relatively simple operation with fewer complications, and allows for simultaneous management of the coexisting ossified ligamentum flavum. For larger, long-segmented TOPLL, anterior decompression surgery is difficult to operate and the risk of spinal cord injury is high, and posterior decompression surgery is a safe and effective surgical approach.

26.8.2.3 Combined Anterior and Posterior Circumferential Decompression

Huge TOPLL or with OLF can lead to severe compression of the spinal cord, and it is difficult to obtain ideal decompression by anterior or posterior decompression alone, so circumferential decompression can be considered. Tomita et al. [62] first began to use circumferential decompression to treat TOPLL combined with OLF, with one-stage posterior enlarged laminectomy and two-stage anterior resection of a part of the vertebral body and the ossified posterior longitudinal ligament, and obtained satisfactory results (improvement rate of 56% ~ 100%). With the development of surgical techniques, many scholars have advocated one-stage surgery to complete circumferential decompression in recent years. One-stage cricoid decompression surgery is thorough, but it is difficult to operate and has a high complication rate. Takahata et al. [59] retrospectively analyzed a group of cases of one-stage posterior cricoid decompression, among which the prognosis of short-segmented cases was good and the prognosis of patients who had five or more segments was poor. Postoperative kyphosis, intervertebral micromovement, and excessive vascularization in long-segmented decompression could lead to a poor prognosis. Kato et al. [63] modified this procedure by completely removing the posterior structures of decompressed segments, which resulted in better intraoperative visualization and easier reduction of kyphosis after removal of the transverse processes and pedicles. It can be used for all thoracic segments, but it is prone to ischemic injury; thus, only continuous OPLLs ≤ 3 segments can be used. Yang et al. [64] achieved circumferential decompression through a posterior posterolateral approach, which is less traumatic, with adequate operative field, and is suitable for patients with large, single isolated posterior longitudinal bodies, and for patients with large, single isolated posterior longitudinal bodies, which may lead to poor prognosis.

Surgical treatment of TOPLL has always been one of the difficulties in spinal surgery. With the continuous development of surgical techniques and medical devices, a variety of different surgical styles have emerged. Different decompression methods have their own advantages and disadvantages, and there is no consensus on the choice of surgical methods. The choice of surgical approach should be based on the actual condition of the patient and the surgical experience of the surgeon. Therefore, no matter which surgical method is chosen, surgical safety is the first priority, and intraoperative manipulation must be performed meticulously to prevent aggravation of spinal cord injury.

26.8.3 OLF

Surgical decompression therapy is more effective than non-surgical treatment when TOLF patients present with clinical symptoms of spinal stenosis and spinal cord compression [65]. Operative access is usually posterior since the ligamentum flavum is located posterior to the spinal cord. As the standard procedure for the treatment of TOLF, traditional open laminectomy is considered to achieve adequate nerve decompression and symptomatic improvement, but the procedure has the disadvantages of high trauma, high bleeding and high complication rate [66] (Fig. 26.7). In recent years, spinal endoscopic technology has been rapidly developed, and now, scholars around the world also apply spinal endoscopic technology to treat TOLF and achieve excellent results [67].

26.8.3.1 Laminectomy

Laminectomies include double-door total laminectomy, total laminectomy, and hemilaminectomy. Studies have shown that double-door total laminectomy is safe and effective in the treatment of TOLF, but care must be taken to minimize damage to the posterior column of the thoracic spine. Double-door total laminectomy is not suitable for those with severe ligamentous ossification. A simple total laminectomy is suitable for

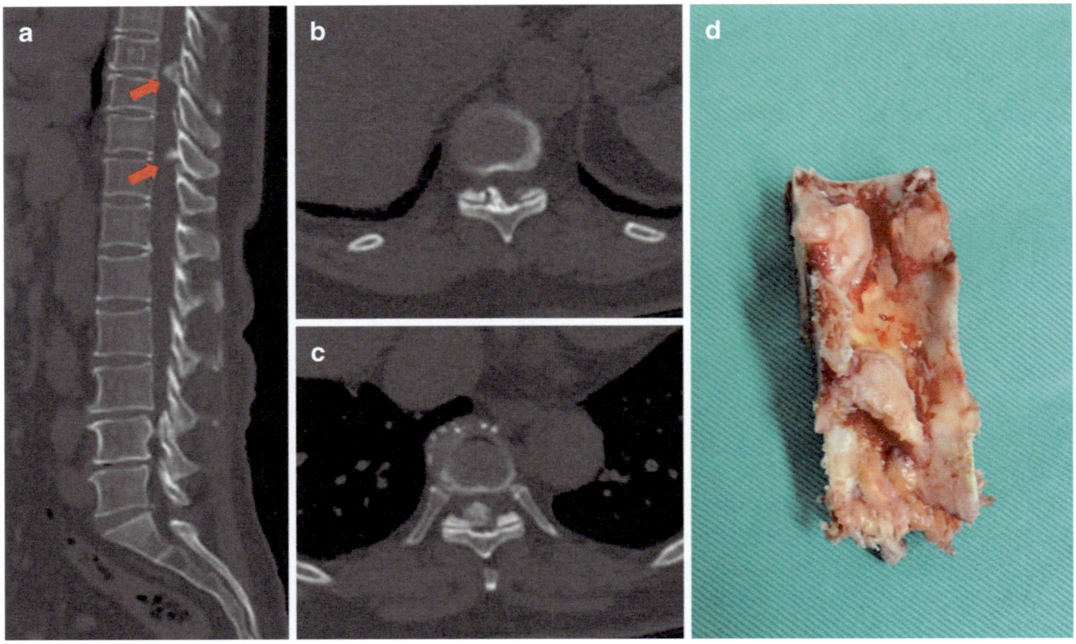

Fig. 26.7 Posterior approach thoracic laminectomy for the treatment of TOLF. (**a, b, c**) Preoperative sagittal and axial CT images demonstrating OLF. (**d**) The OLF was completely resected during the operation

patients whose ossification does not involve the dura, and the ossification can be peeled away from the dura after freeing the laminae. After the ossification has progressed to the dura, total laminectomy with dural resection and patch transplantation can be used [68]. Zhang et al. [69] conducted a retrospective study on patients with TOLF treated with laminectomy and pedicle screw internal fixation, and concluded that internal fixation after total laminectomy can effectively maintain the stability of the thoracic spine, avoiding the re-compression of the spinal cord due to the spinal instability, which may lead to deterioration of neurological function. Hemilaminectomy can effectively increase the volume of the spinal canal and relieve spinal cord compression, and has less impact on the stability of the posterior column of the thoracic spine than total laminectomy [70]. In addition, there is no universally accepted standard for whether or not fusion should be performed at the same time as hemilaminectomy [35, 71].

26.8.3.2 Laminoplasty

Laminoplasty causes relatively less damage to the posterior spinal column structures compared to laminectomy, accomplishing effective decompression of the spinal canal while avoiding extensive disruption of spinal stability. Currently, commonly used laminoplasty procedures include single- and double-door laminoplasty. In terms of maintaining the position of the vertebral plate and preventing reclosure, some studies [72] have shown that both titanium plate fixation and conventional wire fixation are effective in preventing reclosure, but loss of spinal curvature and axial symptoms occur less frequently after titanium plate fixation. Both single and double door opening can increase the spinal canal volume, but they differ in terms of surgical results, indications, and postoperative complications. If the TOLF is more severe and the spinal canal is severely stenotic, single-door laminoplasty is recommended for treatment [73].

26.8.3.3 Microendoscopic Technique

Microendoscopic-assisted spinal decompression was initially used to treat lumbar degenerative diseases. With the gradual development of technology, some scholars have tried to apply it to the treatment of TOLF. Ikuta et al. [74] used microendoscopy to treat a case of thoracic spondylotic myelopathy caused by ossification of the ligamentum flavum. During the operation, posterior decompression was carried out through the interpositional approach, and after resecting the superior spinous processes, a spreader was placed, and the laminectomy was performed under the supervision of microendoscopy to remove part of the vertebral plate and ossified ligamentum flavum, with virtually no bleeding and no complications. The patient's postoperative nerve compression symptoms were significantly reduced. This method achieves full decompression of spinal nerves by removing the bilateral ossified ligamentum flavum, which results in little damage to the paravertebral muscles, demonstrating the clinical value of the microscopic endoscopic treatment of TOLF.

26.8.3.4 Percutaneous Transforaminal Endoscopic Technique

The percutaneous transforaminal endoscopic technique under water media is widely used in clinical treatment with the continuous improvement of spinal endoscopy and minimally invasive surgical instruments. According to the different surgical access and decompression methods, this technique can be divided into percutaneous transforaminal endoscopic decompression (PTED), percutaneous interlaminar endoscopic decompression (PIED), and percutaneous laminar endoscopic decompression (PLED) [75].

Regarding PTED: this procedure establishes a working channel through the lateral posterior approach to the external foraminal opening, removes the lateral and ventral portions of the articular synchondrosis under intervertebral foraminal surveillance, and reveals and resects the ossified ligamentum flavum. PIED: This procedure establishes a working channel through the posterior intervertebral plate space to the dorsal vertebral surface of the ossified ligamentum flavum, removes the bony material overlying the dorsal aspect of the lesion under intervertebral foraminal surveillance, and then reveals and resects the ossified ligamentum flavum, which is similar to the procedure used for the percutaneous laminar endoscopic decompression [76]. PLED: this procedure establishes a working channel through a posterior approach, creates a 6–8 mm diameter bone window in the vertebral plate, and removes the ossified ligamentum flavum under intervertebral foraminoscopic surveillance. PLED does not require the stripping of paravertebral muscles and the destruction of the lesser articular eminence, and it does not require the pulling of the dura mater and nerve roots, so it has the advantages of being less invasive and having fewer complications. Compared with PIED, PLED maintains the integrity of the upper and lower margins of the vertebral plate, resulting in better postoperative spinal stability [75].

26.8.3.5 Unilateral Biportal Endoscopy (UBE)

The UBE establishes 2 independent entrances through 2 small incisions, which serve as the observation and operation channels, respectively. An endoscopic irrigation system is placed in the observation channel to monitor and continuously irrigate the surgical area, and a variety of surgical instruments are placed in the operation channel to perform the operation. With the gradual increase in the use of UBE technology in cervical and lumbar spine disorders [77], some scholars have attempted to use this technology for the treatment of TOLF and have obtained satisfactory results [78]. Deng et al. [67] compared the clinical results of using UBE-assisted ULBD with conventional open decompression fusion for the treatment of TOLF, and the results showed that the efficacy of the two groups was comparable. And the authors concluded that UBE maximizes the preservation of normal bone and achieves adequate decompression while maintaining spinal stability, sparing patients from surgical treatment for fusion. Although UBE decompression for TOLF has the advantages of good results, less invasiveness, and faster postoperative recovery, it is technically demanding and is recommended to be performed only in experienced centers with strict control of surgical indications.

26.8.3.6 Computer-Assisted Minimally Invasive Spinal Surgery (CAMISS)

Tian et al. [79] proposed CAMISS for the first time, which combines computerized navigation technology and minimally invasive spine surgery (MISS), in which an immediate three-dimensional navigation system combined with a high-speed grinder drill was used to complete ligamentum flavum resection and dural decompression under the direct vision of a monitor. The margins of the ligamentum flavum were visualized in the navigation, and the supraspinous ligament, most of the spinous processes, and the interspinous ligament were preserved. The vertebral plate above the ossified ligamentum flavum was ground out of the groove to the contralateral cortex with a high-speed grinding drill, and the bone around the ossified foci was removed with a spatula and vertebral plate biting forceps. The foci were separated from the ossified foci using a nerve peeler and then removed in one piece. The CAMISS maximizes the preservation of all of the supraspinous ligament, most of the spinous processes and interspinous ligaments, which reduces the disruption of the stability of the spine, and the impact on the original biomechanics is smaller, and therefore internal fixation is not used. CAMISS is less invasive and less costly than traditional procedures, but requires a higher level of skill and equipment [80].

26.9 Complications

26.9.1 TOPLL Procedure

Postoperative complications of TOPLL include spinal cord injury, cerebrospinal fluid leakage, intestinal obstruction, dural injury, neurological deterioration and epidural hematoma [81]. The common causes of spinal cord injury, as the most serious complication of TOPLL surgery, are as follows: improper instrumentation and errors during decompression. After decompression surgery, the spinal cord is soaked in an ice sterile 0.9% sodium chloride solution for an insufficient period of time, resulting in increased spinal cord tension and reperfusion injury. Improper fixation position of internal fixation, resulting in direct injury to the spinal cord. The OPLL sometimes adheres severely to the dura mater, and improper separation during decompression leads to dura mater tears [82]. Anterior surgery using a trans-abdominal thoracic approach to the anterior organs is prone to disturbances such as bowel obstruction and other complications. The incidence of postoperative neurological deterioration is considerable, and the mechanism of its occurrence has not been unanimously determined, so MRI examination should be performed immediately to find the cause of postoperative neurological deterioration. Since there are abundant blood vessels in the vicinity of the spine, if the venous plexus is not completely hemostatized during the operation, an epidural hematoma may be caused, and once it is clear that the deterioration is caused by the hematoma, immediate surgery should be performed to remedy the problem.

26.9.2 COPLL Procedure

The onset of the disease is chronic and insidious, and the spinal canal is highly adaptable to chronic compression. Once symptoms appear, the rate of spinal stenosis caused by ossified material is more than 50% in most cases. Therefore, the surgery is complicated, especially for inexperienced anterior surgeons. In the same group of patients who underwent anterior and posterior surgery, the rate of nerve deterioration was higher in the posterior approach than in the anterior approach, which was mainly determined by the characteristics of the pathology. The incidence of C5 nerve root palsy in patients who underwent posterior surgery was 4–5 times higher than that in patients who underwent anterior surgery, especially in cases with loss of cervical lordosis and multiple segmental ossification [83]. However, the incidence of cerebrospinal fluid leakage is 2–3 times

Table 26.1 Complications and advantages/disadvantages of anterior and posterior cervical spine surgery

Methods	Anterior approach	Posterior approach
Complications	Dural cerebrospinal fluid leak, hoarseness, dysphagia, dysarthria	C_5 nerve syndrome, axial pain, cervical instability
Advantages	Direct decompression, minimal tissue dissection	Low recurrence rate, low technical requirements
Disadvantages	Limited visibility, complex anterior anatomy, technical difficulty	Indirect decompression, high complication rate

higher in anterior than in posterior surgery [84], mainly in cases with ossification of the dural sac (Table 26.1).

26.9.3 TOLF Procedure

It can be categorized into early postoperative complications and late complications. Early complications include postoperative cerebrospinal fluid leakage, epidural hematoma, and deep vein thrombosis of the lower extremities, and transient deterioration of neurological function due to reperfusion after sudden decompression of the spinal cord [85]. Zhong et al. [86] reported 22 TOLF patients who underwent simple laminectomy and decompression surgery, and the patients recovered neurological function well after the operation, but the rate of complications was higher. There were 5 cases of dural tear, 1 case of cerebrospinal fluid leakage, 1 case of neurological deterioration, 1 case of epidural hematoma, and 1 case of incision infection [86]. The most significant late complication was kyphotic deformity. Due to excessive resection of the vertebral plate and posterior column-related supporting structures such as the small joints, postoperative instability and posterior convex deformity often ensue, leading to worsening of postoperative neurological symptoms. Therefore, Wang et al. [87] suggested that for single-segment laminectomies, especially in the middle and upper thoracic segments, internal fixation may not be necessary due to the supportive role of the ribs and thoracic contour, while internal fixation is necessary in the lower thoracic and lumbar segments; if two segments are involved, it can be determined according to the patient's specific situation; if multiple segments are involved, posterior pedicle screws for internal fixation and posterior posterolateral fusion with implantation are necessary. Patients should actively perform back stretching exercises postoperatively, which can effectively prevent the occurrence of kyphosis. With the development of MISS and digital orthopedics, the safety of surgery has been improved, and few studies have reported deterioration of neurological function in patients after MISS, which may be closely related to the safety of MISS and its high selectivity for patients.

26.10 Conclusion

In summary, OSL is characterized by the combination of multiple pathologies and multi-segmental stenosis, which leads to complex clinical manifestations and is prone to misdiagnosis and mismanagement. Currently, there is still a lack of effective instruments to define the responsible pathology or responsible segment of spinal ligamentous ossification; therefore, it is necessary to continue to study the correlation between its imaging instruments and clinical features, in order to establish a simple and accurate method to determine whether spinal ligamentous ossification is involved in spinal cord damage. In recent years, a series of encouraging advances have been made in basic research, diagnosis and treatment of OSL, such as diagnosing the disease based on big data, artificial intelligence and other united imaging. However, a consensus needs to be established on how to achieve early diagnosis and how to standardize the classification of ligamentous ossification in various parts of the spine by combining pathological, anatomical, imaging, and specific molecular expression. For spinal ligamentous ossification, drug treatment and prevention have limited effect, and surgery is regarded as the main treatment. With the continuous innovation of new surgical and imaging instruments, the preventive and therapeutic methods are also advancing. For example, microendoscopy and computer-assisted navigation are characterized by less trauma, less impact on spinal stability, shorter operation time and less bleeding compared with traditional surgery.

In conclusion, there is no standardized surgical treatment strategy for OSL, and various surgical procedures have their own indications, advantages and disadvantages. The choice of surgery should be based on a comprehensive assessment of the patient's condition, spinal cord compression, patient tolerance, imaging characteristics, and the surgeon's experience, in order to select the most appropriate surgical procedure for the patient.

References

1. Inamasu J, Guiot BH, Sachs DC. Ossification of the posterior longitudinal ligament: an update on its biology, epidemiology, and natural history. Neurosurgery. 2006;58(6):1027–39; discussion 1027–39.
2. Ikegawa S. Updates on ossification of posterior longitudinal ligament. Genetic approach to the susceptibility genes for ossification of posterior longitudinal ligament of the spine (OPLL) and for its molecular pathogenesis. Clin Calcium. 2009;19(10):1457–61.
3. Kawaguchi Y. Biomarkers of ossification of the spinal ligament. Global Spine J. 2019;9(6):650–7.
4. Matsunaga S, Sakou T. Overview of epidemiology and genetics. In: OPLL: ossification of the posterior longitudinal Ligament. Springer; 2006. p. 7–9.
5. Daniels AH, McDonald CL, Basques BA, Kuris EO. Ossified Ligamentum Flavum: epidemiology, treatment, and outcomes. J Am Acad Orthop Surg. 2022;30(12):e842–51.
6. Kim SI, Ha KY, Lee JW, Kim YH. Prevalence and related clinical factors of thoracic ossification of the ligamentum flavum-a computed tomography-based cross-sectional study. Spine J. 2018;18(4):551–7.
7. Kawaguchi Y, Nakano M, Yasuda T, Seki S, Hori T, Suzuki K, Makino H, Kimura T. Characteristics of ossification of the spinal ligament; incidence of ossification of the ligamentum flavum in patients with cervical ossification of the posterior longitudinal ligament – analysis of the whole spine using multidetector CT. J Orthop Sci. 2016;21(4):439–45.
8. Matsunaga S, Yamaguchi M, Hayashi K, Sakou T. Genetic analysis of ossification of the posterior longitudinal ligament. Spine (Phila Pa 1976). 1999;24(10):937–8; discussion 939.
9. Koike Y, Takahata M, Nakajima M, Otomo N, Suetsugu H, Liu X, Endo T, Imagama S, Kobayashi K, Kaito T, Kato S, Kawaguchi Y, Kanayama M, Sakai H, Tsuji T, Miyamoto T, Inose H, Yoshii T, Kashii M, Nakashima H, Ando K, Taniguchi Y, Takeuchi K, Ito S, Tomizuka K, Hikino K, Iwasaki Y, Kamatani Y, Maeda S, Nakajima H, Mori K, Seichi A, Fujibayashi S, Kanchiku T, Watanabe K, Tanaka T, Kida K, Kobayashi S, Takahashi M, Yamada K, Takuwa H, Lu HF, Niida S, Ozaki K, Momozawa Y; Genetic Study Group of Investigation Committee on Ossification of the Spinal Ligaments; Yamazaki M, Okawa A, Matsumoto M, Iwasaki N, Terao C, Ikegawa S. Genetic insights into ossification of the posterior longitudinal ligament of the spine. Elife. 202312:e86514.
10. Kobashi G, Washio M, Okamoto K, Sasaki S, Yokoyama T, Miyake Y, Sakamoto N, Ohta K, Inaba Y, Tanaka H, Japan collaborative epidemiological study Group for Evaluation of ossification of the posterior longitudinal ligament of the spine risk. High body mass index after age 20 and diabetes mellitus are independent risk factors for ossification of the posterior longitudinal ligament of the spine in Japanese subjects: a case-control study in multiple hospitals. Spine (Phila Pa 1976). 2004;29(9):1006–10.
11. Hou Y, Liang L, Shi GD, Xu P, Xu GH, Shi JG, Yuan W. Comparing effects of cervical anterior approach and laminoplasty in surgical management of cervical ossification of posterior longitudinal ligament by a prospective nonrandomized controlled study. Orthop Traumatol Surg Res. 2017;103(5):733–40.
12. Chesher D, Oddy M, Darbar U, Sayal P, Casey A, Ryan A, Sechi A, Simister C, Waters A, Wedatilake Y, Lachmann RH, Murphy E. Outcome of adult patients with X-linked hypophosphatemia caused by PHEX gene mutations. J Inherit Metab Dis. 2018;41(5):865–76.
13. Kawaguchi Y, Nakano M, Yasuda T, Seki S, Suzuki K, Yahara Y, Makino H, Kitajima I, Kimura T. Serum biomarkers in patients with ossification of the posterior longitudinal ligament (OPLL): inflammation in OPLL. PLoS One. 2017;12(5):e0174881.
14. Zhang B, Yuan L, Chen G, Chen X, Yang X, Fan T, Sun C, Fan D, Chen Z. Deciphering obesity-related gene clusters unearths SOCS3 immune infiltrates and 5mC/m6A modifiers in ossification of Ligamentum Flavum pathogenesis. Front Endocrinol (Lausanne). 2022;13:861567.
15. Convente MR, Chakkalakal SA, Yang E, Caron RJ, Zhang D, Kambayashi T, Kaplan FS, Shore EM. Depletion of mast cells and macrophages impairs heterotopic ossification in an Acvr1R206H mouse model of Fibrodysplasia Ossificans Progressiva. J Bone Miner Res. 2018;33(2):269–82.
16. Tsukamoto N, Maeda T, Miura H, Jingushi S, Hosokawa A, Harimaya K, Higaki H, Kurata K, Iwamoto Y. Repetitive tensile stress to rat caudal

vertebrae inducing cartilage formation in the spinal ligaments: a possible role of mechanical stress in the development of ossification of the spinal ligaments. J Neurosurg Spine. 2006;5(3):234–42.
17. Sorkin M, Huber AK, Hwang C, Carson WF 4th, Menon R, Li J, Vasquez K, Pagani C, Patel N, Li S, Visser ND, Niknafs Y, Loder S, Scola M, Nycz D, Gallagher K, McCauley LK, Xu J, James AW, Agarwal S, Kunkel S, Mishina Y, Levi B. Regulation of heterotopic ossification by monocytes in a mouse model of aberrant wound healing. Nat Commun. 2020;11(1):722.
18. Ikuta M, Kaito T, Fujimori T, Kitahara T, Furuichi T, Bun M, Hirai H, Ukon Y, Kanie Y, Takenaka S, Okada S. Review of basic research about ossification of the spinal ligaments focusing on animal models. J Clin Med. 2023;12(5):1958.
19. Cai HX, Yayama T, Uchida K, Nakajima H, Sugita D, Guerrero AR, Yoshida A, Baba H. Cyclic tensile strain facilitates the ossification of ligamentum flavum through β-catenin signaling pathway: in vitro analysis. Spine (Phila Pa 1976). 2012;37(11):E639–46.
20. Uchida K, Yayama T, Cai HX, Nakajima H, Sugita D, Guerrero AR, Kobayashi S, Yoshida A, Chen KB, Baba H. Ossification process involving the human thoracic ligamentum flavum: role of transcription factors. Arthritis Res Ther. 2011;13(5):R144.
21. Zhong ZM, Chen JT. Phenotypic characterization of ligamentum flavum cells from patients with ossification of ligamentum flavum. Yonsei Med J. 2009;50(3):375–9.
22. Yayama T, Uchida K, Kobayashi S, Kokubo Y, Sato R, Nakajima H, Takamura T, Bangirana A, Itoh H, Baba H. Thoracic ossification of the human ligamentum flavum: histopathological and immunohistochemical findings around the ossified lesion. J Neurosurg Spine. 2007;7(2):184–93.
23. Moon SH, Park SR, Kim H, Kwon UH, Kim KH, Kim HS, Lee HM. Biologic modification of ligamentum flavum cells by marker gene transfer and recombinant human bone morphogenetic protein-2. Spine (Phila Pa 1976). 2004;29(9):960–5.
24. Kim HN, Min WK, Jeong JH, Kim SG, Kim JR, Kim SY, Choi JY, Park BC. Combination of Runx2 and BMP2 increases conversion of human ligamentum flavum cells into osteoblastic cells. BMB Rep. 2011;44(7):446–51.
25. Le HV, Wick JB, Van BW, Klineberg EO. Ossification of the posterior longitudinal ligament: pathophysiology, diagnosis, and management. J Am Acad Orthop Surg. 2022;30(17):820–30.
26. Sakai K, Yoshii T, Arai Y, Hirai T, Torigoe I, Inose H, Tomori M, Sakaki K, Matsukura Y, Okawa A. Impact of preoperative cervical sagittal alignment for cervical myelopathy caused by ossification of the posterior longitudinal ligament on surgical treatment. J Orthop Sci. 2022;27(6):1208–14.
27. Cao B, Chen J, Yuan B, Sun Y, Zhou S, Zhao Y, Xu Z, Tang Y, Chen X. Comparison of the outcome after anterior cervical ossified posterior longitudinal ligament en bloc resection versus posterior total laminectomy and fusion in patients with ossification of the cervical posterior longitudinal ligament: a prospective randomized controlled trial. Bone Joint J. 2023;105-B(4):412–21.
28. Fujimura Y, Nishi Y, Nakamura M, Toyama Y, Suzuki N. Long-term follow-up study of anterior decompression and fusion for thoracic myelopathy resulting from ossification of the posterior longitudinal ligament. Spine (Phila Pa 1976). 19971;22(3):305–11.
29. Epstein N. Diagnosis and surgical management of cervical ossification of the posterior longitudinal ligament. Spine J. 2002;2(6):436–49.
30. Yonenobu K, Ebara S, Fujiwara K, Yamashita K, Ono K, Yamamoto T, Harada N, Ogino H, Ojima S. Thoracic myelopathy secondary to ossification of the spinal ligament. J Neurosurg. 1987;66(4):511–8.
31. Barrios-Anderson A, Wang EJ, Sastry R, Fridley JS. Ossification of the posterior longitudinal ligament in the cervical, thoracic, and lumbar spine. Cureus. 2021;13(3):e14041.
32. Fan T, Sun C, Chen G, Jiang S, Li W, Chen Z. Clinical progression of ossification of the ligamentum flavum in thoracic spine: a 10- to 11-year follow-up study. Eur Spine J. 2023;32(2):495–504.
33. Feng FB, Sun CG, Chen ZQ. Progress on clinical characteristics and identification of location of thoracic ossification of the ligamentum flavum. Orthop Surg. 2015;7(2):87–96.
34. Xu M, Liu Y, Yang J, Liu H, Ding C. Ossification of the cervical anterior longitudinal ligament is an underdiagnosed cause of difficult airway: a case report and review of the literature. BMC Anesthesiol. 2020;20(1):161.
35. Ohara Y. Ossification of the ligaments in the cervical spine, including ossification of the anterior longitudinal ligament, ossification of the posterior longitudinal ligament, and ossification of the Ligamentum Flavum. Neurosurg Clin N Am. 2018;29(1):63–8.
36. Resnick D, Guerra J Jr, Robinson CA, Vint VC. Association of diffuse idiopathic skeletal hyperostosis (DISH) and calcification and ossification of the posterior longitudinal ligament. AJR Am J Roentgenol. 1978;131(6):1049–53.
37. Chang H, Kong CG, Won HY, Kim JH, Park JB. Inter- and intra-observer variability of a cervical OPLL classification using reconstructed CT images. Clin Orthop Surg. 2010;2(1):8–12.
38. Yang H, Yang L, Chen D, Wang X, Lu X, Yuan W. Implications of different patterns of "double-layer sign" in cervical ossification of the posterior longitudinal ligament. Eur Spine J. 2015;24(8):1631–9.
39. Ogawa T, Yoshii T, Oyama J, Sugimura N, Akada T, Sugino T, Hashimoto M, Morishita S, Takahashi T, Motoyoshi T, Oyaizu T, Yamada T, Onuma H, Hirai T, Inose H, Nakajima Y, Okawa A. Detecting ossification of the posterior longitudinal ligament on plain radiographs using a deep convolutional neural network: a pilot study. Spine J. 2022;22(6):934–40.

40. Fong SY, Wong HK. Thoracic myelopathy secondary to ligamentum flavum ossification. Ann Acad Med Singap. 2004;33(3):340–6.
41. Parekh HC, Gurusinghe NT, Perera SS, Prabhu SS. Ossification of the ligamentum flavum in a Caucasian: case report. Br J Neurosurg. 1993;7(6):687–90.
42. Liao CC, Chen TY, Jung SM, Chen LR. Surgical experience with symptomatic thoracic ossification of the ligamentum flavum. J Neurosurg Spine. 2005;2(1):34–9.
43. Hirasawa A, Wakao N, Kamiya M, Takeuchi M, Kawanami K, Murotani K, Matsuo T, Deie M. The prevalence of diffuse idiopathic skeletal hyperostosis in Japan - the first report of measurement by CT and review of the literature. J Orthop Sci. 2016;21(3):287–90.
44. Boody BS, Lendner M, Vaccaro AR. Ossification of the posterior longitudinal ligament in the cervical spine: a review. Int Orthop. 2019;43(4):797–805.
45. Calvanese F, Capo G, Picart T, Durieux E, Vukusic S, Di Carlo D, Barrey CY. Coexistence of flavum ligament ossification with diffuse idiopathic skeletal hyperostosis in the cervical spine: review of literature and technical note starting from a rare case. Neurochirurgie. 2022;68(6):637–47.
46. Kwok SSS, Cheung JPY. Surgical decision-making for ossification of the posterior longitudinal ligament versus other types of degenerative cervical myelopathy: anterior versus posterior approaches. BMC Musculoskelet Disord. 2020;21(1):823.
47. Nakashima H, Imagama S, Yoshii T, Egawa S, Sakai K, Kusano K, Nakagawa Y, Hirai T, Wada K, Katsumi K, Fujii K, Kimura A, Furuya T, Kanchiku T, Nagamoto Y, Oshima Y, Nagoshi N, Ando K, Takahata M, Mori K, Nakajima H, Murata K, Matsunaga S, Kaito T, Yamada K, Kobayashi S, Kato S, Ohba T, Inami S, Fujibayashi S, Katoh H, Kanno H, Li Y, Yatsuya H, Koda M, Kawaguchi Y, Takeshita K, Matsumoto M, Yamazaki M, Okawa A, Japanese multicenter research Organization for Ossification of the spinal ligament. Comparison of laminoplasty and posterior fusion surgery for cervical ossification of posterior longitudinal ligament. Sci Rep. 2022;12(1):748.
48. Kahaer A, Chen R, Maitusong M, Mijiti P, Rexiti P. Zero-profile implant versus conventional cage-plate construct in anterior cervical discectomy and fusion for the treatment of single-level degenerative cervical spondylosis: a systematic review and meta-analysis. J Orthop Surg Res. 2022;17(1):506.
49. Guo J, Jin W, Shi Y, Guan Z, Wen J, Huang Y, Yu B. Is the zero-P spacer suitable for 3-level anterior cervical discectomy and fusion surgery in terms of sagittal alignment reconstruction: a comparison study with traditional plate and cage system. Brain Sci. 2022;12(11):1583.
50. Barot K, Ruiz-Cardozo MA, Singh S, Trevino G, Kann MR, Brehm S, Bui T, Joseph K, Patel R, Hardi A, Yahanda AT, Jauregui JJ, Cadieux M, Pennicooke B, Molina CA. A meta-analysis of surgical outcomes in 25727 patients undergoing anterior cervical discectomy and fusion or anterior cervical Corpectomy and fusion for cervical deformity. Glob Spine J. 2024:21925682241270100.
51. Wang M, Yang G, Zhou B, Cao Z, Li Y, Tan J, Long Z, Xiao Z, Luo M. Anterior cervical controllable Antedisplacement and fusion (ACAF) versus anterior cervical Corpectomy and fusion (ACCF) for ossification of the cervical posterior longitudinal ligament (OPLL) in Chinese population: a systematic review and meta-analysis. Neurosurg Rev. 2024;47(1):783.
52. Sun J, Shi J, Xu X, Yang Y, Wang Y, Kong Q, Yang H, Guo Y, Han D, Jiang J, Shi G, Yuan W, Jia L. Anterior controllable antidisplacement and fusion surgery for the treatment of multilevel severe ossification of the posterior longitudinal ligament with myelopathy: preliminary clinical results of a novel technique. Eur Spine J. 2018;27(6):1469–78.
53. Li C, Wang Z, Tang J, Li D, Tian Y, Yuan S, Wang L, Liu X. Comparison of clinical outcomes of cervical Laminoplasty for cervical Spondylotic myelopathy: double-door with lamina staple, single-door with Miniplate, and double-door with spacer-a 2-year follow-up study. Neurosurgery. 2023;92(6):1259–68.
54. Ng BW, Tan JA, Sabri S, Baharuddin A, Muhamad Ariffin MH. Surgical Management of Cervical Ossification of posterior longitudinal ligament: the treatment algorithm and outcome. Cureus. 2023;15(3):e36517.
55. Mizuno J, Nakagawa H. Ossified posterior longitudinal ligament: management strategies and outcomes. Spine J. 2006;6(6 Suppl):282S–8S.
56. Hirabayashi S, Kitagawa T, Yamamoto I, Yamada K, Kawano H. Surgical treatment for ossification of the posterior longitudinal ligament (OPLL) at the thoracic spine: usefulness of the posterior approach. Spine Surg Relat Res. 2018;2(3):169–76.
57. Yamazaki M, Okawa A, Fujiyoshi T, Furuya T, Koda M. Posterior decompression with instrumented fusion for thoracic myelopathy caused by ossification of the posterior longitudinal ligament. Eur Spine J. 2010;19(5):691–8.
58. Kim CH, Renaldo N, Chung CK, Lee HS. Use of an ultrasonic Osteotome for direct removal of beak-type ossification of posterior longitudinal ligament in the thoracic spine. J Korean Neurosurg Soc. 2015;58(6):571–7.
59. Takahata M, Ito M, Abumi K, Kotani Y, Sudo H, Minami A. Clinical results and complications of circumferential spinal cord decompression through a single posterior approach for thoracic myelopathy caused by ossification of posterior longitudinal ligament. Spine (Phila Pa 1976). 2008;33(11):1199–208.
60. Yamazaki M, Mochizuki M, Ikeda Y, Sodeyama T, Okawa A, Koda M, Moriya H. Clinical results of surgery for thoracic myelopathy caused by ossification of the posterior longitudinal ligament: operative indication of posterior decompression with instrumented fusion. Spine (Phila Pa 1976). 2006 Jun 1;31(13):1452–60.

61. Maruyama J, Furuya T, Maki S, Inoue T, Yunde A, Miura M, Shiratani Y, Nagashima Y, Shiga Y, Inage K, Eguchi Y, Orita S, Takahashi H, Koda M, Yamazaki M, Ohtori S. Posterior decompression and fixation for thoracic spine ossification: a 10-year follow-up study. J Clin Med. 2023;12(17):5701.
62. Tomita K, Kawahara N, Baba H, Kikuchi Y, Nishimura H. Circumspinal decompression for thoracic myelopathy due to combined ossification of the posterior longitudinal ligament and ligamentum flavum. Spine (Phila Pa 1976). 1990;15(11):1114–20.
63. Kato S, Murakami H, Demura S, Yoshioka K, Hayashi H, Tsuchiya H. Novel surgical technique for ossification of posterior longitudinal ligament in the thoracic spine. J Neurosurg Spine. 2012;17(6):525–9.
64. Yang C, Bi Z, Fu C, Zhang Z. A modified decompression surgery for thoracic myelopathy caused by ossification of posterior longitudinal ligament: a case report and literature review. Spine (Phila Pa 1976). 2010;35(13):E609–13.
65. Kovacs FM, Urrútia G, Alarcón JD. Surgery versus conservative treatment for symptomatic lumbar spinal stenosis: a systematic review of randomized controlled trials. Spine (Phila Pa 1976). 2011;36(20):E1335–51.
66. Bian F, Zhang J, Bian G, Wang D, Chen B, An Y. Comparison of the short-term efficacy of percutaneous endoscopic thoracic decompression and laminectomy in the treatment of thoracic ossification of the Ligamentum Flavum. World Neurosurg. 2023;170:e666–72.
67. Deng Y, Yang M, Xia C, Chen Y, Xie Z. Unilateral biportal endoscopic decompression for symptomatic thoracic ossification of the ligamentum flavum: a case control study. Int Orthop. 2022;46(9):2071–80.
68. Miyashita T, Ataka H, Tanno T. Spontaneous reduction of a floated ossification of the ligamentum flavum after posterior thoracic decompression (floating method); report of a case (abridged translation of a primary publication). Spine J. 2013;13(8):e7–9.
69. Zhang JT, Lei T, Yang L, Lin YS, Wang ZH, Cao JM. Subsection laminectomy with pedicle screw fixation to treat thoracic ossification of Ligamentum Flavum: a comparative analysis with lamina osteotomy and the replantation technique. Ther Clin Risk Manag. 2020;17(16):311–9.
70. Xie T, Qian J, Lu Y, Chen B, Jiang Y, Luo C. Biomechanical comparison of laminectomy, hemilaminectomy and a new minimally invasive approach in the surgical treatment of multilevel cervical intradural tumour: a finite element analysis. Eur Spine J. 2013;22(12):2719–30.
71. Li Z, Ren D, Zhao Y, Hou S, Li L, Yu S, Hou T. Clinical characteristics and surgical outcome of thoracic myelopathy caused by ossification of the ligamentum flavum: a retrospective analysis of 85 cases. Spinal Cord. 2016;54(3):188–96.
72. Yu B, Xia YP, Du WJ, Li HN, Gao JW, Zhou LJ. A control study of C5 palsy after expansive open-door laminoplasty with miniplate or suture/anchor fixation. Chin J Orthop. 2015;35(1):7.
73. Hirabayashi S, Kitagawa T, Yamamoto I, Yamada K, Kawano H. Development and achievement of cervical Laminoplasty and related studies on cervical myelopathy. Spine Surg Relat Res. 2019;4(1):8–17.
74. Ikuta K, Tarukado K, Senba H, Kitamura T, Komiya N, Fukutoku Y, Shidahara S. Decompression procedure using a microendoscopic technique for thoracic myelopathy caused by ossification of the ligamentum flavum. Minim Invasive Neurosurg. 2011;54(5–6):271–3.
75. Zheng C, Liao Z, Chen HZ. Percutaneous endoscopic posterior decompression for therapy of spinal cord compression due to ossification of the Ligamentum Flavum: a Long-term follow-up. World Neurosurg. 2021;156:e249–53.
76. He DW, Miao XX, Wu TL, Cheng XG. Minimally invasive percutaneous endoscopic spine surgery for thoracic ossification of ligamentum flavum. Orthopedic J China. 2019;27(11):4.
77. Heo DH, Ha JS, Jang JW. Biportal endoscopic posterior cervical Foraminotomy for adjacent 2-level Foraminal lesions using a single approach (sliding technique). Neurospine. 2023;20(1):92–8.
78. Kang MS, Chung HJ, You KH, Park HJ. How i do it: biportal endoscopic thoracic decompression for ossification of the ligamentum flavum. Acta Neurochir. 2022;164(1):43–7.
79. Tian W, Liu Y, Fan M, Zhao J, Jin P, Zeng C. CAMISS concept and its clinical application. Adv Exp Med Biol. 2018;1093:31–46.
80. Otomo N, Funao H, Yamanouchi K, Isogai N, Ishii K. Computed tomography-based navigation system in current spine surgery: a narrative review. Medicina (Kaunas). 2022;58(2):241.
81. Sun J, Du P, Shen Y. Risk factors for poor outcomes of thoracic ossification of Ligamentum Flavum after laminectomy. Med Sci Monit. 2022;28:e935711.
82. Baaj AA, Smith DA, Vale FL, Uribe JS. Surgical approaches to thoracic ossification of the posterior longitudinal ligament. J Clin Neurosci. 2012;19(3):349–51.
83. Zhang Y, Huang Z, Xu P, Xu Z, Xing X, Xin Y, Gao M, Li X, Xiao Y. Comparison of anterior controllable Antedisplacement and fusion versus Laminoplasty in the treatment of multisegment ossification of cervical posterior longitudinal ligament: a meta-analysis of clinical. World Neurosurg. 2024;185:193–206.
84. Yoshii T, Morishita S, Inose H, Yuasa M, Hirai T, Okawa A, Fushimi K, Fujiwara T. Comparison of perioperative complications in anterior decompression with fusion and posterior decompression with fusion for cervical ossification of the posterior longitudinal ligament: propensity score matching analysis using a nation-wide inpatient database. Spine (Phila Pa 1976). 2020;45(16):E1006–12.
85. Osman NS, Cheung ZB, Hussain AK, Phan K, Arvind V, Vig KS, Vargas L, Kim JS, Cho SK. Outcomes and complications following laminectomy alone for thoracic myelopathy due to ossified Ligamentum

Flavum: a systematic review and meta-analysis. Spine (Phila Pa 1976). 2018;43(14):E842–8.

86. Zhong ZM, Wu Q, Meng TT, Zhu YJ, Qu DB, Wang JX, Jiang JM, Lu KW, Zheng S, Zhu SY, Chen JT. Clinical outcomes after decompressive laminectomy for symptomatic ossification of ligamentum flavum at the thoracic spine. J Clin Neurosci. 2016;28:77–81.
87. Wang CH, Cui WL, Xue JL, Liao Z. Transforaminal en bloc resection for the treatment of thoracic ossification of the ligamentum flavum: retrospective cohort study. Int J Surg. 2018;54(Pt A):278–84.

Rupture of the Transverse Ligament of the Atlas

27

Fang Wang and Fuyou Guo

27.1 Introduction

In 1908, Vincenzo Quercioli, an Italian surgeon from Siena, described four symmetrical fracture lines of the atlas during an autopsy. He emphasized the importance of the integrity of the atlantoaxial ligaments, particularly the transverse ligament, for the stability of the atlas ring [1]. The transverse atlantal ligament (TAL) maintains the odontoid process of C2 close to the C1 ring, allowing rotational movement of the craniocervical junction. Multiple other ligaments, including the capsular, alar, apical, anterior longitudinal ligament, and tectorial membrane, assist the TAL in providing cervical stability, but the TAL plays the most crucial role in C1-C2 articulation [2].

Barker et al. were the first to describe a bony avulsion of the TAL, describing an uncommon fracture entity associated with a fracture of the medial wall of the lateral mass of C1. By an unknown fracture mechanism, they postulated that the bone fragment resulted from a combination of TAL stretching and pressure on the lateral mass caused by neck muscle contraction [3]. Recognizing TAL injury is crucial for preventing late instability or nonunion of an atlas fracture. Rupture or avulsion of this ligament leads to atlantoaxial instability, which carries a high risk of neurologic injury and disability. Using health-related quality of life questionnaires, previous studies have shown that patients with residual atlantoaxial instability after an atlas fracture had worse outcomes than those without instability [4]. The stiff and inelastic cruciate ligament, as demonstrated in vitro, fails suddenly, resulting in anterior C1 on C2 subluxation. It tears as an "all-or-nothing" event and cannot be repaired once torn [2].

Early diagnosis of TAL injury is challenging due to its high risk but rare clinical occurrence. It is often overlooked, especially when multiple injuries are present. TAL injury is usually accompanied by associated bone injury. If the spinal cord is not involved at the moment of injury and appropriate treatment is obtained, delayed spinal cord compression can be prevented. Early appropriate diagnosis is crucial to ensure effective treatment and prevent later neurological impairment.

27.2 Anatomy and Function of the Transverse Ligament of the Atlas

The TAL is a strong, thick, horizontally oriented ligamentous band that extends posterior to the C2 dens and inserts along the medial C1 tubercles. It

F. Wang · F. Guo (✉)
Department of Neurosurgery, The First Affiliated Hospital of Zhengzhou University, Zhengzhou, Henan, China

International Joint Laboratory of Nervous System Malformations, Zhengzhou, Henan Province, China
e-mail: chyou666@hotmail.com

M. Turgut et al. (eds.), *Ligaments of the Vertebral Column*,
https://doi.org/10.1007/978-3-032-09070-6_27

is the major component of the cruciform ligament at C1–C2, composed of transverse and vertical parts forming a cross behind the dens [5]. The transverse part, the TAL, arches across the ring of the atlas behind the dens and attaches to a tubercle on the medial side of the lateral masses of the atlas. The TAL is the principal component of the cruciate ligamentous complex responsible for atlantoaxial stability. It exists in two distinct layers: the superficial one, posterior to the alar ligaments, and hidden by the inferior margin [6, 7]. Once the superficial layer is removed and the alar ligaments reflex superiorly, the fibers of the deep layer and their attachment can be seen. The ligament passes the dens 5 mm below the origin of the apical and alar ligaments; its length is 21.9 mm, and its midportion thickness is 2.5 mm [8]. A small synovial capsule exists between the dens and the TAL, which—along with the smooth anterior fibrocartilaginous surface of the TAL—facilitates rotational movement between C1 and C2 (Fig. 27.1).

Histological analysis shows that the ligament consists almost exclusively of collagen fibers, with minimal elastic fiber content. The collagen fibers interweave in the central part of the TAL to form a network structure, and the angle between the fibers is 30°. Therefore, the collagen fiber content and arrangement determine the mechanical characteristics of high stiffness and low elasticity [2].

The atlantoaxial joints have biconvex surfaces that improve flexion and extension of the skull while permitting a wider range of axial rotation and lateral bending than the atlantooccipital joints [5]. This anatomical configuration affixes the atlas more to the skull than to C2, predisposing the atlas to rotate more in conjunction with the skull base. The atlantoaxial joints allow for as much as 40° of unilateral rotation, the widest range of motion of any cervical vertebra [9]. Unlike the lower cervical spine (C2–C7), C0, C1, and C2 do not contain intervertebral discs, and the ligament complex is the main structure maintaining atlantoaxial stability. The ligament complex comprises the TAL and alar ligaments [2]. Atlantoaxial stability is traditionally thought to be maintained by the TAL because it possesses the most volume, thickness, and strength. As part of the lateral masses of the atlas, the TAL restricts odontoid movement and prevents anterior dislocation of the atlas along with the anterior arch [10]. The TAL plays the most important role in ensuring axial rotation and lateral bending of the C1–2 joints and restraining the flexion of the head during physiological motion and trauma. Its

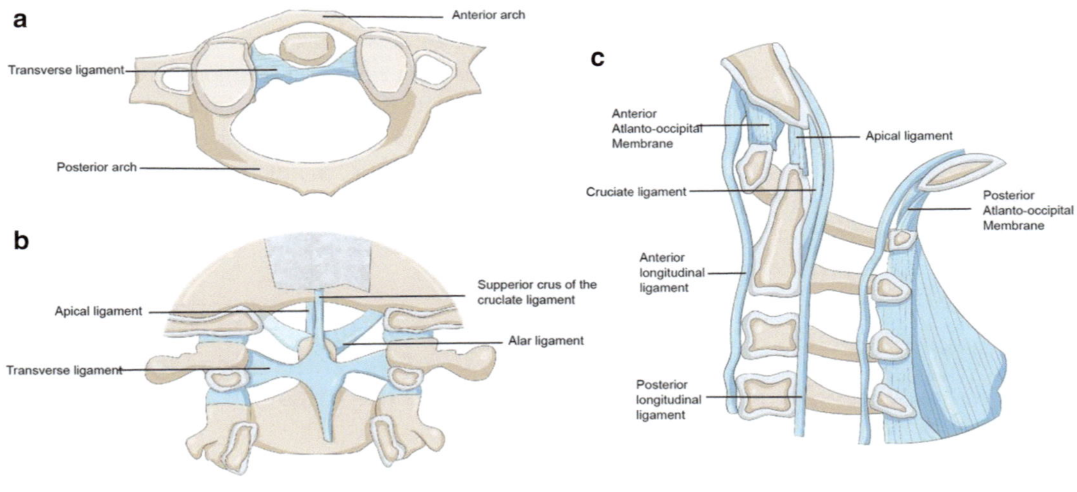

Fig. 27.1 (**a**) Diagram showing the morphology of the first cervical vertebra. (**b**) Diagram showing a view of the cranial-cervical junction from the back, with the posterior elements removed. The cruciate, alar, and apical ligaments are demonstrated. (**c**) Diagram showing a lateral view of the cranial-cervical junction. The cruciate, anterior and posterior atlanto-occipital, and apical ligaments are demonstrated. (Riascos et al. [27])

function as a restraining band on the dens is analogous to that of a seat belt restraining a passenger in an automobile [2].

27.3 Biomechanics of the Transverse Atlantal Ligament

The mobility of the atlantoaxial joints, combined with their critical location at the craniospinal junction, generates high stress on the ligamentous structures that maintain bony alignment and integrity. The TAL is a soft-tissue structure of paramount importance for maintaining physiological alignment between C1 and C2, allowing safe rotation of the spine. The TAL is a tight band that acts as a sling holding the dens against the anterior arch of the atlas. However, since the TAL arises from and inserts into the medial aspect of the C1 lateral mass, it is at risk of injury with bursting fractures [11].

There are some reports on the biomechanical properties of the TAL, which conclude that the ultimate tensile load the TAL can withstand is a significant indicator of its biomechanics [12–14]. Spence et al. investigated the biomechanical properties of the TAL and suggested that final failure loads range from 380 to 1040 N [15]. It has also been tested that the ultimate load of the TAL is between 117 and 1765 N [16]. Dvorak et al. applied a shock acceleration of 1.5 mm/s to the TAL, with a fracture range of 170 to 700 N [17]. In a recent study, a finite element model consisting of bony structures along with cartilage, intervertebral discs, and all ligaments was developed based on CT and MRI images. The effect of head weights (compressive load) of 30 N to 57 N was investigated in cases of intact and ruptured transverse ligament joints. A TAL tear increases the flexion angle of the head and vertebrae, as well as the atlas–dens interval. The atlas–dens interval reaches a critical value when the compressive load exceeds 40 N [18].

27.4 Injury Mechanism of the Transverse Atlantal Ligament

The occipito-atlantal and atlantoaxial articulations contribute significantly to flexion and rotation in the cervical spine, respectively, accounting for 50% of these movements. Given their high degree of motion, these bony segments are among the most commonly injured in adults, particularly prone to fractures. Any fracture involving the atlas necessitates a thorough examination of the ligamentous structures between C0 and C1 and between C1 and C2 [19]. The cervical spine can be subjected to severe injury through various types of accidents and/or extreme movements. Motor vehicle accidents and falls are common causes. However, many other factors could result in fractures or injuries to cervical spine structures, bones, and soft tissues, including multiple ligament injuries, from activities such as athletics and activities or violent physical contact [18]. The rupture of the TAL is one such injury caused by a fall with a blow to the occiput involving an anteriorly directed force to the back of the head with forced flexion, resulting in excessive relative anterior displacement of C1 against C2 [20]. When the head and neck are subjected to flexion violence, the TAL, which moves forward, is "cut" by the armature odontoid process and breaks.

The atlas-dens interval (ADI), defined as the distance between the anterior portion of the atlas and the dens of the axis, exceeding 3 mm in adults, is an indication of failure of either or both the TAL and the alar ligament [21, 22]. Some suggest that the ADI should not exceed 3 to 3.5 mm. In fact, the ADI is often used to assess cervical spine trauma, as an increased value can indicate a TAL rupture. The increase in ADI results in posterior displacement of the dens relative to the atlas, reducing the space available for the spinal cord. This can be recognized by the posterior atlanto-dental interval, which in turn compresses the spinal cord [23].

27.5 Clinical Presentation of Transverse Atlantal Ligament Rupture

The rupture of the TAL is a very serious and dangerous injury. Its consequences are far more severe than those caused by other types of atlantoaxial instability, such as inflammation. Patients with TAL rupture and dislocation may die at the scene of injury due to the impact on the vital center of the medulla oblongata. Even if they are taken to a hospital, their diagnosis is often missed. Sometimes it is not discovered until an autopsy is performed [24].

Additionally, neurological signs and symptoms vary widely, and the clinical manifestations of ligament injury mainly depend on the degree of anterior atlantoaxial dislocation after the ligament injury and whether it causes spinal cord compression. Patients with mild damage may present with only local symptoms, such as suboccipital pain, neck stiffness, and limited movement. They may feel weakness and instability in the occipital neck, accompanied by headache, dizziness, blurred vision, and dysphagia. The vertebral artery, fixed in the transverse foramen, may experience compression or traction due to excessive atlantoaxial displacement, leading to dizziness, fainting, and blurred vision. Symptoms of spinal cord compression can range from pain or lameness in the lower or upper extremities to severe paralysis and even breathing difficulties, which may result in death [25, 26].

27.6 Imaging Assessments of Transverse Atlantal Ligament Rupture

The special anatomical structure of the TAL makes diagnosing the injury challenging. Diagnosis of a TAL rupture is based on clinical presentation, history, and imaging findings. Since the TAL is not visible on X-ray, plain radiographs can only provide indirect evidence. For an accurate diagnosis, a CT scan is mandatory. To distinguish between stable and unstable atlas injury, it is necessary to evaluate the integrity of the TAL using MRI and to classify the TAL lesion [27].

27.6.1 X-Ray Examination

X-ray do not directly reflect the TAL injuries but can reveal bone structure damage or atlantoaxial dynamic instability, which helps infer transverse ligament injury. The lateral spread of the atlantal lateral masses in relation to the lateral limits of C-2, as measured on a transoral radiograph, can be used to infer TAL impairment. The criterion for suspecting a ruptured TAL is a spread of 7 mm or more [15]. However, more studies have found that a distance of ≥ 7 mm is not an accurate method for diagnosing TAL impairment. Using this criterion, approximately 61% of TAL injuries are missed [28, 29].

Another widely used measurement to assess TAL integrity is the ADI, which is the distance between the anterior arch of C-1 and the odontoid process, as measured on lateral cervical radiographs. Oda et al. proposed a 3-mm limit for a normal ADI on a lateral flexion cervical radiograph [15]. An ADI of 3–5 mm can indicate a torn ligament and atlantoaxial instability, while an ADI of 5–10 mm suggests a transverse ligament rupture, possibly with other auxiliary ligament ruptures. An ADI of 10–12 mm can be diagnosed as a complete ligament rupture. In a recent study, the mean ADI for a TAL injury was found to be 1.8 mm (range 0.9–3.9 mm). Furthermore, the mean ADI in patients with atlas fractures without TAL injuries was 1.3 mm, and no significant difference was found in the ADI with or without TAL injury [29]. Thus, using X-ray alone to identify a TAL injury may lead to incorrect diagnoses.

27.6.2 CT Examination

Compared with MRI, CT is a rapidly obtained test, more accessible worldwide, and more cost-effective during the initial evaluation of trauma patients. A CT scan can help increase the accuracy of bone injury assessment and is widely used to diagnose atlas fractures with TAL rupture [29]. High-resolution CT scans can show the location of the TAL, which lies behind the odontoid process and appears as a high-density structure on CT. Sometimes, avulsion fractures of the TAL at the lateral mass attachment of the atlas can also be seen on CT [30]. However, due to its limited ability to distinguish soft tissue, CT images cannot directly reconstruct the TAL structure. One study reviewed cervical CT and MRI exams for 26 patients to evaluate anterior and lateral atlantodens interval widening, lateral C1 mass offset, C1–C2 rotatory subluxation, and TAL injuries on MRI.

They concluded that an anterior atlantodens interval greater than 2 mm is an unreliable method for screening trauma patients for TAL injuries and atlantoaxial instability (Fig. 27.2). Additionally, C1 lateral mass offset, lateral atlantodens asymmetry, and atlantoaxial rotation measured by CT were poor predictors of TAL tears [31].

27.6.3 MRI Scan

A normal ligament appears as a uniform dark band on standard spin-echo pulse sequences. Increased signal intensity or an irregular contour indicates structural damage (Fig. 27.3). MRI is the gold standard imaging modality for assessing TAL integrity [32].

However, MRI may not always accurately identify the TAL, as the anterior atlantal space is often filled with soft tissue that blends with the ligament [2, 28]. Furthermore, MRI may not be available or of sufficient quality in all hospitals. Jongpil Eun et.al compared the radiologic param-

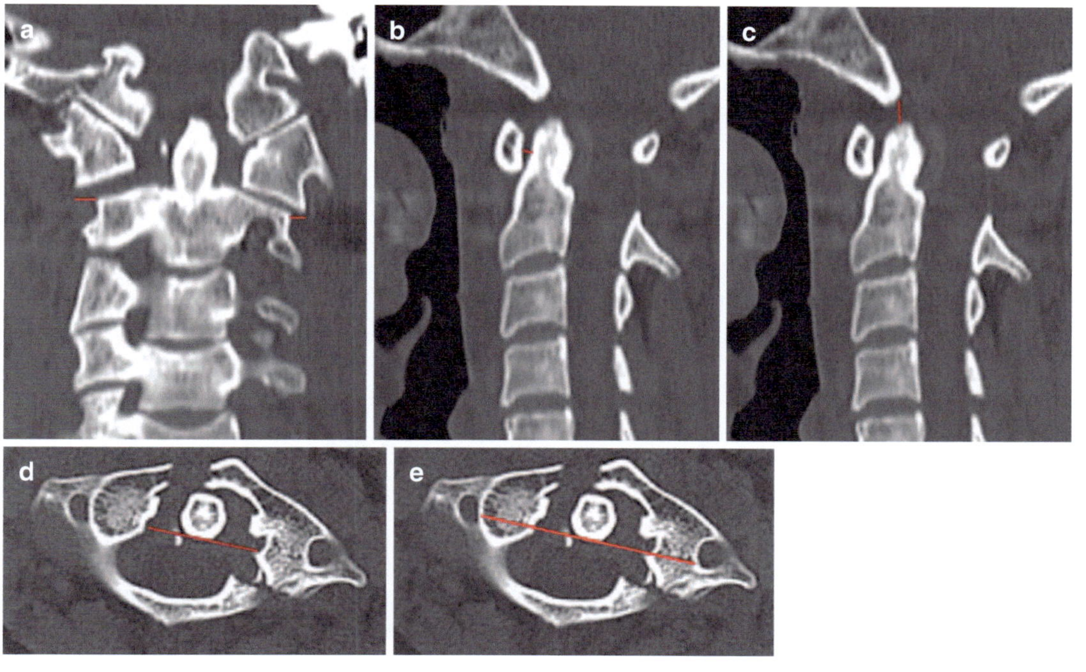

Fig. 27.2 Measurement of radiologic parameters. (**a**) LMD, (**b**) ADI, (**c**) BDI, (**d**) ILM, and (**e**) ELM. *LMD* lateral mass displacement, *ADI* atlanto-dental interval, *BDI* basion-dens interval, *ILM* internal lateral mass displacement, *ELM* external lateral mass displacement. (Eun and Oh [33])

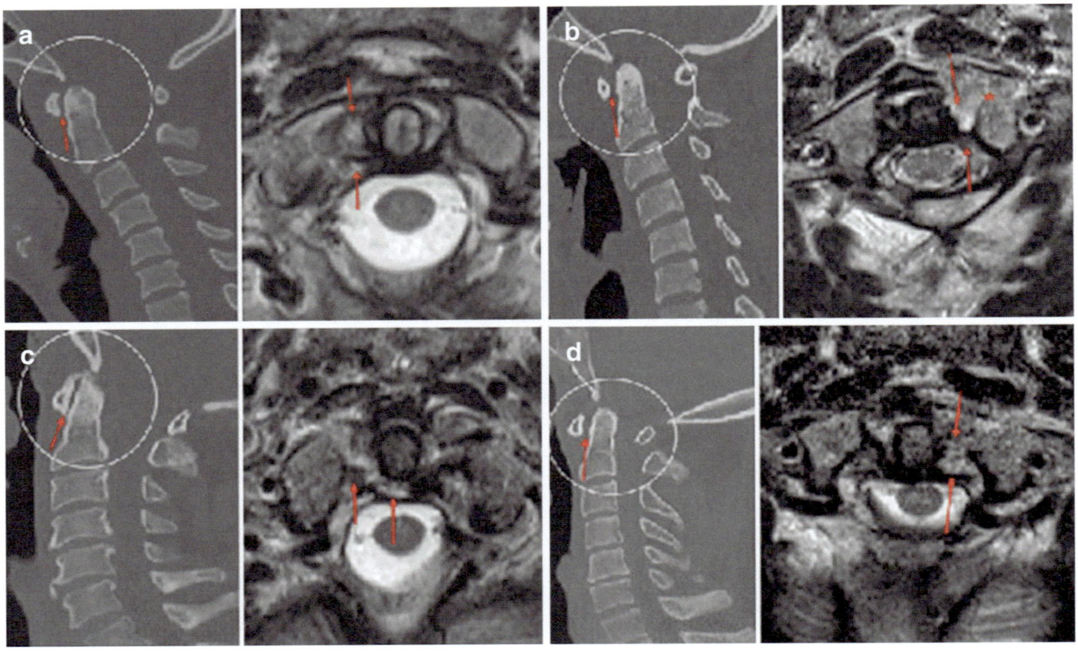

Fig. 27.3 (**a**) The anterior atlantodens interval, measured by CT, is within normal limits at less than 2 mm (red arrow). The MRI (right) demonstrates a full-thickness tear in the right TAL (red arrow). (**b**) The anterior atlantodens interval, measured by CT, is at the upper limits of normal at 2 mm (red arrow). The MRI (right) shows a left posterior arch and lateral mass C1 fracture (red star) along with a full-thickness tear in the left TAL. (**c**) The anterior atlantodens interval is not widened (red arrow). Moderate atlantoaxial osteoarthritis is also present. The MRI (right) reveals a full-thickness tear in the central and right TAL (red arrow). (**d**). The CT shows widening of the anterior atlantodens interval measuring 3 mm (red arrow). The MRI demonstrates a full-thickness tear in the left TAL (red arrow). (Fiester et al. [31])

eter (LMD) associated with TAL injury as detected using MRI. They concluded that LMD is a reliable method for predicting the presence of TAL injury when MRI is unavailable [33].

27.7 The "Rule of Spence" in Transverse Atlantal Ligament Rupture

In 1970, Spence et al. studied the axial load and lateral mass displacement required to disrupt the TAL in 10 human cadaver specimens. They concluded that if the sum of displacement of the lateral mass exceeds 6.9 mm after an atlas fracture, the TAL is disrupted [15]. Clinicians have applied this finding, commonly referred to as the "rule of Spence," to plain radiographic studies to determine whether the TAL is ruptured.

Nowadays, the "rule of Spence" has been shown to be inaccurate for assessing the integrity of the TAL. Studies have reported little correlation between bony displacement of atlas fractures on CT scans and TAL stability. Instead, MRI should be used to evaluate TAL injuries. Dickman et al. demonstrated that 60% of patients with a TAL rupture would not have meet the "rule of Spence" criteria for a TAL injury [34]. Another criterion for instability is the widening of the anterior ADI to more than 3 mm on functional lateral X-rays, indicating translational atlantoaxial instability [35]. Heller et al. investigated the role of X-ray magnification in open-mouth (odontoid) views based on the rule of Spence and redefined this value to 8.1 mm [36]. Since the Heller study, the modified "Rule of Spence" has commonly been used to assess the integrity of the TAL after atlas fractures [32].

27.8 "Dickman Classification" of Transverse Atlantal Ligament Rupture

In 1996, Dickman et al. summarized 39 clinical cases of transverse ligament injury of the atlas. Injuries of the upper cervical spine were assessed with plain radiographs, thin-section computed tomography, and magnetic resonance imaging. The injuries were classified as disruptions of the ligament substance (Type I injuries) or as fractures and avulsions involving the tubercle for insertion of the transverse ligament on the C1 lateral mass (Type II injuries) [28] (Fig. 27.4). He proposed that type I injuries, involving rupture of the ligament substance, have poor prognosis due to atlantoaxial instability and should be treated with early surgery. Type II injuries, involving an avulsion fracture at the TAL insertion site, have a greater chance of healing without sequelae.

Dickman's reports on TAL injuries have been regarded as landmarks in the diagnosis and treatment of atlas fractures, providing a reasonable treatment protocol. In a recent study, Liu Peng et al. analyzed the association of the "rule of Spence," the Dickman classification of TAL injury, and clinical outcomes such as final atlantoaxial stability, suboccipital pain, and cervical spine mobility affecting quality of life. They found that the Dickman classification was much more accurate than the "rule of Spence" in predicting atlantoaxial stability. They also observed a high success rate (100%) in type IIA TAL injuries treated nonoperatively, whereas a relatively lower success rate (66.7%) in type IIB TAL injuries [37]. Patrick et al. reported a 100% success rate in treating three pediatric patients with avulsion TAL injuries (type IIB) [38]. However, the Dickman classification does not encompass all TAL injuries. Kaiser et al. reported a case of

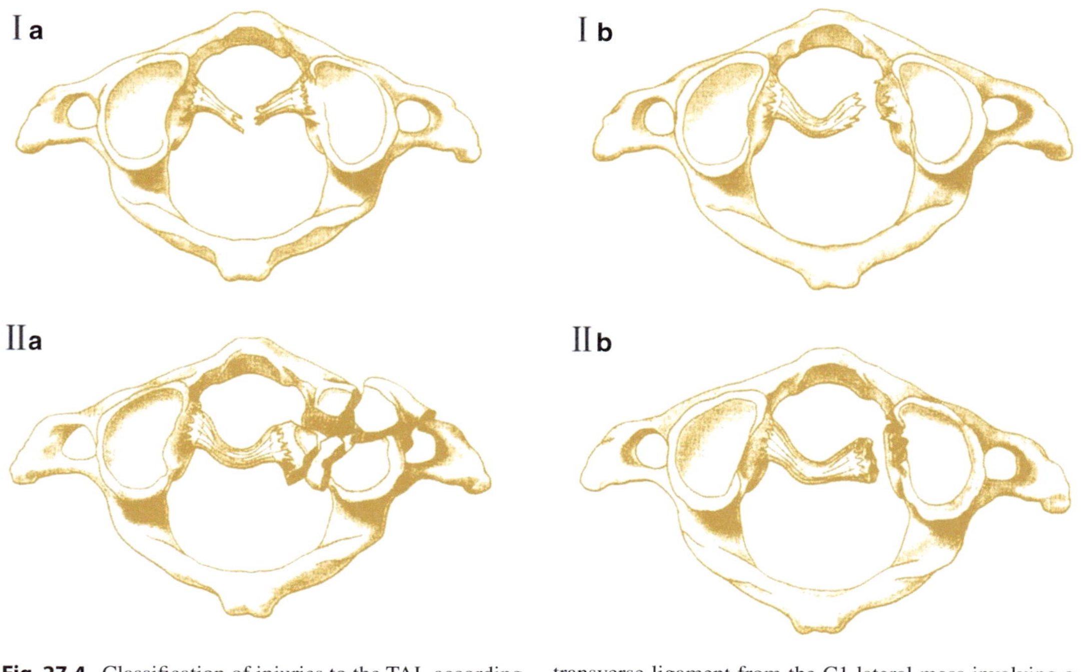

Fig. 27.4 Classification of injuries to the TAL according to Dickman. Type I injuries disrupt the ligament substance in its midportion (IA) or at its periosteal insertion (IB). Type II injuries disconnect the tubercle for insertion of the transverse ligament from the C1 lateral mass involving a comminuted C1 lateral mass (IIA) or avulsing the tubercle from an intact lateral mass (IIB). (Dickman et al. [28])

transverse tear of the TAL, which was not included in this classification [26].

27.9 Atlas Fractures and Transverse Atlantal Ligament Rupture

Atlas fractures, or Jefferson fractures, are common in cervical spine trauma, accounting for approximately 25% of craniocervical injuries, 3–13% of cervical spine injuries, and 1.3–2% of all spinal injuries [39]. Most atlas fractures result from compression forces and are often combined with fractures of the axis, particularly the odontoid process. Multiple classification systems for atlas fractures have been described. Jefferson reviewed 42 patients with atlas fractures and classified them into different patterns, ranging from isolated anterior ring fractures, isolated posterior ring fractures, lateral mass fractures, multiple ring fractures (unilateral or bilateral), and combinations thereof [40]. The most common category was an isolated fracture of the posterior arch, followed by a burst fracture type (Jefferson fracture). While isolated arch fractures (anterior or posterior) are considered stable due to an intact TAL, a burst fracture (Jefferson) may cause instability of the atlantoaxial complex due to diastasis of the lateral masses [41]. Atlas fractures are classified as stable or unstable based on the integrity of the TAL [32].

Gehweiler divided atlas fractures into 5 subgroups (Fig. 27.5). A type 1 atlas fracture is an isolated fracture of the anterior arch, while a type 2 atlas fracture is an isolated, predominantly bilateral fracture of the posterior atlas ring. The combined injury of the anterior and posterior arch of the atlas, the "Jefferson-fracture," corresponds to a Gehweiler type 3 fracture. It is important to distinguish between stable and unstable injuries. In stable injuries, the TAL is intact (type 3a), while unstable injuries are associated with a TAL lesion (so-called type 3b). Type 4 fractures involve the lateral mass, and type 5 fractures are isolated fractures of the C1 transverse process.

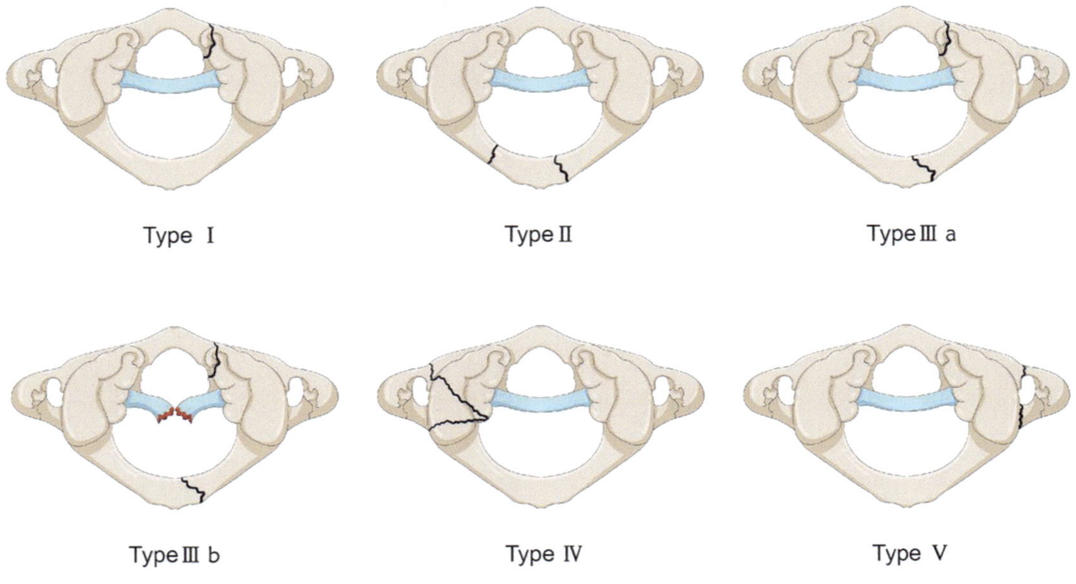

Fig. 27.5 Classification of atlas fractures. (Kandziora F, Scholz M, Pingel A, et al. Treatment of Atlas Fractures: Recommendations of the Spine Section of the German Society for Orthopaedics and Trauma (DGOU). Global Spine J. 2018;8(2 Suppl):5S–11S)

27.10 Treatments for Rupture of Transverse Atlantal Ligament

At present, there is no reliable method for directly repairing the TAL. The primary goal of treating a TAL rupture is to relieve spinal cord compression, restore stability to the occipital and cervical regions, and prevent secondary nerve damage caused by atlantoaxial instability [19, 26]. The optimal treatment of TAL rupture remains controversial and is typically influenced by the presence of other cervical spine injuries. No uniform and established management standards are currently available.

27.10.1 Conservative Management

It is generally believed that type II injury (Fig. 27.4) can be treated non-surgically as a primary option, and most patients experience symptom relief and restored atlantoaxial stability following traction and plaster fixation. Since there is no evidence to suggest the superiority of any specific form of external immobilization (Halo, hard collar, or soft collar), the one with the lowest complication rate may be the best choice [26].

Some recent reviews advocate 6–12 weeks of halo-fixator traction for managing unstable atlas fractures, predominantly with Dickman type II lesions. The advantage of halo-traction is that it provides external stabilization without the need for surgery, thereby avoiding potential surgical complications. Additionally, it may prevent the need for atlantoaxial fusion. However, halo-traction is an invasive form of conservative fracture management and is not without risks for the patient [42].

Patrick reported 3 cases of children with TAL rupture who received conservative management. All children were treated with external immobilization (two with halo vests and one with a Sterno-Occipito-Mandibular Immobilizer brace) for 6 to 12 weeks. Follow-up CT scans demonstrated reattachment of the avulsed osseous tubercle, and dynamic cervical spine radiographs revealed the absence of C1–2 instability. These cases suggest a positive role for external immobilization in treating osseous avulsion injuries of the TAL in children [38].

There is no consistently effective nonoperative method for reliably stabilizing the atlantoaxial joint, and conservative treatment can lead to complications such as superficial infections, pressure sores, and dysphagia. Strohm et al. evaluated halo-fixator treatment in 41 patients with upper cervical spine fractures and reported complications such as fracture redislocation (20%), screw loosening (15%), pin screw infection (10%), skin necrosis (5%), and intracranial screw penetration (2.5%) [43]. Surgical treatment should be considered in the early stages for all type I and type II patients who experience nonunion and persistent instability after 3–5 months of immobilization.

27.10.2 Surgical Management

For unstable type 3b fractures (Fig. 27.5) with minimally displaced bony avulsion of the transverse ligament, direct osteosynthesis is recommended. Osteosynthesis of the atlas can be performed by an anterior–transoral, isolated posterior, or combined posterior/anterior-transoral approach (Fig. 27.6). Isolated atlas osteosynthesis is not recommended in older patients due to their age-related reduced bony healing capability, particularly in cases of severely displaced bony avulsion of the transverse ligament (type Dickman II, Fig. 27.4, [26]).

For displaced type 3b atlas fractures and intraligamentous rupture (type I according to Dickman), atlantoaxial fusion is recommended due to the assumed unlikelihood of ligamentous healing and the potential post-traumatic atlantoaxial instability. Depending on the anatomical situation and the feasibility of intraoperative reduction, posterior atlantoaxial fusion via the Magerl/Gallie or Goel/Harms is a viable treatment option.

In isolated posterior atlas osteosynthesis, atlas repositioning is the key point of the osteosynthesis and may be achieved through a combination

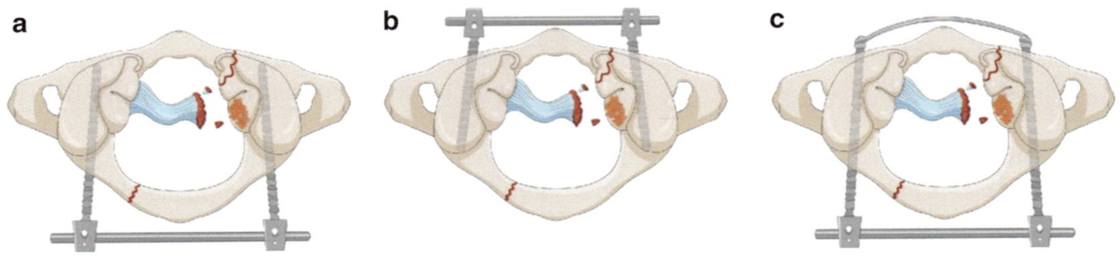

Fig. 27.6 Different treatment strategies for isolated atlas osteosynthesis: (**a**) Posterior fixation; (**b**) Transoral Anterior fixation; (**c**) Combined posterior and anterior fixation. (Kandziora F, Scholz M, Pingel A, et al. Treatment of Atlas Fractures: Recommendations of the Spine Section of the German Society for Orthopaedics and Trauma (DGOU). Global Spine J. 2018;8(2 Suppl):5S–11S)

of monoaxial screws, dedicated repositioning tools, and manual bilateral external neck compression. Final fixation is completed with a screw-and-rod connection. Bicortical lateral mass screws are highly recommended as their pull-out strength is significantly higher compared to monocortical C1 lateral mass screws [44]. The posterior–anterior atlas osteosynthesis described by Böhm combines posterior screw fixation with intentionally longer bicortical C1 lateral mass screws and additional transoral wiring between the screw tips to close the C1 ring anteriorly and posteriorly [45]. The anterior-transoral atlas osteosynthesis, described by Ruf, is performed using a standard transoral approach [46].

Posterior atlantoaxial fusion techniques are widely used to stabilize the atlantoaxial complex, including posterior wiring Wxation, posterior ApoWx laminar clamps Wxation, Magerl technique, etc. [47]. Magerl introduced transatlantoaxial joint space screw internal fixation, which limits C1–2 articular rotation. Biomechanical tests indicate that this Wxation method provides optimal mechanical stability. However, as a Wxation method, assistance from the Gallie or Brooks methods is still needed to complete the atlantoaxial posterior structure stabilization and bone transplant [48, 49]. The C1 lateral mass screw combined with the C2 vertebral pedicle screw Wxation provides superior biomechanical stability [47]. Guo et.al reported 12 cases of Jefferson fractures with TAL rupture. All patients underwent posterior atlantoaxial fusion using bilateral atlas laminar hooks combined with transarticular screw Wxation following atlantoaxial joint reduction, and all achieved good bony fusion after 12–24 months of follow-up [47].

Damage to the odontoid and transverse ligaments of the C1–C2 complex may result in atlantoaxial instability. Currently, this type of instability is corrected using anterior and/or posterior atlantoaxial fusion. However, such fusion leads to considerable motion loss in the head and neck, potentially affecting the patient's quality of life. To address this issue, Cai et.al have designed a novel total atlanto-odontoid joint arthroplasty system that not only stabilizes the atlantoaxial complex but also preserves movement in all directions of the C1–C2 segment. This system can be implanted onto the defect created by anterior decompression [50].

27.11 Conclusion

The TAL plays a vital role in stabilizing the cranio-cervical junction region. TAL rupture is typically associated with fall trauma, where a blow to the occiput directs force anteriorly, causing forced flexion and excessive anterior displacement of C1 relative to C2. The primary risk of TAL injury is spinal cord compression. Early diagnosis of TAL rupture is crucial in patients with trauma and clinical symptoms involving the cranio-cervical junction. Appropriate imaging modalities, such as X-rays, CT examination, and MRIs, should be utilized for precise assessment of TAL injury. The primary goal of treatment for TAL rupture is to restore atlantoaxial stability while minimizing complications. Therefore, management, whether conservative or surgical, should be tailored individually based on the type of fracture and patient comorbidities.

References

1. Domenicucci M, Dugoni DE, Mancarella C, D'Elia A, Missori P. Vincenzo Quercioli (1876-1939), researcher and pioneer of the atlas fracture. J Neurosurg Spine. 2015;22(3):253–8.
2. Debernardi A, D'Aliberti G, Talamonti G, Villa F, Piparo M, Collice M. The craniovertebral junction area and the role of the ligaments and membranes. Neurosurgery. 2015;76(Suppl 1):S22–32.
3. Barker EG Jr, Krumpelman J, Long JM. Isolated fracture of the medial portion of the lateral mass of the atlas: a previously undescribed entity. AJR Am J Roentgenol. 1976;126(5):1053–8.
4. Dvorak MF, Johnson MG, Boyd M, Johnson G, Kwon BK, Fisher CG. Long-term health-related quality of life outcomes following Jefferson-type burst fractures of the atlas. J Neurosurg Spine. 2005;2(4):411–7.
5. Tubbs RS, Hallock JD, Radcliff V, Naftel RP, Mortazavi M, Shoja MM, et al. Ligaments of the craniocervical junction. J Neurosurg Spine. 2011;14(6):697–709.
6. Panjabi MM, Oda T, Crisco JJ 3rd, Oxland TR, Katz L, Nolte LP. Experimental study of atlas injuries. I. Biomechanical analysis of their mechanisms and fracture patterns. Spine (Phila Pa 1976). 1991;16(10 Suppl):S460–5.
7. Fiester P, Rao D, Soule E, Orallo P, Rahmathulla G. Anatomic, functional, and radiographic review of the ligaments of the craniocervical junction. J Craniovertebr Junction Spine. 2021;12(1):4–9.
8. Krakenes J, Kaale BR, Rorvik J, Gilhus NE. MRI assessment of normal ligamentous structures in the craniovertebral junction. Neuroradiology. 2001;43(12):1089–97.
9. Panjabi M, Dvorak J, Crisco JJ 3rd, Oda T, Wang P, Grob D. Effects of alar ligament transection on upper cervical spine rotation. J Orthop Res. 1991;9(4):584–93.
10. Koller H, Resch H, Tauber M, Zenner J, Augat P, Penzkofer R, et al. A biomechanical rationale for C1-ring osteosynthesis as treatment for displaced Jefferson burst fractures with incompetency of the transverse atlantal ligament. Eur Spine J. 2010;19(8):1288–98.
11. Kopparapu S, Mao G, Judy BF, Theodore N. Fifty years later: the "rule of Spence" is finally ready for retirement. J Neurosurg Spine. 2022;37(2):149–56.
12. Brolin K, Halldin P. Development of a finite element model of the upper cervical spine and a parameter study of ligament characteristics. Spine (Phila Pa 1976). 2004;29(4):376–85.
13. Yoganandan N, Kumaresan SC, Voo L, Pintar FA, Larson SJ. Finite element modeling of the C4-C6 cervical spine unit. Med Eng Phys. 1996;18(7):569–74.
14. Zhang QH, Teo EC, Ng HW. Development and validation of a CO-C7 FE complex for biomechanical study. J Biomech Eng. 2005;127(5):729–35.
15. Spence KF Jr, Decker S, Sell KW. Bursting atlantal fracture associated with rupture of the transverse ligament. J Bone Joint Surg Am. 1970;52(3):543–9.
16. Heller JG, Amrani J, Hutton WC. Transverse ligament failure: a biomechanical study. J Spinal Disord. 1993;6(2):162–5.
17. Dvorak J, Schneider E, Saldinger P, Rahn B. Biomechanics of the craniocervical region: the alar and transverse ligaments. J Orthop Res. 1988;6(3):452–61.
18. Mesfar W, Moglo K. Effect of the transverse ligament rupture on the biomechanics of the cervical spine under a compressive loading. Clin Biomech (Bristol, Avon). 2013;28(8):846–52.
19. Kim D, Viswanathan VK, Munakomi S, Menger RP. C1 Fractures. StatPearls. Treasure Island (FL) ineligible companies. Disclosure: Vibhu Krishnan Viswanathan declares no relevant financial relationships with ineligible companies. Disclosure: Sunil Munakomi declares no relevant financial relationships with ineligible companies. Disclosure: Richard Menger declares no relevant financial relationships with ineligible companies. 2024.
20. Fielding JW, Cochran G, Lawsing JF 3rd, Hohl M. Tears of the transverse ligament of the atlas. A clinical and biomechanical study. J Bone Joint Surg Am. 1974;56(8):1683–91.
21. Hein C, Richter HP, Rath SA. Atlantoaxial screw fixation for the treatment of isolated and combined unstable Jefferson fractures – experiences with 8 patients. Acta Neurochir. 2002;144(11):1187–92.
22. Kontautas E, Ambrozaitis KV, Kalesinskas RJ, Spakauskas B. Management of acute traumatic atlas fractures. J Spinal Disord Tech. 2005;18(5):402–5.
23. Oda T, Yonenobu K, Fujimura Y, Ishii Y, Nakahara S, Matsunaga S, et al. Diagnostic validity of space available for the spinal cord at C1 level for cervical myelopathy in patients with rheumatoid arthritis. Spine (Phila Pa 1976). 2009;34(13):1395–8.
24. Domenicucci M, Mancarella C, Dugoni ED, Ciappetta P, Paolo M. Post-traumatic collet-Sicard syndrome: personal observation and review of the pertinent literature with clinical, radiologic and anatomic considerations. Eur Spine J. 2015;24(4):663–70.
25. Deliganis AV, Baxter AB, Hanson JA, Fisher DJ, Cohen WA, Wilson AJ, et al. Radiologic spectrum of craniocervical distraction injuries. Radiographics. 2000.;20 Spec No:S237-50;20:S237.
26. Kandziora F, Chapman JR, Vaccaro AR, Schroeder GD, Scholz M. Atlas fractures and atlas Osteosynthesis: a comprehensive narrative review. J Orthop Trauma. 2017;31(Suppl 4):S81–S9.

27. Riascos R, Bonfante E, Cotes C, Guirguis M, Hakimelahi R, West C. Imaging of Atlanto-occipital and atlantoaxial traumatic injuries: what the radiologist needs to know. Radiographics. 2015;35(7):2121–34.
28. Dickman CA, Greene KA, Sonntag VK. Injuries involving the transverse atlantal ligament: classification and treatment guidelines based upon experience with 39 injuries. Neurosurgery. 1996;38(1):44–50.
29. Perez-Orribo L, Snyder LA, Kalb S, Elhadi AM, Hsu F, Newcomb AG, et al. Comparison of CT versus MRI measurements of transverse atlantal ligament integrity in craniovertebral junction injuries. Part 1: a clinical study. J Neurosurg Spine. 2016;24(6):897–902.
30. Perez-Orribo L, Kalb S, Snyder LA, Hsu F, Malhotra D, Lefevre RD, et al. Comparison of CT versus MRI measurements of transverse atlantal ligament integrity in craniovertebral junction injuries. Part 2: a new CT-based alternative for assessing transverse ligament integrity. J Neurosurg Spine. 2016;24(6):903–9.
31. Fiester P, Orallo P, Soule E, Rao D, Tavanaiepour D. Utility of anterior Atlantodens interval widening on cervical spine CT for assessing transverse Atlantal ligament injury. Global Spine J. 2023;13(8):2319–26.
32. Radcliff KE, Sonagli MA, Rodrigues LM, Sidhu GS, Albert TJ, Vaccaro AR. Does C(1) fracture displacement correlate with transverse ligament integrity? Orthop Surg. 2013;5(2):94–9.
33. Eun J, Oh Y. The relationship between radiologic parameters and transverse atlantal ligament injury obtained from MRI scans in patients with an isolated atlas burst fracture: a retrospective observational study. Medicine (Baltimore). 2021;100(49):e28122.
34. Dickman CA, Mamourian A, Sonntag VK, Drayer BP. Magnetic resonance imaging of the transverse atlantal ligament for the evaluation of atlantoaxial instability. J Neurosurg. 1991;75(2):221–7.
35. Bransford R, Falicov A, Nguyen Q, Chapman J. Unilateral C-1 lateral mass sagittal split fracture: an unstable Jefferson fracture variant. J Neurosurg Spine. 2009;10(5):466–73.
36. Heller JG, Viroslav S, Hudson T. Jefferson fractures: the role of magnification artifact in assessing transverse ligament integrity. J Spinal Disord. 1993;6(5):392–6.
37. Liu P, Zhu J, Wang Z, Jin Y, Wang Y, Fan W, et al. "Rule of Spence" and Dickman's classification of transverse Atlantal ligament injury revisited: discrepancy of prediction on atlantoaxial stability based on clinical outcome of nonoperative treatment for atlas fractures. Spine (Phila Pa 1976). 2019;44(5):E306–E14.
38. Lo PA, Drake JM, Hedden D, Narotam P, Dirks PB. Avulsion transverse ligament injuries in children: successful treatment with nonoperative management. Report of three cases. J Neurosurg. 2002;96(3 Suppl):338–42.
39. Pryputniewicz DM, Hadley MN. Axis fractures. Neurosurgery. 2010;66(3 Suppl):68–82.
40. Jefferson G. Remarks on fractures of the first cervical vertebra. Br Med J. 1927;2(3473):153–7.
41. Levine AM, Edwards CC. Fractures of the atlas. J Bone Joint Surg Am. 1991;73(5):680–91.
42. Longo UG, Denaro L, Campi S, Maffulli N, Denaro V. Upper cervical spine injuries: indications and limits of the conservative management in halo vest. A systematic review of efficacy and safety. Injury. 2010;41(11):1127–35.
43. Strohm PC, Muller CA, Kostler W, Reising K, Sudkamp NP. Halo-fixator vest–indications and complications. Zentralbl Chir. 2007;132(1):54–9.
44. Eck JC, Walker MP, Currier BL, Chen Q, Yaszemski MJ, An KN. Biomechanical comparison of unicortical versus bicortical C1 lateral mass screw fixation. J Spinal Disord Tech. 2007;20(7):505–8.
45. Bohm H, Kayser R, El Saghir H, Heyde CE. Direct osteosynthesis of instable Gehweiler type III atlas fractures. Presentation of a dorsoventral osteosynthesis of instable atlas fractures while maintaining function. Unfallchirurg. 2006;109(9):754–60.
46. Ruf M, Melcher R, Harms J. Transoral reduction and osteosynthesis C1 as a function-preserving option in the treatment of unstable Jefferson fractures. Spine (Phila Pa 1976). 2004;29(7):823–7.
47. Guo X, Ni B, Wang M, Wang J, Li S, Zhou F. Bilateral atlas laminar hook combined with transarticular screw fixation for an unstable bursting atlantal fracture. Arch Orthop Trauma Surg. 2009;129(9):1203–9.
48. Marcon RM, Cristante AF, Teixeira WJ, Narasaki DK, Oliveira RP, de Barros Filho TE. Fractures of the cervical spine. Clinics (Sao Paulo). 2013;68(11):1455–61.
49. Brooks AL, Jenkins EB. Atlanto-axial arthrodesis by the wedge compression method. J Bone Joint Surg Am. 1978;60(3):279–84.
50. Cai X, He X, Li H, Wang D. Total atlanto-odontoid joint arthroplasty system: a novel motion preservation device for atlantoaxial instability after odontoidectomy. Spine (Phila Pa 1976). 2013;38(8):E451–7.

Odontoid Fractures

28

Yuchao Zuo, Yuanhao Lou, and Fuyou Guo

28.1 Introduction

The odontoid fracture is the most common type of cervical fracture in individuals over 65 years old and the most common fracture of the second cervical vertebra (axis). As an important bony connective structure in the upper cervix, the odontoid process is anatomically restricted to a limited range of movement by the transverse ligament to ensure that the atlantoaxial joint is stabilized. Owing to the presence of comorbidities in geriatric patients and the complexity of the anatomical location, the treatment of odontoid fractures poses a significant challenge for surgeons.

Odontoid fracture is reaching epidemic proportions among older patients. Its incidence is growing faster than that of any other spine fracture, but the optimal treatment strategy remains unclear [1]. These fractures are particularly challenging because they entail potential deterioration in function, and the morbidity group mainly comprises older adult patients. In addition, the incidence of odontoid fracture is frequently related to age and the mode of fall [2]. Interventions include operative and conservative treatments, and the risk factors for nonunion—age and comorbidities—must be considered in determining the optimal strategy [3].

28.2 Embryology of the Odontoid Process

28.2.1 Primary Ossification Centers

The armature is the second vertebral body of the cervical spine, consisting of the vertebral body, vertebral arch, transverse arch, and odontoid process. The odontoid process was historically considered part of the atlas body, but is now believed to have separated from the anterior part of the atlas between the sixth and seventh weeks of gestation and to have migrated caudally to fuse with the body of the axis [4]. This important structure originates in the axial portion of the occipital and upper two cervical sclerotomes: caudally from the atlas and cephalically from the axis. The development of ossification in the armature involves the odontoid process, two pairs of transverse arches, and four ossification centers of the vertebral body (Fig. 28.1).

The odontoid process fuses with the vertebral body between the ages of 3 and 6 years. This location can be seen as a translucency on radiographs up to 11 years of age. However, in one-third of adults, this anatomical entity can still

Y. Zuo (✉) · F. Guo
Department of Neurosurgery, The First Affiliated Hospital of Zhengzhou University, Zhengzhou, Henan, China

International Joint Laboratory of Nervous System Malformation, Zhengzhou, China
e-mail: zuoyuchao328@126.com

Y. Lou
Department of Neurosurgery, The First Affiliated Hospital of Zhengzhou University, Zhengzhou, China

M. Turgut et al. (eds.), *Ligaments of the Vertebral Column*,
https://doi.org/10.1007/978-3-032-09070-6_28

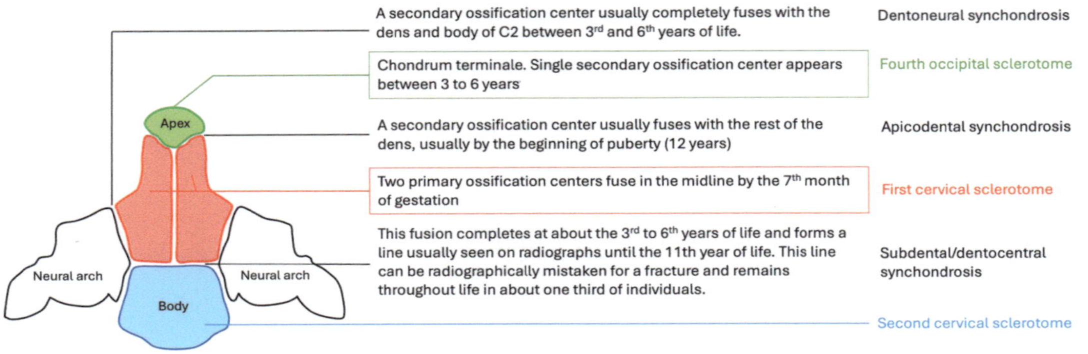

Fig. 28.1 Coronal view of the C2 vertebra showing its embryological fusion sites

be observed and is sometimes misdiagnosed as a cervical fracture. Two additional primary ossification centers of the odontoid process are located laterally and fused in the midline by the eighth month of fetal life [4, 5].

28.2.2 Secondary Ossification Centers

The secondary ossification center develops at the apex of the odontoid process (Fig. 28.1) and merges with it at age 12. This secondary ossification center is referred to as the ossiculum terminale or summit epiphysis. Each transverse arch merges with the vertebral body between the ages of 3 and 6 years. These individual ossification centers are not always fully fused until the onset of puberty. The tip of the odontoid process extends from the apex of the dens to the apicodental junction. The apex gives origin to the apical ligament, which extends rostral to the basion. The anterior arch of the atlas articulates with the odontoid process on its anterior surface. The broad posterior groove and the posterolateral surfaces are attachment sites for the transverse and alar ligaments. The ligaments of the atlantoaxial region develop first, forming during the eighth week of gestation [5–7].

The prevertebral region of the loose hard core of the first cervical vertebra forms the base segment of the odontoid process, and the hard core of the second cervical vertebra forms the axial body. Essentially, the odontoid process is resegmented and consists of a canine segment from the caudal anterior process, an abutment segment from the first cervical dura, and an axial body from the second cervical dura [4].

28.2.3 Synchondrosis

The ossification centers are separated by the synchondroses: the dentocentral synchondrosis lies between the dens and the body of the axis. In contrast, the neurocentral synchondrosis is located between the neural arches and the body of the axis. These synchondroses typically fuse between the ages of 3 and 6 years. The remnant of the dentocentral synchondrosis can occasionally be seen on magnetic resonance imaging (MRI) as a hypointense line between the inferior part of the dens and the superior part of the axis. Of note, ligaments of the atlantoaxial region develop first, forming by the eighth week of gestation [4, 5].

28.3 Odontoid Process Anatomy

28.3.1 Gross Anatomy

Anatomically, the odontoid process has a unique feature: there is an extended constriction where it attaches to the vertebral body. The apex of the odontoid process is pointed, serving as an attachment for the apical ligament. Below the apex, the odontoid process enlarges, and the alar ligaments on both sides are attached to it.

These ligaments connect the odontoid process to the occipital bone. On the anterior surface is an oval articular surface that acts on the joint with the anterior arch of the atlas. There is a superficial groove for the transverse ligament on the posterior surface, sometimes called the lumbar of the odontoid process. Above this level, the odontoid process widens and then tapers to the vertex [8].

The odontoid process can adopt one of three shapes: straight, lordotic, or kyphotic [9, 10]. The odontoid process is located at the center of a rich network of arteries. Arterial penetration is apparent around the base and apex of the odontoid process. In addition to the alar ligament, there is a vascular connection between the ligament and the bone [11].

28.3.2 Articulation Anatomy

The atlas and axis are highly specialized in comparison to the other cervical vertebrae. The axis is composed primarily of three parts: the odontoid process superiorly, the pedicle, and the body. Unique to the atlas and axis articulation is the absence of an intervertebral disc, which allows for greater freedom of rotation and eliminates the risk of herniation. Fifty percent of the rotation-and-flexion, extension (10–20%), and rotation (5–10%) of the cervical spine occurs at the atlas and axis. The skull rests upon the atlas and articulates with the odontoid process of the axis in a pivot joint. This articulation is posterior to the anterior arch of the atlas and projects vertically, making it difficult to assess any pathology [1, 3].

28.3.3 Anatomy of Ligaments

The odontoid process is secured to the anterior arch of the atlas by the cruciate ligament, which is made up of ascending and descending fibers (Fig. 28.2a). Most of the stability of the upper cervical spine is provided by the internal and external craniocervical ligaments, with the contribution of the internal predominating. Included among these ligaments are the tectorial membrane, the apical and alar ligaments, and the transverse atlantal ligament. The tectorial membrane is an extension of the posterior longitudinal ligament, which originates along the posterior

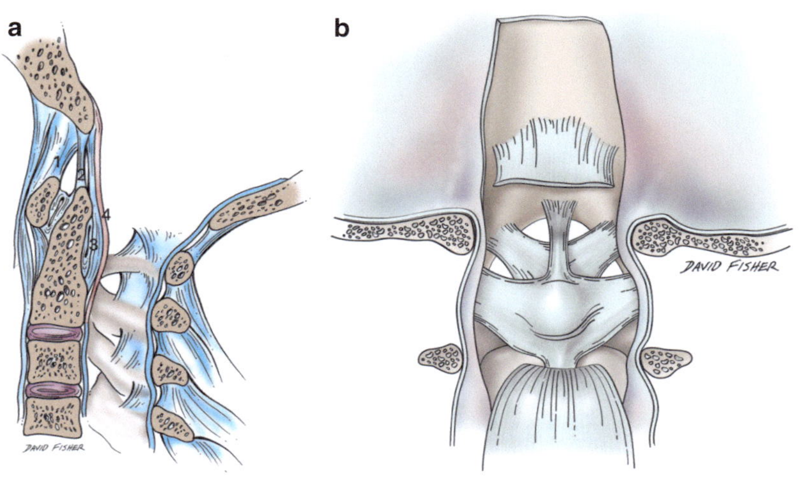

Fig. 28.2 Surrounding ligaments related to the odontoid process. (**a**) Sagittal illustration showing the surrounding ligaments related to the odontoid process. *1* anterior atlanto-occipital membrane, *2* apical ligament, *3* transverse atlantal ligament, *4* tectorial membrane. (**b**) Posterior view illustrating from superficial to deep, the cut tectorial membrane (cut and reflected), the cruciate ligament, and the alar ligaments

surface of the axis and inserts onto the anterolateral aspect of the foramen magnum (Fig. 28.2b). The paired alar ligaments attach just below the tip of the dens and extend laterally to the medial aspect of the occipital condyles, where they function to preclude excessive external rotation. The transverse atlantal ligament, together with associated ascending and descending fibers, is referred to as the cruciate ligament [1, 4, 5, 12].

28.3.4 Vascular Supply

The anterior and posterior ascending branches of the vertebral arteries supply the base of the dens with blood via the accessory ligaments and reach the tip by running cephalad at the periphery. Poor healing is often attributed to impairment of the blood supply to the dens caused by disruption to the perforator vessels, resulting in high rates of nonunion following a dens fracture [1, 3]. In addition to the ascending branches of the vertebral arteries, the arterial arcade above the odontoid process also accepts branches from the ascending pharyngeal, internal and external carotid arteries [11] (Fig. 28.3). The internal carotid artery can provide branches that feed the anterior surface of the odontoid process before entering the carotid canal. Venous drainage of the odontoid is into the surrounding vertebral venous plexus [4].

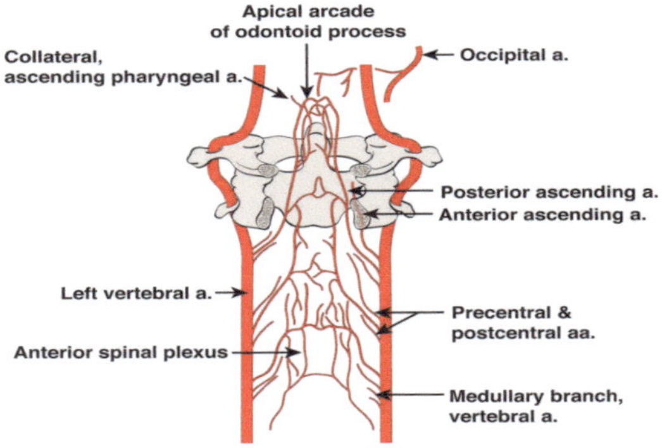

Fig. 28.3 Schematic drawing of the arterial blood supply to the odontoid process

28.4 Variant Anatomy

28.4.1 Absent or Hypoplastic Odontoid Process

It is very rare for the odontoid process to be completely absent or underdeveloped in both segments. Agenesis of the apical segment is the most common anomaly of the odontoid process. Partial absence or hypoplasia of the odontoid is usually associated with spondyloepiphyseal dysplasia, mucopolysaccharidosis, and dwarfism. This anomaly predisposes the craniovertebral junction to dislocation and cord compression owing to the absence of the apical and alar ligaments [1, 13].

28.4.2 Os Odontoideum

Os odontoideum is the separation of the odontoid tip, a derivative of the fourth occipital sclerotomes (the proatlas), from the body of the axis, resulting in a smooth and separate caudal portion of the odontoid process. It is a rare radiographic diagnosis, most often found incidentally [14].

It has been argued that ligament laxity leads to instability and hypermobility, generating abnormal shear stresses during chondrogenesis that interfere with ossification and allow subsequent transverse ligament intervention, thereby establishing nonunion with hypermobility. This overactivity results in repetitive microtrauma, causing dehiscence of the odontoid tip, which retains apical fragments due to the blood supply from the odontoid process [15–17].

28.4.3 Ossiculum Terminale

Bergman's ossicles are usually a benign condition, though in rare cases, they present with clinical symptoms such as neck pain and neurological problems. They can be associated with Down syndrome and cause atlantoaxial instability [6].

According to Greenberg's theory of terminal bone origin, the failure of the apical secondary ossification center to fuse results in persistent terminal ossicles, also known as Bergman ossicles, leading to a shortened pivotal segment and predisposing individuals to atlantoaxial subluxation and high cord compression [4, 18].

28.5 Biomechanics of the Odontoid

28.5.1 Morphometry of the Odontoid

The size of the odontoid process cannot be predicted from a patient's weight, height, or any other measured dimension of the axis. Men tend to have larger dimensions than women [19]. The minimum transverse diameter at the narrowest part of the structure was 9.0 mm, and two 3.5 mm cortical screws could be placed [20]. The minimum intramedullary diameter observed in the cross-section was 4.4 mm, and only one 3.5 mm screw could be placed. Understanding the trabecular anatomy within the odontoid process is essential for better understanding and treatment of fractures. Surgically, understanding the internal anatomy of the odontoid process aids in determining the number of screws that can be placed during surgical fixation of fractures.

The fully formed odontoid process is tooth-like or peg-shaped, with a curved superior surface. It deviates slightly to the left or right in approximately 14-26% of the population. It averages 15.5 mm (±1.8 mm) in males and 14.6 mm (±1.5 mm) in females, with an antero-posterior diameter of 10.3 (±0.7 mm) in males and 9.6 (±0.9 mm) in females. The sagittal and transverse diameters are approximately 10.5 and 10 mm, respectively. The anterior articular surface of the dens is circular or elliptical, measuring approximately 10 × 9 mm. The posterior angulation (retroflexion) of the odontoid process can be influenced by sex, with females exhibiting higher angulation grades [4].

28.5.2 Biomechanics of the Odontoid Process

Studies have shown that two groups of joints control movements of the atlantoaxial joint, which can be divided into anterior and posterior atlanto-axial joints. This structural feature confers a large range of axial rotation and a certain degree of flexion and extension on the atlantoaxial joint; however, the range of lateral flexion is limited [21]. Axial rotation between the atlantoaxial joints is regulated and limited by the alar ligaments; the transverse ligaments limit the forward sliding of the atlantoaxial joints in flexion. Recent studies investigating the mechanism of odontoid process fractures have revealed that the primary factors are the magnitude and direction of the load, shear stress, and bone parameters [8].

A finite element model was used to apply a variable directional load to the odontoid process. In the direction tested, the odontoid process is most vulnerable when subjected to upward and transverse load vectors. Head stretching, combined with force loading in lateral shear, compression, and axial rotation, can lead to different types of fractures. Additionally, the finite element model indicates that the stress-bearing contribution of cancellous bone in the vertebral body is relatively small [22, 23].

Bone mineral density declines with age, and low-density trabecular bone, extending anteriorly and posteriorly upward, reaches the base of the odontoid process, resulting in sparse trabecular bone and thin cortex in areas of mechanical weakness at the posterior edge of that base. The underlying healing of fracture patterns that reach this area is poor [24]. The direction of loading has a secondary role in traumatic fractures of the odontoid process, and bone mineral density and biomechanical results have a significant correlation. Thus, we can conclude that odontoid fracture results from the interaction between load size and bone mass [25].

28.5.3 Mechanism of Injury

In most cases, the kinetic energy transmitted to the upper cervical spine is directed through the odontoid process [26]. Many studies have shown that odontoid fractures have a bimodal age distribution, occurring in younger patients with high-energy trauma and older patients after relatively low-energy accidents such as ground falls [1]. Falls and motor vehicle collisions are the cause of most odontoid C2 fractures [27]. In falls and motor vehicle crashes, low-impact trauma from a standing position is the most common cause [28–30].

Ivancic et al. [31] determined that impingement at the midline of the upper forehead was the mechanism underlying odontoid process fractures and associated atlanto-vertebral and ligament injuries, similar to those observed in real life. Dynamic odontoid fractures are caused by rapid deceleration of the head, resulting in downward transfer of loads, coupled with sustained trunk momentum that leads to spinal compression, anterior incisional forces, and anterior displacement of the axis relative to the atlas.

28.6 Clinical Manifestation

28.6.1 Classification

The classification system of odontoid fractures has evolved significantly, the classic being the system of Anderson and D'Alonzo [32]. This is also the most widely adopted and remains in use today. The authors proposed in 1974 that odontoid fractures can be classified into three types, designated as type I, type II, and type III (Fig. 28.4), based on their anatomical location. Type I fractures are the least common and occur at the tip of the odontoid process; type II fractures are the most common, accounting for 65–74%, and occur at the base of the alveolar system, resulting in C2 subluxation. Type III fractures occur at the junction between the odontoid process and the front of the axis, extending to the side of the body [32]. In general, types I and III fractures are more stable, have limited nerve involvement, and are usually treated noninvasively.

In 1979, Althoff [33] proposed four fracture types based on the anatomical level. Type A is a fracture above the neck; type B is a fracture through the neck that includes the uppermost part of the C2 body; type C includes the medial aspect of an upper articular process; and type D is a fracture through the C2 body that includes the medial aspect of the bilateral superior articular process.

A simplified classification system has recently been proposed, based on the embryology and anatomy of C2 vertebral development, which provides accurate descriptions of odontoid fractures (Fig. 28.5). This system divides the odontoid process into zone I (extending from the apex to the junction of the primary and secondary ossification centers, i.e., the upper one fourth of the odontoid process) and zone II (extending from this junction to the lower three fourths of the chondral symphysis), and divides odontoid fractures into type A and type B (anteroposterior displacement, or angulation of the odontoid process) depending on whether the odontoid process is displaced or angled [7, 34].

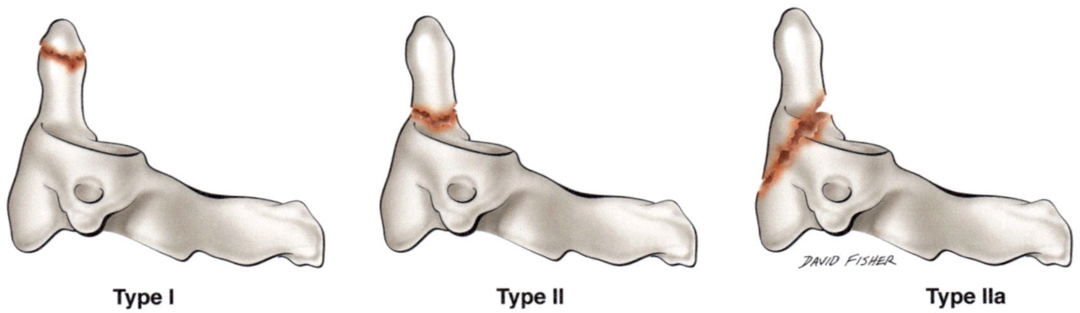

Fig. 28.4 Schematic drawing showing the three types of odontoid fracture according to the Anderson and D'Alonzo classification system

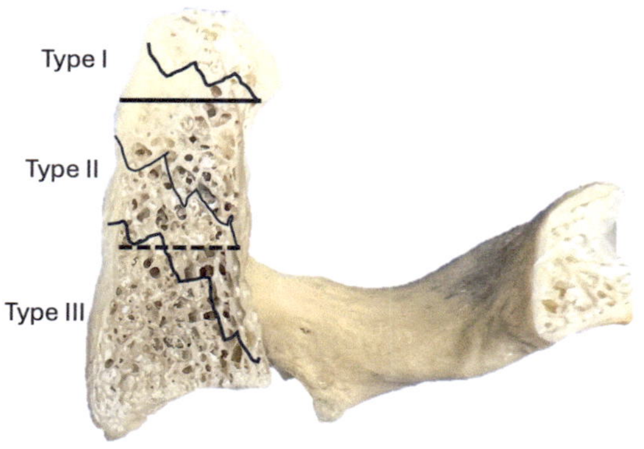

Fig. 28.5 Sagittal section through the C2 vertebra. The dotted line represents the synchondrosis between the odontoid process and the body of C2. Using this line, the odontoid process can be divided into an upper fourth and lower three-fourths. Type I represents fractures through the upper fourth (i.e., apex). Type II fractures involve the lower three-fourths and type III fractures are type II fractures that also involve the body of C2

28.6.2 Clinical Manifestation

Occipital and neck pain is common, often accompanied by limited head and neck movement, and patients are forced to support their head with their hands to relieve symptoms. In severe cases, symptoms may include upper limb weakness, numbness, muscle weakness, loss of fine motor control, difficulty walking, or even paralysis of the lower limbs, along with hyperreflexia of the limb tendons, positive pathological signs, and abnormal urinary and bowel function [21].

Neck instability usually develops when a fracture occurs at the base of the odontoid process. The C1 vertebral body slides forward or backward relative to C2, causing it to move in relation to C2, which can lead to injury and compression of the spinal cord. This injury can occur immediately at the time of the fracture, in which case the patient usually dies, or it can develop when there is repeated trauma from sports or regular daily activities, resulting in varying degrees of paralysis. Often, the only immediate symptom after an injury is severe pain in the neck.

The pain associated with these injuries can be localized or diffuse; however, it is typically severe and immediate in the upper part of the neck or the back of the head, accompanied by muscle spasms that are aggravated by even the slightest movement. Neurological involvement can occur immediately from the initial injury or be delayed for weeks or years, secondary to advanced or progressive subluxation [35–37].

28.6.3 Physical Examination

Most patients with odontoid fractures have a clear history of trauma, such as falls and car accidents, with occipitocervical region pain accompanied by limited movement of the head and neck; patients are forced to support the head with their hands to relieve the symptoms. In severe cases, upper limb weakness, skin numbness, and muscle weakness of the limbs, as well as difficulty with fine motor abilities, walking, or even paralysis of the lower limbs, hyperreflexia of the limbs, and positive pathological signs, may be observed. Additionally, abnormal bowel and urine function may be present. Suspicion of odontoid fractures should be strengthened if there are signs of head trauma.

The initial assessment of the cervical spine is important. When an odontoid process fracture is suspected, a thorough physical examination of the neck and cervical spine is mandatory. Patients typically present with neck pain and a feeling of instability between the head and spine. The examination should include the Romberg test, gait assessment, and evaluation of brainstem and cerebellar function. Cervical tenderness should be assessed. Any other relevant abnormalities should also be emphasized during the examination. A C2 neurological assessment should be performed, including motor, sensory, and reflexes. Clinically significant cervical spine injury is unlikely if the patient presents with no neck pain, no tenderness on examination, no loss of consciousness, no neurological deficits or significant impairment, and a good mental status examination.

Typical findings on physical examination include spinal shock: weakness, reflexes, loss of anal sphincter tone, fecal incontinence, erection, and loss of the bulbocavernosus reflex. Neurogenic shock: hypotension, ectopic bradycardia, redness, dryness, and fever of the surrounding skin. Autonomic dysfunction: intestinal obstruction, urinary retention, and hyperthermia [3].

28.6.4 Imaging Evaluation

28.6.4.1 X-ray Examination

According to Canada's cervical spine rules, an age greater than 65 years is a criterion for the use of X-rays; among young people, X-rays are primarily used for motor vehicle collisions [38]. X-rays reveal most type I and type II odontoid fractures and almost all type III fractures (Fig. 28.6). Initial studies showed that a standard set of lateral, anteroposterior (AP), and open-mouth radiographs was sufficient to detect 93% of cervical injuries. Lateral X-rays usually show a major displaced fracture, and if the patient is alert and cooperative, they can also assist with voluntary, gentle flexion or extension of the neck. However, in cases of acute injury, even such cautious maneuvers can be dangerous.

Currently, imaging of the cervical spine typically consists of an initial screening using lateral cross-table X-rays, followed by one or more additional views, including an AP open-mouth odontoid view, a lower cervical AP view, a swimmer's view, and possibly an oblique view. The tip of the odontoid process should be within 1–2 mm of Wackenheim's line, which is a straight line from the posterior caudal process to the superior cervical vertebra (Fig. 28.7) [39]. Radiological evaluation of suspected odontoid dysplasia also usually begins with anteroposterior and lateral plain radiographs.

28.6.4.2 CT and MRI Examination

Computed tomography (CT) can provide detailed images of the skeletal cervical spine and the atlantoaxial joints (Fig. 28.8). Open-mouth X-rays or coronal CT images should be assessed for signs of fracture or instability that suggest transverse atlantal ligament injury. The odontoid process should be symmetrically located between the occipital condyles; a slight lateral roll could be the only radiographic evidence of occult fracture injury [1].

CT is indicated for traumatic injuries, though significant injuries to the cervical spine can be missed and identified on plain radiographs. CT often misses fractures through the pedicles, articular processes, spinous processes, and nondisplaced odontoid fractures. Direct or reformatted sagittal scans are recommended, but direct axial scans are not advised. Uniaxial CT can miss transverse fractures that are not displaced [1, 3, 39, 40].

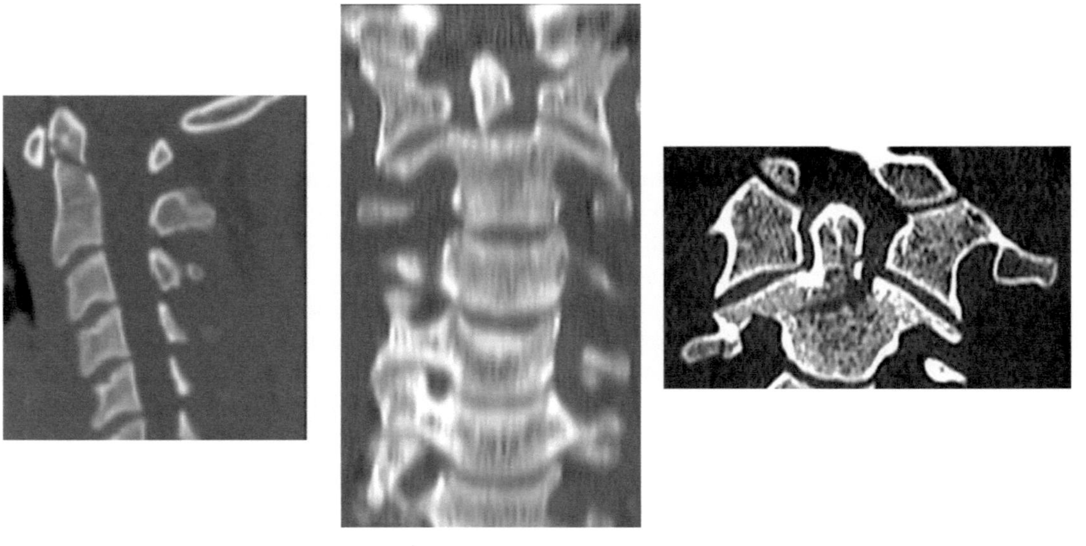

Fig. 28.6 Examples of odontoid fractures as seen on X-ray examination

The role of MRI in spinal trauma is to help characterize injuries to soft tissues, nerve elements, and intervertebral discs, and it can fully visualize pathological changes in the spinal cord. It is therefore particularly advantageous for patients with neurological deficits. MRI is also indicated for patients with hyperextension injury, vascular occlusion (vertebral artery), or post-traumatic disc herniation. Although most patients have prevertebral hematomas, hyperextension injuries are often not noticed on radiography, making MRI essential for evaluating neurological deficits, spinal cord injuries, and ligament injuries in trauma patients. A detailed evaluation of soft tissues by MRI can also help identify associated ligament injuries [1, 3, 39–41].

Due to its detailed anatomical information and ability to distinguish among various tissues, MRI usefully complements traditional plain X-ray examinations for evaluating the odontoid process. It is also often more effective in analyzing soft tissues and cancellous bone [42].

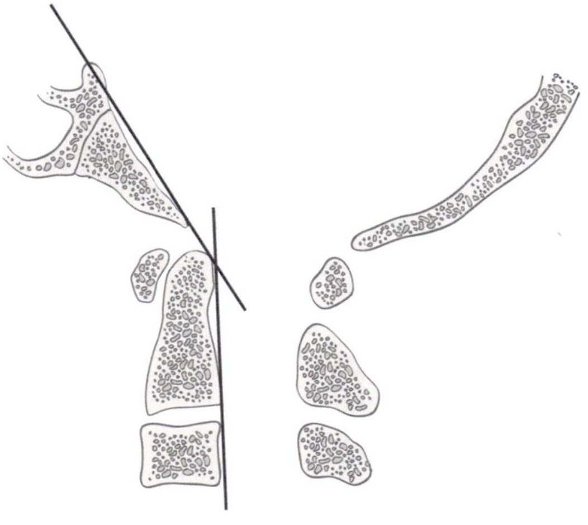

Fig. 28.7 Schematic drawing illustrating Wackenheim's line and the posterior vertebral line (George's line), both used to verify the correct position of the odontoid process in cases of suspected fracture

28.7 Treatment

Treatment options for odontoid fractures depend on the type of fracture and the individual patient's evaluation. The options are conservative treatment (external fixation device) and surgical treatment (posterior fusion, internal fixation, or anterior screw fixation) (Fig. 28.9) [39, 43].

28.7.1 Conservative Treatment

There is considerable controversy regarding the indications for conservative treatment of odontoid fractures. However, most experts and scholars believe that in the absence of occipital-atlantoaxial instability, atlantoaxial instability or

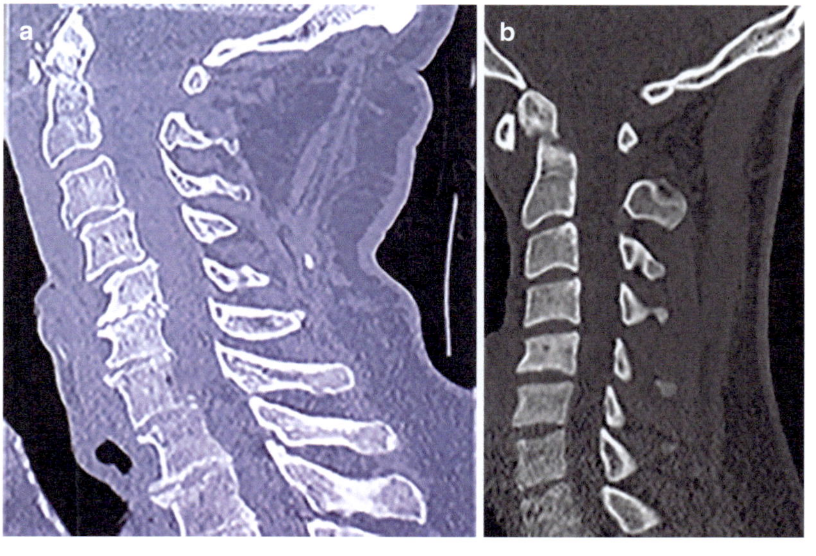

Fig. 28.8 (**a**) Sagittal CT of the cervical spine, noting a fracture of the odontoid process that is nondisplaced. (**b**) Sagittal CT of the cervical spine illustrating a displaced odontoid process fracture

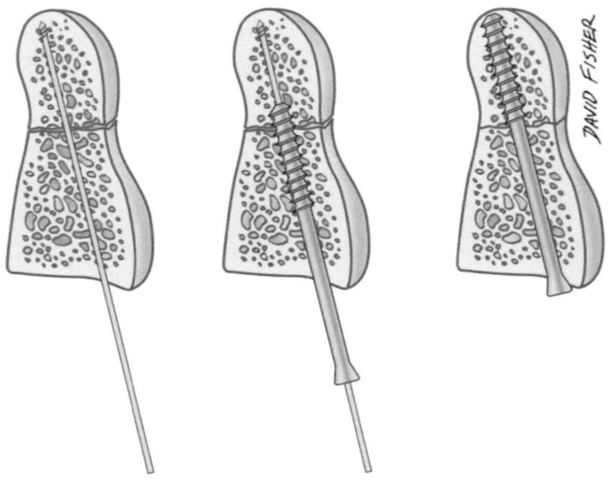

Fig. 28.9 Schematic drawing of the placement of an anterior screw for treating fractures of the odontoid process

other concomitant unstable cervical fractures, the two types of odontoid fractures (types I and III odontoid fractures) have better healing rates, supporting the option of conservative treatment. For some individuals, such as patients with many underlying diseases, poor tolerance of surgery, older age, and severe osteoporosis, the choice of surgery is not wise, and conservative treatment is generally adopted [2].

Conservative observation is indicated for patients without significant instability or radiographic evidence. Conservative treatment for such symptomatic patients includes rigid or semi-rigid neck sleeves, cervicothoracic orthoses, cranial traction, external fixation of the head, neck, and chest cast, external fixation of the halo-vest brace, and external fixation of the neck circumference. Among these, the halo-vest has a good therapeutic effect on type I fractures while limiting the three-dimensional movement of the neck. Before the widespread use of halo-vest treatment, many patients were treated with traction in cranial forceps. However, the long fixation time required for halo-vest treatment makes it difficult to identify healing or stability actively, and prolonged immobilization can lead to cervical stiffness [1–3, 44, 45].

28.7.2 Surgical Treatment

If the odontoid fracture is severely unstable or causes severe instability of the atlantoaxial joint movement, surgery is required to meet the criteria for cure. Most experts and scholars generally diagnose the fracture type before determining whether surgery is indicated. Type I fractures are inherently stable, and conservative treatment should be chosen if there is no atlantoaxial or atlanto-occipital instability. Muller et al. defined type II and type III fractures as stable if they have a displacement of <2 mm, a posterior separation from the vertebral body of <5 mm. Of course, if the odontoid fracture is combined with severe neurological impairment, or there are pathological fractures due to malignancy, metabolic disease, or fractures with old long-term nonunion, these also require surgery [2].

Alessandro's study summarized the treatment of type II fractures as follows: all odontoid fractures without dislocation should be treated with rigid external fixation (preferably with a "halo-vest"). Surgery should be considered for all odontoid fractures with a dislocation of >5 mm. Surgery should also be selected for type II fractures in patients over 50 years of age, while conservative management of type II fractures for those under 50 is preferable [46].

28.7.2.1 Anterior Surgical Treatment

Direct fixation of the odontoid fracture at the base with anterior screws is recommended (Fig. 28.9). Anterior odontoid screw fixation (AOSF) is a safe and effective treatment for type II and rostral type III odontoid fractures. Since 1980, when anterior hollow screw fixation was first reported for treating odontoid process fractures, it has gradually gained acceptance due to its effectiveness. Its main advantage is that it directly fixes the odontoid process fracture and exerts compression on the fracture end, promotes fracture healing, and has little trauma; and cervical spine function is basically not lost after surgery.

AOSF uses intervertebral screws to compress fractures, aiming to achieve primary bone healing. Typically, the lower Smith-Robinson approach is employed, which is anatomically superior and provides exposure to C2. For patients with an adaptable fracture type, AOSF is an effective treatment option for odontoid process fractures, with a successful healing rate of up to 80–100%.

Percutaneous screw internal fixation has also been proposed by some experts and scholars, extending the concept of reducing trauma through precise guidance and positioning. Some assistive technologies have also been applied to anterior surgery such as ISO-C 3D navigation, 3D printing, and endoscopic treatment technology. This method should not be used when there are other concomitant fractures of the upper cervical spine [1–3, 47, 48].

28.7.2.2 Posterior Cervical Instrumented Fusion

Posterior C1-2 internal fixation (PCIF) provides much more stable results than odontoid screw fixation. It can be used for any fracture type, including comminuted or irreducible fractures, symptomatic pseudarthrosis, and severe osteoporosis, in most cases where AOSF is contraindicated. The main disadvantage of posterior fusion is the loss of about 50% of cervical rotation capacity. The posterior surgical technique is also more invasive, which increases the amount of intraoperative bleeding and the risk of postoperative wound complications.

The anterior screw technique is complicated. For certain types of odontoid fractures, such as oblique fractures accompanied by transverse ligament rupture and pathological fractures, anterior screw internal fixation may not achieve ideal atlantoaxial stability. Therefore, posterior atlantoaxial fusion cannot be entirely replaced in clinical applications [1–3, 49].

28.8 Complications

Odontoid fractures can contribute to spinal cord shock, neurogenic shock, complete and incomplete spinal cord syndromes, prespinal syndromes, central spinal cord syndromes, Brown Sequard syndrome, high cervical spinal cord syndrome, Horner syndrome, posterior cerebellar artery syndrome, and craniofacial injury [3]. Non-surgical treatment options for type II fractures have a high rate of nonunion, especially in older patients [50]. In non-surgical cases, progressive instability is the most significant complication and can lead to the development of severe, irreversible neurological problems.

28.9 Conclusions

28.9.1 Summary of Key Points in the Anatomy and Histology of the Odontoid Process

28.9.1.1 Morphometry

The dens is composed of dense cortical and trabecular bone, whereas the anterior part of the body of the axis consists of hypodense trabecular bone. Owing to the distinctive microarchitecture of the base of the odontoid process, this region offers less resistance to fractures.

28.9.1.2 Anatomy of the Odontoid Process

The odontoid has an extended narrow part that attaches it to the body of the vertebra. The apex of the odontoid process acts as an attachment for the apical ligament. The odontoid process is secured to the anterior arch of C1 by the cruciate ligament, which is made up of ascending and descending fibers.

28.9.1.3 Biomechanics

The finite element model shows that the odontoid process is most vulnerable when subjected to upward and transverse load vectors; moreover, the stress-bearing contribution of cancellous bone in the vertebral body is relatively small. There is a significant correlation between bone mineral density and biomechanical characteristics; odontoid fractures result from the interaction between load size and bone mass.

28.9.2 Importance of This Knowledge in Clinical Practice

Understanding the morphometry, anatomy and biomechanics of the odontoid is the cornerstone of clinical practice across a diverse range of medical disciplines. This knowledge underpins precise diagnosis, optimal treatment strategies, and improved results.

28.9.2.1 Precision in Diagnosis and Assessment

A deep understanding of the complex anatomical structure of the odontoid enables healthcare professionals to make precise diagnoses in clinical settings. A thorough investigation of the embryological and phenotypic variations of the odontoid process is the foundation for informed clinical decision-making in the assessment and management of the numerous disorders associated with C2 that affect all stages of life.

28.9.2.2 Tailored Treatment Strategies

Insights gained from developmental changes throughout life enable the creation of tailored treatment plans, thereby optimizing patient outcomes. Neurosurgeons proactively intervene in cases of odontoid fractures. Armed with a deep understanding of growth dynamics, plastic and reconstructive surgeons create precise and individualized corrective procedures to address complex atlantoaxial anomalies.

28.9.2.3 Promoting Multidisciplinary Collaboration

Collaborative healthcare guided by multidisciplinary expertise is fundamental to addressing complex conditions involving the atlantoaxial joint. A culture of information sharing and interdisciplinary collaboration ensures the delivery of comprehensive and holistic patient care, emphasizing the overall health and well-being of the individual.

In summary, an in-depth understanding of the developmental anatomy and biomechanics of the odontoid process extends beyond academic knowledge and is central to clinical practice. It equips healthcare professionals with the tools needed to make informed decisions, provides highly personalized patient management, and promotes medical advances.

References

1. Nourbakhsh A, Hanson ZC. Odontoid fractures: a standard review of current concepts and treatment recommendations. J Am Acad Orthop Surg. 2022;30(6):e561.
2. Chengxin K, Bo Y, Huiyi L, Yuanguang PU, Chuqiang Q, Dongyan LU. Research progress of treatment of odontoid fractures. China Mod Med. 2023;30(12):38–43.
3. Good AE, Ramponi DR. Odontoid/dens fractures. Adv Emerg Nurs J. 2024;46(1):38–43.
4. Akobo S, Rizk E, Loukas M, Chapman JR, Oskouian RJ, Tubbs RS. The odontoid process: a comprehensive review of its anatomy, embryology, and variations. Childs Nerv Syst. 2015;31(11):2025–34.
5. Ishak B, Dhaliwal G, Rengifo R, McCormack E, Mathkour M, Iwanaga J, Bui CJ, Dumont AS, Tubbs RS. The retroverted dens: a review of its anatomy, terminology, and clinical significance. World Neurosurg. 2020;137:304–9.
6. Johal J, Loukas M, Fisahn C, Oskouian RJ, Tubbs RS. Bergmann's ossicle (ossiculum terminale persistens): a brief review and differentiation from other findings of the odontoid process. Childs Nerv Syst. 2016;32(9):1603–6.
7. Mathkour M, Cardona JJ, Chaiyamoon A, Glynn RM, Jenkins S, Graham RA, Johal J, Gardner B, Iwanaga J, Dumont AS, Tubbs RS. Classifications of odontoid process fractures: a systematic review and proposal of a new simplified classification system based on embryology. Cureus. 2022;14(12):e32520.

8. Jenkins S, Bordes S, Aly I, Jeyamohan S, Ishak B, Iwanaga J, Loukas M, Tubbs RS. Internal morphology of the odontoid process: anatomic and imaging study with application to C2 fractures. World Neurosurg. 2019;127:e1120–6.
9. Koebke J. Morphological and functional studies on the odontoid process of the human axis. Anat Embryol. 1979;155(2):197–208.
10. Doherty BJ, Heggeness MH. Quantitative anatomy of the second cervical vertebra. Spine. 1995;5(20):513–7.
11. Althoff B, Goldie IF. The arterial supply of the odontoid process of the axis. Acta Orthop Scand. 1977;48(6):622.
12. Tubbs RS, Grabb P, Spooner A, Wilson W, Oakes WJ. The apical ligament: anatomy and functional significance. J Neurosurg. 2000;92(2 Suppl):197–200.
13. Pang D, Thompson DNP. Embryology and bony malformations of the craniovertebral junction. Childs Nerv Syst. 2011;27(4):523–64.
14. Klimo JP, Coon V, Brockmeyer D. Incidental os odontoideum: current management strategies. Neurosurg Focus. 2011;31(6):E10.
15. William Fielding J, Hawkins RJ. Os odontoideum. J Bone Joint Surg. 1980;3(62-A):376–83.
16. Dou H, Xie C, Wang X, Huang Q. Image measurements of os odontoideum in children. Transl Pediatr. 2021;10(2):388–93.
17. Goel A, Patil A, Shah A, Dandpat S, Rai S, Ranjan S. Os odontoideum: analysis of 190 surgically treated cases. World Neurosurg. 2020;134:e512–23.
18. Greenberg AD. Atlanto-axial dislocations. Brain. 1968;4(91):655–84.
19. Heller JG, Alson MD, Schaffler MB, Gartin SR. Quantitative internal dens morphology. Spine Phila Pa 1976. 1992;17(8):861–6.
20. Nucci RC, Seigal S, Merola AA, Gorup J, Mroczek KJ, Dryer J, Zipnick RI, Haher TR. The normal adult odontoid. Spine. 1995;3(20):264–70.
21. Yuan W. Research progress on odontoid process fracture and its biomechanics. Chin J Spine Spinal Cord. 1998;8(1):47–9.
22. Puttlitz CM, Goel VK, Clark CR, Traynelis VC. Pathomechanisms of failures of the odontoid. Spine Phila Pa 1976. 2000;25(22):2868–76.
23. Graham RS, Oberlander EK, Stewart JE, Griffiths DJ. Validation and use of a finite element model of C-2 for determination of stress and fracture patterns of anterior odontoid loads. J Neurosurg. 2000;93(1 Suppl):117.
24. Korres DS, Karachalios T, Roidis N, Lycomitros V, Spiliopoulou CA, Lyritis G. Structural properties of the axis studied in cadaveric specimens. Clin Orthop Relat Res. 2004;418(418):134–40.
25. Benca E, Zderic I, van Knegsel KP, Caspar J, Hirtler L, Fuchssteiner C, Strassl A, Gueorguiev B, Widhalm H, Windhager R, Varga P. Biomechanical assessment of fracture loads and patterns of the odontoid process. Spine. 2022;17(47):1212–20.
26. Bakhsh A, Alzahrani A, Aljuzair AH, Ahmed U, Eldawoody H. Fractures of C2 (Axis) vertebra: clinical presentation and management. Int J Spine Surg. 2020;14(6):908–15.
27. Malik SA, Murphy M, Connolly P, O'Byrne J. Evaluation of morbidity, mortality and outcome following cervical spine injuries in elderly patients. Eur Spine J. 2008;17(4):585–91.
28. Coleman N, Chan HH, Gibbons V, Baker JF. Comparison of hard and soft cervical collars for the management of odontoid peg fractures in the elderly. Geriatr Orthop Surg Rehabil. 2022;13:1781188809.
29. De Bonis P, Iaccarino C, Musio A, Martucci A, De Iure F, Donati R, Cultrera F, Tosatto L, Servadei F, Alesi D, Cavallo MA, Ghadirpour R, Molinari F, Lofrese G. Functional outcome of elderly patients treated for odontoid fracture. Spine. 2019;44(13):951–8.
30. Golob JF, Claridge JA, Yowler CJ, Como JJ, Peerless JR. Isolated cervical spine fractures in the elderly: a deadly injury. J Trauma. 2008;64(2):311–5.
31. Ivancic PC. Odontoid fracture biomechanics. Spine. 2014;39(24):E1403–10.
32. Anderson LD, D'Alonzo RT. Fractures of the odontoid process of the axis. J Bone Joint Surg Am. 1974;8(56-A):1663–74.
33. Althoff B. Fracture of the odontoid process. An experimental and clinical study. Acta Orthop Scand Suppl. 1979;177(50):1–95.
34. Johal J, Fisahn C, Burgess B, Loukas M, Chapman J, Oskouian RJ, Tubbs RS. The dens: a review of its diverse nomenclature and a recommended simplified terminology. Curēus (Palo Alto, Ca). 2017;9(1):e981.
35. Southwick WO. Current concepts review management of fractures of the dens (odontoid process). 1980;3(62-A):482–6.
36. Marar BC, Tay CK. Fracture of the odontoid process. 1976;3(47):231–6.
37. Griswold DM, Albright JA, Schiffman E, Johnson R, Southwick WO. Atlanto-axial fusion for instability. 1978;3(60-A):285–92.
38. Stiell IG, Clement CM, McKnight RD, Brison R, Schull MJ, Rowe BH, Worthington JR, Eisenhauer MA, Cass D, Greenberg G, MacPhail I, Dreyer J, Lee JS, Bandiera G, Reardon M, Holroyd B, Lesiuk H, Wells GA. The Canadian C-spine rule versus the NEXUS low-risk criteria in patients with trauma. N Engl J Med. 2003;349(26):2510–8.
39. Mackey RA, Bancroft LW. Your diagnosis? Displaced odontoid fracture and radiographic imaging. Orthopedics. 2011;4(34):318–21.
40. Peter Pech MD, Kilgore DP, Pojunas KW, Haughton VM. Cervical spinal fractures: CT detection. Radiology. 1985;1(157):117–20.
41. Davis SJ, Teresi LM, Bradley WG Jr, Ziemba MA, Bloze AE. Cervical spine hyperextension injuries: MR findings. Radiology. 1991;1(180):245–51.
42. Perdikakis E, Skoulikaris N. The odontoid process: various configuration types in MR examinations. Eur Spine J. 2014;23(5):1077–83.
43. Shears E, Armitstead CP. Surgical versus conservative management for odontoid fractures (Review). Cochrane Database Syst Rev. 2010;11:1–11.

44. Apuzzo ML, Heiden JS, Weiss MH, Ackerson TT, Harvey JP, Kurze T. Acute fractures of the odontoid process. An analysis of 45 cases. J Neurosurg. 1978;1(48):85–91.
45. Maiman DJ, Larson SJ. Management of odontoid fractures. Neurosurgery. 1982;4(11):474–6.
46. Di Paolo A, Piccirilli M, Pescatori L, Santoro A. Single institute experience about 108 consecutive cases of type II odontoid fractures: surgery versus conservative treatment. Turk Neurosurg. 2014;24(6):891–6.
47. Jenkins JD, Coric D, Branch JCL. A clinical comparison of one- and two-screw odontoid fixation. J Neurosurg. 1998;89(3):366.
48. Wang C, Liu C, Zhou Z, Qingping, Zheng L. Surgical treatment of odontoid process fractures. Chin J Bone Joint Injury. 2006;11(21):860–2.
49. Wang Q, Liao Y. Research progress in cervical myelopathy. Mod Pract Med. 2015;27(10):1257–8.
50. Govender S, Maharaj JF, Haffajee MR. Fractures of the odontoid process. J Bone Joint Surg. 2000;8(82-B):1143–7.

29 Facet Joint Sprain/Dislocation

Mitchell W. Couldwell and Pate J. Duddleston

29.1 Introduction

The facet joints, also known as zygapophysial joints, of the spine are synovial joints between the superior and inferior articulating processes of two adjacent vertebrae [1]. They coordinate flexion and extension of the spine while limiting rotation, whereas spinal ligaments contribute to the stability of the vertebrae. Facet joint subluxations or dislocations are rare injuries, usually involving spinal trauma or degenerative disease of the spine. Facet dislocations occur throughout the cervical, thoracic, and lumbar regions and often present as neurosurgical emergencies, necessitating prompt treatment depending on the severity and associated neurological deficits [2–5]. Medical professionals need to comprehend the mechanics of injury, the anatomy of the facet joint, diagnostic tools, and treatment options.

29.2 Anatomy

The facet joints of the spine are located between the pedicles and the laminae of the vertebrae. They are true synovial joints, distinct from the articulation of the fibrocartilaginous vertebral disc. This articulation provides structural stability to the vertebral column. At every spinal level apart from C1 to C2, a three-joint complex is formed from two adjacent vertebral bodies: the intervertebral disc in the anterior column and two facet joints in the posterior column; together, this unit is known as the motion segment. The posterior aspect of the motion segment contains the posterior ligamentous complex, which stabilizes the spine and consists of the supraspinous ligament, the interspinous ligament, the articular facet capsules, and the ligamentum flavum [2]. The functions of this complex include keeping the facet joints in contact with each other, therefore keeping the vertebrae in a stable alignment [6].

The motion segment guides spinal movement posteriorly, guided by the plane of facet articulation. The orientations of facet joints differ among locations along the spine. In the cervical spine, the facet joints are oriented in the frontal plane and inclined roughly 45° from horizontal; in the thoracic spine, they are angled even more towards the frontal plane, about 60° from horizontal and rotated 20° in the axial plane; in the lumbar spine, they are nearly 90° or vertical in the sagittal plane. These differences in anatomy and orientation dictate the biomechanics of segmental areas of the spinal column [7–9]. The cervical spine allows for a wide range of motion, including flexion, extension, lateral flexion, and rotation. The thoracic spine supports more lateral flexion and

M. W. Couldwell (✉) · P. J. Duddleston
Department of Neurosurgery, Tulane University School of Medicine, New Orleans, LA, USA
e-mail: mcouldwell@tulane.edu

M. Turgut et al. (eds.), *Ligaments of the Vertebral Column*,
https://doi.org/10.1007/978-3-032-09070-6_29

rotation while restricting flexion and extension. The lumbar spine facilitates flexion and extension while limiting rotation. The facet joint surfaces in the cervical and thoracic spine are reciprocally convex and concave, while those in the lumbar spine become less planar. In the cervical spine, the facet articulation surface area is approximately two-thirds the area of the vertebral end plate, compared to the lumbar spine, where the facet joints are relatively small compared to the vertebral bodies.

The facet joints are true synovial joints, characterized by articular cartilage that covers the articulating surfaces of each adjacent facet, and subchondral bone is covered by a synovial membrane that envelops the cartilaginous portions of the joint. Each facet joint capsule is filled with fat at its superior and inferior aspects. The fibrous joint capsule regulates the internal microenvironment of the joint to facilitate nutrition and immune cell function [6, 10, 11]. A small meniscus consisting of synovium, which encases fat, blood vessels, and collagen, projects into the inferior and superior aspects of the joint. It increases the contact surface area during motion and allows sliding during flexion and extension of the joint and articular surfaces [12].

Arterial vascularization is provided by branches of the ascending cervical artery in the cervical spine, branches from the thoracic aorta in the thoracic spine, and branches from the abdominal aorta in the lumbar spine. Venous drainage is via the internal and external venous plexuses, intervertebral and basivertebral veins [13–15]. The facet joints are innervated by pairs of nerve branches, known as medial branches, which originate from the same spinal level and the level above [6, 16–18].

29.3 Pathophysiology

Facet dislocation is most commonly caused by traumatic high-energy injuries, in which simultaneous multidirectional compressive, distractive, and rotational forces are transmitted across the spinal elements, leading to translational and rotational instability of the spinal column [3]. Facet joint dislocation is rare, occurring in less than 3% of thoracolumbar spine injuries. Common injury patterns include unilateral facet dislocation, bilateral facet dislocation, and fracture/dislocation. Facets are often described as "perched" when the inferior articulating process is sitting on top of the superior articulating process of the vertebrae below, or "jumped" when the inferior articulating process is locked in front of the superior articulating process of the level below (Fig. 29.1) [19, 20].

Unilateral cervical facet dislocations account for upwards of 5% of spinal injuries and usually present with neurological deficits, posterior spinal fractures, disc injury, and ligament injury. Bilateral facet dislocation is relatively uncommon and typically results from flexion and distraction-type injuries, with the mid to lower cervical levels being most often affected [18–20].

Osteoarthritis and spinal degeneration lead to functional changes within the motion unit. Degeneration of the disc, facet joints, or injury to the posterior spinal structures can lead to instability of vertebral segments and the combined three-joint complex can fail [6, 21]. Instability at one level of the spinal column can lead to pathological changes in motion units above or below [22]. During changes associated with disc degeneration, transmission of force across the facet joint is increased because the disc supports less force. In severe cases of disc-space narrowing, up to 70% of axial load can be carried by the facet joints, in contrast to roughly 33% in a healthy motion unit [23, 24]. These changes in biometric forces can lead to increased facet strain. Degenerative spondylolisthesis causes subluxation of facet joints due to progressive loss of cartilage and remodeling of the articulation surface as osteoarthritic changes progress. Changes associated with osteoarthritis and spondylolisthesis lead to alterations in facet joint orientation; the joints become more oriented in the sagittal plane, allowing forces to displace the superior vertebra in the motion segment anteriorly. These changes have been most widely reported at the L4-L5 vertebral level [25, 26].

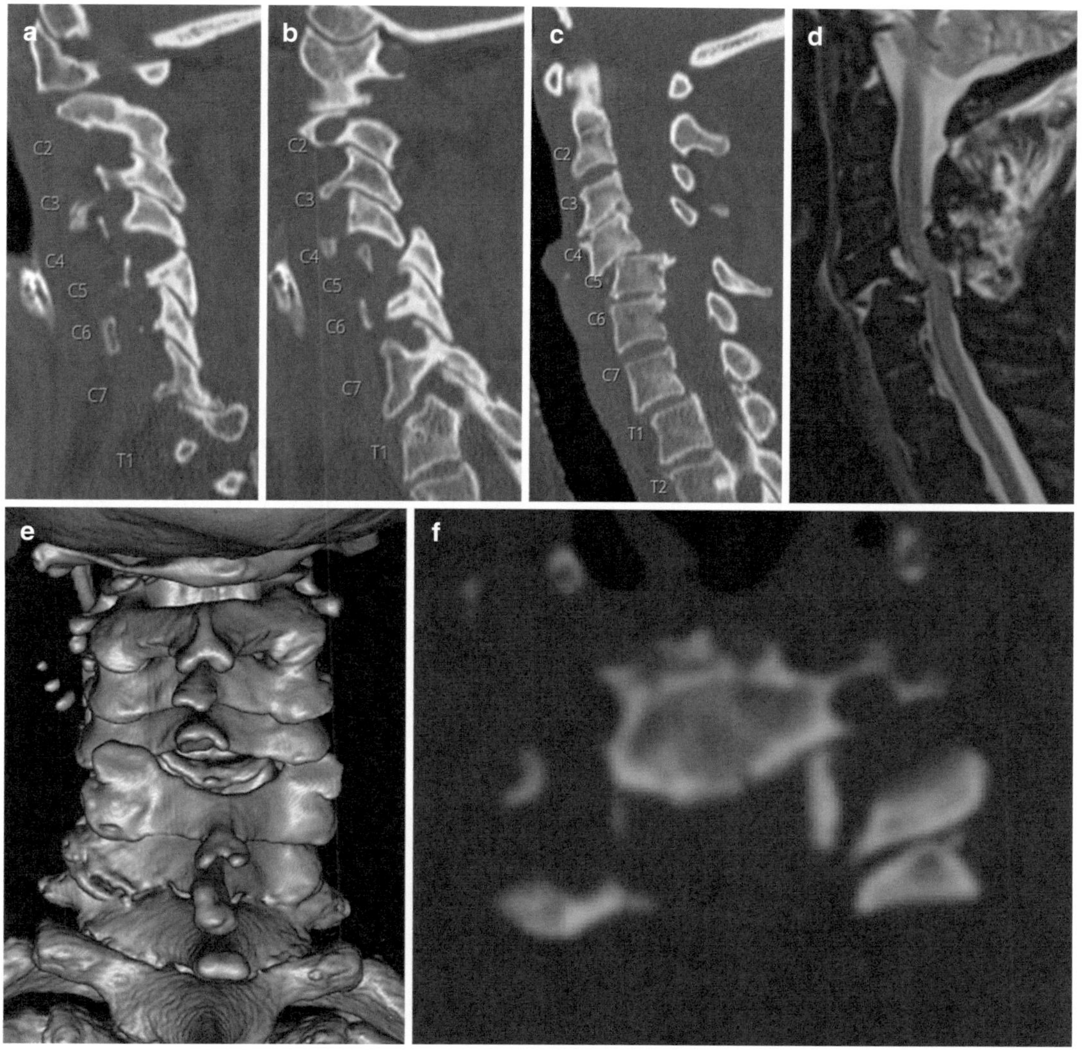

Fig. 29.1 Perched and jumped facets. (**a**) CT showing unilateral perched facet at C4/C5 (**b**) CT showing unilateral jumped (locked) facet at C4/C5 (**c**) CT showing anterolisthesis of C4 on C5 (**d**) MRI STIR sequence showing C4/C5 dislocation with cord compression and injury to the discoligamentous complex and posterior elements (**e**) 3D image, posterior view showing perched facet at C4/C5 on the right and jumped facet on the left (**f**) "reverse hamburger sign" of a locked facet

29.4 Diagnosis

Patient history, symptoms, physical examination, and imaging are used to assess suspected facet injuries. Pertinent history includes a history of trauma due to a flexion-distraction mechanism, ankylosing spondylitis, previous spinal surgeries, or osteoarthritis. Symptoms of facet dislocation injury include pain, particularly in the setting of traumatic flexion-distraction mechanisms, as well as numbness, tingling, or weakness in the limbs. Physical examination can reveal gross misalignment and/or symptoms of spinal cord injury such as changes in neurological reflexes, motor, and sensory function, necessitating a thorough neurological examination [1].

29.5 Imaging

Radiographs are often used in the initial survey of the spinal column. X-rays with anteroposterior, lateral, and oblique views can help to diagnose facet dislocation. Lateral views show subluxation of vertebral bodies, soft tissue swelling, widening of interspinous distance, and changes in sagittal alignment at the level of the injury. Flexion-extension radiographs can also be used for diagnosis, but must be used at the clinician's discretion when dealing with potentially unstable injuries. Facet joints are best visualized on oblique views. Computed tomography (CT) is acquired during most spinal surveys and can reveal the bony anatomy of injury, malalignment, and associated bony fractures (Figs. 29.2 and 29.3). This is the most accurate method for assessing bone pathologies [16]. CT is the most commonly used imaging modality due to its sensitivity and speed (Fig. 29.2). On a CT scan, the superior and inferior facets should be visible equally on each slice with flat articular surfaces opposing each other. This is known as the "hamburger sign" owing to its resemblance of the top and bottom of a hamburger bun (Fig. 29.1). If the facets are dislocated or "jumped," they can be seen as a "reverse hamburger sign" as it appears the hamburger buns are flipped upside down and on top of each other; the two convex portions of the facets are now in contact instead of the normal flat articular surfaces. This can be seen in cervical, thoracic, and lumbar facet dislocations [27].

Magnetic resonance imaging (MRI) enables the resolution of soft tissue with greater sensitivity, allowing non-osseous structures and changes such as soft tissue edema, neurovascular structures, and synovitis to be visualized more clearly (Figs. 29.1d and 29.3e) [6]. Various MRI sequences can be used to improve the sensitivity and specificity of facet joint pathology, including fat-suppressed sequences, which can visualize subchondral bone edema, or contrast agents such as gadolinium, which make it easier to evaluate changes in the facet joint [4, 16]. MRI can be

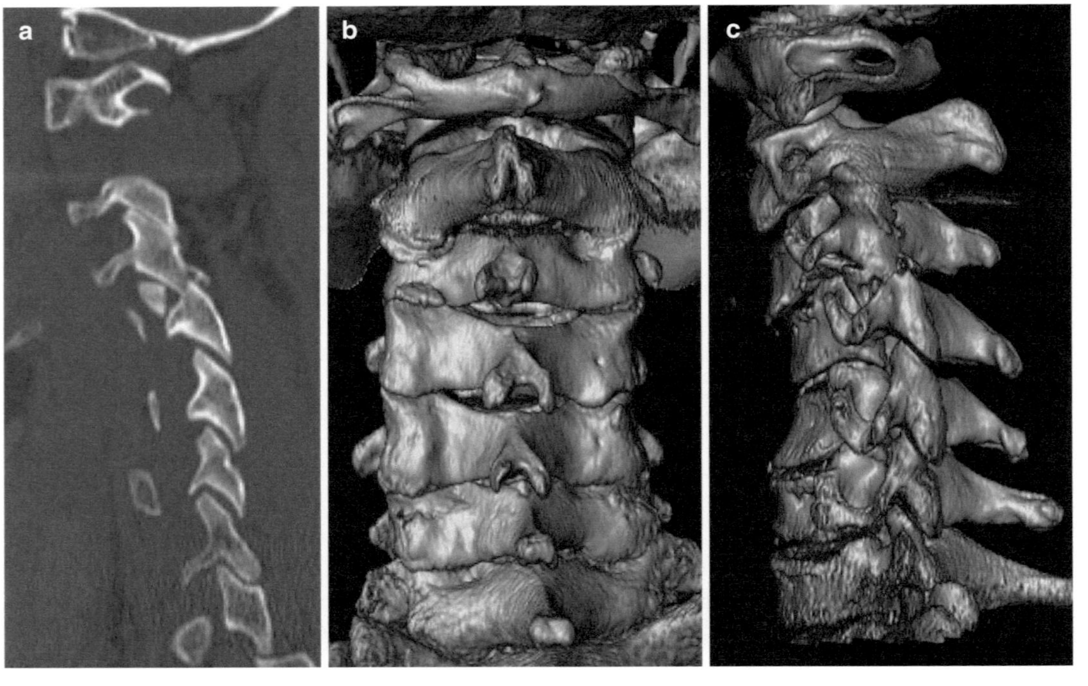

Fig. 29.2 Fracture dislocation. (**a**) CT of a fracture dislocation of unilateral facet (**b**) 3D image, posterior view of unilateral fracture dislocation (**c**) 3D image, sagittal view of fracture dislocation

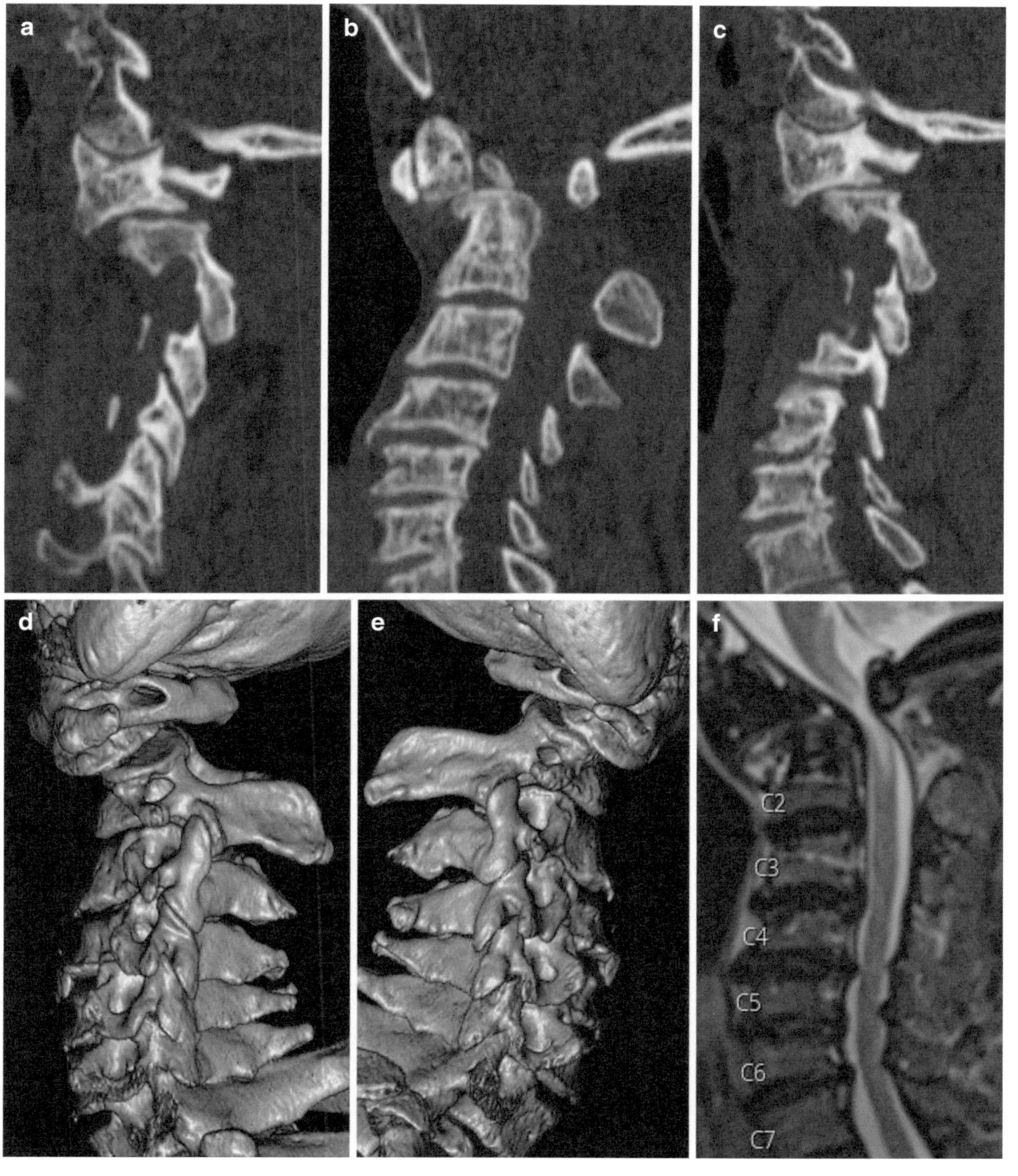

Fig. 29.3 Chronic type II odontoid fracture resulting in C1/C2 subluxation (**a**) right sided parasagittal view of C1/C2 subluxation (**b**) chronic type II odontoid fracture with anterolisthesis of odontoid tip (**c**) left sided parasagittal view of C1/C2 subluxation (**d**, **e**) 3D images of C1/C2 subluxation (**e**) MRI STIR sequence showing severe central stenosis with cord signal change at the level of C1/C2

used to assess injury to the spinal elements in cases of acute facet dislocation in patients with altered mental status before reduction and stabilization. MRI can show soft tissue injury such as disc herniation, posterior ligament injury, sprain or disruption of the posterior facet joint capsules, spinal cord compression, or spinal cord hematoma. It can sometimes identify an injury in patients with negative CT findings. MRI is often used to assess for disc herniation before open reduction. MRI indications include any new neurological deficit observed at presentation or during closed reduction, as well as surgical planning to evaluate for soft tissue or ligamentous injury [4, 19].

29.6 Treatment

The aim of facet dislocation treatment is to restore proper spinal alignment and function of the spinal cord by stabilizing the spine and decompressing neural elements [28]. Cervical facet dislocation can be treated either operatively or non-operatively. In non-operative treatment, closed reduction is the mainstay. Contraindications include uncooperative patients, altered mental status or unreliable neurological exam, or those with disc prolapse and bony fragmentation, which can pose threats to the spinal cord [29–32]. Skull traction tongs, developed by Gardner in 1973, are one of the most common devices used to achieve closed reduction. Timing for traction is essential; most studies suggest that closed reduction within 4 h of injury is necessary to maintain neurological function [33]. Non-operative management approaches using the halo traction device and cervical collar are not as common as they once were, owing to reportedly high rates of spinal instability, delayed neurological injury, and morbidity from pain and disability later in life [34].

Open reduction and cervical fusion are indicated when traction is contraindicated or closed reduction has failed, and it is the gold standard of treatment for facet dislocation in many cases. Options for surgical intervention remain debated, and cervical spine facet dislocations can include anterior cervical decompression and fusion, which is indicated when intervertebral disc injury compromises the spinal cord. Anterior decompression is then needed before facet reduction. It also preserves the native mechanical stability of the injured spine by reducing tension on the posterior spinal components [35]. Posterior cervical reduction and fusion are also used to treat facet dislocation and offer benefits such as direct visualization and reduction of the dislocation. They also allow for direct decompression of bony impingement upon the spinal canal and biomechanically stronger fixation of the tension-holding side of the spine [36].

Combined approaches to the anterior and posterior cervical spine can also be used when a single approach has failed to achieve adequate decompression and fixation or a more robust fixation is desired. However, combined approaches involve greater surgical risk, and cervical spinal movements can be further restricted [3, 37]. Treatment often follows a similar approach in the thoracic and lumbar spine, with most cases being treated with open reduction and fixation in a timely manner in view of associated neurological deficits secondary to spinal cord injury. Most open reductions and fixations in the lower spine are posterior reductions, aiming to reduce the facet dislocations through distraction mechanisms followed by fixation with hardware [38].

References

1. Curtis L, Shah N, Padalia D. Facet joint disease. In: StatPearls. Treasure Island: StatPearls; 2025.
2. Jaumard NV, Welch WC, Winkelstein BA. Spinal facet joint biomechanics and mechanotransduction in normal, injury and degenerative conditions. J Biomech Eng. 2011;133(7):71010. https://doi.org/10.1115/1.4004493.
3. Pavešić J, Jelić M, Dokuzović S, et al. Thoracic fracture dislocation with bilateral locked facet joints: a novel reduction technique. Preprints Published online 2023. https://doi.org/10.20944/preprints202308.0659.v1.
4. Chilvers G, Janjua U, Choudhary S. Blunt cervical spine injury in adult polytrauma: incidence, injury patterns and predictors of significant ligament injury on CT. Clin Radiol. 2017;72(11):907–14. https://doi.org/10.1016/j.crad.2017.06.122.

5. Ganjeifar B, Keykhosravi E, Bahadorkhan G, et al. Predictive value of computed tomography scan for posterior ligamentous complex injuries in patients with thoracolumbar spinal fractures. Arch Bone Jt Surg. 2019;7(4):321–4.
6. Gellhorn AC, Katz JN, Suri P. Osteoarthritis of the spine: the facet joints. Nat Rev Rheumatol. 2013;9(4):216–24. https://doi.org/10.1038/nrrheum.2012.199.
7. White AA, Panjabi MM. Clinical biomechanics of the spine. Lippincott; 1990. https://books.google.com/books?id=hDFsQgAACAAJ
8. Farfan HF, Cossette JW, Robertson GH, Wells RV, Kraus H. The effects of torsion on the lumbar intervertebral joints: the role of torsion in the production of disc degeneration. J Bone Joint Surg Am. 1970;52(3):468–97.
9. Asano S, Kaneda K, Umehara S, Tadano S. The mechanical properties of the human L4-5 functional spinal unit during cyclic loading. The structural effects of the posterior elements. Spine (Phila Pa 1976). 1992;17(11):1343–52. https://doi.org/10.1097/00007632-199211000-00014.
10. O'Leary SA, Paschos NK, Link JM, Klineberg EO, Hu JC, Athanasiou KA. Facet joints of the spine: structure-function relationships, problems and treatments, and the potential for regeneration. Annu Rev Biomed Eng. 2018;20:145–70. https://doi.org/10.1146/annurev-bioeng-062117-120924.
11. Kalichman L, Hunter DJ. Lumbar facet joint osteoarthritis: a review. Semin Arthritis Rheum. 2007;37(2):69–80. https://doi.org/10.1016/j.semarthrit.2007.01.007.
12. Tischer T, Aktas T, Milz S, Putz RV. Detailed pathological changes of human lumbar facet joints L1-L5 in elderly individuals. Eur Spine J. 2006;15(3):308–15. https://doi.org/10.1007/s00586-005-0958-7.
13. Sioutas G, Kapetanakis S. Clinical anatomy and clinical significance of the cervical intervertebral foramen: a review. Folia Morphol (Warsz). 2016;75(2):143–8. https://doi.org/10.5603/FM.a2015.0096.
14. Gkasdaris G, Tripsianis G, Kotopoulos K, Kapetanakis S. Clinical anatomy and significance of the thoracic intervertebral foramen: a cadaveric study and review of the literature. J Craniovertebr Junction Spine. 2016;7(4):228–35. https://doi.org/10.4103/0974-8237.193266.
15. Gkasdaris G, Kapetanakis S. Clinical anatomy and significance of the lumbar intervertebral foramen: a review. J Anat Soc India. 2015;64(2):166–73. https://doi.org/10.1016/j.jasi.2015.10.003.
16. Perolat R, Kastler A, Nicot B, et al. Facet joint syndrome: from diagnosis to interventional management. Insights Imaging. 2018;9(5):773–89. https://doi.org/10.1007/s13244-018-0638-x.
17. Binder DS, Nampiaparampil DE. The provocative lumbar facet joint. Curr Rev Musculoskelet Med. 2009;2(1):15–24. https://doi.org/10.1007/s12178-008-9039-y.
18. Anaya JEC, Coelho SRN, Taneja AK, Cardoso FN, Skaf AY, Aihara AY. Differential diagnosis of facet joint disorders. Radiographics. 2021;41(2):543–58. https://doi.org/10.1148/rg.2021200079.
19. Zhou Y, Zhou Z, Liu L, Cao X. Management of irreducible unilateral facet joint dislocations in subaxial cervical spine: two case reports and a review of the literature. J Med Case Rep. 2018;12(1):74. https://doi.org/10.1186/s13256-018-1609-z.
20. O'Shaughnessy J, Grenier J-M, Stern PJ. A delayed diagnosis of bilateral facet dislocation of the cervical spine: a case report. J Can Chiropr Assoc. 2014;58(1):45–51.
21. Suri P, Miyakoshi A, Hunter DJ, et al. Does lumbar spinal degeneration begin with the anterior structures? A study of the observed epidemiology in a community-based population. BMC Musculoskelet Disord. 2011;12:202. https://doi.org/10.1186/1471-2474-12-202.
22. Ruberté LM, Natarajan RN, Andersson GB. Influence of single-level lumbar degenerative disc disease on the behavior of the adjacent segments—a finite element model study. J Biomech. 2009;42(3):341–8. https://doi.org/10.1016/j.jbiomech.2008.11.024.
23. Dunlop RB, Adams MA, Hutton WC. Disc space narrowing and the lumbar facet joints. J Bone Joint Surg Br. 1984;66(5):706–10. https://doi.org/10.1302/0301-620X.66B5.6501365.
24. Adams MA, Hutton WC. The mechanical function of the lumbar apophyseal joints. Spine (Phila Pa 1976). 1983;8(3):327–30. https://doi.org/10.1097/00007632-198304000-00017.
25. Kalichman L, Suri P, Guermazi A, Li L, Hunter DJ. Facet orientation and tropism: associations with facet joint osteoarthritis and degeneration. Spine (Phila Pa 1976). 2009;34(16):E579–85. https://doi.org/10.1097/BRS.0b013e3181aa2acb.
26. Wang J, Yang X. Age-related changes in the orientation of lumbar facet joints. Spine (Phila Pa 1976). 2009;34(17):E596–8. https://doi.org/10.1097/BRS.0b013e3181abbf1e.
27. Daffner SD, Daffner RH. Computed tomography diagnosis of facet dislocations: the "hamburger bun" and "reverse hamburger bun" signs. J Emerg Med. 2002;23(4):387–94. https://doi.org/10.1016/s0736-4679(02)00577-2.
28. Joaquim AF, Patel AA. Subaxial cervical spine trauma: evaluation and surgical decision-making. Glob Spine J. 2014;4(1):63–70. https://doi.org/10.1055/s-0033-1356764.
29. Cotler JM, Herbison GJ, Nasuti JF, Ditunno JFJ, An H, Wolff BE. Closed reduction of traumatic cervical spine dislocation using traction weights up to 140 pounds. Spine (Phila Pa 1976). 1993;18(3):386–90. https://doi.org/10.1097/00007632-199303000-00015.
30. Grant GA, Mirza SK, Chapman JR, et al. Risk of early closed reduction in cervical spine subluxation injuries. J Neurosurg. 1999;90(1 Suppl):13–8. https://doi.org/10.3171/spi.1999.90.1.0013.

31. Lu K, Lee TC, Chen HJ. Closed reduction of bilateral locked facets of the cervical spine under general anaesthesia. Acta Neurochir. 1998;140(10):1055–61. https://doi.org/10.1007/s007010050214.
32. Newton D, England M, Doll H, Gardner BP. The case for early treatment of dislocations of the cervical spine with cord involvement sustained playing rugby. J Bone Joint Surg Br. 2011;93(12):1646–52. https://doi.org/10.1302/0301-620X.93B12.27048.
33. Dvorak M, Vaccaro AR, Hermsmeyer J, Norvell DC. Unilateral facet dislocations: is surgery really the preferred option? Evid Based Spine Care J. 2010;1(1):57–65. https://doi.org/10.1055/s-0028-1100895.
34. Ordonez BJ, Benzel EC, Naderi S, Weller SJ. Cervical facet dislocation: techniques for ventral reduction and stabilization. J Neurosurg. 2000;92(1 Suppl):18–23. https://doi.org/10.3171/spi.2000.92.1.0018.
35. Dvorak MF, Fisher CG, Fehlings MG, et al. The surgical approach to subaxial cervical spine injuries: an evidence-based algorithm based on the SLIC classification system. Spine (Phila Pa 1976). 2007;32(23):2620–9. https://doi.org/10.1097/BRS.0b013e318158ce16.
36. Kim S-M, Lim TJ, Paterno J, Park J, Kim DH. A biomechanical comparison of three surgical approaches in bilateral subaxial cervical facet dislocation. J Neurosurg Spine. 2004;1(1):108–15. https://doi.org/10.3171/spi.2004.1.1.0108.
37. Mubark I, Abouelela A, Hassan M, Genena A, Ashwood N. Sub-axial cervical facet dislocation: a review of current concepts. Cureus. 2021;13(1):e12581. https://doi.org/10.7759/cureus.12581.
38. Wang F, Zhu Y. Treatment of complete fracture-dislocation of thoracolumbar spine. J Spinal Disord Tech. 2013;26(8):421–6. https://doi.org/10.1097/BSD.0b013e31824e1223.

30 Sacroiliitis

Mitch Hungerpiller and Daniel Denis

30.1 Introduction

Sacroiliitis is inflammation of one or both sacroiliac (SI) joints and is a common cause of low back and buttock pain. The SI joint is a combined synovial plane and fibrous joint that joins the sacrum to the ilium of the pelvis and forms the union between the upper and lower body. Sacroiliitis has many etiologies, including but not limited to osteoarthritis, spondyloarthropathies (SpA), pregnancy, and trauma. Diagnosis requires a thorough history, physical examination, laboratory testing, and imaging, if warranted. Several provocative tests can also be used if sacroiliitis is suspected. Data on the prevalence of sacroiliitis vary widely, some studies suggesting it occurs in 10–25% of those with low back pain [1]. Management is primarily medical. The aim of treatment is to address the underlying etiology of the patient's SI joint dysfunction. Surgery can be offered in the setting of chronic pain that is refractory to medical management.

30.2 Anatomy

The SI joint is one of two paired C- or L-shaped joints formed from the auricular surfaces of the sacrum and ilia (Figs. 30.1, 30.2, 30.3, and 30.4). Its cranial portion is shorter than its caudal portion. It is unique because it includes both fibrous and synovial components. The superior portion of the cranial segment is fibrous, and the inferior portions of the cranial and caudal segments are plane synovial (Fig. 30.4). The joint correlates with the first three sacral vertebrae (S1-S3), with the S1 segment accounting for the most significant proportion of the joint surface (Fig. 30.1). In the sagittal plane with a patient standing, the S1 segment lies mostly vertically, and the remaining surface is oriented anterosuperior to posteroinferior. When viewed from the coronal plane, the

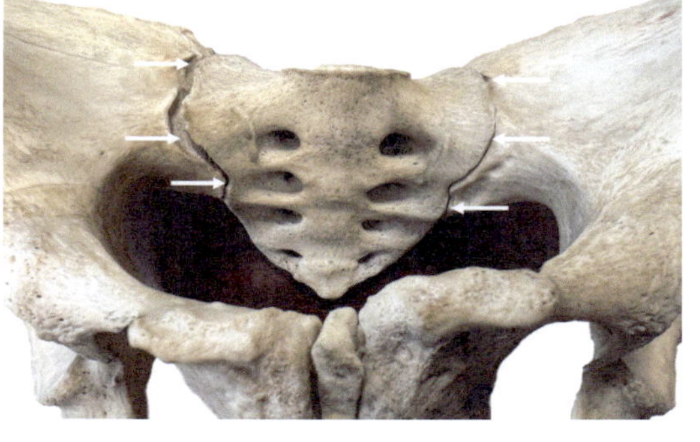

Fig. 30.1 Anterior view of the human pelvis illustrating the sacroiliac (SI) joints (arrows)

M. Hungerpiller (✉)
Department of Surgery, Ochsner Lafayette General Medical Center, Lafayette, LA, USA
e-mail: ralph.hungerpiller@ochsner.org

D. Denis
Ochsner Health, Kenner, LA, USA

M. Turgut et al. (eds.), *Ligaments of the Vertebral Column*,
https://doi.org/10.1007/978-3-032-09070-6_30

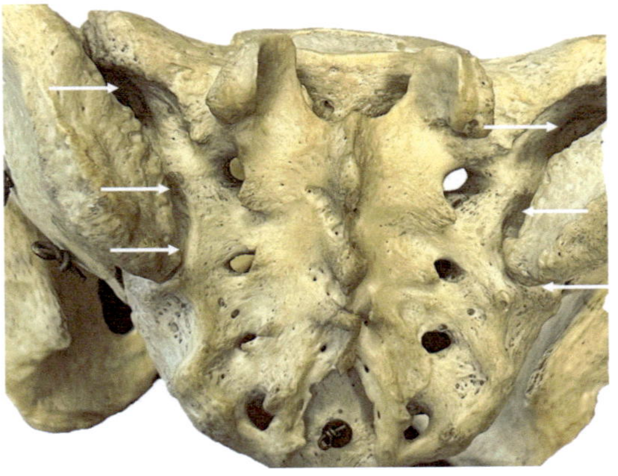

Fig. 30.2 Posterior view of the human pelvis illustrating the SI joints (arrows)

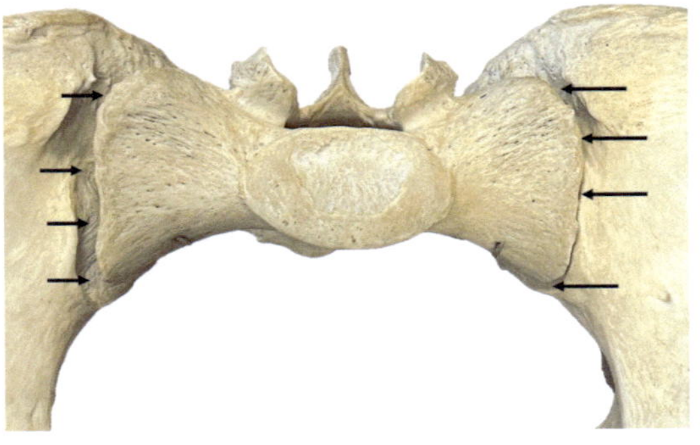

Fig. 30.3 Superior view of the human pelvis illustrating the SI joints (arrows)

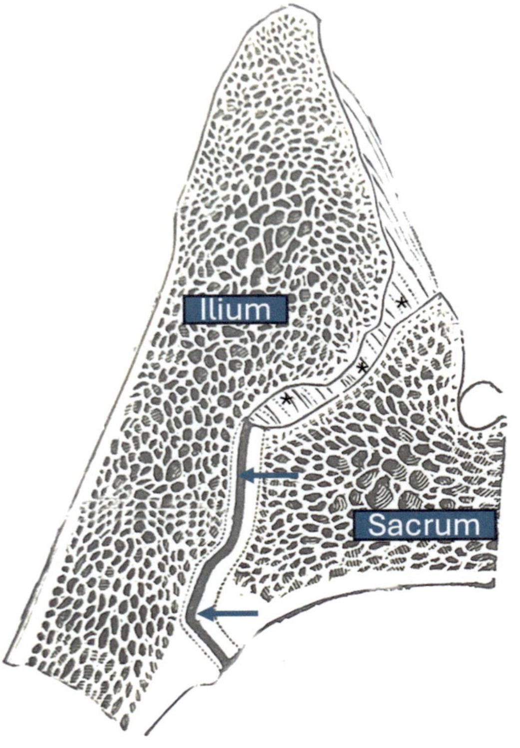

Fig. 30.4 Schematic drawing of a cross section through the SI joint, noting the fibrous (*) and synovial parts (arrows). (After Testut)

joint's inferior portion follows the inferiorly directed taper of the triangular sacrum. The joint space usually measures 0.5–4 mm with a capsule that adheres closely to the articular margins [2, 3]. The auricular surfaces of the SI joint contain two types of cartilage: hyaline on the sacral portion and fibrocartilage on the iliac portion.

Anterior and posterior divisions of the blood supply and the venous drainage of the SI joint can be distinguished. Anteriorly, the joint is supplied by the iliolumbar artery, which mostly originates from the posterior division of the internal iliac artery. Posteriorly, it receives blood from the median and lateral sacral arteries. Venous drainage is closely related to the arterial supply and ultimately enters the internal iliac vein.

Innervation of the SI joint varies widely among individuals and includes the anterior rami of L4 and L5, the superior gluteal nerve, and the posterior rami of L5-S2. Because of this innervation pattern, sacroiliitis can present with referred pain in the dermatomal distributions of the parent nerves. It is now easy to see why sacroiliitis can be difficult to diagnose initially. A patient presenting with low back or buttock pain could have SI joint dysfunction. There should be a high index of suspicion for sacroiliitis in such patients, and they should always be subjected to provocative maneuvers.

The SI joints require strong ligamentous and muscular support. This entails a minimal range of motion: about 3° in flexion-extension, 1.5° axially, and 0.8° in lateral bending [4]. The primary function of the ligamentous architecture of these joints is to prevent rotational, shearing, and distraction forces. There are five main ligaments in the SI joint complex (Figs. 30.4, 30.5 and 30.6):

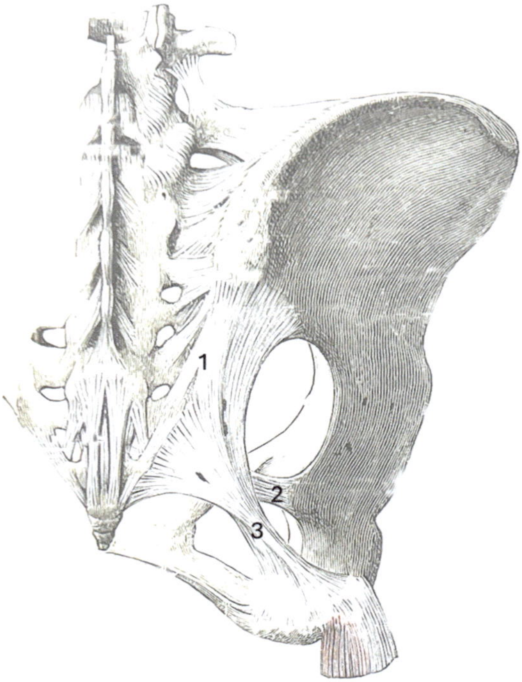

Fig. 30.5 Schematic drawing of the lower spine and pelvis with associated ligaments. Note the posterior SI (1), sacrospinous (2), and sacrotuberous (3) ligaments. (After Testut)

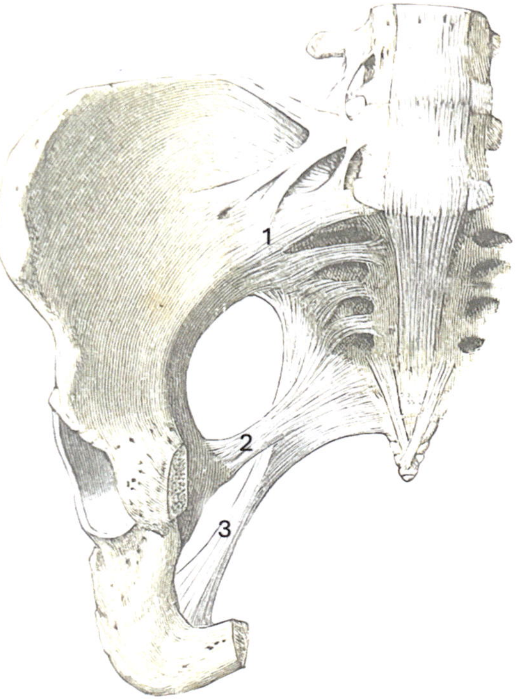

Fig. 30.6 Schematic drawing of the lower spine and pelvis with associated ligaments. Note the anterior SI (1), sacrospinous (2), and sacrotuberous (3) ligaments. (After Testut)

1. Anterior sacroiliac.
2. Posterior sacroiliac.
3. Sacrotuberous.
4. Sacrospinous.
5. Interosseous sacroiliac.

The anterior sacroiliac ligament is the least well-defined of the five and can be described as an anterior-inferior thickening of the SI joint capsule. It is quite thin and prone to injury, which makes it a common source of SI joint pain.

The remaining ligaments are found posteriorly. The posterior sacroiliac ligament connects the posterior superior iliac spine (PSIS) to the sacral tubercles. It comprises long (extrinsic) and short (intrinsic) segments. Its primary function is to limit sacral extension. The PSIS and sacrum are connected to the ischial tuberosity via the sacrotuberous ligament, which limits sacral flexion; it is the inferior boundary of the lesser sciatic foramen (Fig. 30.5). The sacrospinous ligament connects the apex of the sacrum to the ischial spine. It also limits sacral flexion (Figs. 30.5 and 30.6). This ligament is of great clinical importance as it divides the greater and lesser sciatic foramina. The interosseous sacroiliac ligament is extremely strong and prevents shearing forces across the SI joint (Fig. 30.4).

Several muscles stabilize the SI joint but do not act directly on it. They include the erector spinae, multifidus, gluteus maximus, piriformis, biceps femoris, transversus abdominis, iliacus, and pelvic floor muscles (levator ani and coccygeus).

30.3 Pathophysiology

As previously discussed, sacroiliitis has many etiologies. Most forms of the condition involve SI joint erosion and sclerosis. The SI joint is a relatively small, confined space with a limited range of motion. It supports the upper body and is acted on by three levers: the spine, the right lower limb, and the left lower limb. These levers exert tremendous multidirectional forces on the joint daily. An autoimmune inflammatory condition, abnormal joint architecture, or increased stress due to the patient's body habitus or pelvic anatomy can easily irritate the SI joint and cause it to begin degenerating.

30.4 Osteoarthritis

Osteoarthritis (OA) of the SI joint develops much the same way as in any other joint in the human body. Risk factors include older age, female sex, obesity, previous trauma, and abnormal joint surface anatomy. OA begins with erosion and degradation of cartilage. This initial cartilaginous injury worsens joint mechanics and leads to further degradation of the articular surface. Eventually, this degradation extends down to the bone. Microscopically, the type II collagen forming the articular cartilage is damaged, and chondrocytes begin proliferating to rectify this destruction. While new cartilage can be formed, the constant stress on the joint induces a phenotypic change in chondrocytes that causes new bone to form. This leads to the classic osteophyte formation seen on imaging in a patient with advanced OA.

Sustained joint stress also causes chondrocytes to undergo apoptosis and impairs mineralization. Subchondral sclerosis and rare bone cysts can also occur [6]. Recent studies suggest that inflammatory mediators such as IL-1β, TNF-α, and IL-6 are also involved in the progression of OA [5].

30.5 Seronegative Spondyloarthropathies (SpA)

Sacroiliitis can occur in the setting of seronegative spondyloarthropathies (also called spondyloarthritis), where, along with spine involvement, it is referred to as axial spondyloarthritis (axSpA). The many relevant associations will be discussed later in this chapter. The pathophysiology of sacroiliitis secondary to spondyloarthritis is not fully understood, and several hypotheses have been proposed. Genetically, patients with major histocompatibility complex (MHC) class I antigen HLA-B27 are at a higher risk than the rest of the population for developing spondyloarthritis. MHC class I antigens are found on all nucleated cells and platelets in humans. They interact with CD8+ T cells (cytotoxic T cells).

A leading hypothesis concerning HLA-B27 pathogenicity is the "arthritogenic peptide" hypothesis. This proposes that HLA-B27 presents several antigenic peptides, leading to cross-reactivity with cytotoxic T cells and a subsequent inflammatory response. This inflammatory response affects selected joints and tissues. Another hypothesis is the "unfolded protein response." According to this, HLA-B27 inherently folds slowly and frequently misfolds. Misfolded proteins accumulate in the endoplasmic reticulum (ER), leading to an unfolded protein response (UPR). The UPR activates pro-inflammatory cytokines, including but not limited to IL-17, IL-23, and IFN-γ. A third hypothesis proposes that HLA-B27 forms homodimers at the cell surface, acting as ligands for an autoimmune response and activating natural killer (NK) and T cells, which leads to the upregulation of IL-17, a pro-inflammatory cytokine. Evidence suggests that ER aminopeptidase 1 (ERAP1), which is responsible for optimizing the sizes of peptides for antigen presentation, plays a significant role in the pathogenesis of spondyloarthritis. Loss of function of ERAP1 can lead to intracellular accumulation of heavy chains and a subsequent pathological response [7].

30.6 Pregnancy

Pregnancy causes sacroiliitis in two main ways: increased stress on the SI joint and the release of relaxin. During pregnancy, the center of gravity shifts forward, causing more stress on the SI joints, hips, and spine. The sacrum is flexed (nutated), leading to ligamentous stretching and inflammation. During the postpartum period, ligaments surrounding the SI joints remain inflamed, which causes the familiar low back and buttock pain. Relaxin is a member of the insulin-like superfamily of protein hormones. It is normally produced by the corpus luteum and breast as well as the placenta, chorion, and decidua during pregnancy. It acts on many tissues throughout the body; its role in pregnancy is to soften the pubic symphysis and ripen the cervix in preparation for labor. In sacroiliitis during pregnancy, the effects of relaxin on the bone and ligaments require discussion. The hormone acts on osteoclasts, increasing bone resorption by enabling osteoclast progenitor cells to differentiate and mature. Resorption softens and weakens the architecture of bones, making them more susceptible to stress-related injuries. The SI joint, which is subject to considerable daily stress because of its anatomical location and function, is vulnerable to changes in the bony framework. The effect of relaxin on ligamentous stretching is attributable to its well-established collagenolytic effect. The hormone increases the expression of matrix metalloproteinases, collagenase, and plasminogen activator. As mentioned, the SI joint is supported and strengthened by a highly robust and voluminous ligamentous framework. Relaxin acts on this framework during pregnancy, effectively "loosening" and widening the joint. Combined with the stress added by the newfound center of gravity, this makes the joint more vulnerable to inflammation and degeneration [8].

30.7 Lumobosacral Fusion

Lumbar fusion ending to the sacrum increases the SI joint range of motion, a form of adjacent segment degeneration [15]. Sacroiliac joint pain incidence increases with the number of levels fused to the sacrum [16]. Stabilizing the sacroiliac joints during long-segment fusion has been shown to reduce sacroiliac joint range of motion [18], which may lead to a decrease in SI joint pain after surgery [17, 19].

30.8 Diagnosis

Sacroiliitis should always be included in the list of differential diagnoses for patients complaining of low back pain. The clinical diagnosis is called SI joint dysfunction and is presumed to be related to abnormal or increased SI joint range of motion. The incidence of SI joint dysfunction in patients presenting with low back pain is thought to vary between 15% and 30% [21] and is more frequent in female patients [22]. Suspicion should be high if the pain worsens after sitting for long periods or with rotational movements. The pain can often radiate down the lower limbs. As with any complaint, an accurate diagnosis of sacroiliitis starts with a focused history and physical examination. Attention should be given to the timing, onset, and characteristics of the pain. A thorough family history should also include possible inflammatory or autoimmune conditions. Additionally, an exhaustive review of systems should be conducted to rule out systemic illness. "Red flag" signs and symptoms include but are not limited to fever, night sweats, unintended weight loss, changes in bowel habits, and urinary incontinence.

A methodical physical exam is of utmost importance when sacroiliitis is suspected. It should start with a careful visual examination of the patient in sitting and standing positions. Note any pelvic or lower limb asymmetry. Any assumed leg-length discrepancy should be followed up with lower limb measurements. Gait should also be assessed carefully. An antalgic gait is most likely. Neurological evaluation, strength testing, and active and passive ranges of motion should be performed on the lower extremities. Special provocative testing is beneficial if the clinician has a high index of suspicion for sacroiliitis. Sacroiliitis or SI joint dysfunction is most likely if the patient's pain is reproduced by at least three of the following provocative maneuvers [20, 21]:

- FABER (Patrick's) test: pain is reproduced from passively abducting and externally rotating the patient's hip on the affected side.
- "Fortin finger sign": deep palpation over the SI joint(s) reproduces the pain.
- Gaenslen test: The hip on the unaffected side is flexed while the patient is seated. The hip on the affected side is maximally extended off the examination table. Downward pressure is then applied to the extended lower limb. A positive test is the reproduction of pain.
- Iliac compression test: pain is reproduced after downward pressure is applied to the superior aspect of the iliac crest.
- Sacral distraction (gapping) test: the patient lies supine as the examiner applies posteriorly-directed forces bilaterally to the anterior superior iliac spine (ASIS). Reproduction of pain is a positive test.
- Sacral thrust test: pain is reproduced when an anteriorly-directed force is applied through the sacrum of the prone patient.
- Thigh thrust (posterior pelvic pain provocation) test: the patient lies supine with their thigh flexed to 90°. Posterior force is applied along the length of the femur with one hand while the other supports the sacrum.

If the history and physical exam, complete with provocation testing, strongly point to sacroiliitis, the diagnosis is usually confirmed with selective SI joint blocks under fluoroscopic guidance [23]. There is good evidence that SI joint dysfunction can be diagnosed with dual SI joint blocks, resulting in pain relief above 70% for the duration of the block [24].

In the absence of trauma or suspected inflammatory disorders, imaging and lab testing are not required. Sacroiliitis is a clinical diagnosis. Lab testing will be needed to support and confirm the diagnosis if the clinician suspects an inflammatory disorder. Imaging is also warranted; the various modalities will be discussed later. Several lab tests should be ordered in the setting of a presumed inflammatory disorder such as SpA. These include WBC count, erythrocyte sedimentation rate (ESR), C-reactive protein (CRP), HLA-B27, and rheumatoid factor (RF). WBC count is usually not elevated unless a pyogenic cause of sacroiliitis is suspected. ESR and CRP are markers of inflammation and are elevated if sacroiliitis is secondary to an inflammatory condition. HLA-B27 is present in 50–92% of patients with ankylosing spondylitis. RF will be negative in ax-SpA ("seronegative").

The Assessment of Spondyloarthritis International Society (ASAS) criteria for the classification of axSpA in patients less than 45 years of age is the gold standard for diagnosing sacroiliitis objectively. To use this assessment tool properly, patients must have had back pain for at least 3 months. They are then diagnosed using either an "imaging arm" or a "clinical arm." If the imaging arm is chosen, magnetic resonance imaging (MRI) with active inflammation or definite radiographic sacroiliitis must be present, along with at least one SpA feature. If the clinical arm is chosen, the patient must be positive for HLA-B27 along with at least two SpA features, which can include:

- Arthritis.
- Crohn's/colitis.
- Dactylitis.
- Elevated CRP.
- Enthesitis (heel).
- Family history for SpA.
- Good response to NSAIDs.
- HLA-B27.
- Inflammatory back pain.
- Psoriasis.
- Uveitis.

30.9 Imaging

Sacroiliitis secondary to trauma or a suspected inflammatory condition warrants further imaging workup. Four primary imaging modalities are used to diagnose sacroiliitis: plain radiography (Fig. 30.7), computed tomography (CT), magnetic resonance imaging (MRI), and nuclear medicine bone scanning.

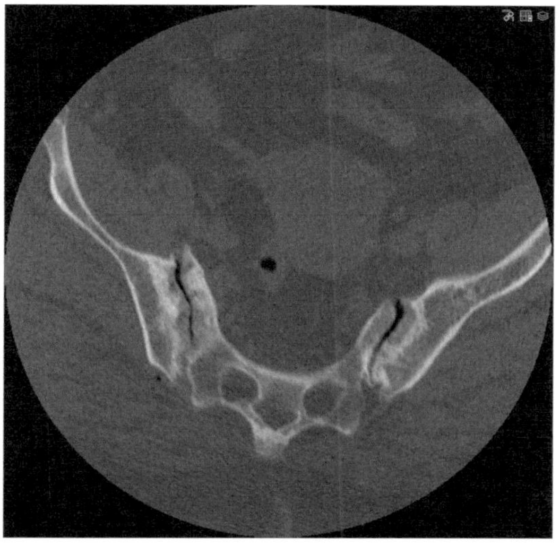

Fig. 30.7 Radiography example of a patient with sacroiliitis. Note the SI joints as the bilateral hypodense curvilinear structures

30.10 Plain Radiography

First-line imaging is anteroposterior plain radiography of the pelvis and lumbar spine. For bilateral disease, the patient should be supine with the central ray placed in the midline 5 cm below the ASIS and angled cephalad 30° in males and 35° in females [9]. For unilateral SI joint dysfunction, an AP oblique view should be obtained. The affected side should be raised approximately 25–30°. The central ray should be centered 2.5 cm medial and 4 cm distal to the ASIS with a cephalad angle of 20–25° [10]. Radiographic findings in sacroiliitis include sclerosis of endplates, widening or narrowing of the joint space, erosions, and ankylosis. Furthermore, sacroiliitis can be graded using the New York criteria:

- Grade 0: normal.
- Grade I: suspicious changes.
- Grade II: minimum abnormality (small areas of erosion or sclerosis; no change in joint width).
- Grade III: unequivocal abnormality (moderate or advanced disease with erosions, sclerosis, widening or narrowing of the joint space, or partial ankylosis).
- Grade IV: severe abnormality (complete ankylosis).

Sacroiliitis should be diagnosed if the score is at least grade II bilaterally or at least grade III unilaterally.

30.11 Computed Tomography

Computed tomography (CT) provides a much more detailed view of the SI joints and can reveal pathology more clearly than plain radiographs. When the examiner suspects SI joint dysfunction and the plain radiograph is negative, a pelvic CT scan should be ordered. CT scan findings in sacroiliitis are similar to those on plain radiographs.

30.12 Magnetic Resonance Imaging (MRI)

Magnetic resonance imaging is considered the gold standard for diagnosing sacroiliitis. Not only can it detect early inflammatory changes in the SI joint, but it can also visualize the surrounding soft tissues. Enthesitis, characterized by inflammation of the insertion points of ligaments and tendons on bones, is a common feature of axSpA and is pathognomonic for the condition. It can only be seen on MRI. Active inflammation in and around the SI joint appears as increased signal intensity on axial T2-weighted MRI. This increased signal intensity results from tissue swelling (edema), indicating an active disease process. As with plain radiography and CT scans, MRI can reveal necessary information about joint space width and bone defects. Widening of the SI joint space suggests an effusion, which indicates acute disease; the joint space is narrowed in chronic disease. T1-weighted MRI is more helpful in visualizing bone defects such as erosions and sclerosis.

The Spondyloarthritis Research Consortium of Canada (SPARCC) Magnetic Resonance Index is a useful scoring system when axSpA is suspected. This index relies on Short Tau Inversion Recovery (STIR) sequence MRI imaging to grade the severity of inflammation in spondyloarthritis of the SI joints. STIR is a fat suppression technique. SPARCC uses six coronal images of the SI joint with a maximum score of 72. Three criteria are included: (1) "bone marrow edema," (2) "intense edema," and (3) "deep edema."

- Bone marrow edema: each SI joint is divided into upper iliac, lower iliac, upper sacrum, and lower sacrum. Any increased signal in each quadrant is recorded. The maximum score is eight if bilateral disease is present, giving a maximum score of 48 (six coronal slices x maximum eight points for each slice = 48).
- Intense edema: if a bone lesion is classed as "intense" in any SI joint quadrant, a score of one is given for unilateral disease and two for bilateral disease. Therefore, a maximum score of 12 is possible (two points for each slice x six coronal slices = 12).
- Deep edema: a lesion is considered "deep" if it extends at least 1 cm from the articular surface. Two points maximum per slice if bilateral disease is present. A maximum score of 12 is possible (two points per slice x six coronal slices = 12).

Mild sacroiliitis is indicated by a score of less than 24 overall. Moderate sacroiliitis has a score of 24–48. A score of 49–72 indicates severe sacroiliitis [11].

30.13 Nuclear Medicine Bone Scanning

Nuclear medicine scans help identify areas of active inflammation in the SI joints and the rest of the body. They should be ordered when the physician suspects a systemic inflammatory condition such as SpA. These scans provide a comprehensive view of the skeletal system, helping to locate focal areas of inflammation. In inflammatory sacroiliitis, bones can be scanned before or after SpA is diagnosed. The most common nuclear medicine technique for diagnosing sacroiliitis is the Technetium-99 m bone scan. Technetium-99 m-labeled methylene diphosphate is given to the patient undergoing single-photon emission computed tomography (SPECT) imaging. Areas of high bone turnover ("hot spots") detected by the scanner can indicate inflammation. The pros of this technique are its relative straightforwardness, comprehensive (whole-body) image, and ability to detect active inflammation. The cons are its cost and radiation exposure.

30.14 Associations

Sacroiliitis is associated with several rheumatological conditions, which can be classified into a family of disorders called seronegative spondyloarthropathies (SpA). They include ankylosing spondylitis (AS), psoriatic arthritis (PsA), inflammatory bowel disease (IBD)-associated arthritis, reactive arthritis (formerly Reiter syndrome; ReA), and undifferentiated SpA. Patients with SpA present with inflammatory joint pain along with the SpA features described in the "Diagnosis" section. These conditions can be differentiated into non-radiographic axial SpA (nr-axSpA), peripheral SpA, and juvenile-onset SpA. There is a correlation between HLA-B27 and SpA, strongest in ASa and weakest in IBD-associated arthritis. Worldwide, the prevalence of SpA ranges from 0.5% to 1.9% [12]. AS and nr-axSpA are its most common forms in the United States [13]. Overall, ReA is rare. It follows enteric or urogenital infections with Chlamydia, Campylobacter, Salmonella, Shigella, and Clostridium difficile. ReA patients classically present with the triad of urethritis, arthritis, and conjunctivitis or uveitis. Enthesitis is pathognomonic of SpA.

It is essential to recognize that several conditions can mimic sacroiliitis; however, a thorough workup will reveal that they are, in fact, distinct entities. A keen clinician can easily avoid falsely associating these conditions with true sacroiliitis. Diffuse idiopathic skeletal hyperostosis (DISH) is characterized by abnormal calcification of the ligaments and soft tissue around the spine. It most commonly involves the anterior longitudinal ligament. Rarely is the superior ligamentous complex of the SI joint affected, mimicking sacroiliitis. Osteitis condensans ilii is a non-inflammatory condition caused by abnormal bone deposition and sclerosis of the ilium adjacent to the SI joint. Radiographic imaging reveals bilateral, symmetrical, sharply demarcated areas of subchondral sclerosis without erosion. This condition usually presents in childbearing women with low back pain. Finally, hyperparathyroidism leading to osteitis fibrosa cystica can cause low back and buttock pain and can be mistaken for sacroiliitis. Typically, patients complain of other symptoms associated with hyperparathyroidism. These include, but are not limited to, abdominal pain, nephrolithiasis, polyuria, and psychiatric disturbances.

30.15 Treatment

Treatment of sacroiliitis depends entirely on its etiology. Treatment modalities range from very conservative to surgery. First, the clinician must recognize sacroiliitis secondary to conditions that require immediate and emergent intervention. Septic sacroiliitis is a bacterial infection of the SI joint(s) that requires prompt recognition and treatment with IV antibiotics. Joint aspiration with culture is necessary to narrow the antibiotic coverage. In rare cases, open SI joint debridement is required, but this is associated with high morbidity.

The first-line therapy for both osteoarthritic sacroiliitis and inflammatory sacroiliitis is exercise, physical therapy, and nonsteroidal anti-inflammatory drugs (NSAIDs). Muscle relaxants can be used to treat acute exacerbations. NSAIDs must be prescribed in high-dose formulations for treating inflammatory sacroiliitis. Biologics are the next step in treating ax-SpA when a patient fails at least two NSAID trials. TNF-α inhibitors such as infliximab, etanercept, adalimumab, golimumab, and certolizumab are the first-line biologics used to treat SpA. Contraindications to treatment with biologics are active or latent tuberculosis, advanced heart failure, lupus, multiple sclerosis (MS), and cancer. Systemic glucocorticoids should be reserved for patients with sacroiliitis secondary to IBD-associated arthritis. ReA usually has a short course, so treatment with NSAIDs is most likely to suffice. Disease-modifying anti-rheumatic drugs (DMARDs) have no role in treating ax-SpA.

Conservative management of SI joint pain also includes therapeutic image-guided SI joint injections. Usually, a mixture of anesthetic and corticosteroid is injected. Ultrasound (US), CT, or fluoroscopy can be used for guidance. In patients with narrow joint spaces, fluoroscopic-guided injection can be challenging, but it is easier than US, which should be reserved for thin patients. CT is the imaging modality of choice for patients with severely narrowed joint spaces. SI joint injection has shown short- and long-term clinical efficacy (Fig. 30.8) [14]. Corticosteroids should not be injected into patients with inflammatory sacroiliitis, as it can lead to worsening of enthesitis and possible ligamentous tearing.

The last resort treatment of sacroiliitis is surgery in the form of minimally invasive SI joint fusion (Fig. 30.9) [25]. This is reserved for patients with severe, chronic disease who have

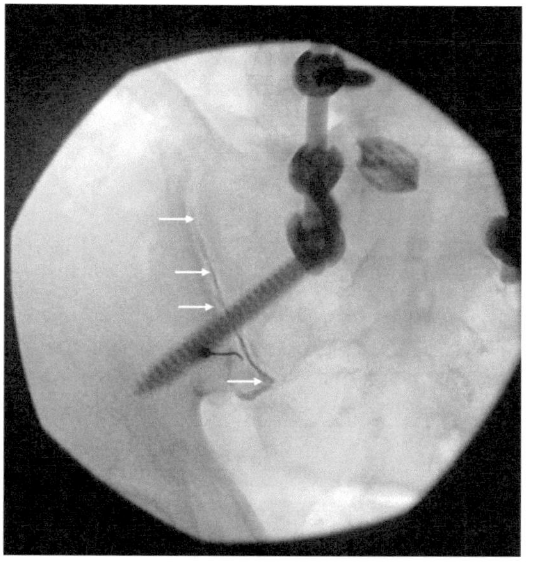

Fig. 30.8 Fluoroscopy of a patient undergoing diagnostic injection of the right SI joint (arrows) for suspected sacroiliitis. Note the injection needle between the lower two arrows and the previous surgical hardware placement

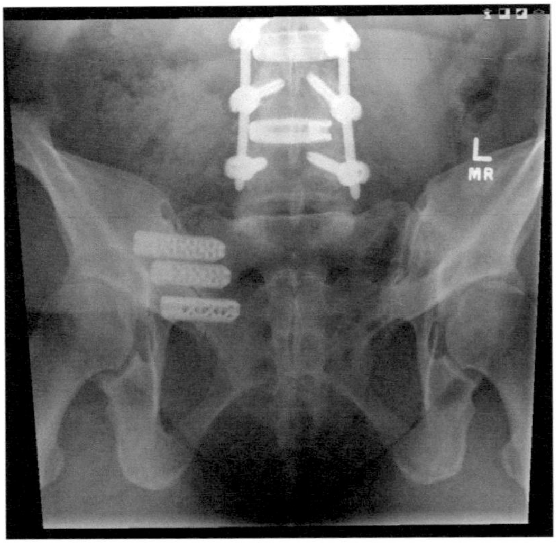

Fig. 30.9 Anteroposterior radiograph of a patient with fusion of the right SI joint. Note the previous lumbar spine fusion procedure hardware

failed medical management and obtained no sustained relief from SI joint therapeutic injections. The procedure is performed under general anesthesia, utilizing fluoroscopy or CT guidance. A small, 2–3 cm incision is made in the lateral aspect of the buttock. Implants (made from titanium or a hollow modular anchorage screw filled with bone matrix) are then screwed into place. Three implants are usually placed (two in S1 and one in S2) to fuse the SI joint.

References

1. Buchanan BK, Varacallo M. Sacroiliitis. [Updated 2023 Aug 8]. In: StatPearls [Internet]. Treasure Island (FL): StatPearls; 2024. Available from: https://www.ncbi.nlm.nih.gov/books/NBK448141/
2. Vleeming A, Schuenke MD, Masi AT, Carreiro JE, Danneels L, Willard FH. The sacroiliac joint: an overview of its anatomy, function and potential clinical implications. J Anat. 2012;221(6):537–67. https://doi.org/10.1111/j.1469-7580.2012.01564.x.
3. Stallmeyer M, Zoarski GH. Sacroiliac joint injection. In: Johnson BA, Staats PS, Wetzel FT, Mathis JM, editors. Image-guided spine interventions. New York: Springer; 2004. https://doi.org/10.1007/0-387-21794-0_13.
4. Kiapour A, Joukar A, Elgafy H, Erbulut DU, Agarwal AK, Goel VK. Biomechanics of the sacroiliac joint: anatomy, function, biomechanics, sexual dimorphism, and causes of pain. Int J Spine Surg. 2020;14(Suppl 1):3–13. Published 2020 Feb 10. 10.14444/6077
5. Scanzello CR. Chemokines and inflammation in osteoarthritis: insights from patients and animal models. J Orthop Res. 2017;35(4):735–9. https://doi.org/10.1002/jor.23471.
6. Sen R, Hurley JA. Osteoarthritis. [Updated 2023 Feb 20]. In: StatPearls [Internet]. Treasure Island (FL): StatPearls; 2024. Available from: https://www.ncbi.nlm.nih.gov/books/NBK482326/
7. Sharip A, Kunz J. Understanding the pathogenesis of spondyloarthritis. Biomolecules. 2020;10(10):1461. Published 2020 Oct 20. https://doi.org/10.3390/biom10101461.
8. Dehghan F, Haerian BS, Muniandy S, Yusof A, Dragoo JL, Salleh N. The effect of relaxin on the musculoskeletal system. Scand J Med Sci Sports. 2014;24(4):e220–9. https://doi.org/10.1111/sms.12149.
9. Steward A, Murphy A, Fahrenhorst-Jones T, et al. Sacroiliac joint (AP sacrum view). Reference article, Radiopaedia.org. Accessed 4 Oct 2024. https://doi.org/10.53347/rID-49976.
10. Steward A, Tan W, Murphy A, et al. Sacroiliac joint (AP oblique view). Reference article, Radiopaedia.org. Accessed 4 Oct 2024. https://doi.org/10.53347/rID-49974.
11. Maksymowych WP, Inman RD, Salonen D, et al. Spondyloarthritis Research Consortium of Canada magnetic resonance imaging index for assessment of sacroiliac joint inflammation in ankylosing spondylitis. Arthritis Rheum. 2005;53(5):703–9. https://doi.org/10.1002/art.21445.
12. Bakland G, Nossent HC. Epidemiology of spondyloarthritis: a review. Curr Rheumatol Rep. 2013;15(9):351. https://doi.org/10.1007/s11926-013-0351-1.
13. Strand V, Rao SA, Shillington AC, Cifaldi MA, McGuire M, Ruderman EM. Prevalence of axial spondyloarthritis in United States rheumatology practices: assessment of SpondyloArthritis International Society criteria versus rheumatology expert clinical diagnosis. Arthritis Care Res (Hoboken). 2013;65(8):1299–306. https://doi.org/10.1002/acr.21994.
14. Braun J, Bollow M, Seyrekbasan F, Häberle HJ, Eggens U, Mertz A, Distler A, Sieper J. Computed tomography-guided corticosteroid injection of the sacroiliac joint in patients with spondyloarthropathy with sacroiliitis: clinical outcome and followup by dynamic magnetic resonance imaging. J Rheumatol. 1996;23:659–64.
15. Mushlin H, Brooks DM, Olexa J, Ferrick BJ, Carbine S, Hayward GM, Bucklen BS, Sansur CA. A biomechanical investigation of the sacroiliac joint in the setting of lumbosacral fusion: impact of pelvic fixation versus sacroiliac joint fixation. J Neurosurg Spine. 2019;31(4):562–7. https://doi.org/10.3171/2019.3.SPINE181127. PMID: 31200368
16. Unoki E, Abe E, Murai H, Kobayashi T, Abe T. Fusion of multiple segments can increase the incidence of sacroiliac joint pain after lumbar or lumbosacral

fusion. Spine (Phila Pa 1976). 2016;41(12):999–1005. https://doi.org/10.1097/BRS.0000000000001409. PMID: 26689576
17. Unoki E, Miyakoshi N, Abe E, Kobayashi T, Abe T, Kudo D, Shimada Y. Sacropelvic fixation with S2 alar iliac screws may prevent sacroiliac joint pain after multisegment spinal fusion. Spine (Phila Pa 1976). 2019;44(17):E1024–30. https://doi.org/10.1097/BRS.0000000000003041. PMID: 31415028
18. de Andrada Pereira B, Lehrman JN, Sawa AGU, Lindsey DP, Yerby SA, Godzik J, Waguespack AM, Uribe JS, Kelly BP. Biomechanical effects of a novel posteriorly placed sacroiliac joint fusion device integrated with traditional lumbopelvic long-construct instrumentation. J Neurosurg Spine. 2021;35(3):320–9. https://doi.org/10.3171/2020.11.SPINE201540. PMID: 34144523
19. Polly D, Mundis G, Eastlack R, Leveque JC, Elder BD, Martin C, Kent R, Snowden R, Kim HJ, Sembrano J, Herzog J, Lieberman I, Matheus V, Buchholz A, Franke J, Lee R, Shaffrey C, SILVIA Investigator Group. Randomized trial of augmented pelvic fixation in patients undergoing thoracolumbar fusion for adult spine deformity: initial results from a multicenter randomized trial. World Neurosurg. 2024;187:e15–27. https://doi.org/10.1016/j.wneu.2024.01.156. Epub 2024 Feb 3. PMID: 38310950
20. Telli H, Telli S, Topal M. The validity and reliability of provocation tests in the diagnosis of sacroiliac joint dysfunction. Pain Physician. 2018;21(4):E367–76. PMID: 30045603
21. Szadek KM, van der Wurff P, van Tulder MW, Zuurmond WW, Perez RS. Diagnostic validity of criteria for sacroiliac joint pain: a systematic review. J Pain. 2009;10(4):354–68. https://doi.org/10.1016/j.jpain.2008.09.014. Epub 2008 Dec 19. PMID: 19101212
22. Madani SP, Dadian M, Firouznia K, Alalawi S. Sacroiliac joint dysfunction in patients with herniated lumbar disc: a cross-sectional study. J Back Musculoskelet Rehabil. 2013;26(3):273–8. https://doi.org/10.3233/BMR-130376. PMID: 23893142
23. Maigne JY, Aivaliklis A, Pfefer F. Results of sacroiliac joint double block and value of sacroiliac pain provocation tests in 54 patients with low back pain. Spine (Phila Pa 1976). 1996;21(16):1889–92. https://doi.org/10.1097/00007632-199608150-00012. PMID: 8875721
24. Simopoulos TT, Manchikanti L, Singh V, Gupta S, Hameed H, Diwan S, Cohen SP. A systematic evaluation of prevalence and diagnostic accuracy of sacroiliac joint interventions. Pain Physician. 2012;15(3):E305–44. PMID: 22622915
25. Polly DW, Cher DJ, Wine KD, Whang PG, Frank CJ, Harvey CF, Lockstadt H, Glaser JA, Limoni RP, Sembrano JN, INSITE Study Group. Randomized controlled trial of minimally invasive sacroiliac joint fusion using triangular titanium implants vs nonsurgical management for sacroiliac joint dysfunction: 12-month outcomes. Neurosurgery. 2015;77(5):674–90.; discussion 690-1. PMID: 26291338; PMCID: PMC4605280. https://doi.org/10.1227/NEU.0000000000000988.

Part IX

Other

31 Medicolegal Problems Regarding Spinal Ligaments

Mehmet Turgut

31.1 Introduction

The spinal cord ligaments are strong fibrous strips of tissue composed of collagen fibers that attach to bones. The spine is a very complex and important anatomical structure, and the ligaments connecting the head to all parts of it stabilize it. Various lesions of the spinal ligaments from the craniocervical junction (CCJ) to the lumbosacral region, such as traumatic lesions, calcifications, ossifications, thickenings, degenerative cysts, and infections or neoplastic lesions of neighboring tissues, are pretty common clinical conditions. They can potentially lead to various forensic legal problems [25]. They can be diagnosed by neuroimaging studies such as X-rays, computed tomography (CT), or magnetic resonance imaging (MRI) using special imaging protocols. Radiologically, CT is useful for diagnosing calcification/ossification and cysts of some ligaments that can cause various neurological deficits in the human spine. At the same time, MRI provides excellent imaging of spinal ligaments in traumatic lesions, thickenings, degenerative cysts, infections, and neoplastic lesions of neighboring tissues. When a conservative approach is not indicated, early and appropriate surgical intervention can be necessary in cases of spinal cord instability and/or neurological deficit due to pressure on the spinal cord and/or nerve roots and in spinal canal stenosis. Such cases should be evaluated cautiously by a team of clinicians comprising neurosurgeons, orthopedic spinal surgeons, physical therapists, rehabilitation physiotherapists, and neuroradiologists.

A literature review revealed that case reports and case series provide various results concerning the appropriate treatment of patients with different lesions involving spinal ligaments. We shall focus here on these interesting but complex issues, which can entail allegations of malpractice owing to delayed or inadequate imaging and/or consequent improper clinical management. Traumatic, neoplastic, or infectious lesions of the spine that do not involve spinal ligaments will be excluded from this section.

Basic legal concepts such as medical negligence, medical practice error, patient interviews, informed consent, parents' right to information, and common medical conditions related to spinal ligaments as potential sources of forensic problems are discussed in detail below. From a medical law perspective, every healthcare provider needs to recognize and appreciate that any negligent action or lack of care in such a clinical situation can lead to an allegation of malpractice in

M. Turgut (✉)
Department of Neurosurgery, Aydın Adnan Menderes University Faculty of Medicine, Aydın, Aydın, Türkiye

Department of Histology and Embryology, Aydın Adnan Menderes University Health Sciences Institute, Efeler, Aydın, Türkiye
e-mail: drmturgut@yahoo.com

M. Turgut et al. (eds.), *Ligaments of the Vertebral Column*,
https://doi.org/10.1007/978-3-032-09070-6_31

the handling of patients with various lesions involving the spinal ligaments from the CCJ to the lumbosacral region, as described in detail below.

31.2 Common Medical Conditions Involving the Spinal Ligaments as Potential Sources of Medicolegal Problems

There is an ongoing debate about various aspects of treating different pathologies involving spinal ligaments, from the CCJ to the lumbosacral region. This chapter will only briefly explain the common medical conditions that are sources of potential forensic legal problems, such as traumatic lesions, calcifications, ossifications, thickenings, degenerative cysts, infections, and neoplastic lesions of neighboring tissues. Each of these entities will be covered in detail in the respective chapters. Those most relevant to the present chapter are given in detail in, e.g., Chapters 6, 7 and 8.

31.2.1 Lesions of the Spinal Ligaments from Craniocervical Junction to Lumbosacral Region

31.2.1.1 Diagnosis of "Spinal Instability" Caused by the Involvement of Osseous and Ligamentous Structures

The spine is stabilized by important anatomical structures such as firm spinal ligaments and complex spinal bones that extend from the CCJ to the lumbosacral region. In clinical practice, "spinal instability" develops when the bone and ligamentous structures lose their ability to maintain normal alignment in a physiological load. It can result from various lesions involving the spinal ligaments, such as traumatic lesions, thickenings, calcifications, ossifications, degenerative cysts, infections, and neoplastic lesions of the neighboring tissues as a cause of neurological deficits [5].

For lesions involving the CCJ, which account for 1/3 of all spinal lesions, the following information should be considered for accurate radiological diagnosis and appropriate treatment of spinal instability. Instability develops when the spinal ligaments lose their ability to maintain normal alignment under a physiological weight. In traumatic lesions involving the CCJ, atlanto-occipital (C1-C0) dissociation (distraction) injuries include dislocations (usually fatal) and subluxations (rarely fatal) [19, 29]. From a radiological point of view, regardless of the imaging method used, lesions in the CCJ area should be investigated using the following criteria for the correct diagnosis of potential instability: (a) Basion-axial interval (BAI), the length between the basion and the posterior axial line drawn on the posterior cortex of the C2 body and extending cranially, with typical values ≤12 mm; an increased BAI distance indicates anterior subluxation of C0-C1 [20–22, 28]; (b) The basion-dens interval (BDI), the length from the postero-inferior end of the basement to the upper direction of the dens of C2, with typical values ≤12 mm; an increased BDI indicates the decomposition (distraction) of C0-C1, dislocation or subluxation [20, 21, 28, 46]; (c) Clivo-axial angle (CXA), the angle between the bony part of the skull base and the posterior part of the dens of C2 with typical values in the range of 139–172°; a decrease in CXA (<135°) indicates compression of the anterior brainstem, medulla oblongata and upper spinal cord with kyphosis [22]; (d) The Grabb-Oakes line (GOL) is a line drawn from the end of the skull base to the lower-rear direction of the body of C2; its typical values are <9 mm; an increased length indicates a high risk of ventral compression of the brainstem and upper spinal cord [22]; (e) For radiological evaluation of the C1-C2 relationship, the "anterior" atlantodental interval (ADI) has typical values <3 mm in men and < 2.5 mm in women (up to 5 mm in children); the "posterior" ADI has typical values >18 mm. Increasing or decreasing distance in the anterior or posterior ADI, respectively, indicates failure of the transverse ligament [23, 28, 46]; (f) Powers' ratio is the ratio of the length from the basion (B) to the posterior arch of C1 (C) to the distance between the anterior aspect of the dens of C2 (A) and the opisthion (O); an increased ratio of anterior C1-C0 decoupling (distraction) and instability of C1/C2 is indicated when the BC/AO value is <1 [42, 46]; and (g) any crossing of McRae's line [the foramen magnum (FM) line joining the basion to the opisthion] by the apex of the dens of C2, crossing of the McGregor's line (line drawn from the posterosuperior margin of the hard palate to the lowest point of the midline of the occipital bone) by the apex of the dens of C2 > 4 mm, or crossing of the Chamberlain's line (line drawn from the posterior tip of the hard palate to the posterior margin of the FM) >6 mm indicates "basilar invagination" [37].

For lesions involving the subaxial cervical, thoracic, and lumbar regions, which account for 2/3 of all spinal lesions, spinal instability is determined according to the concept of "three columns": the anterior, middle, and posterior. This applies to injuries involving parts of the spine other than the CCJ, as described by Denis [11, 57]. Anatomically, the spine comprises (a) the anterior column composed of the anterior vertebral body, the anterior longitudinal ligament (ALL), and the anterior anulus fibrosus; (b) the middle column composed of the posterior vertebral body, the posterior longitudinal ligament (PLL), and the posterior anulus fibrosus; and (c) the posterior column composed of the posterior elements of the spine, the ligamentum flavum (LF), interspinous ligaments (ISLs), supraspinous ligaments (SSLs), and facet joint capsules [11]. A "compression fracture" develops when hyperextension injures the anterior column with or without a middle column injury or when hyperflexion injures the middle and posterior columns [5]. Axial and rotational forces can cause a "burst fracture"; a bilateral interfacet dislocation or tear fracture develops due to the deterioration of all three columns [5]. Biomechanically, an unstable spine requiring surgical stabilization is thought to prevent further injury if the two contiguous columns, including the middle column, are injured. Radiologically, the following findings lead to suspicion of spinal instability: involvement of two adjacent columns, including the middle column, >2 mm translation, expansion of the facet joint and interspinous distance, deterioration of the line of the posterior vertebral body, and > 50% loss of height of vertebral body or > 20° of kyphosis [57].

Surgical intervention for various lesions involving the spinal ligaments, from the CCJ to the lumbosacral region, focuses on cases with neurological problems associated with "spinal instability," such as persistent pain, motor weakness, or sphincter disturbances. Technically, the type of surgery performed depends on its objective and includes conventional or microscopic discectomy, partial or complete laminectomy, corpectomy, foraminotomy, and spinal instrumentation for fusion. Each of these techniques is diverse and can be accomplished by various means. From a medical law perspective, the critical issue for surgical intervention is whether the problem will lead to a much more critical issue, such as a progressive neurological disorder if left untreated [25].

31.2.1.2 Importance of "Dynamic Imaging" for Diagnosis of Lesions of the Spinal Ligaments

Radiologically, the diagnosis of spinal instability in patients with subluxation uses "static" imaging techniques, but "dynamic" imaging of the spine in flexion and extension is necessary for the correct diagnosis of cases involving the CCJ, C3-C7 subaxial segments, the thoracic, and lumbar spine [45]. Specifically, dynamic imaging of the CCJ region with neck rotation is helpful for accurate diagnosis in cases with traumatic lesions of the spinal ligaments [45]. Otherwise, X-rays, CTs, or MRIs of patients with instability in the CCJ can be mistakenly diagnosed as normal, and potential medico-legal consequences can arise when such injuries are not identified and managed quickly.

31.2.1.3 Ideal "Imaging Time" for Radiological Diagnosis of Lesions of the Spinal Ligaments

In general, X-ray and CT using coronal and sagittal reformatted thin-section axial source data are obtained, preferably three-dimensional reformatted images of the CCJ, C3-C7 subaxial segments, thoracic, and lumbar spine [41]. Importantly, CT angiography should also be used to investigate possible vascular injuries, especially in cases with traumatic injuries of the CCJ adjacent to the internal carotid arteries (ICAs) and vertebral artery (VA) [41]. In cases with traumatic lesions of the spinal ligaments, MRI indications are: (a) Patients whose X-rays and CT are negative but have neurological symptoms or constant neck and/or back pain; (b) Patients who cannot be evaluated for "more than 48 hours" owing to a change in their consciousness level; (c) X-rays or radiological findings on CT indicating a ligamentous injury such as facet dislocation, enlargement of the IVD cavity or interspinous cavity, bone fractures adjacent to the spinal ligaments, and prevertebral swelling such as facet dislocation, enlargement of the intervertebral disc (IVD) cavity or interspinous cavity; (d) Patients with a spinal fracture or unstable trauma on X-ray or CT; and (e) MRI before closed facet reduction or open surgery helps diagnose possible IVD herniation or extradural/subdural hematoma [57].

MRI is the best option for imaging spinal ligament injuries from the CCJ to the lumbosacral region, especially in patients with neurological deficits whose CT is normal [5, 57]. However, MRI should be reviewed with conventional imaging tools such as X-rays and CT [57]. More importantly, acute injuries to the spinal ligaments are readily detected by an increased T2/STIR signal due to edema or bleeding. In contrast, the ligaments are commonly T1 and T2 hypointense on MRI, and this decreases after 72 h. Therefore, in the radiological evaluation of the spinal ligaments, the optimum period between the injury and MRI should be "less than 72 hours" [48, 49]. Within 72 h after injury, T2 signal hyperintensitivity caused by edema or blood leakage into traumatized extradural tissues improves the imaging of low signal intensity ligaments in all MRI sequences, providing an excellent contrast agent effect [5]. However, resolution of edema or bleeding beyond this period will lessen the sensitivity of MRI in revealing the effects of the traumatic event [5].

Technically, the selection of appropriate sequence parameters, field of view, slice thickness, and standard signal to equalize the effects on signal-to-noise ratio and spatial resolution consistent with the strength of the field or gradient, coil design, and software potentials of the MRI system is important for diagnosing lesions of the spinal ligaments from the CCJ to the lumbosacral region [5]. A standardized MRI practice for evaluating spinal ligament injury should include T1-weighted, fast spin-echo T2-weighted, GRE, and fast spin-echo inversion-recovery sequences in the sagittal plane [5]. In the axial plane, the protocol should include GRE or T2-weighted MRIs for optimal imaging of the spinal ligaments. In contrast, T1-weighted MRIs provide excellent anatomical detail, show the alignment clearly, and are essential for detecting bone fractures [5]. From the radiological point of view, MRI has high sensitivity for detecting PLL (93%) and interspinous (100%) injuries, but it is less sensitive for ALL (71%) and LF (67%) injuries [17]. ALL injury occurs when the ligaments are separated from the underlying bone by linear T2/STIR hyperintensity of the PLL, fluid, or discontinuity [57]. These ligament injuries are accompanied by fractures of the posterior spinal structures. The spinous fractures are useful indicators of the expansion of the interspinous space at each ledge. However, there is potential for more destruction than the amount of ligament injury to be estimated, leading to unnecessary surgical intervention [57].

31.2.1.4 Role of "Posterior Ligamentous Complex" in the Development of Postoperative Spinal Deformity

Anatomically, there are three main ligaments in the subaxial cervical, thoracic, and lumbar spine: (a) The LF or yellow ligaments are fibrous bands throughout the spine extending from C2 to S1. These are paired structures that cover between the laminae of neighboring vertebrae, 5 mm thick in the anterior to the posterior direction. (b) The ALL, the tissue at the front of the vertebrae, resembles a length of tape placed anteriorly to hold the spinal bodies in place and avoid nonessential movement. (c) The PLL is a long fiber along the posterior aspect of the vertebrae that helps keep the IVDs in anatomical position and ensures the spine's stability [25].

From a surgical point of view, the posterior ligamentous complex (PLC) is involved in retaining spinal activity and preventing spinal deformity, abnormal movement, and neighboring segment degeneration after surgical intervention [26]. In vitro biomechanical examination has shown that the spine becomes less stable with progressive resection of the PLC [1, 35]. The PLC, which extends as a "back tension band" on the dorsal part of the vertebral body from the CCJ to the sacrum, provides cervical stability and limits flexion, lateral bending, and rotation [2, 34, 60]. Surgical resection of it can cause complications such as cerebrospinal fluid leakage and compression of the spinal cord [30, 54]. It is, therefore, necessary to protect the PLC to ensure spinal stability and avoid complications during the postoperative period. As a precaution, the application of "laminoplasty" instead of laminectomy can preclude postoperative complications such as scar tissue formation, spinal instability, kyphotic deformity, adhesions of the perineural region, and late nerve injury [24]. It is technically recommended because it has advantages such as preservation of cervical spine movement, support of the integrity of the back muscles, and prevention of epidural scarring after surgical intervention [59, 60]. Spinal deformities are more frequent following laminoplasty, especially in children whose bones are immature; protection of the PLC during decompression can prevent the degeneration of neighboring segments [26, 60]. The PLC is crucial for maintaining spinal stability and preventing spinal deformities and progressive neural injury [56].

31.2.1.5 Adverse Effects of Chiropractic Manipulation for Various Lesions of Spinal Ligaments

Chiropractic spinal manipulation, manual therapy provided by chiropractic specialists, is an alternative treatment for neuromusculoskeletal disorders affecting the spine. It includes the application of a high-speed, low-amplitude force to a spinal segment to treat acute and chronic back and neck pain involving the spinal ligaments. Spinal manipulation has various adverse effects and significant complications, including vascular accidents, which can cause permanent disability or death. However, the frequency of serious adverse effects of problematic manipulation therapy is unknown [13]. Some chiropractors report the relative frequency of important side effects as five in 10^6 manipulations of the CCJ and upper cervical spine and one in 10^7 manipulations of the lower cervical spine. Still, these are unreliable statistics because reporting these patients is incomplete [51]. On the other hand, the efficacy of spinal manipulation for managing back and/or neck pain involving spinal ligaments is not convincing, so caution regarding upper cervical spinal manipulation is becoming more routine [13, 14, 58]. Some therapists have begun to advocate the investigation of patients for various risk factors before starting treatment [9, 36, 44]. If there are arteriosclerotic changes such as calcified arterial walls, vascular folds, or high homocysteine levels, the stretching and/or compressive effects of the rotational spinal manipulation could result in a vascular accident, including arterial dissection [8, 10, 12, 13, 15, 55].

In summary, chiropractic spinal manipulation, especially on the CCJ and subaxial cervical spine, can cause serious complications, although the incidence is unknown [8, 10, 12, 13, 15]. Therefore, informed consent should be mandatory for all therapists who use spinal manipulation for spinal ligament lesions from the CCJ to the lumbosacral region [13, 33].

31.3 Medicolegal Aspects of Medical Conditions Involving the Spinal Ligaments

31.3.1 Failure to Identify Ligamentous Injury in the Absence of Osseous Fractures

It is critical to remember that ligament injury can occur in cases with trauma involving the CCJ, C3-C7 subaxial segments, thoracic, and lumbar spine in both pediatric and adult populations, even though there are no fractures in bony structures. In particular, traumatic injuries to the CCJ involving the spinal ligaments and traumatic injuries to the PLC in the subaxial C3-C7 segments, thoracic and lumbar spine, can be acutely symptomatic and have longer-term sequelae if not identified acutely and managed appropriately, albeit conservatively in many cases, leading to the development of spinal deformity. There are potential medicolegal consequences if such injuries are not diagnosed and treated quickly, owing to the factors detailed below. To the best of my knowledge, although there are very few malpractice lawsuits regarding failure to identify ligamentous injury in the absence of fractures of skeletal structures, almost all of them were ruled against by the medical staff or hospital administration, and the court ordered a significant amount of compensation.

31.3.2 Delayed Imaging of Spinal Ligaments Following Traumatic Event

Because traumatic soft tissue edema appearing as a high-intensity signal on T2-weighted MRI can decrease "after 72 hours," MRI should be performed "within 72 hours after injury" as a delayed exam could give a false negative result for acute injury [32, 40]. It is forensically critical to know that "delayed" imaging of spinal ligaments after 72 h can yield a false negative result and that such diagnostic failure can lead to a malpractice lawsuit.

31.3.3 Inadequate Imaging of Spinal Ligaments Following Traumatic Event

In addition to "static evaluation" of the CCJ, C3-C7 subaxial segments, the thoracic and lumbar spine, "dynamic evaluation" of the entire spine in flexion and extension positions is crucial for correct diagnosis and adequate management of cases with traumatic injury to the spinal ligaments, as mentioned above [45]. Without such evaluation, patients with spinal instability as a result of spinal ligament injury can be incorrectly diagnosed as normal. Such "misdiagnosis" can have potential medical-legal consequences.

31.3.4 Limitations of Imaging of Spinal Ligaments Following Traumatic Event

The number of patients admitted to hospitals because of spinal ligament injury has increased significantly in recent years. Identifying an abnormality on MRI only in the ligaments from the CCJ to the lumbosacral region is not always clinically significant because such findings occur in asymptomatic people [25]. The problem is that many diagnostic findings are associated with asymptomatic degenerative changes related to aging [25]. Some studies suggest that 20–30% of the population who are asymptomatic have numerous abnormalities on CT of the spine [25]. Interestingly, some studies show that, no matter which imaging study is used, an important pathology can be observed in the spines of people with no history of a clinical syndrome [25]. Therefore, legally, the consultant must agree that an abnormality detected on imaging should not be accepted as diagnostic "unless it corresponds to a clinical syndrome" [25]. In other words, for an abnormality detected on imaging to be deemed medically significant, it must be supported by clinical findings [25].

31.3.5 Inadequate or Non-existence of Informed Consent Regarding Results of Diagnostic and Therapeutical Approaches for Lesions of Spinal Ligaments

Almost all therapeutic procedures performed for problems involving the subaxial cervical, thoracic, and lumbar spine, including different surgical approaches and chiropractic manipulation for various lesions of the spinal ligaments, can cause serious complications [13]. From a forensic perspective, it is a legal obligation for medical staff, including physicians and all therapists, to comply strictly with the "informed consent principles" for various lesions of the spinal ligaments and, after providing all necessary information, to obtain consent from the patient and their relatives concerning the examination and treatment procedures to be applied [13, 33]. Legally, not knowing these circumstances would not represent an acceptable defense in court. The vast majority of malpractice claims in spinal surgery today result from insufficient or absent communication between the orthopedic spine surgeon or neurosurgeon and the patient, in addition to incorrect patient selection, and have nothing to do with surgical errors.

31.4 Basic Legal Concepts Regarding Lesions Involving the Spinal Ligaments

As described above, most lesions affecting the spinal ligaments and causing related forensic legal problems involve spinal surgery, neurosurgery, orthopedic surgery, neuroradiology, and physical therapy. These surgical disciplines are the subspecialties listed with the highest number of malpractice cases worldwide [25, 27, 53]. It is impossible for the vast majority of spine surgeons, neurosurgeons, orthopedic surgeons, neuroradiologists, physical therapists, and rehabilitation physiotherapists to avoid a malpractice claim at some point in their careers. Unfortunately, the average time taken to resolve a claim is reported to be at least 2 years, and the average annual probability of malpractice litigation is around 20% [47]. Physicians are not insured against the indirect expenses of litigation related to the amount of time spent, intense stress, additional work, and loss of reputation. However, malpractice insurance can partially protect them against potential compensation payments [3, 27]. Of course, the increasing responsibility of "defensive medicine" affects tax practices, and there are concerns that it could lead to higher hospital admission fees [53].

From a legal point of view, physicians and other medical staff are responsible for harm caused by carelessness in their efforts to achieve the expected outcome [4, 18, 31, 38]. It is widely accepted that they are at fault for the smallest mistakes [31]. As a legal requirement, patients and their relatives have the right to expect their physicians and other medical personnel to act meticulously and carefully at every stage in treating patients with lesions affecting the spinal ligaments. The physician must consider the patient's concomitant medical diseases, such as diabetes, mellitus, hypertension, and heart disease, and refer the patient to the relevant specialist(s) without wasting time for further treatment [16]. In particular, a physician or other medical personnel must inform patients and their relatives about the possible risks and benefits of the surgical procedure. As a basic principle, in resolving any medical practice error case involving a negligence claim, it should be considered whether the behavior of the physician or other medical personnel violated the standard of medical care and whether an affirmative answer is relevant to the harm to the plaintiff patient [6]. In most medical practice error cases, the main focus is on whether there is negligence on the part of the physician or other medical personnel, and the issue of patient harm is generally accepted. Nevertheless, the type of damages claimed by the plaintiff necessitates more scrutiny, as it is uncommon to put it simply.

31.4.1 Medical Malpractice Litigation Process

Today, cases related to surgery involving the spinal ligaments cause many malpractice allegations, serious financial exposure, and a heavy emotional burden, threatening the future of this type of surgical intervention [25]. Surgical intervention covers various complex procedures, not always involving a medical error, surgical error, or misconduct, with associated risks and natural complications [25]. This kind of surgical procedure is usually the last option for the patient, and the doctor cannot reconstruct the intact spine [25]. Therefore, consultants and insurance professionals need to have logical expectations regarding spinal surgery to better interpret a claim's validity [25]. Medical malpractice litigation entails the competing interests of physicians who think they are facing a malpractice disaster that mandates defensive medicine, and opposing counsel that defend patients from medical mistakes in a strategy impenetrable to regulations [25].

For an action of medical malpractice, the following issue must be legally proven: (a) the treatment is not consistent with the principles of standard medical care; (b) the patient is injured because of negligence; and (c) the injury leads to the patient's disability or death [18, 25]. In medical negligence, unlike "medical malpractice" by health personnel, the provider is aware of the possible consequences of their action or inaction. In malpractice, patients do not want to see themselves hurt; it is not because the individual is at risk of harm due to intentional injury or knowing that such an action is regarded as the cause. If medical standard(s) have been violated in a procedure, the patient and/or their relatives can file a malpractice lawsuit claiming improper treatment [18]. Studdert et al. found that about 40% of claims were unrelated to medical errors [52]. Some authors argue that current legal regulations are important for improving the quality of care. In contrast, others strongly argue that they fail to compensate many patients with preventable medical injuries and harm not caused by medical negligence when some medical personnel, such as physicians, are placed in untenable situations [3, 4, 7, 18]. Regardless of perspective, the significant increases in malpractice premiums in recent years and the significant increases in the number and magnitude of claims awarded to plaintiffs have caused an increased interest in the malpractice liability organization, resulting in an imbalance between the cost of malpractice liability and the quality of care [3, 39].

31.4.2 Tort of Negligence in Medical Care

"Medical negligence" refers to something that an accused medical person, such as a doctor, should or should not do in certain situations in accordance with the principles of "tort law" [43, 50]. To demonstrate at first glance that negligence has occurred, the patient must provide the four components ("four Ds") of medical malpractice -"d"uty, "d"ereliction (deviation from the standard of care, negligence), "d"amages, and "d"irect cause [43]. The physician establishes a trusting relationship with his patient as a requirement of his duties towards that patient [18, 31]. In clinical practice, neglect of duty (violation) occurs if the physician provides services below the accepted standard of care, for example, if the patient is given insufficient informed consent. If informed consent is inadequate, it is accepted that there is a violation of the patient's rights to health through neglect of duty if the patient suffers complications or injury after surgery [25]. Finally, damage owing to complications should have a direct causal link with neglect of duty [18, 31]. It should not be forgotten that there is no intent in medical negligence; there has been accidental harm to the patient because the healthcare provider fails to notice something (ignorance) or take action at the necessary time and place [50]. Although the action or omission is strictly medical negligence, it is not considered a medical practice error due to the medical provider's failure to perform the action with the intention of causing harm or the ability to predict that the patient could be harmed [4, 50].

31.4.3 Informed Consent Process as a Prerequisite for Medical Procedure

Legally, the "informed consent process" is a prerequisite for every medical procedure, including surgical procedures for lesions involving the spinal ligaments. Indeed, failure to obtain informed consent constitutes medical negligence [18, 25, 31, 33]. It must be ensured that the patient fully understands the situation and possible solutions, the course and consequences of the situation, the nature of the options proposed for treatment, the additional treatment options required, and any available alternative management methods. The approximate cost of the treatment procedure, the possible risks of alternative treatment methods or procedures recommended by the physician to the patient, the likely outcome of the treatment and the chances of success or failure, the timeline of events, and pre- and postoperative services are all part of the informed consent process [4, 25]. Obtaining consent from the patient essentially means entering into a contractual obligation covering the duty of care to the patient. Still, it also means that the patient has consented and signed a comprehensive consent form for the procedure(s). This form does not mean that patients and their relatives will be prevented from making malpractice claims against the physician if things go badly and there is a judicial issue [25, 33]. If a complication develops, the surgeon, neuroradiologist, physical therapist, or rehabilitation physiotherapist must prove that it occurred despite strict adherence to medical standards and not because of a deviation from the work and procedures that an average physician should perform.

31.5 Conclusions

A lesion involving the spinal ligaments can be treated incorrectly; misdiagnoses are frequent, leading to delayed or inappropriate treatment. For this reason, there are often mistakes in managing patients with various problems involving the spinal ligaments, such as traumatic lesions, thickenings, calcifications, ossifications, degenerative cysts, and involvement of infections and neoplastic lesions in neighboring tissues. From a forensic medicine perspective, physicians, including neurosurgeons, orthopedic spine surgeons, neuroradiologists, physical therapists, and other medical personnel, often recognize that any medical negligence and carelessness at any stage of treatment will lead to different errors of medical practice in treating various lesions involving the spinal ligaments. Randomized, controlled, multicenter, prospective trials and evidence-based medicine will be needed to reach reliable conclusions.

Acknowledgments The author would like to thank Atty. Sabri Güleç for his guidance and support on the legal interpretation of the potential problems regarding various spinal ligament lesions.

References

1. Alanay A, Yazici M, Acaroglu E, Turhan E, Cila A, Surat A. Course of nonsurgical management of burst fractures with intact posterior ligamentous complex: an MRI study. Spine. 2004;29(21):2425–31.
2. Aryal V, Jimenez A. Anatomy, back, posterior longitudinal ligament. In: StatPearls [Internet]. Treasure Island (FL): StatPearls; 2022.
3. Baicker K, Fisher ES, Chandra A. Malpractice liability costs and the practice of medicine in the Medicare program. Health Aff (Millwood). 2007;26(3):841–52.
4. Bal BS. An introduction to medical malpractice in the United States. Clin Orthop Relat Res. 2009;467(02):339–47.
5. Benedetti PF, Fahr LM, Kuhns LR, Hayman LA. MR imaging findings in spinal ligamentous injury. AJR Am J Roentgenol. 2000;175:661–5.
6. Berlin L. Proximate cause. AJR Am J Roentgenol. 2002;179:569–73.
7. Brennan TA, Leape LL, Laird NM, Hebert L, Localio AR, Lawthers AG, Newhouse JP, Weiler PC, Hiatt HH. Incidence of adverse events and negligence in hospitalized patients. Results of the Harvard medical practice study I. N Engl J Med. 1991;324(6):370–6.
8. Cagnie B, Barbaix E, Vinck E, D'Herde K, Cambier D. Atherosclerosis in the vertebral artery: an intrinsic risk factor in the use of spinal manipulation? Surg Radiol Anat. 2006;28:129–34.
9. Cagnie B, Vinck E, Cambier D. Side and adverse effects of spinal manipulation. Tijdschrift voor Geneeskunde. 2002;58:1317–23.
10. Coulter ID. Efficacy and risks of chiropractic manipulation: what does the evidence suggest? Integr Med. 1998;1:61–6.
11. Denis F. The three-column spine and its significance in the classification of acute thoracolumbar spinal injuries. Spine. 1983;8:817–31.
12. Dupeyron A, Vautravers P, Lecocq J, Isner-Horobeti ME. Complications following vertebral manipulation-a survey of a French region physicians. Ann Readapt Med Phys. 2002;46:33–40.
13. Ernst E. Adverse effects of spinal manipulation: a systematic review. J R Soc Med. 2007;100(7):330–8.
14. Ernst E, Canter P. A systematic review of systematic reviews of spinal manipulation. J R Soc Med. 2006;99:192–6.
15. Gevers-Montoro C, Provencher B, Descarreaux M, Ortega de Mues A, Piché M. Clinical effectiveness and efficacy of chiropractic spinal manipulation for spine pain. Front Pain Res (Lausanne). 2021;2:765921.
16. Gilbert M. Agreements, coercion, and obligation. Ethics. 1993;103(04):679–706.
17. Goradia D, Linnau KF, Cohen WA, Mirza S, Hallam DK, Blackmore CC. Correlation of MR imaging findings with intraoperative findings after cervical spine trauma. Am J Neuroradiol. 2007;28:209–15.

18. Hakeri H. Distiction between malpractice and complication in medical law (in Turkish). Toraks Cerrahisi Bülteni. 2014;1:23–8.
19. Harris JH Jr. The cervicocranium: its radiographic assessment. Radiology. 2001;218:337–51.
20. Harris JH Jr, Carson G, Wagner L. Radiologic diagnosis of traumatic occipitovertebral dissociation: 1. Normal occipitovertebral relationships on lateral radiographs of supine subjects. Am J Roentgenol. 1994;162:881–6.
21. Harris JH Jr, Carson GC, Wagner LK, Kerr N. Radiologic diagnosis of traumatic occipitovertebral dissociation: 2. Comparison of three methods of detecting occipitovertebral relationships on lateral radiographs of supine subjects. AJR Am J Roentgenol. 1994;162(4):887–92.
22. Henderson F Sr, Rosenbaum R, Narayanan M, Mackall J, Koby M. Optimizing alignment parameters during craniocervical stabilization and fusion: a technical note. Cureus. 2020;12:e7160.
23. Hinck VC, Hopkins CE. Measurement of the atlanto-dental interval in the adult. Am J Roentgenol Radium Therapy Nucl Med. 1960;84:945–51.
24. Hirabayashi K, Watanabe K, Wakano K, Suzuki N, Satomi K, Ishii Y. Expansive open-door laminoplasty for cervical spinal stenotic myelopathy. Spine. 1983;8(7):693–9.
25. Hodge SD Jr. A medical-legal guide to spinal surgery. J Health Biomed Law. 2021;17:169–208.
26. Huang YP, Du CF, Cheng CK, Zhong ZC, Chen XW, Wu G, Li ZC, Ye JD, Lin JH, Wang LZ. Preserving posterior complex can prevent adjacent segment disease following posterior lumbar interbody fusion surgeries: a finite element analysis. PLoS One. 2016;11(11):e0166452.
27. Jena AB, Seabury S, Lakdawalla D, Chandra A. Malpractice risk according to physician specialty. N Engl J Med. 2011;365(7):629–36.
28. Kassem MW, Tubbs RS. Injuries to the craniocervical ligaments: radiological diagnosis. In: Tubbs RS, Iwanaga J, Loukas M, Oskouian RJ, editors. Clinical anatomy of the ligaments of the craniocervical junction. London: Cambridge Scholars; 2019. p. 89–110.
29. Kassem MW, Tubbs RS. The cruciform ligament. In: Tubbs RS, Iwanaga J, Loukas M, Oskouian RJ, editors. Clinical anatomy of the ligaments of the craniocervical junction. London: Cambridge Scholars; 2019. p. 155–85.
30. Kilitci A, Asan Z, Yuceer A, Aykanat O, Durna F. Comparison of the histopathological differences between the spinal material and posterior longitudinal ligament in patients with lumbar disc herniation: a focus on the etiopathogenesis. Ann Saudi Med. 2021;41(2):115–20.
31. Kök N. Malpractice and complication distinction. In: Kalkan E, Serel TA, Yilmaz EN, editors. Legal guide for physicians, Turkish neurosurgery academy publications no:1. Ankara: Sage; 2018. p. 109–39. in Turkish.
32. Krakenes J, Kaale B, Rorvik J, Gilhus N. MRI assessment of normal ligamentous structures in the craniovertebral junction. Neuroradiology. 2001;43:1089–97.
33. Langworthy JM, le Fleming C. Consent or submission? The practice of consent within UK chiropractic. J Manip Physiol Ther. 2005;28:15–24.
34. Le HV, Wick JB, Van BW, Klineberg EO. Ossification of the posterior longitudinal ligament: pathophysiology, diagnosis, and management. J Am Acad Orthop Surg. 2022;30(17):820–30.
35. Li Y, Shen Z, Huang M, Wang X. Stepwise resection of the posterior ligamentous complex for stability of a thoracolumbar compression fracture: an in vitro biomechanical investigation. Medicine. 2017;96(35):e7873.
36. Mann T, Refshauge KM. Causes of complications from cervical spine manipulation. Aust J Physiother. 2001;47:255–66.
37. Marathe NA, Dahapute AA, Desai JR, Dhole KP, Bhaladhare S, Shah S. X-ray and computed tomography scan-based morphometric analysis of skull baselines in Indian population. Asian J Neurosurg. 2019;14(4):1116–21.
38. Marcus P. Book review of medical malpractice law: a comparative law study of civil responsibility arising from medical care. Hastings Int Comp Law Rev. 1981;5:235–43.
39. Mello MM, Studdert DM, Brennan TA. The new medical malpractice crisis. N Engl J Med. 2003;348(23):2281–4.
40. Mirvis SE, NessAiver M. The radiology of acute cervical spine trauma. Baltimore: William and Wilkins; 1996.
41. Offiah CE, Day E. The craniocervical junction: embryology, anatomy, biomechanics and imaging in blunt trauma. Insights Imaging. 2017;8:29–47.
42. Powers B, Miller MD, Kramer RS, Martinez S, Gehweiler JA Jr. Traumatic anterior Atlanto-occipital dislocation. Neurosurgery. 1979;4(1):12–7.
43. Preskorn SH. Clinical psychopharmacology and medical malpractice: the four Ds. J Psychiatr Pract. 2014;20(05):363–8.
44. Refshauge KM, Parry S, Shirley D, Larsen D, Rivett DA, Boland R. Professional responsibility in relation to cervical spine manipulation. Aust J Physiother. 2002;48:171–9.
45. Riascos R, Bonfante E, Cotes C, Guirguis M, Hakimelahi R, West C. Imaging of atlanto-occipital and atlantoaxial traumatic injuries: what the radiologist needs to know. Radiographics. 2015;35:2121–34.
46. Rojas CA, Bertozzi JC, Martinez CR, Whitlow J. Reassessment of the craniocervical junction: normal values on CT. Am J Neuroradiol. 2007;28:1819–23.
47. Seabury SA, Chandra A, Lakdawalla DN, Jena AB. On average, physicians spend nearly 11 percent of their 40-year careers with an open, unresolved malpractice claim. Health Aff (Millwood). 2013;32(11):111–9.
48. Selden NR, Quint DJ, Patel N, d'Arcy HS, Papadopoulos SM. Emergency magnetic resonance

imaging of cervical spinal cord injuries: clinical correlation and prognosis. Neurosurgery. 1999;44:785–92.
49. Shen P, Nidecker A. Magnetic resonance imaging of the craniovertebral junction ligaments: normal anatomy and traumatic injury. J Neurol Surg Part B Skull Base. 2016;77:388–95.
50. Sohn DH. Negligence, genuine error, and litigation. Int J Gen Med. 2013;6:49–56.
51. Stevinson C, Honan W, Cooke B, Ernst E. Neurological complications of cervical spine manipulation. J R Soc Med. 2001;94:107–10.
52. Studdert DM, Mello MM, Gawande AA, Gandhi TK, Kachalia A, Yoon C, Puopolo AL, Brennan TA. Claims, errors, and compensation payments in medical malpractice litigation. N Engl J Med. 2006;354(19):2024–33.
53. Studdert DM, Mello MM, Sage WM, DesRoches CM, Peugh J, Zapert K, Brennan TA. Defensive medicine among high-risk specialist physicians in a volatile malpractice environment. JAMA. 2005;293(21):2609–17.
54. Sugita D, Nakajima H, Kokubo Y, Takeura N, Yayama T, Matsumine A. Cyclic tensile strain facilitates ossification of the cervical posterior longitudinal ligament via increased Indian hedgehog signaling. Sci Rep. 2020;10(1):7231.
55. Thanvi B, Munshi SK, Dawson SL, Robinson TG. Carotid and vertebral artery dissection syndromes. Postgrad Med J. 2005;81:383–8.
56. Vaccaro AR, Lehman RA Jr, Hurlbert RJ, Anderson PA, Harris M, Hedlund R, Harrop J, Dvorak M, Wood K, Fehlings MG, Fisher C, Zeiller SC, Anderson DG, Bono CM, Stock GH, Brown AK, Kuklo T, Oner FC. A new classification of thoracolumbar injuries: the importance of injury morphology, the integrity of the posterior ligamentous complex, and neurologic status. Spine. 2005;30(20):2325–33.
57. Vassiou K, Eftichia K, Marinos K, Kotrogianni F, Fanariotis M, Fezoulidis I, Arvanitis D. Magnetic resonance imaging of the ligaments of the craniocervical region at 3Tesla magnetic resonance unit: quantitative and qualitative assessment. J Biomed Sci Eng. 2012;5:901–9.
58. Vautravers P. Cervical spine manipulation and the precautionary principle. Joint Bone Spine. 2000;67:272–6.
59. Wang J, Wo J, Wen J, Zhang L, Xu W, Wang X. Laminoplasty versus laminectomy with fusion for treatment of multilevel cervical compressive myelopathy: an updated meta-analysis. Postgrad Med J. 2022;98(1163):680–8.
60. Yin X, Luo K, Jin Y, Liu Y, Wang Y, Liu M, Liu P. Role of posterior longitudinal ligament complex in spinal deformity secondary to surgical resection of the intradural tumor. Orthop Surg. 2023;15(3):819–28.

MIX
Papier aus verantwortungsvollen Quellen
Paper from responsible sources
FSC® C105338

If you have any concerns about our products,
you can contact us on
ProductSafety@springernature.com

In case Publisher is established outside the EU,
the EU authorized representative is:
Springer Nature Customer Service Center GmbH
Europaplatz 3, 69115 Heidelberg, Germany

Printed by Libri Plureos GmbH
in Hamburg, Germany